Textbook of
Nuclear Medicine
Volume I: Basic Science

JOHN HARBERT, M.D.

Professor of Medicine and Radiology
Department of Radiology
Georgetown University Medical School
Washington, D.C.

and

ANTONIO FERNANDO GONÇALVES DA ROCHA, M.D.

Director, Centro de Medicina Nuclear
da Guanabara
Advisor, Comissão Nacional de Energia Nuclear
Rio de Janeiro

Second Edition

LEA & FEBIGER • 1984 • *Philadelphia*

Lea & Febiger
600 Washington Square
Philadelphia, PA 19106-4198
U.S.A.
(215) 922-1330

Library of Congress Cataloging in Publication Data
Main entry under title:

Textbook of nuclear medicine. Volume I: Basic Science

   Bibliography: p.
   Includes index.
   1. Nuclear medicine. I. Harbert, John
II. Rocha, Antonio Fernando Gonçalves da. [DNLM:
1. Nuclear medicine. WN 440 T3548]
R895.T48   1984   616.07′57   83-25594
ISBN 0-8121-0891-4

Printed in the United States of America

Print Number: 5 4 3 2 1

PREFACE

Technologic advances are faster paced in nuclear medicine than in most specialties of medicine—partly because it is a young medical science and partly because so many participants from such other fields as physics, chemistry, engineering, and energy provide us with sophisticated technology needing merely to be adapted to medical use. We have tried in this second edition to reflect these advances while retaining all of the important elements that form the basic science of nuclear medicine.

The numerous changes in the technologic aspects of nuclear medicine that have occurred since publication of the first edition in 1978 (and it companion volume, *Textbook of Nuclear Medicine: Clinical Applications,* in 1979) have been carefully reviewed and constitute most of the changes in the second edition. Noteworthy advances are contained in the chapters on imaging systems, computer systems, and radiopharmaceutical chemistry. New developments are reflected in the complementary imaging disciplines of computed tomography and ultrasound. New chapters covering MR, digital radiography, and the elements of image perception have been added because of substantial developments in these areas. The chapters on counting statistics and production of radionuclides have been completely rewritten. A new chapter on cerebral blood flow studies with Xe-133 has been added. Finally, several useful tables have been added as appendices. The result, we believe, is a more useful general textbook for physicians, residents, and students of nuclear medicine and reference for active laboratory scientists with nuclear counting and radioassay problems.

Washington, D.C.
Rio de Janeiro

JOHN HARBERT
ANTONIO F. G. da ROCHA

ACKNOWLEDGMENTS

The task of writing and compiling as much information as is contained herein required the collaboration of many colleagues, all of whom have the editors' deep gratitude. For their invaluable assistance with manuscripts, we particularly want to thank Drs. Guido Heidendal, Kenneth Mossman, Warren Schadt, Edward Grant, Sheldon Levin, William Eckelman, Stanley Levenson, Robert Pollina, Jack Coffey, Evelyn Watson, and Seong Ki Mun.

The staffs at both the Centro de Medicina Nuclear da Guanabara and Georgetown Division of Nuclear Medicine have our sincere thanks.

J.H.

A.F.G.R.

Parts of Chapter 11 were written under Interagency Agreement Nos. FDA 224-75-3016 and DOE 40-286-71 and contract DE-AC05-760R00033.

Parts of Chapter 10 contain material contributed by Dr. Manuel Tubis to the first edition.

The section on echocardiography in Chapter 19 was coauthored by Dr. Pravin Shah, Veterans Administration, Wadsworth Medical Center, Los Angeles.

CONTRIBUTORS

Roger L. Aamodt, Ph.D.
Division of Grants Associates
National Institutes of Health
Bethesda, Maryland

Robert H. Ackerman, M.D.
Associate Professor of Radiology
Harvard Medical School
Director, Cerebral Blood Flow and Metabolism
  Laboratory and Carotid Evaluation Labora-
  tory
Associate Radiologist and Neurologist
Massachusetts General Hospital
Boston, Massachusetts

Nathaniel M. Alpert, Ph.D.
Assistant Professor of Radiology
Harvard Medical School
Associate Physicist
Massachusetts General Hospital
Boston, Massachusetts

Stephen L. Bacharach, Ph.D.
Adjunct Associate Professor
Department of Radiology
Uniformed Services University of the Health
  Sciences
Physicist, Department of Nuclear Medicine
National Institutes of Health
Bethesda, Maryland

Edwaldo E. Camargo, M.D.
Associate Professor of Nuclear Medicine
Director, Center of Nuclear Medicine and
  Radioisotope Service, Heart Institute
São Paulo University School of Medicine
São Paulo, Brazil

James C. Carlson, M.S.
Radiological Physicist
Department of Radiology
Hackley Hospital
Muskegon, Michigan

Roger J. Cloutier, M.D.
Program Director, Professional Training Pro-
  grams
Manpower Education, Research, and Training
  Division
Oak Ridge Associated Universities
Oak Ridge, Tennessee

Jack L. Coffey, B.S.
Scientist, Medical and Health Sciences Divi-
  sion
Oak Ridge Associated Universities
Oak Ridge, Tennessee

Stanton H. Cohn, Ph.D.
Professor of Medicine (Clinical Physiology)
State University of New York
Stony Brook, New York
Head, Medical Physics Division
Medical Research Center
Brookhaven National Laboratory
Upton, Long Island, New York

Lelio G. Colombetti, Sc.D.
Professor of Pharmacology
Stritch School of Medicine
Loyola University
Chicago, Illinois

John A. Correia, Ph.D.
Associate Professor of Radiology
Harvard Medical School
Associate Applied Physicist
Physics Research Laboratory
Massachusetts General Hospital
Boston, Massachusetts

William C. Eckelman, Ph.D.
Head, Section of Radiopharmaceutical Chemistry
Department of Nuclear Medicine
National Institutes of Health
Bethesda, Maryland

Jon J. Erickson, Ph.D.
Associate Professor of Radiology and Radiological Sciences
Vanderbilt University School of Medicine
Department of Radiology and Radiological Sciences
Vanderbilt Medical Center
Nashville, Tennessee

John Harbert, M.D.
Professor of Medicine and Radiology
Department of Radiology
Georgetown University Medical School
Washington, D.C.

Homer B. Hupf, Ph.D.
Head, Department of Radionuclide Production
Cancer Therapy Institute
King Faisal Specialist Hospital
Riyadh, Saudi Arabia

A. Everette James, Jr., Sc.M., J.D., M.D.
Professor and Chairman
Department of Radiology and Radiological Sciences
Professor of Medical Administration
Lecturer in Legal Medicine
Senior Research Associate
Professor of Biomedical Engineering
Vanderbilt Institute for Public Policy Studies
Vanderbilt University Medical School
Nashville, Tennessee

Steven M. Larson, M.D.
Professor, Department of Radiology
Uniformed Services University of Health Sciences
Chief, Department of Nuclear Medicine
Clinical Center
National Institutes of Health
Bethesda, Maryland

Paulo Roberto Leme, Ph.D.
Head, Physics Section
Radioisotope Service
Hospital do Servidor Público Estadual
São Paulo, Brazil

Sheldon G. Levin
Senior Statistician
Armed Forces Radiologic and Research Institute
Bethesda, Maryland

Michael Lincoln, M.D.
Division of Nuclear Medicine
Georgetown University Hospital
Washington, D.C.

Stuart Mirell, Ph.D.
Research Physicist
Nuclear Medicine/Ultrasound Service
Veterans Administration Medical Center, Wadsworth Division
Los Angeles, California

Kenneth L. Mossman, Ph.D.
Associate Professor and Director
Graduate Program in Radiation Science
Department of Radiation Medicine
Georgetown University Medical Center
Washington, D.C.

C. Leon Partain, M.D., Ph.D.
Associate Professor of Radiology, Radiological Sciences, and Biomedical Engineering
Vanderbilt University School of Medicine
Director, Nuclear Medicine Division and NMR Project
Vanderbilt University Medical Center
Nashville, Tennessee

Dennis D. Patton, M.D.
Professor of Radiology
Director, Division of Nuclear Medicine
Arizona Health Sciences Center
University of Arizona
Tucson, Arizona

Gerald D. Pond, M.D.
Associate Professor of Radiology
Arizona Health Sciences Center
University of Arizona
Tucson, Arizona

Antonio Fernando Gonçalves da Rocha, M.D.
Director, Centro de Medicina Nuclear da Guanabara
Advisor, Comissão Nacional de Energia Nuclear
Rio de Janeiro, Brazil

Val M. Runge, M.D.
Department of Radiology
Vanderbilt University Medical Center
Nashville, Tennessee

Walton W. Shreeve, M.D., Ph.D.
Professor of Medicine and Radiology
State University of New York
Stony Brook, New York
Chief, Nuclear Medicine Service
Veterans Administration Medical Center
Northport, New York

Evelyn E. Watson
Program Manager, Radiopharmaceutical Internal Dose Information Center
Manpower Education, Research and Training Division
Oak Ridge Associated Universities
Oak Ridge, Tennessee

Martin A. Winston, M.D.
Associate Professor of Radiological Sciences
UCLA School of Medicine
Chief, Section of Ultrasonography
Assistant Chief, Nuclear Medicine Service
Veterans Administration Medical Center, Wadsworth Division
Los Angeles, California

CONTENTS

Chapter 1

ATOMIC AND NUCLEAR STRUCTURE

ANTONIO F. G. DA ROCHA

MATTER AND ENERGY

Structure of Matter

Although the corpuscular nature of matter had been postulated in antiquity, an understanding of matter was only philosophic and provided no basis for experimental proof. At the end of the eighteenth century, Lavoisier postulated the existence of molecules of definite chemical composition, which could be reduced to simpler substances that were not further reducible by classic chemical methods.

In the following century, Dalton verified that the ratio of elements within molecules varied discretely and that the numeric relationship between elements in molecules represented whole numbers. For example, in the group of hydrocarbons, 12 g of carbon and 4 g of hydrogen form one mole of methane, 24 g of carbon and 6 g of hydrogen form a mole of ethane, and 24 g of carbon and 4 g of hydrogen form a mole of ethylene.

Subsequent developments that reinforced the concept of the atom were contributed by Gay-Lussac (law of gas volumes, 1809), Avogadro (Avogadro's number, 1811), Faraday (electrolysis, 1833), Cannizzaro (atomic weights, 1858), Meyer and Mendeleev (periodic table, 1870), and Perrin (Brownian motion, 1908).

Based initially on atomic weights, Mendeleev's classification of the elements indicated a periodic recurrence of similar chemical properties. This categorization reveals an admirable degree of precision when one considers that Mendeleev was without knowledge of several important facts about matter, particularly data derived from mass spectrometry. Inconsistencies in the periodic chart were later clarified by arraying the elements in order of increasing atomic number rather than weight.

Rutherford's Atom

The understanding of matter further evolved following experiments by Lord Rutherford in 1911. He directed a narrow beam of alpha particles at a thin gold foil and observed that some of the alpha particles passed through in a straight line while others were deflected through large scattering angles. This suggested to Rutherford that matter is discontinuous, that the atom is positively charged, and that the charge is localized to a small volume whose size he was able to estimate from the alpha particle charge and the scattering angle.

The atom imagined by Rutherford was

analogous to a solar system, which is still a useful comparison. The atom may be thought of as having a small, dense, central nucleus consisting of Z protons—each with unit positive charge—and N neutrons, the sum of which equals the *atomic mass number* A. The radii of nuclei are related to the atomic mass:

$$r_N \cong 1.45 \times 10^{-15} \, A^{1/3} m$$

The electrons, which contribute negligibly to the atom's mass, are disposed about the nucleus in spherical orbital *shells,* each with unit negative charge and equal in number to the number of protons. The radius of the outer orbital shell of the atom is approximated by:

$$r_a \cong 0.6 \times 10^{-10} \, (A/\rho)^{1/3} m$$

where ρ is the density of the material in its solid form. Thus atoms vary in diameter from about 0.6×10^{-10} m for hydrogen to about 1.7×10^{-10} m for the largest atoms, not a great variation in size. With the mass of an electron $\frac{1}{1836}$ that of a proton, an apt spatial analogy would be a golf ball surrounded by a few pinheads circling one kilometer out in space. By far, the greatest volume of matter, even in solids, is empty space, which helps explain why radiation traveling through matter may go a long way before interacting with an atomic nucleus or electron.

Rutherford's atom presented two large inconsistencies: 1. According to classical mechanics, negatively charged electrons orbiting positively charged nuclei as Rutherford postulated would spiral inward with ever-decreasing radius, decelerate, and emit energy. Clearly this does not happen. 2. Why did the nucleus not disintegrate by repulsion if it were composed of many particles of like charge?

Bohr's Atom

In 1913, Niels Bohr provided a more satisfactory model of the atom, based on quantum mechanics, wherein the electrons occupy positions at well defined distances from the nucleus (stable orbits). Changes in energy state are required for an electron to move from one level to another. Energy is required to raise an electron from an inner, more stable orbit to an outer, less stable orbit. These levels are fixed, so that discrete increments of energy are required to move an electron from one level to another. The energy required is equal to the difference in the *binding energies* of the two orbits between which the electron moves. Bohr determined that this energy difference would be equal to $h\nu$, where h is Planck's constant, or 6.62×10^{-34} joule-sec and ν is the frequency of the emitted radiation in hertz.

The orbital shells are denominated by the principal quantum number n, which relates to the energy state of the electron, and by letters for the orbital shells (Table 1–1). Each orbital shell has a number of subshells, denominated by roman numerals, with the electron capacities shown in Table 1–1 and Figure 1–1. When the atom is at *ground state,* i.e., the state with the least energy, all of the inner orbital shells are filled before the outer shells are filled. The maximum number of electrons found in any shell is a function of the quantum number n and is given by $2n^2$. The outer subshell never contains more than eight electrons. These are termed the *valence electrons* and determine to a large extent the chemical properties of the atom. Other quantum numbers are assigned for the angular momentum, magnetic moment, and spin direction of the electron. According to the *Pauli exclusion principle,* no two electrons in any atomic system have identical values for all four quantum numbers.

Energy

Kinetic energy is the energy that a body or particle possesses by virtue of its movement. Classically, this energy is expressed as:

$$T = \frac{1}{2} mv^2$$

This expression applies when the ve-

TABLE 1–1. *Denomination and Capacity of Electron Shells*

Principle quantum number n	Primary shell	Electrons per subshell							Total capacity
		I	II	III	IV	V	VI	VII	
1	K	2	—	—	—	—	—	—	2
2	L	2	2	4	—	—	—	—	8
3	M	2	2	4	4	6	—	—	18
4	N	2	2	4	4	6	6	8	32
5	O	2	2	4	4	6	6	8	32
6	P	2	2	4	4	x	x	x	32
7	Q	2	x	x	x	x	x	x	32

x These subshells are available to electrons in excited states, but are not needed by atoms in the ground state.

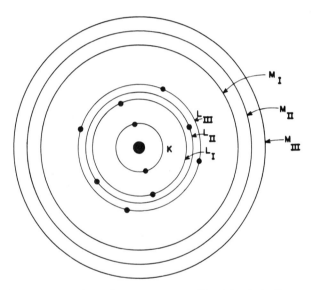

Fig. 1–1. Schematic representation of a neon atom. The M subshells contain only electrons in excited states.

locity v is small compared with that of light. As a particle approaches the speed of light, the variation of mass with velocity becomes appreciable, the mass increasing with increasing velocity:

$$m = \frac{m_o}{\sqrt{1 - v^2/c^2}}$$

where m_o is the rest mass. Mass and energy are equivalent, related by Einstein's equation:

$$E = mc^2$$

The total energy of a particle, then, is the sum of the energy that it has by virtue of its mass and its kinetic energy:

$$E = \frac{m_o c^2}{\sqrt{1 - v^2/c^2}}$$

As the velocity of a particle approaches the speed of light, the mass increases by an amount equal to the increase in T. The variation of mass with velocity is important when dealing with such accelerated particles as protons or deuterons in cyclotrons.

Units of Mass and Energy

In the *International System of Units* (SI), the basic unit of mass is the kilogram (kg) and the derived unit of energy is the joule (J), or that amount of energy required to accelerate 1 kg to a velocity of 1 m/sec (Appendix A). For events occurring on the atomic scale, however, more appropriate units are used. Energy of particles and of electromagnetic radiation is most often expressed in units of electron volts (eV), which correspond to the energy acquired by an electron accelerated across a potential difference of 1 volt (1.6×10^{-19} J). The basic unit of mass is the *universal mass unit* (u), which by convention is defined as 1/12 the mass of C-12 including its electrons.*

The equivalence between mass and energy cannot be determined by classic chemistry because the variation in mass that occurs in chemical reactions is extremely small. One must observe the larger mass changes encountered in nuclear reactions to appreciate these differences. Thus the classic concept of conservation of matter has been replaced by the law of conservation of energy and the law of the equivalence between mass and energy, which are expressed in Einstein's equation $E = mc^2$ where c is the velocity of light in a vacuum $\simeq 3 \times 10^8$ m/sec. The transformation of 1 u into energy yields 931.5 MeV, and an electron at rest is equivalent to 0.511 MeV. Appendix A lists several additional units, constants, and useful conversion formulae.

The energy released by mass conversion occurs most often in the form of electromagnetic radiation, especially *photons.* These are oscillating electrical and magnetic fields without mass, traveling in a vacuum at the speed of light. Electromagnetic radiation is characterized by wavelength λ and frequency v related by

$$\lambda v = c$$

where λ is expressed in Angstrom units (10^{-10} m). Photon energy is represented by the following equation:

$$E(keV) = 12.4/\lambda(Å)$$

By convention, photons that arise from nuclear transformations are called *gamma (γ) rays,* and photons that arise from extranuclear sources are called *x-rays.*

Electrons

J.J. Thomson demonstrated in 1895 that cathode-ray tubes function by means of a flux of very small particles with a negative electrical charge—now known to be electrons. The mass of the electron is 9.1×10^{-28} g, with a charge of 1.602×10^{-19} coulombs. A similar particle, with equal mass but with a positive charge, was discovered by Anderson in 1932 and called a positive electron, or *positron.* The positron does not exist free in nature, because soon after being formed, it combines with an electron, both of which undergo *annihilation* to produce two photons of 0.511 MeV each.

Electron Energy Levels

Electrons are bound to the atom within their various orbital shells. Each shell and subshell has a characteristic binding energy, which can be determined by nuclear spectrometry. In an atom at the ground state, the electron energy level is at a minimum and said to be stable. In a hydrogen atom, the binding energy of its single electron is given by

$$E_b = \frac{-13.6}{n^2} \text{ eV}$$

where the value -13.6 is the *mean ionization potential* and n is the principal quantum number (Table 1–1). In the case of hydrogen, which has a single orbital

---

*A slightly different unit, the *atomic mass unit* (amu), is used frequently in chemistry and is based upon the average weight of the isotopes of oxygen. One universal mass unit equals 1.00083 amu.

shell, n equals 1 and E_b equals -13.6 eV. The mean ionization potential I represents the mean energy required to remove an orbital electron (ionization), which forms an *ion pair* consisting of the negatively charged electron and the positively charged atom. Because ionization occurs most frequently in the outer orbital shells of multielectron atoms, where the binding energies are less, any specific ionizing event may require much less energy than the mean potential.

These concepts are illustrated in Figure 1–2, which depicts the orbital shells of Tc-99m as though they were various levels in a well. The binding energy, given at the right, represents the amount of energy needed to lift an electron at that particular level out of the well. If an electron in the K shell interacts with and acquires the energy of a 20.98 keV photon, it would not

gain enough energy to escape the atom, but would be elevated to the N_I subshell (dotted line). The atom would then be in an *excited* state. Numerous transition patterns exist whereby the atom could "deexcite" and return to its ground state. One possible pattern is depicted in the series of solid arrows showing transitions $N_I \rightarrow M_V \rightarrow L_{II} \rightarrow K_I$. During this process, three photons of 0.18, 2.55, and 18.25 keV, respectively, are given off, representing the energy differences between transitions. This process of deexcitation, in which several photons are emitted in random direction, is called a *cascade* and usually occurs in nanoseconds. Only certain transitions are allowed. Thus if the K electron received only 15 keV, it would not be sufficient to excite the atom. If an L_I electron received this 15 keV, however, it would be ejected from the atom with $15.00 - 3.04$

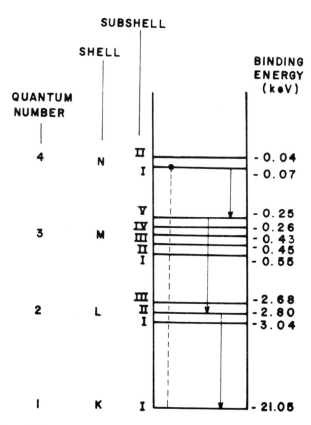

Fig. 1–2. Energy level diagram for Tc-99m.

= 11.96 keV of kinetic energy, which would ionize the atom in the process. Subsequently, this L_I vacancy would be filled by electrons from higher levels, each transition resulting in the emission of a photon equal in energy to the difference between its previous and new levels until the atom deexcites, and emits a total of 3.04 keV energy in the form of photons.

Ionization by removal of an outer electron may require only a few eV whereas to remove an inner electron from a large atom requires many keV (E_b increases with increasing Z). The deexcitation process, however, is the same. Photons emitted in deexcitation between 1.7 and 3.0 eV are in the visible light range. Higher energy photons are called "characteristic" x-rays because their energy identifies the orbital transition that produced them. Characteristic x-rays are also named by the transition process that creates them. If a free electron falls into a K vacancy, a K characteristic x-ray is emitted, and the atom deexcites with a single photon emission. If the K shell vacancy is filled by an L electron, a K_α x-ray is emitted; if filled by an M electron, a K_β x-ray, and so forth. L shell vacancies filled by M and N electrons emit L_α and L_β x-rays, respectively. The outermost shell vacancies are filled by free electrons in the environment.

The excited atom has an alternative means of deexcitation by giving off *Auger electrons*. Part of the energy of excitation may be imparted to an orbital electron (usually in the outer orbits), which, when ejected from the atom, carries with it the energy absorbed minus the binding energy of the vacant subshells:

$$T = E - E_b$$

The Auger process leaves a vacancy, which is filled by an electron from a higher shell or by a free electron, and further emission of characteristic x-rays occurs. The *Auger yield* is the fraction of vacancies that, when filled, result in the emission of Auger electrons versus photons.

This yield is higher with lighter elements. The *fluorescence yield* is the fraction of vacancies that, when filled, result in photon emission. The fluorescence yield increases with increasing Z.*

The Nucleus

In its simplest conceptualization, the nucleus is composed of neutrons and protons, collectively known as *nucleons* (Table 1–2). The nucleus is described in terms of its mass number A, which corresponds to the sum of its neutrons and protons, and its atomic number Z, which is equal to the number of protons and to the number of oribital electrons in the nonionized state. The atom is called a *nuclide* and is symbolized

$$^A_Z X$$

where X is the element symbol. For example, hydrogen is expressed as ^1_1H, and deuterium, which has a proton and a neutron, as ^2_1H. In the medical literature and by convention in this book, the mass number follows the elemental symbol, e.g., H-2, as the nuclide is pronounced. The subscript is often deleted since the atomic number can be determined from the chemical symbol. Nuclides with the same Z but different A are called *isotopes.* Since chemical properties depend upon the atomic number, which determines the number of orbital electrons, isotopes have identical chemical properties. Most elements found in nature have more than one isotope. Some examples of natural isotopes are listed in Table 1–3. Note that the mass units u are different from the *atomic weight* used in chemistry. The latter refers to the average weight in g/mol of an element's isotopes in their natural state.

---

*Auger electrons are denoted by e_{abc} where *a* denotes the shell with the original vacancy, *b* denotes the shell from which the vacancy was filled, and *c* denotes the shell from which the Auger electron was emitted. For example, an Auger electron denoted e_{KLM} arose from the M shell in response to a K-shell vacancy filled by an L-shell electron.

TABLE 1–2. *Mass and Energy Characteristics of Nucleons and Electrons*

Particle	Symbol	Charge	Mass (u)	Energy (MeV)
Proton	p	+1	1.007593	938.211
Neutron	n	0	1.008982	939.505
Electron	e	−1	0.000548	0.511
α-particle	α	+2	4.0028	3727

TABLE 1–3. *Examples of Natural Isotopes*

Element	Isotopes	u	% Abundance
H	$^{1}_{1}H$	1.008145	99.98
	$^{2}_{1}H$	2.014741	0.02
	$^{16}_{8}O$	16.00000	99.759
O	$^{17}_{8}O$	17.00453	0.037
	$^{18}_{8}O$	18.00488	0.204
	$^{35}_{17}Cl$	34.98006	75.4
Cl	$^{37}_{17}Cl$	36.97767	24.6
	$^{234}_{92}U$	234.1129	0.006
U	$^{235}_{92}U$	235.1156	0.712
	$^{238}_{92}U$	238.1241	99.282

The arrangement of nucleons within the nucleus is not yet fully understood. One model, called the *shell model,* depicts the nucleons moving in orbits about one another in a manner similar to the movement of electrons about the nucleus in Bohr's model of the atom. The most stable arrangement for the nucleons is the ground state. When the energy level is raised above the ground state, the nucleus is said to be either *excited* or *metastable.* Excitation is a transient state lasting less than 10^{-12} sec; metastability is an excited state lasting longer, i.e., minutes or hours.

Another way of conceptualizing nuclear energy levels is provided by the energy "well" shown in Figure 1–3. The nucleus has an internal organization of energy levels that are in some respects analogous to, though much higher than, the energy levels of orbital electrons. The nucleus can be excited when a nuclear constituent is raised above its ground energy level. When it falls back to the ground state, en-

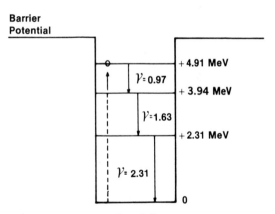

Fig. 1–3. Energy level diagram representing nuclear energy excess.

ergy is liberated in the form of photons with energy equal to the difference between the two nuclear energy levels. Radioactive nuclei may be naturally unstable, or they may be made radioactive by bombardment with high-energy photons or accelerated particles. Figure 1–3 shows N-14 after photon bombardment, which creates an unstable nucleus 4.91 MeV above the ground state. One possible means of deexcitation is *isomeric transition,* in which the cascade of gamma photons is emitted as indicated. *Isomers* possess the same Z and A, but different energy states. Nuclides of the same A but different Z are called *isobars. Isotones* have the same number of neutrons, but different A and Z (Fig. 1–4).

One obstacle of Rutherford's theory of the atom was an explanation of nuclear stability in view of the electrostatic forces exerted by the protons' tending to repel one another. It is now known that this nuclear stability is achieved by nuclear binding forces immensely stronger than electrostatic or gravitational forces, which operate only over very short distances ($\sim 10^{-15}$ m) as found in the nucleus. These forces are thought to be exerted by the newly discovered W particles, which are in perpetual agitation between neutrons and protons. One paradoxical aspect of these strong intranuclear forces is that they do not exert influence outside the nucleus. Furthermore, the nuclear binding energy E_b is equivalent to the atomic *mass defect.* The mass defect is the difference between the weight of the nucleus and the sum of the weight of its component particles. Nuclear binding energy is the mass defect expressed in energy units and can be calculated according to the equation

$$E_b = 931.5 \left[(Zm_p + Nm_n + Zm_e) - M \right]$$

where 931.5 represents MeV/u, Z is the number of protons and electrons, N is the number of neutrons, and M is the atomic mass (not the nuclear mass). As an example, consider the binding energy of $^{16}_{8}$O.

$$
\begin{aligned}
E_b &= 931.5 \, [(8 \times 1.007593 + 8 \\
&\quad \times 1.008982 + 8 \times 0.000548) \\
&\quad - 16.0000] \\
&= 127.601 \text{ MeV}
\end{aligned}
$$

The energy binding the nucleus (and the electrons) is the energy required to separate it into its constituent nucleons. Figure 1–5 presents the mean nuclear binding energy in relation to the mass number.

RADIOACTIVITY

In 1896, Henri Becquerel observed that uranium ore was capable of blackening photographic plates and ionizing gases. In 1898, Marie and Pierre Curie named this phenomenon radioactivity and demonstrated its occurrence in radium, polonium, and thorium besides uranium. Not until some years later did Rutherford and Soddy explain radioactivity as a process of transmutation of an unstable element to another element through the emission of radiation. Alpha particles were detected by Rutherford, who later identified them as helium nuclei.

Natural radionuclides, i.e., those associated with radioactive elements found in

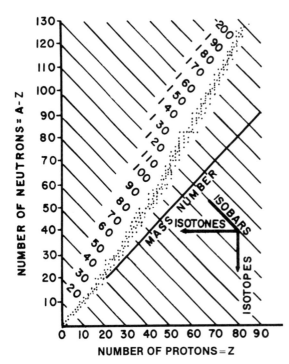

Fig. 1–4. Nuclear composition of the natural elements. The ratio of neutrons to protons increases with increasing atomic number.

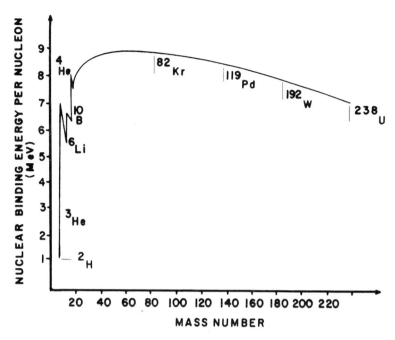

Fig. 1–5. Average nuclear binding energy (MeV) per nucleon as a function of mass number.

nature, all decay with emissions of alpha, beta, or gamma radiation or in some cases, by nuclear fission. Most of these natural radionuclides belong to "radioactive families," which include the actinium, thorium, and uranium families. A family exists when one radionuclide decays to a second radionuclide, and so forth, until a stable nuclide is formed. Parent radionuclides of these families all have atomic numbers greater than 82. These so-called *primordial* radionuclides decay very slowly ($\sim 10^8$–10^{10} yr). It could not be otherwise, since they have existed since the formation of our galaxy and all naturally formed short-lived radionuclides have disappeared. Some radionuclides, such as K-40 (1.3 × 10⁹ yr) and Rb-87 (5.2 × 10¹⁰ yr) do not belong to families, but do have very long half-lives. Several *comogenic* radionuclides have shorter half-lives. An example is C-14 (5730 yr) which is being created continuously in the atmosphere through bombardment of stable carbon nuclei by cosmic rays. This radionuclide forms the basis of carbon dating tech-

niques. When carbon is fixed in terrestrial organic material, the formation of new C-14 ceases. The concentration of C-14 in nonliving matter compared with contemporary concentrations is related by the half-life of C-14 to its age. All other radionuclides found in the environment originate from man-made sources. An excellent discussion of this subject may be found in NCRP Report No. 50.[1]

Radioactive Decay

Radioactive decay is the process whereby a nucleus that contains an excess of energy undergoes a transformation to a more stable state by emitting energy in the form of elementary particles or electromagnetic radiation. For every radioactive nuclide, a probability of decay exists. The relationship between this probability and the number of atoms in a large sample that will decay in some given time is called the "radioactive decay law." It states that the number N_t of atoms that have not decayed after time t is related to the change in time dt and to the proportionality constant λ:

$$-dN = \lambda N \, dt$$

The negative sign indicates that N is decreasing with time. The integral form of this equation gives the radioactive decay law:

$$N_t = N_0 e^{-\lambda t}$$

where N_0 is the number of undecayed atoms at t = 0.

The *half-life* ($T_{1/2}$) is the parameter that is usually measured and may be used to identify a radionuclide. The half-life is the time required to reach $\frac{1}{2} N_0$:

$$\frac{1}{2} N_0 = N_0 e^{-\lambda T_{1/2}}$$

$$T_{1/2} = \frac{\ln 2}{\lambda} = \frac{0.693}{\lambda}$$

and

$$\lambda = \frac{0.693}{T_{1/2}}$$

The average time a radionuclide survives is the *mean life* τ and is given by:

$$\tau = \frac{1}{\lambda} = \frac{T_{1/2}}{0.693} = 1.44 \, T_{1/2}$$

This value is important to radiation dosimetry (Chapter 11).

Activity

The activity A of a radioactive sample is the number of atoms undergoing transformation per unit time dN/dt. Since the activity decreases at the same rate as N_t, a similar relationship exists:

$$A_t = A_0 e^{-\lambda t}$$

The unit of radioactivity is the bequerel (Bq), which corresponds to a decay rate of 1 disintegration per sec. Most quantities of radioactivity in the literature are expressed in curies. The curie (Ci) equals 3.7 $\times$ 10^{10} disintegrations per sec (dps), or 2.22 $\times$ 10^{12} disintegrations per min (dpm). The curie was adopted because it was

thought to represent the activity in exactly 1 g of Ra-226, a readily available radioactive material. As measurements improved, this value was found to be in error by about 1%. Because the Ci is a large amount of activity for the applications encountered in nuclear medicine, the mCi (3.7 $\times$ 10^7 Bq) and μCi (3.7 $\times$ 10^4 Bq) are used more frequently. In this text, activity is expressed in both units.

The mass M of a carrier-free radionuclide represented by an activity of 1 Ci varies with the half-life. It is given by

$$M \, (g/Ci) = \frac{k \cdot T_{1/2} \cdot at \, wt}{N_0}$$

where k is a constant that depends upon the units in which the half-life is expressed and N_0 is Avogadro's number, or 6.025 $\times$ 10^{23}. The *specific activity* expresses the activity of a radionuclide relative to the total elemental mass in a mixture of radioactive and stable atoms (e.g., the amount of I-131 in a mixture with stable I-127) and is usually expressed in curies per gram of the element. For *carrier-free* radionuclides, the decay rate of the sample is

$$dN/dt = \lambda N = 0.693 N / T_{1/2}$$

One gram of the radionuclide contains

$$N = \frac{6.023 \times 10^{23}}{A} \, atoms$$

Then

$$A(Ci/g) = \frac{0.693 \times 6.023 \times 10^{23}}{A \times T_{1/2} \times 3.7 \times 10^{10}}$$

$$= \frac{1.12 \times 10^{13}}{A \times T_{1/2} \, (sec)}$$

$$= \frac{1.86 \times 10^{11}}{A \times T_{1/2} \, (min)}$$

$$= \frac{3.1 \times 10^9}{A \times T_{1/2} \, (hr)}$$

DECAY PROCESSES

All radionuclides used in nuclear medicine are artificially produced in either reactors or particle accelerators (see Chap. 8, "Production of Radionuclides"). The excess nuclear energy that they all contain is eliminated by six different processes, which generically are termed radioactive decay. These processes are described by the *decay scheme*, which is unique for each radionuclide and describes not only the mode of decay, but also the energy carried off with each nuclear transition and the probability of decay by that transition (Appendix B). Since most radionuclides have several possibilities of decay by which they reach ground state, these decay schemes may be extremely complex.

Alpha Decay

Alpha (α) particles are helium nuclei consisting of two neutrons and two protons. They are emitted with discrete energies in the range of 4 to 8 MeV and are often accompanied by photon emissions. The decay of Ra-224, shown schematically in Figure 1–6, is written as

$$^{224}_{88}Ra \rightarrow {}^{220}_{86}Rn + \alpha$$

In this example, alpha particles of two

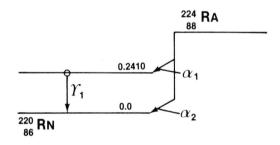

	MEAN NUMBER/ DISINTE-	TRAN- SITION ENERGY
TRANSITION	GRATION	(MEV)
ALPHA 1	0.0520	5.5427
ALPHA 2	0.9480	5.7837
GAMMA 1	0.0520	0.2410

Fig. 1–6. Decay scheme of Ra-224. Half-life = 3.64 d. (From Dillman, L.T., and VonderLage, F.C.[2])

different energies are emitted: α₁ with 5.54 MeV in about 5% of disintegrations and α₂ with 5.78 MeV in about 95% of disintegrations. The particle α₁ is accompanied by a photon emission of 0.241 MeV. In both decay modes, the nucleus loses 5.78 MeV of energy, decreasing its atomic weight by 4 and atomic number by 2. The energetics of alpha disintegration may be generalized for any nuclide X disintegrating to Y:

$$^{A}_{Z}X \rightarrow [{}^{A-4}_{Z-2}Y] + [{}^{4}_{2}\alpha] + E$$

Alpha-emitting nuclides have practically no usefulness in nuclear medicine. They are primarily of interest in that they represent great health hazards if ingested or inhaled. Since radium and radon, the principal alpha emitters in use in medicine, may leak from their containers, it is necessary to be able to detect this radiation and to limit the spread of contamination.

Isobaric Transitions

Most radionuclides are unstable by virtue of a neutron-proton imbalance: either too many neutrons or too many protons. Most nuclei do not have enough energy to eject a nucleon. A much more common mode of decay is to eject a charged electron, either beta particle (β⁻) or positron (β⁺), thus converting neutrons into protons or protons into neutrons respectively. In these transitions, the atomic number changes, but the atomic mass remains the same—thus the denomination *isobaric transitions*. In general, nuclides with excess neutrons transform by beta decay, and nuclides with proton excess decay by positron emission or *electron capture*.

Beta Decay

Beta emission, which was elucidated largely by Fermi in 1934, can be represented by the following notation:

$$^{A}_{Z}X \rightarrow {}^{A}_{Z+1}Y + {}^{0}_{-1}e + E_{\nu} + E_{\beta-}$$

In this case a neutron is transformed into a proton, a negative electron is emitted, and the atomic number increases by 1. Unlike alpha and gamma emissions, beta emissions do not have discrete energies. The kinetic energies of beta particles emitted from the same radionuclide vary from a little above zero to a maximum E_{max}, which is characteristic of the nuclide (Fig. 1–7). Since the total loss of energy by the nucleus in any disintegration must be discrete, an additional process must be postulated. Pauli hypothesized that another, undetected particle emitted with the beta particle must carry the necessary energy to preserve energy conservation. This "particle" ν, called the *neutrino,* has no mass or charge. Hence it interacts weakly with matter and goes unobserved except through elaborate detection techniques. Its half-value thickness in lead is ten times the distance between the moon and the earth!

The mass difference between X and (Y + B) is $E_{max} = E_\beta + E_\nu$. This process of decay is also accompanied by the release of antineutrinos, but they can be neglected because they also go undetected.

The distribution of beta energies is important because they have a short range in tissue and thus deposit their energy close to the atom. For dosimetry purposes, whenever the energy deposited in tissue is calculated, the mean beta energy $\bar{E}_\beta$ is given. This value is usually about 40% of E_{max}.

Decay schemes involving beta emission may be simple, as in the case of C-14 decay (Fig. 1–8), or complex, as in the case of Mo-99, in which beta particles with several E_{max} values may be emitted along with gamma photons in decaying to Tc-99 (Fig. 1–9). In standard nuclear notation:

$$\underset{Z}{\overset{A}{X}} \overset{\beta^-}{\rightarrow} \underset{Z+1}{\overset{A}{Y}}{}^* \overset{\gamma}{\rightarrow} \underset{Z+1}{\overset{A}{Y}}$$

where * refers to a nucleus in an excited state.

In the case of Mo-99, eight beta decay possibilities are shown in Figure 1–9. In every case the Tc-99 nucleus is left in an excited state, i.e., the beta particles and neutrinos have not carried off sufficient energy to reach the ground state. This energy is given off in the form of photons within nanoseconds of the beta emission. In contrast with the beta particles, gamma rays are emitted with discrete energies. In

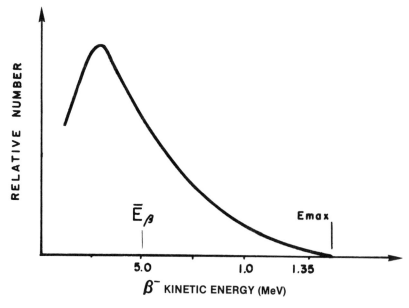

Fig. 1–7. Beta spectrum of K-40.

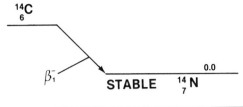

TRANSITION	MEAN NUMBER/ DISINTE- GRATION	TRAN- SITION ENERGY (MEV)
BETA MINUS 1	1.0000	0.1561

Fig. 1–8. Decay scheme of C-14. Half-life = 5730 yr. (From Dillman, L.T., and VonderLage, F.C.[2])

about 87% of disintegrations, the Tc-99 nucleus is left in a metastable state (Tc-99m), decaying with a half-life of 6 hr. Metastable states will be further discussed in this chapter.

Positron Decay

A proton can be converted to a neutron in two ways. One is by the formation and ejection of a β^+ particle, or positron, in which the atomic number decreases by 1. The nuclear transformation is denoted:

$$_Z^A X \xrightarrow{\beta^+} {}_{Z-1}^A Y + {}_{+1}^0 e + E_{\beta^+} + E_\nu$$

The excess nuclear energy is thus reduced by an amount equivalent to the positron mass, 0.511 MeV, plus the kinetic energy of the positron and the neutrino. Any excess energy remaining is then usually given off in the form of photon emissions (Fig. 1–10). Positrons also have a spectrum similar to that of beta particles. The positron cannot exist long in nature, but soon combines with an electron and annihilates to form two 0.511 MeV photons, which are given off at 180-degree angles (see Fig. 1–15).

In order to decay by positron emission, the parent radionuclide must have a mass greater than its daughter by at elast two electron rest masses. In order to form the positron, its antiparticle, an electron, must also be formed. This formation requires the mass equivalence of 1.022 MeV of energy. The vertical line representing positron decay in the decay scheme of Figure 1–10 represents this 1.022 MeV of energy.

Electron Capture

The other mechanism whereby a proton is converted to a neutron is by nuclear capture of an orbital electron. The electrons may be thought of as oscillating in their orbits. In these oscillations, some electrons, particularly those in the inner K and L shells, may be captured by the nucleus, whose charge effectively neutralizes a proton. The excess nuclear energy is given off by the formation and ejection of a neutrino, which goes undetected. As the electron vacancy is filled by electrons from other orbits, deexcitation occurs through emission of characteristic x-rays. Iron-55 and Tungsten-181 are radionuclides that decay in this manner. The kinetics of electron capture may be written:

$$_Z^A X + e^- \longrightarrow {}_{Z-1}^A Y + E_\nu + E_b$$

where E_b is the orbital binding energy of the captured electron.

Neutron-deficient nuclei with less than 1.022 MeV excess energy usually decay exclusively by electron capture. Nuclei with more than 1.022 MeV excess energy may decay by either positron emission or electron capture. In general, nuclei of lighter atomic weight decay by positron emission while heavier nuclei decay by electron capture. In heavier nuclei, the orbital electrons are closer to the nucleus, which increases the probability of capture. In many cases, the nucleus remains in an excited state (designated by an asterisk *) and returns to its ground state through gamma-ray emission:

$$_Z^A X + e^- \longrightarrow {}_{Z-1}^A Y^* \xrightarrow{\gamma} {}_{Z-1}^A Y$$

Medically important radionuclides that decay by electron capture (EC) and by elec-

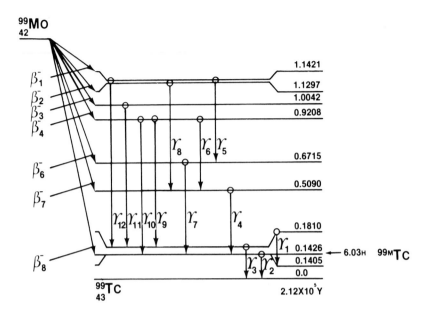

RADIATION		MEAN NUMBER/ DISINTE- GRATION N_i	MEAN ENERGY/ PARTICLE $\bar{E}_i$ (MeV)	RADIATION		MEAN NUMBER/ DISINTE- GRATION N_i	MEAN ENERGY/ PARTICLE $\bar{E}_i$ (MeV)
BETA MINUS	1	0.0012	0.0658	GAMMA	4	0.0143	0.3664
BETA MINUS	3	0.0014	0.1112	GAMMA	5	0.0001	0.3807
BETA MINUS	4	0.1850	0.1401	GAMMA	6	0.0002	0.4115
BETA MINUS	6	0.0004	0.2541	GAMMA	7	0.0005	0.5289
BETA MINUS	7	0.0143	0.2981	GAMMA	8	0.0002	0.6207
BETA MINUS	8	0.7970	0.4519	GAMMA	9	0.1367	0.7397
GAMMA	1	0.0130	0.0405	K INT CON ELECT		0.0002	0.7186
K INT CON ELECT		0.0428	0.0195	GAMMA	10	0.0479	0.7782
L INT CON ELECT		0.0053	0.0377	K INT CON ELECT		0.0000	0.7571
M INT CON ELECT		0.0017	0.0401	GAMMA	11	0.0014	0.8231
GAMMA	2	0.0564	0.1405	GAMMA	12	0.0011	0.9610
K INT CON ELECT		0.0058	0.1194	K ALPHA-1 X-RAY		0.0253	0.0183
L INT CON ELECT		0.0007	0.1377	K ALPHA-2 X-RAY		0.0127	0.0182
GAMMA	3	0.0657	0.1810	K BETA-1 X-RAY		0.0060	0.0206
K INT CON ELECT		0.0085	0.1600	KLL AUGER ELECT		0.0087	0.0154
L INT CON ELECT		0.0012	0.1782	KLX AUGER ELECT		0.0032	0.0178
M INT CON ELECT		0.0004	0.1806	LMM AUGER ELECT		0.0615	0.0019
				MXY AUGER ELECT		0.1403	0.0004

Fig. 1–9. Principal decay scheme of Mo-99. Half-life = 66.7 hr. (From Dillman, L.T., and VonderLage, F.C.[2])

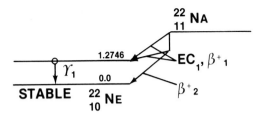

TRANSITION	MEAN NUMBER/ DISINTE- GRATION	TRAN- SITION ENERGY (MEV)
ELECT CAPT 1	0.0940	1.5680
GAMMA 1	1.0000	1.2746
BETA PLUS 1	0.9060	0.5460
BETA PLUS 2	0.0006	1.8210

Fig. 1–10. Principal decay scheme of Na-22. Half-life = 2.6 yr. (From Dillman, L.T., and VonderLage, F.C.[2])

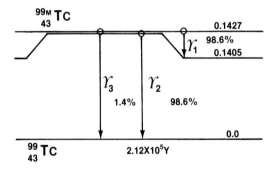

TRANSITION	MEAN NUMBER/ DISINTE- GRATION	TRAN- SITION ENERGY (MEV)
GAMMA 1	0.9860	0.0021
GAMMA 2	0.9860	0.1405
GAMMA 3	0.0140	0.1426

Fig. 1–11. Principal decay scheme of Tc-99m. Half-life = 6.0 hr. (From Dillman, L.T., and VonderLage, F.C.[2])

tron capture plus gamma emission (EC, γ) include Ga-67, In-111, I-123, and I-125.

Isomeric Transitions

As already seen, many radionuclides emit gamma rays to bring the nucleus to its ground state. This is called *isomeric*

transition, because the atoms have the same A and Z before and after decay. When a delay occurs between the first decay event and the second, the nuclide is said to be metastable and is designated with an *m* after the mass number. Technetium-99m is the most common example encountered in nuclear medicine (Fig. 1–11). In the case of Tc-99m, the parent Mo-99, with a half-life of 66.7 hr, decays by beta emission, 82% of which results in Tc-99m with an energy level of 0.142 MeV. This excited nucleus decays with a 6-hr half-life by one of two processes: in 98.6% of disintegrations a two-step cascade yields 2-keV and 140-keV gamma rays; in the other 1.4% of disintegrations, a single 142-keV gamma ray is emitted. Since technetium and molybdenum are chemically different, they can be easily separated to yield a radionuclide that has a short half-life, emits no beta particles, and yields a high percentage of useful gamma photons.

Internal Conversion

This process is an alternative to gamma emission and occurs frequently with metastable radionuclides. The excited nucleus imparts its excitation energy to an orbital electron called a *conversion electron,* which is ejected from the atom. Any excess nuclear excitation energy that exceeds the orbital binding energy is imparted to the conversion electron as kinetic energy. The orbital vacancy is then filled from peripheral or free electrons with the emission of characteristic x-rays or Auger electrons.

As described in the example of Tc-99m, the metastable nuclide can decay by two processes. Internal conversion occurs with both decay schemes. Approximately 10% of the 140-keV gamma rays are converted, and the ratio of orbital electrons undergoing conversion is $K:L:(M + N) = 913:118:39$ per 10^4 disintegrations (see Appendix B). The spectrum of Tc-99m, then, shows not only the 142-, 140- and 2-keV gamma rays, but also the K, L, M, and

N x-rays and a variety of Auger electrons. The latter are important only from a dosimetry standpoint, because while they are not detected externally, they nevertheless contribute to absorbed radiation.

The conversion electron behaves like a beta particle in matter, with energy equal to the nuclear excitation energy minus the orbital binding energy. For Tc-99m, the energy imparted to a K conversion electron is:

$$E_{eK} = 142 - 21 = 121 \text{ keV}$$

or

$$E_{eK} = 140 - 21 = 119 \text{ keV}$$

The observable difference between beta particles and conversion electrons is that the latter are emitted with discrete energies, rather than in a continuous spectrum of energies.

Nuclear Fission

Such heavy radionuclides as U-235, Np-237, Pu-239, and Cf-252 undergo *spontaneous fission,* which results in two smaller nuclei and two or three *fission neutrons.* The masses of the two *fission fragments* occur typically in a 60:40 ratio. For example:

$$^{235}_{92}U + {}^{1}_{0}n \rightarrow [{}^{236}_{92}U] \nearrow {}^{99}_{40}Zr \searrow {}^{135}_{52}Te + 2 {}^{1}_{0}n + E$$

The excess energy E, usually 200 to 300 MeV per fission fragment, is initially imparted to the fragments and neutrons as kinetic energy and ultimately dissipated as thermal energy. Most of the fission fragments have excess neutrons and decay further by beta decay. Fission is of interest to nuclear medicine, first, because most of the fission fragments are radioactive and provide a source of inexpensive, high specific-activity tracer nuclides (e.g., I-131, Xe-133, Mo-99), and second, because the neutrons liberated in the fission process may be used to produce radionuclides by *neutron activation.* These processes are discussed in Chapter 8.

INTERACTION OF RADIATION WITH MATTER

All types of radiation have energy, whether inherent, as in the case of electromagnetic radiation, or kinetic, as in the case of moving particles. When radiation interacts with matter, this energy is transferred to the atoms of the material through which it passes. The mechanisms whereby radiation is absorbed are of fundamental interest, because they form the basis of both radiation detection, and an understanding of the biologic effects of radiation.

The transfer of energy from a particle or photon to the absorbing material occurs primarily through two mechanisms: *ionization* and *excitation.* Ionization is the process whereby an orbital electron is removed from an atom or molecule, resulting in an ion pair: a negative electron and a positively charged atom or molecule. Excitation leaves the atom or molecule in an excited state without ejecting an electron. The end result of excitation is the ultimate dissipation of energy as light, heat, or chemical reactions. In this section, radiation is taken to mean nuclear radiation, either charged particles or gamma rays. Neither accelerated particles nor neutrons are discussed because they have little to do with nuclear medicine, even though many of the principles of interaction are the same.

Alpha and Heavy Charged Particles

Heavy charged particles are those nuclear elements larger than electrons. Most frequently encountered in nuclear medicine are alpha particles, but the same principles apply to such accelerated particles as protons and deuterons. Electrons are considered separately in this chapter.

The forces acting between charged particles and matter are coulomb, or electrostatic, forces. The force F between two particles of charge q and q' is inversely proportional to the square of the distance between them:

$$F = \frac{q\,q'}{d^2}$$

If the charges are alike, the force is repelling; if they are opposite, it is attractive. Thus when a charged particle moves through matter, the interactions with orbital electrons and nuclei are not mechanic collisions, but coulombic deflections. The amount of force exerted on nuclei and electrons is inversely proportional to the distance between them (Fig. 1–12). Since the number of particles per unit volume is proportional to the density, more interactions per unit path length occur in denser materials than in lighter ones. The energy imparted to the absorbing matter through ionization and excitation is ultimately dissipated in the production of characteristic x-rays, light photons, and heat.

The three principal interactions between heavy charged particles and matter are: (1) elastic collision with atomic nuclei, which results in bremsstrahlung radiation (discussed in the next section), (2) excitation of atomic electrons, which results in characteristic x-rays and Auger electrons, and (3) ionization by collision with atomic electrons. Usually, ejected electrons are outer orbital electrons, which require only small amounts of energy to overcome their binding energy. Except for collision with nuclei, which have very small stopping cross sections because of their small size, only a small fraction of the particle's energy is lost with each interaction, principally through ionization. An alpha particle, for example, loses approximately 35 eV per ion pair formed in air. Thus a 2-MeV alpha particle interacts a great many times before slowing down sufficiently to pick up orbital electrons

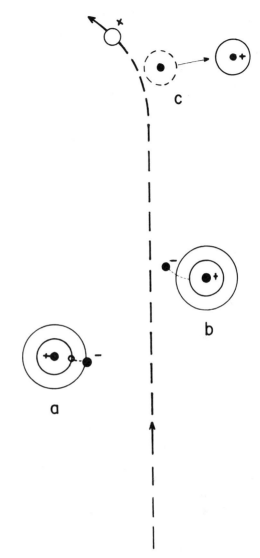

Fig. 1–12. Path of heavy charged particle in matter. Excitation (a) and ionization (b) do not deflect the speeding alpha particle. Close approach to an atomic nucleus (c) causes deflection of the alpha particle and the nucleus, which may in turn produce ionization.

and finally form a neutral helium atom. Occasionally, a *secondary electron* is ejected with sufficient force for it to behave as a beta particle, which causes secondary ionizations. Such particles are referred to as delta (δ) rays.

The loss of energy in a medium gives

rise to a number of important concepts. The *total* energy lost per unit length of path traversed, including both radiation and collisional losses, is the *linear stopping power* (S_l), expressed in MeV/cm. This is closely related to the *linear energy transfer* (LET), which relates to the energy deposited *locally* in the absorber per unit path length. In most biologic materials, little energy is lost by bremsstrahlung production; thus the values of S_l and LET are nearly equal. The LET is important in radiation biology because it reflects the tissue damage done by type of particle. Because of the relatively short path length of heavy charged particles, the LET is high relative to other forms of radiation of the same energy. Alpha particles, for example, travel a few centimeters in air and a few microns in tissue.

The rate of energy loss depends on the particle charge, the density of the medium, and the velocity of the particle. The *specific* ionization (SI) refers to the number of ionization events per unit distance. The increase in specific ionization as the particle slows near the end of its track is known as the *Bragg effect* (Fig. 1–13). The rapid fall in the SI after the Bragg peak represents the sudden decrease in specific ionization as the charge is neutralized by the addition of orbital electrons.

The ratio of linear energy transfer to specific ionization gives the *average energy expended per ionizing event* (W).

$$W = LET/SI$$

The value of W for air is approximately 33.7 eV/event.

Another concept is the *ionization potential* (I), which represents the average energy required to produce ion pairs, an average obtained from all of the orbital electron shells. W is always greater than I because almost half of a particle's energy is dissipated in excitation events that do not result in ionization. Both W and I decrease with increasing Z of the absorber material because of the greater number of

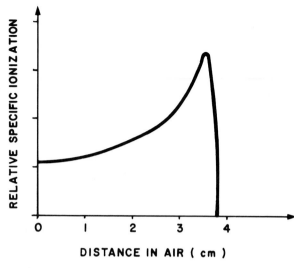

Fig. 1–13. Specific ionization of an alpha particle as a function of path length. The peak just before the end of the particle track is the *Bragg peak.*

orbital electrons of lower binding energy. For example, W = 33.7 eV for air (Z ≅ 7.6) and W = 2.9 for germanium (Z = 32) used in semiconductor detectors. The greater number of ion pairs per MeV of particle energy accounts for the greater detector efficiency of materials with higher Z.

Beta Particles

Electrons undergo the same interactions in matter as heavy charged particles. For considerations in nuclear medicine, beta particles and positrons interact with matter identically, but certain differences occur in the process of energy loss for electrons compared with that for heavy charged particles. First, a larger energy loss per interaction generally occurs because the masses of the incident electron and the orbital electron are the same. The path of an electron is likely to vary greatly, because of a greater likelihood that an interaction will result in a large angular deflection. The path of heavy charged particles, on the other hand, is usually straight and nearly the same for all particles having the same charge and velocity.

Beta particles also lose energy by the production of *bremsstrahlung,* or "braking radiation." When an electron approaches an atomic nucleus, the strong attraction for the nucleus decelerates the particle (Fig. 1–14). When the kinetic energy of a charged particle exceeds its rest mass energy, the excess energy is eliminated through photon emission. This process, which holds for all particles, becomes particularly important for electrons because their rest mass energy is only 0.511 MeV. The intensity of bremsstrahlung production is proportional to the square of the atomic number Z of the material and the particle's charge z and inversely proportional to the square of the particle's mass M or Z^2z^2/M^2. Thus electrons are more likely to produce bremsstrahlung than alpha particles because of their smaller mass, despite their lesser charge. Electrons striking dense material produce more photons than those striking lighter material. This process accounts for the production of x-rays in an x-ray tube. Bremsstrahlung also is used to detect the presence of such highly energetic beta particles as P-32 (E_{max} = 1.71 MeV) in tissue. The bremsstrahlung spectrum is continuous, similar to the distribution shown in Figure 1–7.

The energy depends upon the velocity of the particle and the deceleration produced by each encounter.

Because bremsstrahlung production increases by Z^2 of the absorber, high Z materials do not provide the best shielding for beta-emitting radionuclides. Thus lead should not be used to contain energetic beta emitters because, while the beta particles will not escape, the bremsstrahlung may. Plastic and glass provide better shielding because beta particle absorption is adequate and bremsstrahlung production is minimal.

In any absorbing medium, the path length of beta particles exceeds the range of heavy charged particles. Measured by absorption thickness, the range of beta particles varies even for particles of the same energy (e.g., conversion electrons) because of their irregular track characteristics. For comparison, the maximum ranges of H-3, C-14, and P-32 beta particles are shown in Table 1–4.

Cerenkov radiation also is produced by beta particles. These radiations are light photons, emitted by energetic electrons whose velocity is greater than the speed of light in the medium in which they are travelling. This phenomenon, which is responsible for the bluish white light emitted around the core of swimming pool reactors, is discussed in more detail in Chapter 2.

A third radiation process comes about through positron annihilation. When positrons are emitted from the nucleus, they produce excitation, ionization, bremsstrahlung, etc., just as electrons do. As they slow down, however, they do not

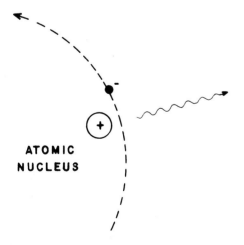

ATOMIC NUCLEUS

Fig. 1–14. Production of bremsstrahlung.

TABLE 1–4. *Beta-Particle Ranges in Air and Water*

	E_{max} (MeV)	Air (cm)	Water (cm)
³H	0.018	5	0.0006
¹⁴C	0.156	22	0.03
³²P	1.70	610	0.8

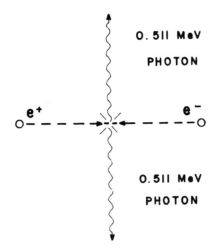

Fig. 1–15. Positron annihilation.

wander freely in the absorbing material as do electrons. They combine with a free electron and annihilate to form two 0.511 MeV photons equal to the rest mass of the two particles. The photons are given off at angles 180 degrees to each other, as shown in Figure 1–15. This phenomenon can be used to detect the location of the positron emitter. The positron travels only a few millimeters in tissue before annihilating; therefore, precise localization can be determined by placing two opposing detectors, connected through a coincidence circuit, on either side of the source. Since the 180-degree directionality of the simultaneous photons is constant, only one of the detectors need be collimated to achieve precise localization.

Photons

The interaction of all uncharged particles, including neutrons, neutrinos, and photons, is largely the same and quite different from interactions involving charged particles. The photons of importance include gamma rays, x-rays, and bremsstrahlung, which have different denominations only by virtue of their origin; gamma rays from nuclei, x-rays from the atom—usually from orbital electrons, and bremsstrahlung from free particles.

While photons appear to be influenced by the electromagnetic fields of electrons and nuclei, their only interaction is by direct impact upon them. Three principal mechanisms explain how photons are absorbed or *attenuated.*

The Photoelectric Effect

This phenomenon occurs when all of the photon's energy is absorbed by an orbital electron, usually from the K or inner shells (Fig. 1–16a). If the incident photon has more energy than the electron's binding energy E_b, it leaves the orbit with kinetic energy:

$$T_e = E\gamma - E_b$$

The atom is ionized and the ejected electron, or photoelectron, then behaves as a beta particle. This vacancy is then filled by higher orbital electrons and by emission of characteristic x-rays and Auger electrons.

The photon energy must exceed the electron binding energy in order to produce a photoelectron. If it does, a definite preference exists for the photon to be absorbed by the innermost electrons. This probability is expressed graphically in Figure 1–17, in which the photoelectric cross section (probability of absorption) in barns is shown as a function of the photon energy in a lead absorber.

The dashed lines represent the absorption cross sections for the K and L orbital shells, and the solid lines represent cross sections for combinations of shells. For example, the binding energy for an L_3 orbital electron is 13 keV. Absorption of photons below this energy by an L_3 electron is practically nil. As the incident gamma-ray energy reaches this energy, the probability of absorption by photoelectric effect increases suddenly and then falls off sharply with increasing energies until the K *edge* or *discontinuity* is reached. At this point, another sudden increase in photoelectric absorption occurs, now by the K electrons with a binding energy of 88 keV. The pho-

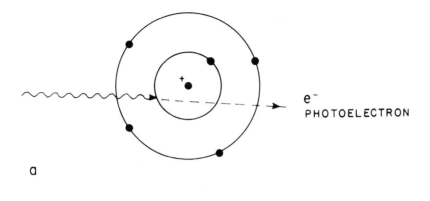

a

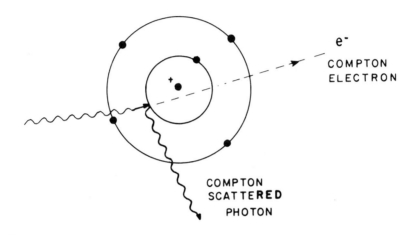

b

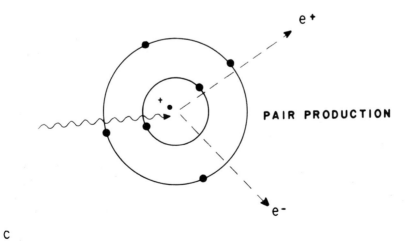

c

Fig. 1–16. Principal photon interactions in matter.

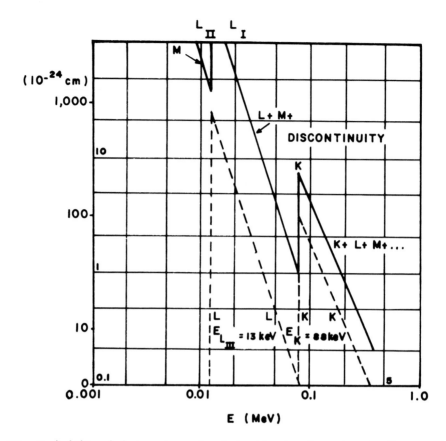

Fig. 1–17. Probability of photon absorption in lead by the photoelectric effect as a function of photon energy.

ton preference is always for the inner electrons.

In Figure 1–18, the linear absorption coefficients are shown for a sodium iodide crystal as a function of gamma-ray energy. It can be seen that the photoelectric effect predominates in sodium iodide crystals for energies below about 250 keV. In general, the photoelectric effect increases with increasing Z of the absorber and decreases with increasing gamma-ray energies. The photoelectric effect is approximately proportional to Z^3/E_γ^3.

The Compton Effect

A second mechanism of gamma absorption is the Compton effect, in which an incident photon is absorbed by an electron, which emits a new, "scattered" pho-

ton and simultaneously gains kinetic energy (Fig. 1–16b). The second photon is emitted in a new angle, and it can be shown that the second photon energy E_γ' is proportional to the angle between the primary and secondary photon:

$$E_\gamma' = \frac{E_\gamma}{\left(1 + \dfrac{E}{m_e c^2}\right)\left(1 - \cos \phi\right)} - E_b$$

where $m_e c^2$ is the electron rest mass energy, or 0.511 MeV, and E_b is the binding energy of the electron. The kinetic energy of the *recoil* electron is then

$$T_e = E_\gamma - E_\gamma'$$

This phenomenon is also called *Compton scattering* although the incident and

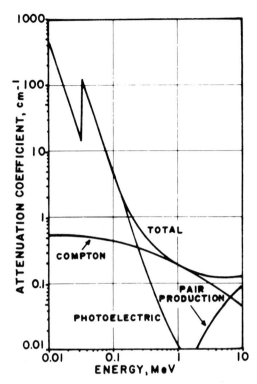

Fig. 1–18. Attenuation coefficients as a function of photon energy in NaI.

scattered photons are different photons. This effect, which is discussed in detail in Chapter 3, is responsible for many of the characteristics of gamma pulse-height spectra. The Compton scatter component decreases slowly with increasing photon energy and with increasing Z of the absorber.

Pair Production

When an energetic photon closely passes an atomic nucleus, the photon may annihilate and form an electron-positron pair (Fig. 1–16c). The minimum energy required for this interaction is $2\ m_e c^2$ or 1.022 MeV. The remaining energy is divided between the two particles as kinetic energy:

$$E_\gamma = 2\ m_e c^2 + T_{e-} + T_{e+}$$

The positron soon combines with an electron in the absorber and annihilates to

form two 0.511 MeV photons, which are given off at 180-degree angles. The cross section of pair production increases with increasing Z of the absorber and logarithmically with the gamma energy (Fig. 1–18).

Of these three processes, only the photoelectric effect results in all or nearly all of the incident photon energy being deposited in the absorber. In Compton scattering, the total energy of the incident photon is absorbed only if the secondary photons are completely absorbed as well. Since the probability of all of these interactions increases with increasing Z, it is evident that high Z materials, such as lead (Z = 82), provide the best shielding for gamma rays.

There are two other photon interactions that are of interest even though they contribute little to gamma-ray attenuation encountered in nuclear medicine. They are *Rayleigh scattering* and *photonuclear reactions.*

Rayleigh Scattering

Rayleigh scattering, or *coherent scattering,* is an interaction between a photon and an atom as a whole. Because of the large atomic mass, there is practically no recoil energy absorbed by the atom. The photon is absorbed and reemitted with approximately the same energy, but in a random direction. Thus this mechanism contributes little to energy absorption but may contribute significantly to the attenuation of a photon beam. It is important to CT scanning. Rayleigh scattering occurs principally at low photon energies (<50 keV).

Photonuclear Reactions

At very high proton energies (>2 MeV), photons may be absorbed by atomic nuclei with the ejection of a nucleon: a proton, neutron, or alpha particle. Since the (γ, n) reaction predominates, neutron-deficient nuclei are formed. These are usually radioactive and decay by positron emission. Photonuclear reactions are of some theoretical interest as a means of radionuclide production but have no importance in photon attenuation in nuclear medicine.

Attenuation of Photon Beams

The measure of photon absorption is given by the *linear attenuation coefficient* μ. The fractional decrease in photon beam intensity $\Delta I/I$ by an absorber of thickness x is given by

$$\frac{\Delta I}{I} = - \mu \, x$$

Integrating for some thickness x:

$$I = I_0 e^{-\mu x}$$

This equation may be expressed in terms of the density of the absorber or the *mass attenuation coefficient* in cm^2/g as

$$I = I_0 e^{-\mu m}$$

since

$$\mu_m = \frac{\mu}{\rho}$$

The linear attenuation coefficient μ represents the cross section of interaction for all three gamma absorption processes illustrated in Figure 1–18. Here the attenuation of gamma rays in cm^{-1} is plotted as a function of gamma-ray energy in MeV. The total attenuation is plotted as a solid line, which is the product of attenuation by photoelectric effect, Compton scattering, and pair production.

REFERENCES

1. NCRP Report No. 50: Environmental radiation measurements. Washington, D.C., National Council on Radiation Protection and Measurements, 1976.
2. Dillman, L.T., and VonderLage, F.C.: MIRD Pamphlet No. 10. Radionuclide Decay Schemes and Nuclear Parameters for Use in Radiation-Dose Estimation. New York, Society of Nuclear Medicine, 1975.

BIBLIOGRAPHY

Avogadro, A.: D'une manière de déterminer les masses relatives des molécules élémentaires des corps, et les proportions selon lesquelles elles entrent dans ces combinaisons. J. Phys., *73*:58, 1811.
Cannizzaro, S.: An abridgement of a course of chemical philosophy given in the Royal University of Genoa. Nuovo Cimento, *7*:321, 1858.
Dalton, J.: Experimental enquiry into the proportions of the several gases or elastic fluids constituting the atmosphere. Mem. Literary Philosophical Soc. Manchester *1*:244, 1805.
Dillman, L.T., and VonderLage, F.C.: MIRD Pamphlet No. 10. Radionuclide Decay Schemes and Nuclear Parameters for Use in Radiation-Dose Estimation. New York, Society of Nuclear Medicine, 1975.
Gay-Lussac, J. : Sur la combinaison des substances gazeuses, les unes avec les autres. Mem. Soc. d'Arcoeil, *2*:207, 1809.
Lederer, C. M., Shirley, V.S. (Eds.): Table of Isotopes. 7th Ed. New York, John Wiley & Sons, 1978.
Mendeleev, D.: The relation between the properties and atomic weights of the elements. J. Russ. Chem. Soc., *1*: 60, 1869.
Meyer, J.: Die Natur der chemischen Elemente als Funktion ihrer Atomgewichte. Ann. Chem., *7*:354, 1870.
Millikan, R.: A new modification of the cloud method of determining the elementary electrical charge and the post probable value of that charge. Phil. Mag., *19*:209, 1910.
Perrin, J.: Atoms. London, Constable, 1923.
Rutherford, E.: The scattering of alpha and beta particles by matter and the structure of the atom. Phil. Mag. *21*:669, 1911.
Thomson, J.: Papers on positive rays and isotopes. Phil. Mag. (6th series), *13* :561, 1907.
Thomson, J.: Cathode rays. Phil. Mag. (5th series), *44*:293, 1897.

Chapter 2

RADIATION DETECTOR SYSTEMS

JOHN HARBERT

The detection of radioactivity is based on the physical interaction of radiation with matter. Detection systems are classified in three ways: (1) by the medium in which the interaction takes place, i.e., liquid, solid, or gas; (2) by the nature of the physical phenomenon produced, i.e., excitation, ionization, or chemical change; or (3) by the type of electronic pulse generated, i.e., amplitude that is constant or proportional to the energy of the incident radiation. Examples of radiation detection systems based on chemical changes include film emulsion and thermoluminescent dosimeters. Along with the associated electronics used to register the interactions, detection systems make up an impressive array of apparatus.

GAS-FILLED DETECTORS

Gas-filled ionization chambers have many important uses in modern nuclear medicine and are among the earliest nuclear radiation detectors. The three most common types are ionization chambers used for personnel dosimeters, radiopharmaceutical dose calibrators, and laboratory monitors; proportional counters for measuring charged particles; and Geiger-Müller tubes for measuring ambient radiation. Their applications are discussed in the next chapter.

These detectors all operate on the same general principle: the ability of ionized gas within an electrically charged enclosure to alter the voltage potential between two electrodes. The general design of these chambers is schematically represented in Figure 2–1. A gas-filled chamber made of some conducting material, which serves as the cathode, is connected to a well-insulated central anode through a resistance-capacitance (R-C) circuit across which a voltage V has been applied. Ionizing radiation entering the chamber produces negative and positive ion pairs from the gas atoms. These are collected by the central anode and chamber walls respectively because of the direction of the electrical field. The change in charge on the capacitor C per radiation detected (pulse height) is proportional to the number of ions collected. The pulse height as a function of the voltage V applied across the electrodes is shown in Figure 2–2 for two charged particles of different energy. The curves reflect the capacitance that would be generated by the two ionizing events as a function of the external voltage applied across the electrodes.

These curves are divided into four recognizable regions. In region I, the voltage

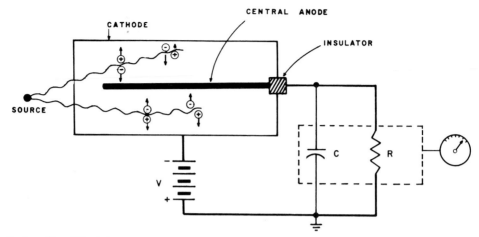

Fig. 2–1.   Gas-filled detector.

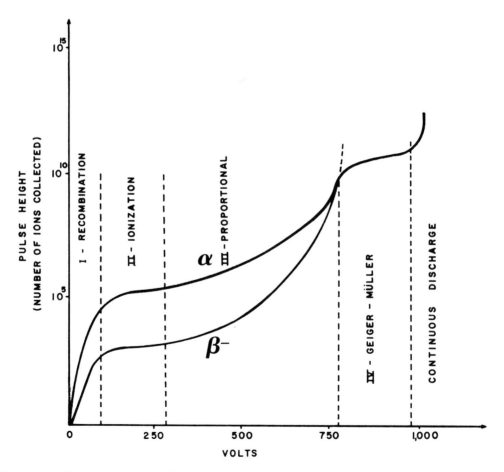

Fig. 2–2.   Characteristic pulse-height curves produced by a beta particle and an alpha particle as a function of applied voltage in a gas-filled detector.

applied produces an electric field too weak to attract many ion pairs to the electrodes before they recombine to neutral atoms. Those that recombine have no effect on the charge collected. As the voltage is increased, the drift velocity of the ions increases, reducing the time available for recombination. The fraction of the charge collected therefore increases. This region has little utility for most detector systems.

In region II, further increases in voltage have little effect upon the pulse height because all of the ions produced by each radiation event are collected and none recombines. This plateau, where the pulse height remains relatively constant with changes in applied voltage, is called the *ionization* region, and the charge necessary for operation in this region is known as the *saturation voltage.* In this region, the pulse height is proportional to the energy deposited in the chamber by the incident radiation, although the signal output requires considerable amplification. For example, the energy expended (W) in producing a single ion pair in air is about 34 eV. A 1-MeV beta particle thus would produce about $10^6/34 \approx 3 \times 10^4$ ion pairs. The total charge generated would be approximately 10^{-15} coulombs. For this reason, detectors operated in this region are seldom used for measuring individual events, but rather used for measuring radiation flux (particles/cm²/sec).

As voltage is increased further, the charge collected is increased by a multiplication factor due to the phenomenon of *gas amplification* (region III, Fig. 2–2). The electrons formed in the primary ionizing event are now accelerated sufficiently to cause secondary ionization of the neutral gas molecules as they speed toward the collecting electrodes and thus add to the collected charge. The secondary ions may also acquire enough energy to ionize more neutral atoms so that a *cascade* effect is produced. The factor by which ionization is increased is called the *gas amplification factor.* It may reach as

high as 10^4 to 10^6. In the portion of region III used for particle detection, the pulse height remains dependent upon the initial energy of the ionizing particle, so this area is called the *proportional* region. As voltage is increased at the upper end of this region, the two curves come together, i.e., the pulse height now becomes more dependent upon the voltage applied than upon the energy of the ionizing event, so this area is called the region of *limited proportionality.* It is not important in the measurement of ionizing radiations.

In region IV, the pulse height is entirely independent of the energy of the original ionizing event. The upper limit of gas amplification is here limited by the type of gas used and the design characteristics of the chambers. A plateau is again reached. This area is known as the Geiger-Müller region. Above this region, *continuous discharge* occurs within the chamber. This phenomenon is discussed in more detail in the next section.

Ionization-Chamber Detectors

The broadest application of ionization-chamber detectors is found in health physics, in which they are used to measure the intensity of environmental radiation or cumulative doses of radiation. These detectors often contain dry air at atmospheric pressure, enclosed within a cylindric chamber, as shown in Figure 2–1. Saturation voltage is maintained between the electrodes, usually by a battery, so that they operate in region II of Figure 2–2. The saturation voltage must be determined for each instrument because it varies with the size and shape of the detector, the spacing of the electrodes, and the type of gas used. Ionization chambers may be used to measure all types of ionizing radiation. Since the pulse height is proportional to the radiation energy, they may be operated in a *pulse mode* in conjunction with electronic equipment designed for pulse-height analysis. They are seldom used in this manner, however, because the time for ion collec-

tion on the electrodes is long (~10⁻³ sec)
and the pulse amplitude is so low that a
high level of noise is inherent in the system. They are most often used in *mean-level* operation to measure radiation of relatively high intensity where the current
measured is proportional to the rate of
radiation emitted from some radiation
source. An example is the "Cutie Pie," a
portable dose ratemeter in which ambient
radiation (exposure rate) is read directly
from a meter calibrated in roentgens per
hour (R/hr) (Fig. 2–3).

The sensitivity of ionization-chamber
survey meters is strongly influenced by
the photon energy. Weak photons are attenuated by the chamber walls and high-energy photons escape absorption by the
detector gas, thereby reducing detector efficiency. A typical survey-meter response
curve is shown in Fig. 2–4.

Another common ionization chamber is
the pocket dosimeter, which measures the

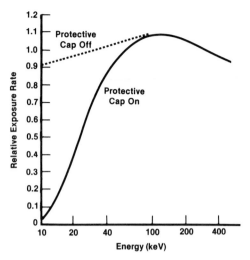

Fig. 2–4. Energy-response curve of an ionization-chamber survey meter with removable protective cap.

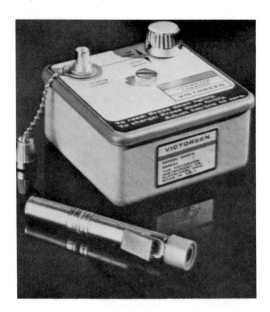

Fig. 2–5. Pocket dosimeter and charging system.

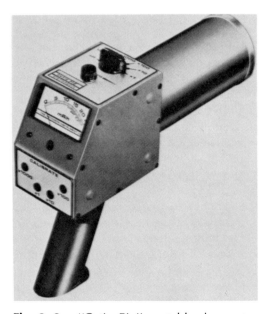

Fig. 2–3. "Cutie Pie" portable dose rate-meter. External voltage is provided by batteries. The cylindric ionization chamber is usually provided with a protective cap that can be removed to measure low penetrating radiation.

quantity of radiation delivered over a certain time period (Fig. 2–5). The dosimeter
is charged to a predetermined voltage V_1
by a battery-powered charging system. As
ions are produced by incident radiation,
they are collected by the electrodes and
they gradually reduce the original voltage
between the electrodes. At the end of the

exposure period, the reduced voltage V_2 is measured by an electrometer, and the difference is proportional to the radiation dose calibrated in rads. Direct-reading dosimeters are modifications of the Lauritzen electroscope, which consists of a gas-filled chamber with heavy-duty enclosure and a specially adapted collecting electrode. The collecting electrode consists of a gold-plated quartz fiber attached to the collector electrode. When the dosimeter is charged by a battery, electrostatic forces repel the quartz fiber from the electrode. As the charge between the electrodes is neutralized by ionizing radiation, the electrostatic forces diminish and the fiber moves toward its resting position. The fiber is viewed through a lens system, which also focuses on a scale calibrated in R or mR. Thus, at any time, the wearer can determine the integrated dose of radiation he has received.

One of the most common gas-filled detectors is the dose calibrator, which consists of a large-volume sealed ionization chamber with a central well large enough to accept vials or syringes of up to about 100-ml capacity for determining the activity to be given patients (Fig. 2–6). Several selector settings are available for particular nuclides so that the readout is given directly in μCi or mCi, automatically correcting for decay scheme and energy of the principal gamma emissions. Special features may be added to give a readout in terms of concentration, e.g., μCi/ml. Most instruments are reasonably accurate over a wide range of activities, from 1.0 μCi to 2.0 Ci.

The *linearity* of activity response, however, must be measured periodically as a part of prudent quality control. This measurement is easily accomplished by counting a large dose of Tc-99m periodically over 48 hours and comparing the values with a decay chart. Significant deviations require repair of the instrument. Dose calibrators are also sensitive to volume changes. Such changes are determined by measuring the output after successive additions of water to a container without varying activity.

These devices are now used almost universally in clinical nuclear medicine laboratories as a check against the manufacturer's assay and/or as a final check upon the accuracy of the dose to be injected into the patient. Actually, ionization chambers are not very sensitive to x-rays or gamma rays. For their usual applications in nuclear medicine, however, this is not a serious limitation.

Proportional Counters

In these detectors, the voltage applied between the collector electrode and the chamber wall is sufficient to produce gas amplification factors as high as 10^6. This produces pulse heights that require less elaborate amplification circuitry than is required for region II counters. Proportionality between radiation energy and pulse height is maintained, allowing highly accurate spectrometry.[1] A common adaptation is the *gas flow proportional counter.* It is used for detecting beta and alpha radiation in samples, which can be inserted directly into the chamber (Fig. 2–7). The gas is supplied from cylinders of compressed gas mixtures, which continuously replenish the gas that escapes from the entry port. These systems are generally operated in the pulse mode and are calibrated against known standards of the same radionuclide as the unknown samples. Their principal application in nuclear medicine is in gas chromatography, in which compounds labeled with H-3 and C-14 are converted to ^3H_2O or $^{14}CO_2$ and passed through the proportional counter for measurement.

Geiger-Müller Tubes

When the ion chamber is operated in region IV, the dependence between radiation energy and pulse height is lost. Electrons now strike the central anode with sufficient force to produce ultraviolet pho-

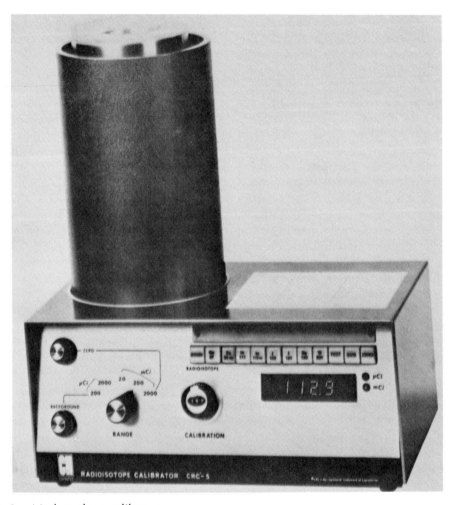

Fig. 2–6. Modern dose calibrator.

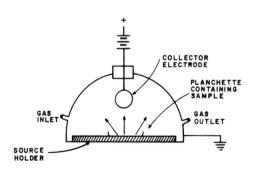

Fig. 2–7. Gas flow proportional counter.

tons. These photons strike other electrons within the gas and walls of the chamber, causing an *avalanche* of billions of ion pairs. Gradually, a barrier of slow-moving positive ions builds up around the central wire anode. This barrier serves to stop the avalanche by capturing additional electrons before they reach the anode. Geiger-Müller tubes are therefore suitable for measuring all types of ionizing radiation, including weak x-rays. They are also useful in detecting low-level radiation from radioisotope spills that occur in the laboratory. The large pulse heights (several volts) require only simple amplifier circuitry. On the other hand, the independence of radiation energy and pulse height does not allow discrimination between various kinds of radiation. Also, the rate of detection is severely limited (about 20,000 counts per sec (cps).

The high sensitivity of the Geiger-Müller (G-M) tube derives from the fact that only a single ion pair is required to trigger the discharge. When this discharge occurs, the avalanche induced proceeds all along the central collecting anode, causing a complete breakdown throughout the tube. In order for the counter to recover, a *quenching* mechanism must be provided to stop the discharge. The most efficient quenching agents are such organic molecules as ethyl alcohol. These molecules are broken down by secondary photons produced in the discharge and consequently absorb sufficient energy to stop it. If the high voltage is increased above the Geiger plateau, the ion pairs receive so much energy that the quenching effect cannot absorb enough and the tube goes into continuous discharge. When this happens, the organic molecules are broken down at a very rapid rate, and the tube may be quickly ruined unless the voltage is reduced.

Even so, tubes containing organic molecules have a limited working life (about 10^{10} pulses). Most modern tubes contain halogen gases as quenching agents, usually chlorine or bromine. In the case of halogen molecules, the atoms recombine upon completion of the discharge, thus reducing or eliminating the problem of depletion and greatly lengthening tube life. There is a tradeoff, however. Because halogens are less effective than organic molecules as quenching agents, the Geiger-Müller plateau is both shortened (from about 300V to 150V) and steepened (from 2 to 10% slope). As a consequence, the sensitivity varies much more sharply with fluctuations in high voltage.

Most G-M tubes used as survey instruments are enclosed in a sturdy case of aluminum or stainless steel. They may have an end- or side-window and frequently have a very thin, low-density window (1.5 mg/cm²) made of mica or mylar so that beta particles can enter the chamber. For detecting gamma rays, the window thickness is generally less critical. The tube is usually on a cord for easy probing while the battery, ratemeter, and audible "clicker" are contained in a convenient carrying case (Fig. 2–8).

Calibration of Ionization Chambers

Most ionization chambers are calibrated in roentgens per hour or in rads. Those with very thin windows operate at atmospheric pressure and require periodic calibration using a standard source of known activity. Several radionuclide sources may be used; Cs-137 and Co-60 are the most common. The ionization chamber is placed at a measured distance d from the source, and the meter deflection is noted. The dose rate I_o in R/hr is determined from the relation:

$$I_o = \frac{\Gamma C}{d^2}$$

where Γ is the specific gamma-ray constant, C is the activity in mCi, and d is the distance in centimeters. The distance used is usually 1 m or sufficient distance between source and detector to consider the source a point source and the detector a point detector. Most ion chambers are purchased with certificates specifying this distance.

Table 2–1 lists values of Γ for several radionuclides. More recently, the *exposure-rate constant* has replaced the specific gamma-ray constant.[2] The exposure-rate constant includes the exposure rates from photons of the characteristic x-rays and internal bremsstrahlung along with the exposure rate from the gamma rays. The specific gamma-ray constant includes only the latter rate. For such encapsulated radionuclides as radium, the exposure rates from all of these radiations are modified by self-attenuation and by attenuation

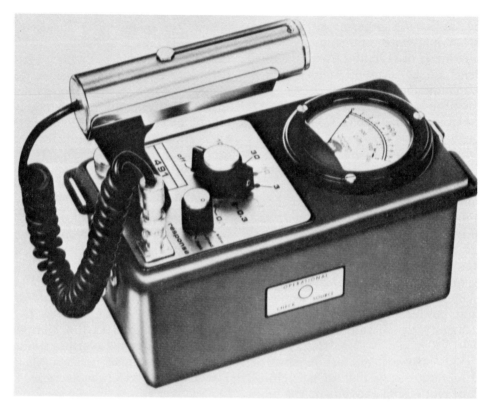

Fig. 2–8.   Survey meter with G-M tube.

TABLE 2–1.   *Specific Gamma-Ray Constants and Exposure-Rate Constants for Selected Gamma-Ray Sources.*

Radionuclide	γ Energies (MeV)	Specific gamma-ray constant (R cm² h⁻¹ mCi⁻¹)	Exposure-Rate constant (R m² h⁻¹ Ci⁻¹)
¹³⁷Cs	0.6616	3.226	0.3275
⁵¹Cr	0.3200	0.1842	0.01842
⁶⁰Co	1.173 − 1.322	13.07	1.307
¹⁹⁸Au	0.4118 − 1.088	2.327	0.2376
¹²⁵I	0.0355	0.0423	0.1326
¹⁹²Ir	0.1363 − 1.062	3.948	0.4002
²²⁶Ra with daughters	0.0465 − 2.440	9.068*	1.015

*This value includes no filtration. The usual value of 8.25 is for a filter of 0.5 mm platinum and includes secondary radiations generated in the platinum filter.
Modified from NCRP Report No. 41[3]

in the wall of the capsule. Note the different units of these two constants.

Integrating dose meters such as the pocket dosimeter are calibrated in the same manner by using a timed exposure measured in rads. For x-rays and gamma rays, roentgens and rads are considered to be roughly equivalent.

SCINTILLATION DETECTORS

In comparison with gas-filled detectors, scintillation detectors have two principal advantages that augment their use in nu-clear medicine: they are capable of much higher counting rates because of fast re-solving times, and they are much more ef-ficient for gamma-ray detection while pre-serving pulse-height proportionality. These detectors have a relatively short his-tory; modern detectors were only intro-duced in the late 1940s. The basic ele-ments of a scintillation detector system using a thallium-activated NaI(Tl) crystal are shown in Figure 2–9. Ionizing radia-tion is absorbed in the scintillator, and its energy is converted to light photons, hence the term *scintillation crystal*. Some

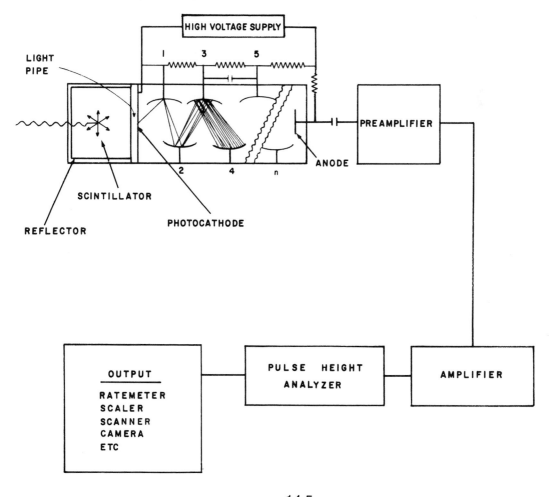

14.5 cms

Fig. 2–9. Scintillation detector system with a light pipe coupling the scintillation crystal to the PM tube.

of these photons strike the photocathode of a photomultiplier (PM) tube. Electrons ejected by the photocathode are amplified by a series of dynodes in the PM tube to form a voltage output pulse proportional in height to the energy of the ionizing event. This signal is then amplified and shaped prior to processing according to several possible display formats. The general system is highly versatile and forms the basis for most radiation detector systems used in nuclear medicine.

Sodium Iodide Crystals

While scintillation crystals may be used for detecting any type of ionizing radiation, this discussion considers primarily gamma-ray detection. Many different materials produce transmittable fluorescence when struck by ionizing radiation, and each has its own particular characteristics, for example, wavelength emission, decay time, and density.[4] Among these materials are anthracene crystals, various plastic and liquid phosphors, and such inorganic crystals as NaI, CsI, LiI, ZnS, and BGO. Plastic scintillators are used when large volume detectors are needed, when particles are to be measured in the presence of gamma rays, and for neutron measurements.[5] Sodium iodide crystals are particularly useful in gamma-ray detection because of their high density, created by high iodine content (85% by weight) with high atomic number (Z = 53). While NaI(Tl) crystals are slower than most organic phosphors, they are sufficiently fast for most nuclear medical applications, and the spectral wavelength emission is well matched to the bi-alkali photocathodes used in most PM tubes.

Gamma rays striking the crystals are absorbed by the three processes described in Chapter 1, namely photoelectric effect, Compton scattering, and pair production. Photoelectric effect predominates at low energies but falls off rapidly above 90 keV (Fig. 1–18). NaI(Tl) crystals are efficient

scintillators, producing ~1 photon for each 30 eV of energy absorbed.

In each photon absorption process, photon energy is imparted to orbital electrons within the crystal lattice. This raises the electron from the valence band to a conduction band, where the electron is free to move from atom to atom across a crystal plane (Fig. 2–10). When an unfilled orbital shell (electron hole) is encountered, the electron quickly returns to the valence band and, in doing so, emits light photons. This process requires approximately 10^{-12} sec. In NaI crystals, this process is greatly aided by the addition of small amounts of impurities or such electron acceptors as thallium, which provide the holes and emit fluorescence.

Since many ion pairs are formed in the ionization process, a single gamma photon is ultimately converted into many light photons (approximately one photon for every 30 to 50 eV of absorbed gamma energy). The number of light photons emitted is directly proportional to the gamma-ray energy, assuming the gamma ray has been completely absorbed within the crystal. If part of the energy escapes from the crystal, as frequently occurs with Compton scattering, fewer light photons will be produced, and the resulting output pulse will be less than the energy of the incident photon. This energy loss creates the Compton region of the gamma-ray spectrum (see Fig. 2–13). The entire deionization process within a NaI(Tl) crystal requires approximately 3×10^{-7} sec.

In the design of crystals, it is important for most of the light produced to reach the photocathode. Because NaI is highly refractive, crystals are often roughened to reduce the reflection between the crystal and the light pipe. Both the crystal and the circmference of the light pipe are coated with a highly reflective substance, usually Al_2O_3 or MgO, to reflect maximum light to the photocathode. NaI(Tl) crystals are hygroscopic and must be hermetically sealed. Absorption of moisture and oxy-

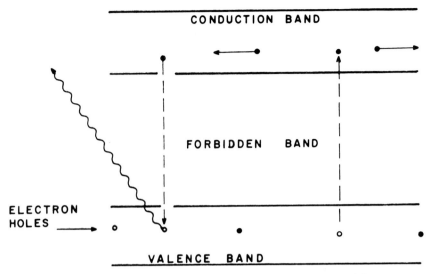

Fig. 2–10. Ionization process in crystal lattice showing mechanism of fluorescence production.

gen discolors the crystal, which causes increased internal light absorption. In many cases, the PM tube is sealed directly to the crystal. In other cases, such as the gamma camera, the PM tube is separated from the crystal. In this case, a plastic light pipe is optically coupled to the crystal and the PM tube with silicone grease.

Photocathodes

The thin coating of semitransparent material applied to the inner surface of the PM tube is the photocathode. Light photons produced in the crystal strike the photocathode and eject loosely bound electrons from the valence band directly into the vacuum of the PM tube. The photocathode usually consists of some alkali metal deposited on the glass window of the PM tube. Most modern PM tubes have a bi-alkali photocathode consisting of Sb-K_2-Cs, which has a high photo-efficiency in the spectral range of NaI(Tl) emissions, i.e., many photocathode electrons are ejected per MeV of incident gamma energy. Even so, only about 10% efficiency is generally achieved. Thus a 0.5-MeV gamma ray produces approximately 10^4 photons within the crystal, which results

in the ejection of about 10^3 electrons from the photocathode. The photocathode must be thick enough to absorb the incident photon efficiently yet thin enough to minimize self-absorption of the ejected electrons. In bi-alkali tubes, the optimal photocathode thickness is about 200 nm.

The photocathode is sensitive to ambient temperature variations, which may affect its efficiency. Also, elevated temperatures may increase electronic noise. With very low activity samples, cooling the PM tube to 0° C may be useful.

Photomultiplier Tubes

Once ejected from the photocathode, the electrons are accelerated toward the first dynode. This is a metal plate covered with the same photoemissive material as the photocathode. It is positively charged with respect to the photocathode. Electrons emitted from the photocathode are accelerated and gain sufficient energy to eject secondary electrons from the dynode. These secondary electrons are then accelerated toward the second dynode, where further multiplication occurs, and so on through 10 to 14 dynodes with an amplification of 10^6 to 10^8 (Fig. 2–9).

A constant gain at each dynode is essential to maintaining proportionality because a small variation at one dynode is amplified by each succeeding dynode, thus magnifying the error and distorting the proportionality between the input scintillation event and the output pulse. Capacitors at higher stages help maintain the stability of charge on each dynode as do protective shields, which minimize the effects of changing magnetic fields.

High-Voltage Supply

The PM tube is almost always energized by a separate voltage source to supply high voltage to the dynodes. Each dynode is charged with progressively higher voltage by a voltage divider circuit (Fig. 2–9). If 1000 V are applied across 10 dynodes, the potential across each dynode is 100 V more than that across the preceding dynode. In this way, the electron direction is always toward the anode, and the amplification between dynodes is approximately equal per incident electron. To maintain proportionality between gamma energy and pulse output, the voltage supply must be very stable. Instability is called *drift* and may be due to temperature changes and alterations in line voltage. If the drift is downward, the pulse output is low relative to the gamma-energy input. If the drift is upward, the pulse output is erroneously high. If the drift becomes too high, another effect may occur: electrons may be pulled off preceding dynodes in the absence of any photon emission (dark current). These electrons are then accelerated through the dynode sequence and produce *thermal emission* noise. This phenomenon can be demonstrated easily in a scintillation counter by increasing the high voltage until the scaler begins to register spontaneous counting rate in the absence of any radioactive source.

Preamplifiers

The output pulses from the PM tube are of low voltage, typically on the order of a few millivolts, and often have undesirable characteristics for subsequent electronic manipulation. Consequently, a preamplifier is inserted between the PM tube and the amplifier. The preamplifier has three essential functions: (1) to amplify the signal, (2) to match electrical impedance between the PM tube and the amplifier, and (3) to shape the signal for optimum handling by the amplifier. Shaping is usually accomplished by an R-C circuit which typically increases the pulse time constant. An essential feature of a preamplifier is linearity, i.e., the signal output must be proportional to the input. Usually, this is not too difficult to accomplish with PM tubes, but it is more exacting when amplifying the weak signals of semiconductor detectors.

The pulse in Figure 2–11 has a rapid rise and a long tail. The rise time is a reflection of: (1) the decay time of the scintillation event within the crystal (usually about 0.25 μsec) and (2) the time required for the electrons to traverse the dynodes in the PM tube. This time varies with the number and structure of the dynodes.[6] The pulse rise generally requires 1 to 2 μsec to complete, and the tail is much longer. If subsequent pulses fall within this tail, the voltage height will be increased and thus distorted. Pulse-shaping circuits, including R-C clipping and delay lines, help to

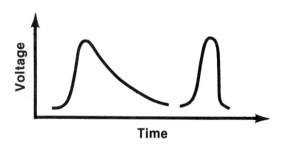

Fig. 2–11. The output pulse from the PM tube has a long tail, which increases the probability of "pulse pileup" at high counting rates. The clipped pulse at right maintains the pulse-height information but eliminates the long tail.

eliminate tailing by producing pulses of 1 μsec or less, thus greatly increasing the pulse pair resolution, i.e., the number of pulses per second that can be separated and correctly discriminated (Fig. 2–12).

Amplifiers

Boyd et al. have listed the characteristics of amplifiers:[7]

1. Shape pulse to decrease resolving time.
2. Increase gain to drive pulse-height analyzers, scalers, etc.
3. Increase signal-to-noise ratio. Noise is any unwanted signal arising anywhere in the system. Noise sources include PM dark current, electrostatic frequencies, arcing of high voltage, and other radiofrequency (RF) sources.
4. Stabilize signal gain to maintain proportionality between pulse height and photon energy deposition in the crystal.
5. Provide proper polarity of the output signal (usually positive).

Most modern amplifiers utilize transistors, which have the advantage of small size, short warm-up time, low heat generation, minimal drift, and low power requirements.

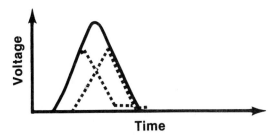

Fig. 2–12. Pulse pileup occurs when two pulses overlap. The resulting output pulse (solid line) is distorted, which causes one of the pulses to go undetected. Subsequent pulse-height analysis may reject the high amplitude pulse, resulting in loss of both counts.

Pulse-Height Analyzers

The pulse height from a linear amplifier is proportional to the radiation energy deposited within the crystal. The implication is that if a monoenergetic beam strikes the crystal and each photon is completely absorbed, all of the output pulses will be the same height. Perfect registry, however, is an elusive goal. Some loss of incident energy occurs through Compton scattering, in which scattered photons escape the crystal, and through the photoelectric effect, when characteristic x-rays, particularly at the edge of the crystal, escape. As a result, a distribution of pulse heights forms around the photopeak value, and the shape of this distribution depends on photon to photoelectric transfer variance; crystal size, composition, and intrinsic rsolution; PM efficiency; and amplifier stability and linearity (Fig. 2–13). Pulse-height analyzers (PHAs) measure the frequency distribution of these pulse *amplitudes.*

The essential components of a single-channel analyzer (SCA) are two *pulse-height discriminators,* which may be set at E and E + ΔE respectively (Fig. 2–14). The upper- and lower-level discriminators consist of electronic circuits called *comparators,* which serve to compare the input pulse amplitude with their own voltage setting. They produce an output only when the input pulse exceeds their voltage setting. The discriminator pulses are sent to an *anticoincidence circuit,* which produces an output pulse when only one of the pulses (lower or threshold) occurs. This *differential* mode of operation then defines a "window," or energy range, equal to ΔE. If the upper discriminator is disabled, all pulses with amplitude greater than E will be counted—the *integral* mode of operation. The output pulses from the SCA are then used to drive scalers, ratemeters, and other devices for count registration.

Most detection devices with SCA's have

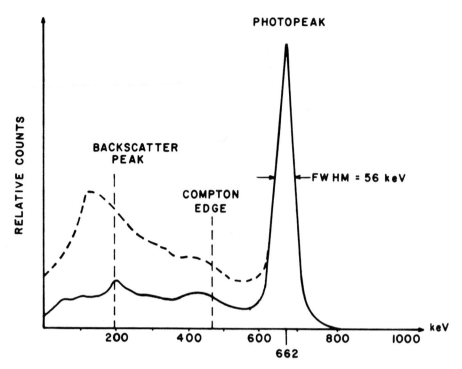

Fig. 2–13. Pulse-height spectrum of Cs-137, using a 5-in. NaI(Tl) detector. The addition of a scattering medium (dotted line) affects primarily the lower end of the spectrum.

two controls for adjusting the discriminators, usually calibrated in keV. The lower-level discriminator is often called the *base level.* In some cases, one determines the center of the window, while the other determines the window width as a percentage of that setting. For example, if Tc-99m (E_γ = 140 keV) were being counted with a symmetric 20% window, the energy range selected would be 140 ± 14 keV, or 126 to 154 keV. In some situations, exclusion of some of the Compton scatter below the 140-keV photopeak is desirable. An "asymmetric window" can be selected merely by increasing the center-line adjustment to 150 keV. If the 20% window is retained, the new range is 150 ± 15 keV, or 135 to 165 keV. Notice that the same "percent window" now encompasses a wider energy range. Most modern detection devices have pushbutton selectors that designate the radionuclides most frequently counted. For special counting

situations, however, it is important to have manual controls that override these automatic selectors.

Some applications of pulse-height analysis require multiple levels of discrimination. An example is gamma-ray spectroscopy (see Chapter 3). Rather than connect numerous SCA's, a *multichannel analyzer* (MCA) is usually employed. The heart of a MCA is a pulse sorting device known as an *analog-to-digital converter* (ADC). Incoming pulses are separated according to amplitude and stored in a series of channels numbering from 128 to as many as 8192, each channel proportional to a preselected energy or amplitude range, ΔE. To accomplish this, the ADC uses either a series of comparators or a *ramp converter.*[8] The multichannel analyzer uses a *digital storage* device that receives and sums pulses selected by the ADC as corresponding to various energy levels. This storage device contains X-Y

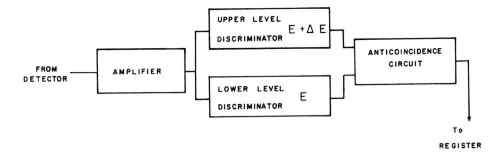

A

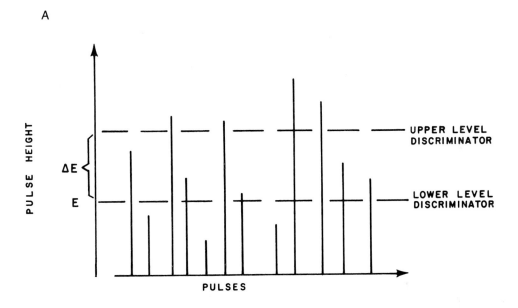

B

Fig. 2–14. *A*. Principles of a single-channel PHA. *B*. In the differential mode, the pulse height analyzer passes only those pulses falling within the window (5 counts). In the integral mode, all pulses with energy greater than E will be counted (9 counts).

locations, usually in a magnetic core in which the X location corresponds to ΔE and the Y location corresponds to the frequency of pulses falling within that window width. Once accumulated, the spectrum may be displayed by an X-Y plotter, cathode-ray tube, line printer, or other readout device.

Gamma-ray spectra can be derived with a single-channel analyzer by serial count-ing with a narrow window and progressively advancing up the energy scale, recording and plotting each count in turn. The advantage of a multichannel analyzer for spectrum analysis is obvious.

From Figure 2–14, it is apparent that the monoenergetic gamma rays of Cs-137 (actually they derive from the short-lived daughter, Ba-137m) result in a distribution of pulse heights. The width of the principal peak at half its value, or full-width-half maximum (FWHM), characterizes the system's resolution, that is, the distribution of pulses around the true photon energy. This distribution determines the detector's ability to differentiate between gamma rays of different energies. Energy resolution is often expressed as a percentage of the peak energy of Cs-137.

% resolution

$$= \frac{^{137}\text{Cs FWHM (keV)}}{662} \times 100$$

Good NaI(Tl) detection systems provide approximately 7 to 9% resolution. The value varies greatly with the size crystal, the type of PM tube, and the detection geometry. For example, for scintillation cameras with several PM tubes, light pipe, and capacitor circuitry, resolutions of about 15% can be expected.[6]

Scalers

The scaler integrates the number of pulses accepted by the analyzer, either mechanically or, more commonly, electronically. Most scalers now read in decimal, using LEDs, although the primary circuitry usually operates in a binary system. Most counting systems are equipped with scaler-timers, which measure both elapsed time and accumulated counts. The scaler-timer permits the detector to count for a *preset time* or until a *preset count* has been scaled.

Ratemeters

The ratemeter provides a direct and continuous measurement of the rate at which accepted pulses are processed, usually by means of a meter that fluctuates continuously with the changing count per unit time. *Analog* ratemeters operate by means of an RC circuit in which the arriving pulses build up on a capacitor and are shunted through a resistor (Fig. 2–15). The time to reach equilibrium is a function of the rate of the pulses and of the RC *time constant* of the circuit. Most ratemeters

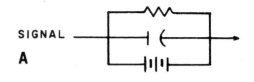

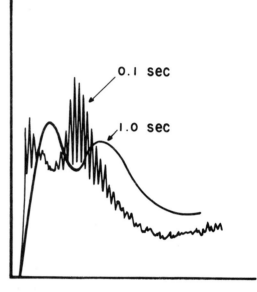

B

Fig. 2–15. Ratemeter circuit (A) and recordings (B) of a radioactive bolus through the heart recorded with 0.1 sec and 1.0 sec time constant. With 1.0 sec time constant, individual heart beats are completely lost.

have several time constants, which may be selected to reflect rapid fluctuations or to average the counts over greater time (long-time constant). The effect is illustrated in Figure 2–15, which represents the passage of a bolus of activity through the heart. With a time constant of 1 sec, it is possible to discern the bolus entering and leaving the right and left chambers. The individual heart beats, however, which are seen easily with a 0.1-sec time constant, cannot be resolved at the longer time constant.

Errors caused by time lag may be avoided by use of a *digital ratemeter*. A scaler is a type of digital ratemeter. After a preset time, the scaler indicates the counts accumulated during that period. A digital ratemeter is merely a constantly resetting scaler. The recycle frequency, however, is in reality a time constant. If long frequency intervals are selected, rapidly changing count rates may go undetected. Very short recycle times may themselves induce some counting error unless some buffering device is used.

The ratemeter output may be recorded in several ways, including a strip-chart recorder, magnetic tape, or magnetic disc. The strip-chart recorder, which reflects the changing rate on paper moving at a predetermined speed, is useful because it is easy to calibrate, simple to operate, versatile, and relatively inexpensive.

SEMICONDUCTOR DETECTORS

Solid-state detectors made of semiconducting materials are becoming increasingly important in radiation detection. Semiconductor detectors operate in a manner analogous to gas-filled detectors, except that they are 2000 to 5000 times more dense and are therefore much more efficient as radiation absorbers. Ordinarily, such semiconducting substances as silicon and germanium are poor electrical conductors. When they are ionized by ionizing radiation, however, the charges generated can be collected by applying a voltage potential across the detector crystal.

Semiconductors take many forms, but they generally consist of a *p-n junction,* made by creating two zones within the semiconductor material: a *p*-type material zone, which acts as an electron acceptor, and an *n*-type material zone, which acts as an electron donor (Fig. 2–16). If an electrical potential or bias is applied to the detector, the electrical field draws electrons toward the *p* side and electron holes (in the valence band) toward the *n* side, thus forming an electrically neutral and insulating *depletion* region between the two. In this depleted region, no current flows. When radiation is absorbed within the depleted region (and only in this region), ion pairs are formed. The electrons are raised from the valence band to the conduction band and drift toward the positive *p* side. The electron holes drift toward the electron donor *n* side, where they are filled. As a result, a small change in the bias develops proportional to the energy deposited in the depletion region. The physical principles thus contain elements analogous to both scintillation crystals and ionization chambers.

Semiconductor detectors have several advantages. The most important is that they have very high resolution and are thus capable of resolving energies only a few electron volts apart. The reason for this capability is that far more electrons are collected per million electron volts of energy absorbed than in ion chambers or scintillation detectors. Germanium requires only 2.9 eV and silicon 3.5 eV to form an ion pair, while NaI(Tl) requires 30 to 50 eV. Furthermore, the variability of the photocathode is eliminated. Thus the energy resolution of semiconductors may be 20 times greater than that of NaI(Tl) crystals (Fig. 2–17).[9] They have a very short response time, so that pulse pair resolution is high. These semiconductors can be made so small that they can be inserted directly into the body, if desired.

Semiconductors also have several disadvantages. Because of the very low energy required to produce a conduction electron, thermal noise may be high. Most applications require liquid nitrogen cooling to reduce this noise both in the detector and in the preamplifier. The bias voltage must be relatively high, which necessitates careful shielding, and the detectors are sensitive to atmospheric moisture. A major problem is encountered in producing detectors with sufficiently large volume to be efficient for gamma-ray detection. Present technology limits the depletion zone to a few millimeters of thickness. Thus they are excellent for detecting charged particles and weak x-rays, but

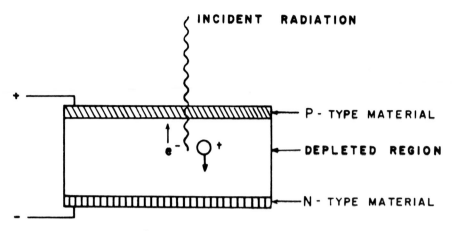

Fig. 2–16. P-N type semiconductor.

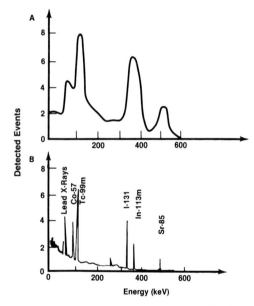

Fig. 2–17. Spectra derived from multichannel analyzer using A, NaI(Tl) crystal, and B, Germanium lithium drifted (GeLi) detector.

gamma rays with sufficient energy to escape the body unattenuated are detected with low efficiency.

LIQUID SCINTILLATION COUNTING

The use of a liquid phosphor offers a singular advantage: it allows complete immersion of the radioactive sample in the detector volume, thereby achieving virtual 4π geometry and eliminating any absorption in the container walls between sample and detector. Liquid scintillation counting is therefore especially suitable for counting such weak beta emitters as H-3 and C-14 as well as most other types of emissions. The counting efficiency for beta particles in many cases approaches 100%.

The basic elements of a liquid scintillation system include:

1. A *solvent*, which mixes with the radioactive sample and absorbs the ionizing radiation.
2. A *primary scintillator*, which converts a fraction of the ionizing radiation dissipated in the solvent into fluorescence. Often a *secondary scintillator* may be used to shift the fluorescence spectrum of the primary scintillator to match the spectral response of the photocathode of the PM tube.
3. Associated PM tube and electronics, which convert the fluorescence into an electrical pulse for measurement and analysis.

Scintillation Solvents

Such aromatic solvents as xylene, toluene, or dioxane are favored because of their high scintillation yield. Toluene is

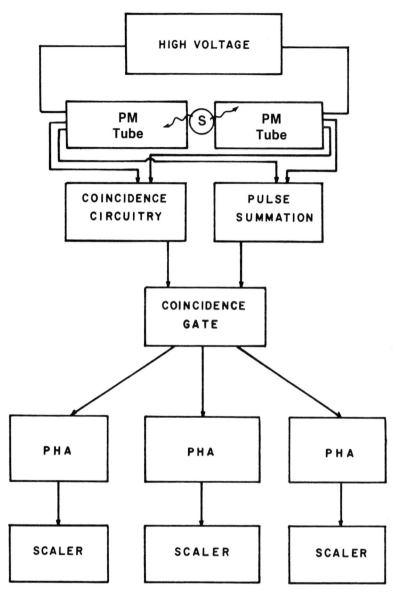

Fig. 2–18. Diagram of three channel liquid scintillation counter electroncs. The sample S is positioned between the two PM tubes.

often chosen because of its relatively low price and intermediate susceptibility to quenching. Dioxane, an aliphatic solvent, is useful because of its greater miscibility with aqueous solutions than the aromatic solvents. Also, alcohol may be added as a secondary solvent to increase water miscibility. Suspensions are often used for counting insoluble or particulate radio-active samples. These suspensions most often consist of a gel formed by suspending colloidal silica in the solvent solution.

Primary Scintillators

These aromatic compounds, such as PPO (2,5-diphenyloxazole), are added to the solvent in 10^{-2}- to 10^{-3}-M concentrations, which serve to convert the excitation of the solvent into photon emissions in the ultraviolet and visible range. These emissions are detectable by standard PM tubes. Because they are electron acceptors, they may be likened to the thallium impurities in a NaI(Tl) detector. Electrons elevated to the conduction band by ionizing radiation return to the valence band when they encounter a scintillator molecule, and they emit light photons in the process. Since the number of photons emitted is proportional to the energy of the ionizing event, spectrometric separation of different radionuclides is possible. Horrocks and Peng list several "fluors" or scintillator solutes in common use.[10] An important part of the art of liquid scintillation counting lies in the appropriate selection of scintillators to achieve the highest fluorescence quantum yield for any particular liquid counting system. This yield determines the number of photocathode electrons emitted per MeV of absorbed energy and thus the energy resolution of the system.

Secondary Scintillators

The function of a secondary scintillator solute is to shift the spectral emission of the primary scintillator to a longer wavelength, thereby providing a better spectral match for the photocathode. The secondary scintillators absorb the photons emitted by the primary scintillator and emit secondary photons of a longer wavelength. One of the most commonly used secondary scintillators, POPOP (1,4-bis[2-(5-phenyloxazolyl)]-benzene), shifts the fluorescence maxima of PPO from about 380 to 440 nm. The latter wavelength was desired in order to match the peak sensitivity of S-11 photocathodes. The currently used bi-alkali photocathodes, however, have a peak sensitivity of 380 to 390 nm, so use of the secondary scintillator is unnecessary.[11] Other considerations, however, such as the size of the liquid solvent volume and the transmission characteristics

of the glass vials, may demand a spectral shift for optimal detection efficiency.

Associated Electronics

Figure 2–18 outlines the basic elements of a liquid scintillation counter and associated electronics.

The sample is lowered into a shielded well viewed by two PM tubes. The output of the two PM tubes is amplified and summed for better resolution (since spectral resolution depends on the efficiency of light collection). The outputs are also coincidence-gated to reduce low-level noise, which is an inherent problem in any system employing high-gain amplification of low-energy signals. A scintillation event must be detected by both PM tubes simultaneously in order to be counted. Thermal and electronic noise originating in one or the other PM tube circuits is random and therefore goes unregistered. A second means of reducing thermal noise is to place the entire system inside a refrigerator with a temperature of approximately $-8°C$.

REFERENCES

1. Snell, A.H. (Ed.): Nuclear Instruments and Their Uses. Vol. 1. New York, John Wiley & Sons, 1962.
2. ICRU Report 19: Specification of High Activity Gamma-Ray Sources. Washington, D.C. International Commission on Radiation Units and Measurements, 1971.
3. NCRP Report No. 41: Specification of Gamma-Ray Brachytherapy Sources. Washington, D.C., National Council on Radiation Protection and Measurements. 1974, p. 8.
4. Price, W.J.: Nuclear Radiation Detection. New York, McGraw-Hill, 1964, p. 162.
5. Watt, D.E., Lawson, R.D., and Clare, D.M.: An experimental appraisal of the validity of neutron dosimetry theory in radiation protection. In Neutron Monitoring. IAEA, Vienna, 1967, p. 27.
6. Cradduck, T.D.: Fundamentals of scintillation counting. Semin. Nucl. Med., 3:205, 1973.
7. Boyd, C.M., and Dalrymple, G.V. (Eds.): Basic Scientific Principles of Nuclear Medicine. St. Louis, C.V. Mosby, 1974.
8. Kowalski, E.: Nuclear Counting Electronics. New York, Springer, 1970.
9. Ter-Pogossian, M.M., and Phelps, M.E.: Semiconductor detector systems. Semin. Nucl. Med., 3:343, 1973.
10. Peng, C.T., Horrocks, D.L., and Alpen, E.L.

(Eds.): Liquid Scintillation Counting. Vols. 1 and 2. New York, Academic Press, 1980.

11. Birks, J.B.: The Theory and Practice of Scintillation Counting. Oxford, Pergamon Press, 1964.

BIBLIOGRAPHY

Bransome, E.D. (Ed.): The Current Status of Liquid Scintillation Counting. New York, Grune and Stratton, 1970.

Crook, M.A., Johnson, P., and Scales, B. (Eds.): Liquid Scintillation Counting. Vols. 1 and 2. London, Heyden and Son, 1972.

ICRU Report 20: Radiation Protection Instrumentation and Its Application. Washington, D.C., In-terntional Commission on Radiation Units and Measurements, 1976.

Kobayashi, Y., and Mandsley, D.V.: Practical aspects of double isotope counting. *In* The Current Status of Liquid Scintillation Counting. Edited by E.D. Bransome. New York, Grune and Stratton, 1970.

Peng, C.T.: A review of methods of quench correction in liquid scintillation counting. *In* The Current Status of Liquid Scintillation Counting. Edited by E.D. Bransome. New York, Grune and Stratton, 1970.

Shonka, F.R., Dose, J.E., and Failla, G.: Conductive plastic equivalent to tissue, air, and polystyrene. In 2nd U.N. International Conference of the Peaceful Uses of Atomic Energy. Vol. 21. New York, United Nations, 1958, p. 184.

Chapter 3

COUNTING RADIOACTIVITY

JOHN HARBERT

It is not particularly difficult to derive meaningful and reproducible results from radioactivity measurements, but careful attention to details is rewarding. Measurement techniques differ greatly depending upon the type of radiation counted and the nature of the radioactive source. Beta- and gamma-ray detection are discussed separately; some principles common to both are considered first.

All radioactivity counting problems involve a source of ionizing radiation and a detector sensitive to the radiation. Few problems in nuclear medicine involve merely the detection of radioactivity; rather, the amount and/or location of the activity must be determined with a manageable degree of error.

Individual radionuclide disintegrations are random, but the rate of transformation can be described by the decay law:

$$\frac{dN}{dt} = -N\lambda$$

where N is the number of radioactive atoms present and λ is the decay constant, or $0.693/T_{1/2}$. If λ is known and every disintegration ($-N \, dt$) is detected, it is possible to calculate the total number of radioactive atoms present. Such fortuity is almost never achieved, however, because

several factors prevent perfect detection efficiency.

COUNTING EFFICIENCY

The overall efficiency of any radiation counting system is defined as the ratio of the counting rate to the number of disintegrations per unit time:

$$E = \frac{cps}{dps}$$

The factors that affect overall efficiency of a counting system are the geometry, absorption, scatter, intrinsic detector efficiency, and fidelity of count registration.

Overall detector efficiency D can be expressed as

$$D = F \times g \times \epsilon \times f$$

where F is a factor accounting for absorbed and scattered radiation, g is the geometric efficiency, ϵ is the intrinsic efficiency of the detector, and f is the fraction of pulses accepted by the pulse-height analyzer.

Geometry

The greatest factors affecting the efficiency of any counting system are the location, size, and shape of the sample in relation to the sensitive volume of the detector. The radiations from a radioactive

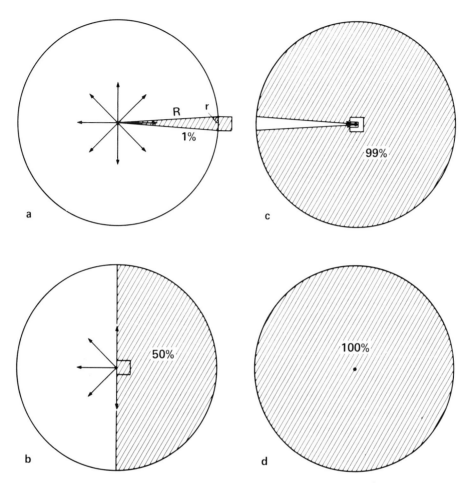

Fig. 3–1. Four different counting geometries: *a*, point source R cm from a cylindric crystal detector of radius *r*; *b*, point source at the detector face; *c*, point source inside well crystal; *d*, 4π geometry as in liquid scintillation counting.

source are emitted isotropically, i.e., equally in every direction. For the case of a point source and detector with radius r located at some distance R from the source (Fig. 3–1a), the area exposed to the sphere of radiation flux emanating from the source is given by:

$$g = \frac{\pi r^2}{4\pi R^2} = \frac{\text{crystal area}}{\text{sphere area}}$$

If the crystal measures 4 cm in diameter and is situated 10 cm from the source, the exposed area is only:

$$g = \frac{3.14 \times 2^2}{4 \times 3.14 \times 10^2} = \frac{12.56}{1256} = 1\%$$

If the same crystal is moved twice this distance away, the geometric factor is less by:

$$g = \frac{12.56}{12.56 \times 20^2} = 0.25\%$$

This example is a simple demonstration of the *inverse square law*, which states that the counting rate decreases by $\frac{1}{R^2}$ as the detector moves away from a point source and increases by the same proportion as it is moved toward the source.

The inverse square law is only an approximation and does not hold for either large detectors or extended sources, such as activity within the human body. Thus, if R is reduced to zero and the source is placed against the detector (Fig. 3–1b), the counting rate does not become infinite; it reaches only about 50% of $\frac{dN}{dt}$. A closer approximation to the true geometric efficiency for cylindric detectors is given by the factor $\frac{1}{2}$ (1 − cos θ) where θ is one-half the angle subtended by the crystal. In the case of Figure 3–1b where θ = 90° and cos θ = 0, the geometric factor becomes 0.5, which represents the actual condition.

Even greater detector efficiency is achieved by placing the source within the crystal as seen in Figure 3–1c, which is the geometry of a well counter. Now only the narrow angle subtended by the well opening allows radiations to escape. Figure 3–2 relates the response of a typical well counter (in percent of gamma rays detected) to the volume of sample measured. The loss of counts is due almost entirely to the decreasing angle subtended by the crystal and only slightly to the increased self-absorption due to increasing volume.

Virtually 100% geometric efficiency can be obtained by suspending the source completely within the detector (Fig. 3–1d). Such 4π geometry is most commonly encountered in liquid scintillation counting.

Absorption

Not all radiations emitted from the radioactive source and subtended by the detector reach the detector. Some are absorbed through interaction with the material of the source *(self-absorption)*, in the medium between the source and the detector, and in the cladding of the detector itself. Self-absorption is more important with particulate radiation than with gamma radiation. Every beta emitter has a *saturation thickness* beyond which adding to the sample fails to increase the detected counts. Absorption outside the detector always decreases counting rate.

The usual method of correcting for external absorption is to count an aliquot of activity with and without the addition of absorber material while keeping all other factors of geometry equal. In general, the fraction of gamma rays that are emitted from a source and undergo absorption before reaching the detector decreases with increasing gamma energy.

Scatter

Scattered photons in the source may either increase or decrease detection efficiency. Figure 3–3 shows a source of photons distributed within a scattering medium. Photons e, g, and h are Compton scattered photons, which increase the counting rate. Photon e has been scattered off the wall of the collimator. Photon g has arisen outside the field of view of the collimator and is scattered into the detector. Photon h has undergone *multiple scattering* to reach the detector. Scattering reduces the photon energy but may increase the total counts observed.

Scattering of gamma photons increases with Z of the material and varies with the energy of the photon, as shown in Figure 3–4. One of the chief functions of pulse-

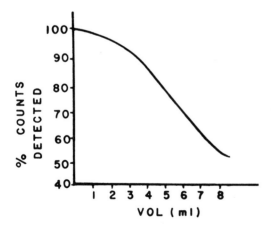

Fig. 3–2. Changing counting rate as a function of source volume in a typical well counter.

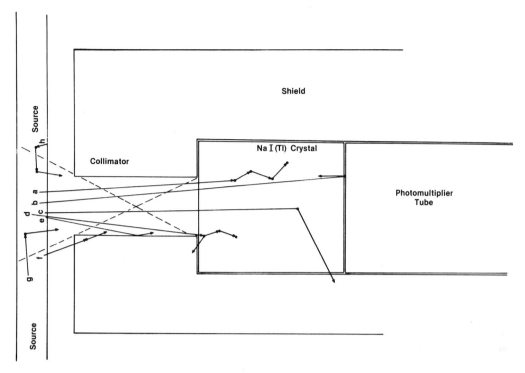

Fig. 3–3. Extended gamma photon source and collimated NaI(Tl) detector. See text for description.

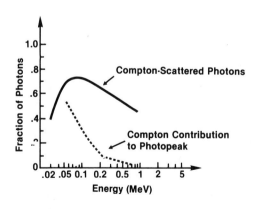

Fig. 3–4. The fraction of gamma rays scattered in tissue medium (solid line) as a function of energy. The fraction appearing in the photopeak (broken line) is calculated for a 20% window and a NaI(Tl) crystal. (Modified from Anger, H.O.[1])

height discrimination in gamma-ray detection is the elimination of scattered photons (particularly in imaging because of the degradation of resolution). Figure 3–4 also plots the contribution of Compton scattering to the photopeak. The reason for decreasing Compton contribution with increasing energy is that the distance between photopeak and *Compton edge* increases. Most analyzer windows are set as a percentage of photopeak energy. Table 3–1 indicates angles of gamma-ray scattering that result in only 10% energy loss for several radionuclides. Gamma rays with 10% less than photopeak energy fall within a 20% analyzer window. Obviously, with lower-energy photons, a significant portion of the counts accepted result from scattered photons.

Scattered beta particles usually increase counting rate, especially with higher energy particles, which scatter from the sample mount back into the detector volume *(backscatter)*.

TABLE 3–1. *The angle of scatter resulting in 10% loss of energy for several radionuclides*

Radionuclide	Incident Gamma-Ray Energy (keV)	Scattering Angle	Scattered Gamma-Ray Energy (keV)
^{125}I	35	152°	32
^{133}Xe	81	68°	73
^{99m}Tc	140	39°	126
^{131}I	364	31°	330
^{137m}Ba	662	22°	600

From Hine, G.J.: Performance characteristics of nuclear instruments. *In* Quality Control in Nuclear Medicine. Edited by B.A. Rhodes. St. Louis, C.V. Mosby, 1977.

Detector Efficiency

The *intrinsic efficiency* of a detector ϵ is defined as the ratio of the number of radiations (photons or particles) that interact in the detector to the total number of incident radiations. Intrinsic efficiency of most detectors is nearly 100% for alpha and beta particles because of their short path length. Intrinsic efficiency for gamma rays, however, depends upon the photon energy and the size, shape, and composition of the sensitive volume of the detector.

If each photon absorbed results in an output signal, the intrinsic efficiency may be represented as follows:

$$\epsilon = 1 - \exp\left[-\mu_l (E)\, x\right]$$

where μ_l is the linear attenuation coefficient of the detector material for photon energy E and x is the detector thickness. The relationship between linear attenuation coefficient μ_l and photon energy is shown in Figure 3–5 for water, sodium iodide, and lead. Detector attenuation, and therefore intrinsic efficiency, decrease nearly logarithmically with increasing energy. For higher-energy photons, larger, denser crystals are usually employed. Germanium crystals are denser than NaI(Tl) crystals by 5.68:3.67 g/cm^3. Ge(Li) crystals, however, are restricted to thicknesses of less than approximately 5 cm because of

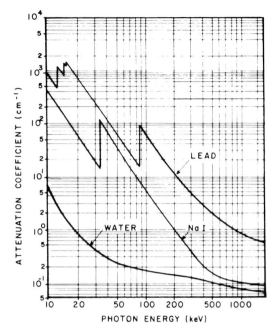

Fig. 3–5. Linear attenuation coefficients for water, NaI, and lead as a function of photon energy.

limitations imposed by the depletion zone (see Chapter 2).

Most gas-filled detectors have efficiencies of less than 1% for the gamma-ray energies encountered in nuclear medicine. Some multiwire proportional counters have been filled with xenon gas under pressure for use as imaging devices, but they are suitable only for radionuclides that emit low-energy gamma-rays and x-rays, such as Ta-178, Xe-133, and Tl-201. One such "camera" containing xenon gas at 10 atm was described by Zimmerman et al.;[2] its intrinsic efficiency was 70% of that of an Anger camera with a 6-mm NaI(Tl) crystal for photons of 60 to 81 keV. With such detector systems, scatter with partial absorption of photons commonly gives rise to escape peaks (see "Gamma-Ray Spectrometry" in this chapter).

Use of a pulse-height analyzer and photopeak counting further reduces the intrinsic efficiency. In this case, only those photons that are completely absorbed in the crystal, the *photofraction,* and meet the energy requirements of the window enclosing the photopeak are counted. The photofraction of any radionuclide depends on the photon energy and the size and composition of the detector, as discussed earlier.

Instrument Deadtime

For all radiation detectors, there are counting rate limitations imposed by the time required to transform the ionizing event into an electronic signal. In the case of GM tubes, this time is relatively long (100 to 500 μsec) because of the time required for the large positive ions to reach the outer cathode. In the case of modern scintillation detectors, this time is very short (nanoseconds) because of fast deexcitation times and efficient PM tubes. In both cases, the electronic signal is produced by the sharp drop in potential dif-

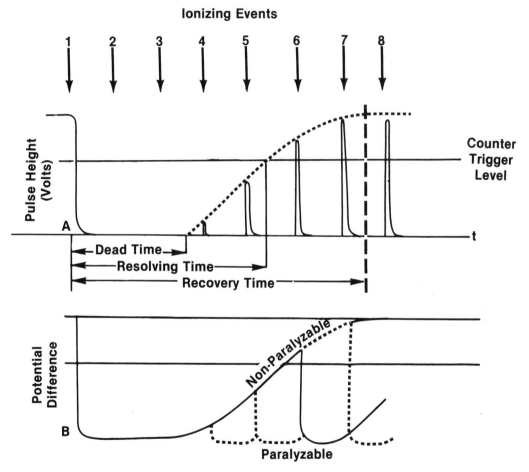

Fig. 3–6. Output pulses from a radiation detector illustrating the effect of coincidence on pulse height in paralyzable and nonparalyzable systems. *A.* The dotted line represents the return of potential difference across the electrodes following an initial pulse. During the deadtime, no pulse results from ionizing events 2 and 3. Pulses 4 to 7 would result in pulses of reduced amplitude. Only event 8, which occurs after the recovery time, will produce a full amplitude pulse. *B.* The potential difference from the detector is represented here as a solid line. In a nonparalyzable system, event 6 would produce a second pulse of reduced amplitude. In a paralyzable system (broken line) only the first event would produce a pulse.

ference between electrodes once the electrons reach the anode. The signal strength, or *pulse height,* is proportional to the change in potential difference across the electrodes (Fig. 3–6B). During the *recovery time,* the potential difference between electrodes is restored. Several terms that refer to this process are defined as follows. The *deadtime* is the period following the first pulse, during which the detector is insensitive to incoming ionizing events. The *resolving time* is the time required for the potential difference to increase sufficiently to produce a pulse that can "trigger" the counter. It is also the shortest time interval by which two pulses must be divided to be detected as separate pulses. The recovery time is the period required for regaining a potential difference sufficient to produce a full amplitude pulse. Ionizing events that enter the detector before the resolving time are lost because of *coincidence.* This loss is called *pulse pileup,* or *deadtime loss.* Ionizing events that occur during the recovery time result in lower pulse heights, or *baseline shift.* Such pulses are lost if they fall below the lower-level discriminator of the PHA.

Counting systems are *paralyzable* if each event introduces a deadtime τ, whether or not the event is counted (dotted lines in Fig. 3–6B). In a nonparalyzable system, an event occurring during the deadtime has no effect on the recovery of potential difference. In such a system, the deadtime equals the resolving time.

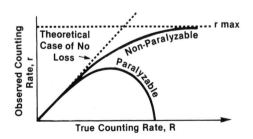

Fig. 3–7. The relationship between true and observed counting rates in paralyzable and nonparalyzable counting systems.

Figure 3–7 demonstrates that as the counting rate increases, coincidence losses produce a variation between the observed counting rate r and the true counting rate R. At low counting rates, the values are identical. But as true counting increases (dashed line), the observed counting rate declines, approaching zero in a *paralyzable* counting system and reaching $r_{max} = 1/\tau$ in a nonparalyzable system. The shape of this curve depends upon the resolvng time and the type of system. For a nonparalyzable system:

$$\frac{R}{r} = \frac{1}{1 - R\tau} \qquad (1)$$

This equation is difficult to solve. Because $1 - R\tau$ is closely approximated by $1 - r\tau$ for the usual counting rates encountered in the laboratory, the above equation can be simplified to:

$$R = \frac{r}{1 - r\tau} \qquad (2)$$

In the case of a paralyzable system, the dead periods are not all the same but dependent on the distribution of intervals between random events. For the paralyzable model:

$$r = Re^{-R\tau}$$

This equation does not permit a direct solution of the true rate R. Instead, an iterative solution is required.

A deadtime τ is determined most often by the paired-source method, wherein the counting rates of two sources are counted separately as r_1 and r_2, and together as r_{12}. Then for a nonparalyzable system for which negligible background is assumed:

$$\tau \cong \frac{r_1 + r_2 - r_{12}}{r_{12}^2 - r_1^2 - r_2^2} \qquad (3)$$

For a paralyzable system:

$$\tau \cong \left[\frac{2r_{12}}{(r_1 + r_2)^2} \right] \ln \left[\frac{r_1 + r_2}{r_{12}} \right] \qquad (4)$$

The sources are counted separately and

simultaneously under constant conditions of geometry, scatter, and absorption. The activity of each source must be selected carefully so that neither source counted by itself induces appreciable coincidence loss, but when counted together, the sources induce about 20% coincidence loss.

A second method, the *decaying source* technique, may be used if a short-lived radioisotope is available in sufficient quantity. Taking advantage of the known change in count rate through decay:

$$R = R_0 e^{-\lambda t}$$

where R_0 is the true counting rate at the beginning of the determination.[3]

Some detectors have built-in coincidence correction circuitry through storage buffers, but in general, these buffers are effective only up to about 30% coincidence loss. While the usual solution to this problem is to avoid coincidence loss by limiting source activity, such a solution is not always possible, and coincidence errors must be corrected by using equation (2) or by graphically using plotted counting rate response as in Figure 3–7. Knowledge of the counting rate response of each instrument used is therefore essential. If the instrument is equipped with a PHA, one must remember that any detected event can cause pulse pileup, whether it falls within the analyzer window or not. To determine the maximum counting rate to be encountered in any experimental situation, the integral mode should be used. The value of τ is determined by the counts from the total spectrum, not merely by those passing the analyzer window.

Standards

The problem of determining absolute activity, which requires knowledge of the overall efficiency, is usually overcome by comparing the counting rate of the unknown source with that of a known standard of the same nuclide:

$$\frac{\text{unknown activity } (\mu Ci)}{\text{standard } (\mu Ci)} = \frac{\text{cps unknown}}{\text{cps standard}}$$

Therefore:

unknown activity (μCi)

$$= \text{standard } (\mu Ci) \times \frac{\text{cps unknown}}{\text{cps standard}}$$

The only criterion for assuring the validity of this relationship is that the same conditions exist for counting both unknown and standard. Usually, this condition is easily fulfilled for samples contained in counting vials, but when the source is located inside the patient, additional problems arise.

When a different radionuclide is used as a standard for counting gamma emissions, the percent abundance of gamma rays per disintegration must be determined for both radionuclides. The activity of the standard must then be corrected to compensate for any difference in abundance; for example, 88% of Tc-99m disintegrations result in emission of a 140-keV gamma photon. If the Tc-99m activity is compared against a Co-57 standard, which yields 122- and 136-keV gamma rays in 96% of disintegrations, the Tc-99m activity must be corrected by 96/88.

Extraneous Counts

An important consideration in many radioactivity measurements, in most in vivo measurements, and in all low-level counting is the occurrence of extraneous counts, which may be defined as counts having any origin other than the radioactive atoms of interest. Two origins of extraneous counts are background counts and interfering radioactivity in the source.

Background

Ambient background radiation derives principally from three sources (Table 3–2):

TABLE 3–2. *Typical environmental radiation field*

Radiation	Energy (MeV)	Source	Absorbed Dose Rate in Free Air (μrad/h)
α	1–9	radon (atm)	2.7
β	0.1–200	radon (atm)	
		K, U, Th, Sr (soil)	3.4
		cosmic rays	
γ	0.8–2.6	K, U, Th, Cs, Rn	5.9
η	0.1–100	cosmic rays	0.1
ρ	10–2000	cosmic rays	0.1
μ	100–30,000	cosmic rays	2.3
		TOTAL	14.5

Modified from NCRP Report No. 50.[4]

1. primordial radionuclides

   The most important of these are uranium and thorium, found in many rocks and soil, and their daughters, K-40 and Rb-87, found in air and ground water.

2. cosmic rays and cosmogenic radionuclides

   These include C-14 and radioberyllium. Cosmic rays derive from radiation of galactic particles upon the upper atmosphere and from the sun, especially during solar flares.

3. man-made radionuclides

   The most notable of these are Sr-90 and Cs-137 from nuclear fallout.

Background radiation varies from location to location, depending upon altitude, building material, construction, and geographic location. Particularly variable background may occur in nuclear laboratories, because of stored radionuclides, ambient contamination, and often, radioactive patients injected with radiopharmaceuticals. Measured background varies directly with the detector volume and inversely with detector shielding. In general, background may be neglected when the source activity is high or when samples and standards are counted with the same geometry and counting times. Under other conditions than these, however, background may cause counting errors if not corrected.

In addition, background may arise from the detector instrumentation in the form of electronic "noise" pulses, which have already been discussed. Usually, background is allowed for by measuring a "dummy," or "blank" sample that is identical to the unknown source in all respects except for its absence of radioactivity.

Interfering Radioactivity

Both source and standard may contain interfering radioactivity. It may be added as a contaminant during sample processing; it may be generated during isotope production; or it may arise merely as a consequence of source geometry. If the interfering nuclide in the unknown source is the same as the radioactive source, it cannot be distinguished by either chemical or physical techniques. An example is the variable blood activity encountered in organ imaging. If the interfering nuclide is a different isotope of the same element, separating them by spectrometry may be possible. For example, the $^{122}Te(d,n)^{123}I$ reaction in a cyclotron produces various quantities of I-130, I-126, and I-124, which are only partially discriminated by spectrometry. If the interfering radioactivity is a different element, it may be distinguished by chemical separation or by physical methods. The most common physical procedure is separation by half-life. For example, Hg-197 ($T_{1/2}$ = 2.7d) contamination of Hg-203 ($T_{1/2}$ = 46.9d) may be reduced by simple decay. Often, beta-emitting radionuclides, which have continuous energy spectra, can be discriminated only by physical separation methods.

COUNTING BETA PARTICLES

The measurement of beta-emitting nuclides presents some special problems not encountered with gamma-emitting nuclides. Beta particles are negatively charged and are emitted in a continuous energy distribution ranging from zero to the maximum energy characteristic of the particular nuclide, E_{max}. Because they are charged, beta particles readily interact with matter and are easily absorbed and scattered.

The most commonly used beta counters are liquid scintillation counters. Their principal advantage over solid-state detectors, Geiger-Müller tubes, and gas flow proportional counters is that the radioactive sample is intimately mixed with the liquid fluor, resulting in high geometric efficiency and good overall efficiency even for such low-energy beta as H-3 and Fe-55. Beta particles may also be counted with Geiger-Müller tubes fitted with thin mica windows. Gas flow proportional counters may be used to count weak-energy beta particles. In the latter instrument, the radioactive sample is placed directly into the sensitive volume of the detector, thus eliminating beta absorption in the detector window.

Samples are prepared by pipetting small amounts (0.1 ml) of a radioactive solution onto a sample counting planchette, usually stamped from copper or aluminum. The sample is then dried and often covered with Scotch tape to prevent loss. Liquid samples are almost never counted because of the changing absorption due to evaporation. It is essential to prepare the samples and standard in an identical manner so that the loss of efficiency due to self-absorption is the same. Also, both samples and standard must be counted on the same type of planchette so that back-scatter will be the same. For example, P-32 mounted on a copper planchette has almost 30% higher counting rate than when counted on paper.

GAMMA-RAY SPECTROMETRY

Gamma-emitting nuclides are preferred to beta emitters in biologic tracer studies because:

1. They are easier to detect and quantitate in patients.
2. They are easier to detect within the environment, which improves radiation protection.
3. They can generally be administered in larger quantities per unit of absorbed dose to the patient.
4. The administered dose is more easily calibrated.

Most applications of gamma-ray detection in nuclear medicine involve the measurement of pulse-height, particularly to identify or separate different radionuclides and to reject scattered radiation for improved resolution of radionuclide images. In the majority of cases, spectrometry is performed with NaI(Tl) crystals for reasons already described. Consequently, the spectra illustrated here are those derived from NaI(Tl) systems.

Photon attenuation or absorption within the scintillation crystal occurs by the three processes of photon interaction described in Chapter 1:

1. In the photoelectric effect, all of the photon energy is transferred directly to an orbital electron, the photoelectron, which behaves as a beta particle, causing secondary ionization over a short path length. The chance that all of the original photon energy

will be deposited within the crystal is high if the crystal is more than a few centimeters in thickness. Each ion pair formed ultimately results in the production of fluorescent light photons. However, the process occurs so quickly that the many individual photons appear as a single flash of light proportional to the incident photon energy.

2. Compton scattering results in only part of the photon energy being imparted to the orbital electron. The scattered photon may interact elsewhere in the crystal and undergo a photoelectric interaction or another Compton scattering. In either case, the processes occur so quickly that the total energy transfer is registered the same as in the photoelectric effect. If the Compton-scattered photon passes out of the crystal, a lesser amount of light is produced and a lower pulse from the PM tube results (photon c, Fig. 3–3).

3. Pair production results in the conversion of 1.022 MeV of the photon energy into an electron and positron, with the remaining photon energy divided between the two particles as kinetic energy. The positron combines with an electron and annihilates to produce two 0.511-MeV photons. Either or both of these photons may interact in the crystal by the preceding two processes. If one or both of these annihilation photons escapes the crystal, the resultant pulse is 0.511 MeV or 1.022 MeV lower than the photopeak. Such losses contribute to *escape peaks* superimposed upon the photopeak. The most probable of these occurrences, however, is total energy transfer.

In a perfect detection system, a monoenergetic gamma source such as Cs-137 should yield a single line photopeak at 662 keV. The spectrum in Figure 3–8 using a

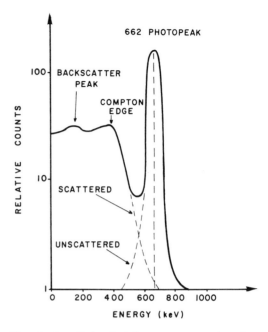

Fig. 3–8. Pulse-height spectrum showing the distribution of unscattered and scattered photons forming the Compton trough, Compton edge, and backscatter peak.

3-in. NaI(Tl) crystal shows a spread of energies about the photopeak with a complex lower-energy component.

The distribution of energies of unscattered photons, i.e., photons completely absorbed within the crystal, stems from several variables operating within the scintillation detection system:

1. Variable amount of absorbed energy converted to heat rather than light photons.
2. Variable self-absorption of light within the crystal.
3. Variable photon absorption caused by nonuniform photocathode thickness.
4. Imperfect dynode amplification.
5. Fluctuating background or electronic noise.
6. Variable amplifier gain.

Most of these variables are random and additive. Therefore, the final spectrum has a photopeak with a more or less Gaussian distribution about a maximum. This spectrum is illustrated in Figure 3–8 by the dashed line extending down from the peak, which represents the theoretic distribution of unscattered photons.

Scattering, which makes up the lower-energy portion of the spectrum, derives from several phenomena, as shown in Figure 3–3. The principal mechanism of photon absorption in NaI above 100 keV is Compton scattering. There is a high probability that the Compton electron will be absorbed and a lesser probability that the Compton-scattered photon will be absorbed: A scattered photon that escapes from the crystal (photon c in Fig. 3–3) results in a pulse that falls into the *Compton plateau* between the *Compton edge* and the *backscatter peak* (Fig. 3–8).

Recall that the maximum energy is imparted to a Compton electron when the electron is scattered at 180 degrees to the incident photon. The Compton edge is determined by the relation:

$$\text{Compton edge (keV)} = \frac{E^2}{E + 256}$$

where E is the photon energy. The backscatter peak occurs at the lower end of the Compton plateau and is caused by photons that pass completely through the crystal unabsorbed, strike the shielding or PM tube, and are scattered back 180 degrees into the crystal, where they are absorbed (photon b, Fig. 3–3). These photons have an energy about equal to the photopeak minus the Compton edge. The backscatter peak can be calculated:

$$\text{Backscatter peak (keV)} = \frac{256E}{E + 256}$$

Other types of scattering that degrade the spectrum include:

1. iodine K escape
   Photon d in Figure 3–3 has undergone Compton scattering. The photoelectron from the K shell leaves an orbital vacancy, which is filled by an outer electron with the emissions of a K-characteristic x-ray. If this x-ray escapes the crystal, a pulse 28 keV lower than the photopeak results. This iodine K x-ray escape usually occurs at the edge of the crystal. The resultant iodine escape peak is apt to be seen only with thin crystals (Fig. 3–9).

2. single and double escape peaks that result from pair production
   These have already been discussed. Following positron annihilation, one or both annihilation photons may escape the crystal, resulting in pulses 0.511 and 1.022 MeV below the photopeak (Fig. 3–10). These escape peaks also decrease with increasing crystal size.

3. scattering within the source
   This is the most common origin of low energy pulses (photons g and h, Fig. 3–3). The scattered photon energy decreases with increasing angle of scatter and the number of scatter events before striking the crystal. It may be desirable to exclude these scattered photons by pulse-height discrimination.

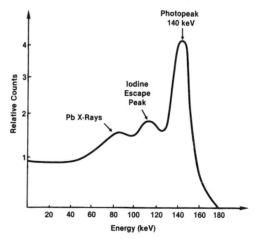

Fig. 3–9. Iodine escape peak in Tc-99m spectrum using a thin crystal.

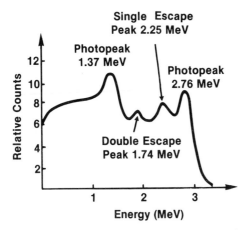

Fig. 3–10. Spectrum of Na-24 showing the two photopeaks and single and double escape peaks below the 2.76-MeV photopeak.

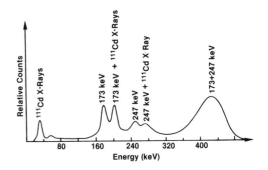

Fig. 3–11. Pulse-height spectrum of In-111 taken from a NaI(Tl) well counter. Coincidence summing occurs with both x- and gamma rays. The probability of summing increases with the geometric efficiency.

4. collimator scatter

This is a source of two different kinds of scatter. The simplest type is represented by photon e in Figure 3–3, in which the incident photon undergoes Compton scattering and the degraded photon strikes the crystal producing a lower-energy pulse. The second is illustrated by photon f, which produces a Compton electron in the collimator with resultant production of a lead x-ray at 73 to 75 keV (Fig. 3–9).

Coincidence Summing

Many radionuclides emit more than one photon in the decay process. Except in the case of metastable radionuclides, multiple emissions are emitted almost simultaneously. The direction of emission is random, so that the probability of two or more photons striking the detector simultaneously increases in proportion with geometric efficiency. When this occurs, the detector output registers a single pulse equal to the sum of the absorbed photon energies (Fig. 3–11). The result may be a dramatic alteration of the radionuclide spectrum. Coincidence sum peaks are encountered in the spectra derived from well

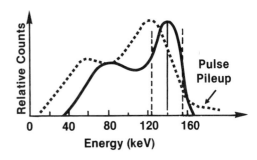

Fig. 3–12. Spectrum of Tc-99m at low (solid line) and high (broken line) counting rates. Pulse pileup causes *tailing* on the upper end of the spectrum while baseline shift causes lowering and broadening of the peak.

counters much more frequently than in those derived from scintillation cameras. One means of identifying sum peaks is to observe the changing spectrum and record successive spectra as a source is raised out of a well counter.

Effects of Counting Rate

Distortions of the energy spectrum are also introduced by high counting rates. The effect is usually manifested by a broadening of the photopeak and by a shift of the photopeak toward lower energies (Fig. 3–12). These changes are caused by pulse pileup and baseline shift, respectively. Since the window does not change, both distortion and shift of the photopeak result in lost counts, which cause errors in counting determinations. Counting rates that result in 3 to 5% deadtime losses should be posted on all instruments being used for quantitative measurements. Samples exceeding these counting rates should be remeasured (along with their standards) after sufficient decay or dilution to reduce the counting rate. Remember that the counting rate of importance is that which includes the entire spectrum, not just the photopeak.

Energy Calibration

Spectrometers with multichannel analyzers and persistence oscilloscopes are easy to calibrate. A source of the radionuclide to be counted is selected, and the upper- and lower-level discriminators are adjusted to straddle the peak. Usually, the discriminators are set so that the ten-turn potentiometer readings correspond to energy in kiloelectron volts (keV). The gain is then adjusted to center the peak within the window (Fig. 3–13). Small changes in

gain cause the peak to shift upward or downward, both of which result in diminished counts and counting errors. The gain settings should be tested against known standards to check for correct gain settings.

If no direct readout is available, the gain settings may be made by adjusting the gain to yield a maximum ratemeter deflection or by plotting the counting rate as a function of gain. Most amplifiers are linear over limited ranges. Thus, in window 2 of Figure 3–13, if the gain is adjusted to center the 364 peak of I-131, the peak of Tc-99m should center on 140 keV without further adjustment. The linearity of every amplifier is limited, however. For example, the above gain settings are not likely to center the peak of I-125 at 35 keV. Rather, increased gain would probably be required.

DUAL-ISOTOPE COUNTING

By means of pulse-height analysis and differential spectrometry, two radionuclides can be easily counted simultaneously provided their photopeaks are reasonably well separated. Figure 3–13 shows the contributions of I-131 and Tc-99m. When counted together, the activity (μCi) of unknown samples containing both I-131 (A_I) and Tc-99m (A_{Tc}) can be determined by counting separate I-131 and Tc-99m standards and by using the relationships:

$$A_I = \frac{n_1 f_2 - n_2 f_1}{C_1 f_2 - C_2 f_1}$$

and

$$A_{Tc} = \frac{n_1 C_2 - n_2 C_1}{C_1 f_2 - C_2 f_1}$$

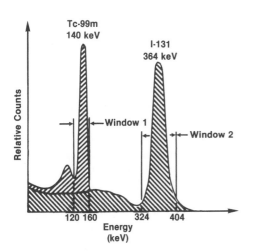

Fig. 3–13. Appropriate window settings for counting Tc-99m and I-131 with a linear amplifier. The contribution of I-131 scattered radiation (crosstalk) within the Tc-99m window is substantial and must be subtracted.

where:

C_1 = cpm/μCi of I in lower window,
C_2 = cpm/μCi of I in upper window,
f_1 = cpm/μCi of Tc in lower window,
f_2 = cpm/μCi of Tc in upper window,
n_1 = counting rate in lower window,
n_2 = counting rate in upper window.

COINCIDENCE COUNTING

Many radionuclides decay with more than one emission. An example is I-131, which decays with beta emission followed by prompt emission of a gamma ray (Appendix C). An effective means of reducing background is to arrange separate beta and gamma detectors so that both emissions are registered simultaneously. The output of these detectors is channeled through coincidence circuitry, which registers a count only if both detectors register counts simultaneously (Fig. 3–14). Extraneous counts that fail to activate both detectors are thus eliminated.

Radionuclides that emit cascades of gamma rays, such as Se-75, In-111, and Te-123m, have been proposed for tomographic scanning.[5]

ABSORPTION-EDGE COUNTING

An ingenious method for measuring the concentration of specific atoms in biologic specimens makes use of the differential absorption of closely separated K x-rays that just straddle the K-shell absorption edge of the atoms to be measured. This technique is based upon the marked decrease in the attenuation coefficient at the

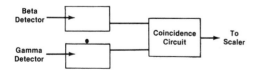

Fig. 3–14. Schematic representation of coincidence counting for low-level detection of beta-emitting radionuclides.

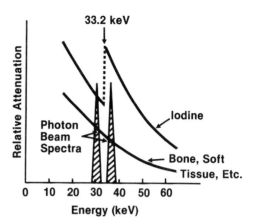

Fig. 3–15. The photon beam from a Ce-139 source contains two photopeaks at 33.0 and 33.4 keV. The 33.4-keV photons are strongly attenuated by iodine in the absorbing medium because of the K-shell absorption edge at 33.2 keV. The 33.0-photopeak is attenuated much less by iodine.

absorption edge for gamma-ray transmission. As an example, Sorenson has used the transmission of Ce-139 x-rays to measure iodine concentration in biologic samples.[6] Cerium-139 decays to La-139 by electron capture with a 140-day half-life. The emissions of interest are the K_α x-rays from the lanthanum daughter, which neatly bracket the 33.2-keV absorption edge at 33.0 and 33.4 keV (Fig. 3–15). Samples containing iodine are exposed to a source of Ce-139, and the transmission of the two x-rays is measured. The difference in x-rays detected is proportional to the concentration of iodine in the sample. The principle behind this technique is that the 33.0-keV x-ray is only slightly attenuated by iodine, but the 33.4-keV x-ray is greatly attenuated.

The relative decrease in absorption of the two x-rays compared with known standards yields the iodine concentration in the unknown. Of course, separating two such closely placed x-ray energies is beyond the capabilities of all but the most sensitive spectrometers. By appropriate use of energy-selection filtration, however, the higher-energy x-ray can be largely eliminated from the source beam. Measuring the transmitted beams with and without filtration then allows calculation of the sample attenuation, even with coarse spectrometric systems employing NaI crystal detectors. The sensitivity of this technique for in vitro samples is approximately 5 µg/ml. The possibility of using this technique for in vivo measurement also exists.

LIQUID SCINTILLATION COUNTING

The basic instrumentation of liquid scintillation counters was discussed in the previous chapter. Preparation of samples prior to counting is somewhat more critical with liquid scintillation counting than with most other detector systems. Along with the usual considerations of sample mixing, container characteristics, and geometry, the chemical composition and optical characteristics of the counting medium must be controlled to avoid *quenching,* a phenomenon that results in reduced counting efficiency.

The amount of water in the sample must be matched to the solubility of the solvent. The content of inorganic salts, heavy metals, oxygen, as well as pH and temperature, must all be controlled. These considerations are reviewed in detail by Bransome, Crook et al. and Peng et al.[7,8,9]

In general, it is not possible to solve every problem induced by sample preparation. The validity of the final count result, however, is most often secured by scrupulously avoiding any difference between treatment of the sample and that of the standard against which it is compared.

Instrument Settings

If one radionuclide is being counted, the instrument setting is simple: the lower discriminator is set near zero, just above the range of instrument noise. The upper discriminator is set at the point that gives the highest signal:background ratio (R_s/R_b).

Since background is largely a function of window width, the ratio can be determined by serially counting background and a standard at various settings of the upper discriminator. A slightly better *figure of merit* can be achieved using the highest value of R_s^2/R_b.

Usually the optimum counting conditions are achieved at *balanced point operation.* If the spectrum is divided into two channels and the counts summed, there is an optimum high voltage setting such that counts in the two channels are approximately equal with the sum of the channels at a maximum (Fig. 3–16). This setting determines the operating conditions corresponding to the highest counting efficiency and the counting condition least susceptible to the effects of quenching. If a sample is quenched, the decreased counts in the upper channel are partially offset by increased counts in the lower channel. The adjustment of instrument settings for dual isotope counting is discussed in the following sections.

Quench Correction

Quenching is of three general types. *Impurity quenching* is due to dissolved substances (e.g., O_2, heavy atoms, inorganic salts) that absorb excitation energy without emitting fluorescence. *Color quenching* is caused by substances that absorb fluorescence and thus reduce the photon collection efficiency. *Photon quenching* is a process whereby the fluorescence yield of the system is reduced. This type of quenching is especially significant in heterogeneous or suspension systems.

There are several means of reducing quenching. Oxygen quenching can be reduced by purging the sample with nitrogen, although this solution is generally impractical. More often, additional secondary solute is added to increase the competition for energy transfer from the solvent molecules. Other types of impurities may be reduced by precipitation, filtration, ion exchange, distillation, and

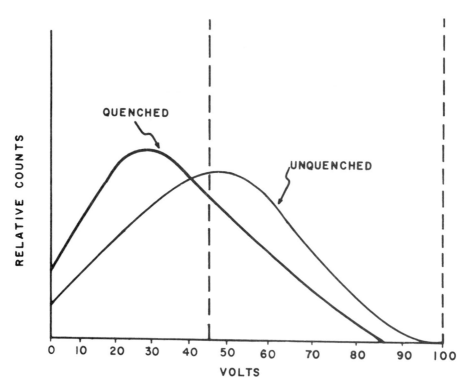

Fig. 3–16. Balance point operation for counting C-14. High voltage is adjusted so that counts of unquenched standard in lower channel (0–45V) equal counts in upper channel (45–100V). At this point, quenching the sample will have least effect on total counts (0–100V).

other sample preparation measures. Color quenching may be reduced by bleaching agents, charcoal filtration, and sample combustion.

Some quenching occurs in all liquid scintillation samples. Therefore, the degree of quenching must be determined. Several methods of quench correction have been reviewed by Peng et al.[9]

Internal Standard

One of the simplest (and most time-consuming) methods is the addition of a known standard S to the unknown sample U. After measuring the sample activity R_u, a small amount of standard is added, a procedure known as "spiking" the sample, which gives a total activity $R_t = R_u + R_s$. Since the absolute activity of the standard A_s is known, the absolute activity of the sample A_u can be calculated:

$$A_u = A_s \frac{R_u}{R_t - R_u}$$

To determine quenching due to the added standard, a chemically identical solution without radioactivity is added to a second unknown sample and the decrease in counting rate R_t noted. This factor is applied to the final calculation of A_u.

External Standard

In this method, a sealed gamma source (usually Ra-226 or Am-241) is used to irradiate the sample after R_u is determined. The secondary Compton and recoil electrons generated in the sample produce a broad fluorescence spectrum, which is channeled by two separate pulse-height analyzers.

The ratio of the counts within the two channels is then used as a correction for R_u. This method is most suitable for quench correcting double isotope samples. The samples must be homogeneous; gel suspensions cannot be quench corrected by this method.

Channels Ratio Method

Quenching shifts the observed spectrum of a radioactive sample to the left (Fig. 3–16). If the spectrum is divided into two adjacent or overlapping channels, quenching causes a shift in the counts in the two channels, and the ratio between them is proportional to the shift. A series of quenched standards is determined, and a curve of the ratio of counts between channels versus the ratio of quenched to unquenched counts is then plotted. The channels should be unequal, with the narrow channel viewing the lower energy range of the spectrum. This method is best employed with only moderately quenched samples with high counting rates. The statistical accuracy is too low for correcting low activity samples.

Background

As with every radiation detector system, background is a constant concern in liquid scintillation counting. Besides all of the contributions to background to which scintillation crystal detectors are subject (cosmic radiation, K-40 in the counting equipment, PM thermal noise), liquid scintillation systems may contain *chemiluminescence.*

This type of phosphorescence is of much longer duration than fluorescence and is caused by chemical reactions in the scintillation media. It is one of several mechanisms, like heat production, of dissipating energy. When chemiluminescence occurs in the spectral range to which the photocathode is sensitive, it contributes to background. One common source of chemiluminescence is exposure to heat and light. Therefore, it is advisable to cool the samples in a dark enclosure before counting. This type of chemiluminescence declines quickly. Other forms, however, are more subtle, e.g., impurities in the solvents and chemical reactions with the counting vial caps.[10] Often, these problems are detected only by serial counts over several hours or days as a means for observing the declining counting rate. Another way of detecting the presence of chemiluminescence is to prepare a blank that contains all of the elements of the assay system except the radionuclide.

Dual-Isotope Counting

Because of the low energy of many of the radiations being measured, the inefficient transfer of photons to the photocathode by quenching and self-absorption, and the broad inherent beta-emission spectrum, the ability of liquid scintillation spectrometry to separate two radionuclides is more limited than, for example, that of proportional counters. Nevertheless, if the energies of the two nuclides are sufficiently different, they can be distinguished when counted simultaneously. Fortunately, an energy difference does exist in the nuclide pairs most commonly used in biomedical research: H-3 and C-14, H-3 and S-35, H-3 and P-32, and C-14 and P-32. In such cases as C-14 and S-35, which have similar spectra, the radionuclides must be chemically separated before counting.

Radionuclide	E_{max} (MeV)
H-3	0.018
C-14	0.155
S-35	0.167
Cl-36	0.714
P-32	1.710

Figure 3–17 shows the relative counts of H-3 and C-14 determined experimentally in a toluene-PPO mixture. It is generally possible to select discriminator settings so that one isotope (in this case H-3) is completely excluded from one channel; however, overlap of spectra will always

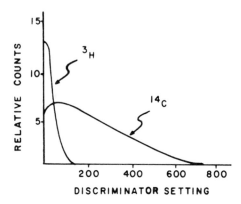

Fig. 3–17. Beta spectra of H-3 and C-14 plotted on a linear scale.

occur in the lower channel, necessitating correction of the counts in the lower channel for the contribution of the more energetic nuclide. Eliminating H-3 from the C-14 channel permits accurate determination of C-14, but also greatly decreases the C-14 counting efficiency.[11] It may be more useful to allow a small "spillover" of H-3 into the C-14 channel to increase the counting efficiency for C-14. In the example of Figure 3–17, H-3 would be completely eliminated from the upper channel if its lower discriminator were set at 170. The C-14 counting efficiency, however, would be only 50%. By lowering the discriminator to 100, the C-14 efficiency increases to 70% while adding only 1% of counts from the H-3 spectrum. In the latter case, simultaneous equations must be used to calculate the H-3 and C-14 activities:

where:

A_C = dpm in C-14 sample

A_H = dpm in H-3 sample

E_{C_u} = C-14 efficiency in upper channel (100% = 1.00)

E_{C_l} = C-14 efficiency in lower channel

E_{H_u} = H-3 efficiency in upper channel

E_{H_l} = H-3 efficiency in lower channel

R_u = net observed counts in upper channel

R_l = net observed counts in lower channel

then $R_u = A_C (E_{C_u}) + A_H (E_{H_u})$ (5)

and $R_l = A_C(E_{C_l}) + A_H (E_{H_l})$ (6)

Solving these equations for A_C and A_H:

$$A_C = \frac{R_u - R_l (E_{H_u}/E_{H_l})}{E_{C_u} - E_{C_l} (E_{H_u}/E_{H_l})} \qquad (7)$$

$$A_H = \frac{R_l - R_u (E_{C_l}/E_{C_u})}{E_{H_l} - E_{H_u} (E_{C_l}/E_{C_u})} \qquad (8)$$

If all of the H-3 is excluded from the C-14, the equations are simplified to:

$$A_C = \frac{R_u}{E_{C_u}} \qquad (9)$$

$$A_H = \frac{R_l - A_C E_{C_l}}{E_{H_l}} \qquad (10)$$

Equations (7) and (8) are general equations that can be applied to any dual isotope counting. These formulae do not take into account quench corrections, which must be performed first. This calculation is usually performed by the channels ratio method, which is applied to the upper channel and then used to correct both upper and lower channels.

Counting on Solid Supports

Solid supports include chromatographic strips, filter paper discs, and wipe test swabs. Radioactivity adhered to these supports is counted by immersing the entire support into the liquid scintillators. Frequently, a liquid scintillation system is more convenient to use than a gas-flow proportional counter for measuring these samples, especially with H-3, which is not counted efficiently in a gas-flow system. The greatest problem involves geometry and absorption of the weak beta emissions by the support substance. Furlong has offered several recommendations for solid support counting.[12]

1. Use an internal standard whenever possible to check sample-to-sample variability. External standards have no meaning whatever for evaluating quenching under these conditions.
2. If the counting problem involves measuring a radioactive substrate and metabolic products, the assay conditions for the two should be identical.
3. The quenching characteristics of filter paper should be determined.

Cerenkov Counting

Cerenkov radiation is a particular form of light emission that beta particles give off as they travel through a liquid medium. Cerenkov radiation is emitted when the velocity of the particle exceeds the speed of light c in the medium, which is c/n where n is the refractive index of the medium. This light is mostly in the ultraviolet range but extends into the visible range and is responsible for the blue-white light surrounding the core in swimming pool reactors. The light is not propagated in all directions but is conical, with the path of the electron at the axis of the cone. The result is analogous to the shock wave caused by supersonic aircraft.

Cerenkov radiation is particularly useful since its detection does not require a scintillator and since it is not quenched by chemical impurities, although it is subject to color quenching. Water, solvents, and even strong acids can be used as counting media. They are only useful, however, for counting strong beta emitters. For water, beta particles must have energy greater than 0.263 MeV. With solvents of very high refractive indices, however, weaker energy betas can be detected. For example, Ross reported efficient detection of C-14 in alphabromonaphthalene.[13] Because no scintillator is required, many samples such as urine (which has been decolorized), waste water, and tissue fluids can be counted directly without the addition of fluors. Color quenching may

be corrected by internal standards, by the channel ratio method, or by external standards, provided the radiation is sufficiently energetic to produce Compton electrons. Thus Ra-226 is suitable whereas Am-241 is not.

IN VIVO MEASUREMENTS

When the radioactivity to be measured is located within the body, additional problems are encountered because of a variable amount of scattering from overlying and surrounding tissues. The most common means of quantitating in vivo activity is constructing a phantom of approximately the same size, dimensions, and elemental composition as the body or organ and placement of a known amount of activity within the phantom to simulate the in vivo distribution. An example is the measurement of radioiodine uptake by the thyroid. The usual neck phantom is made of tissue-equivalent plastic with a hole drilled in the location of the trachea; through this hole, a standard quantity of radioiodine can be inserted to simulate the intrathyroidal radioiodine. This kind of comparison necessarily entails a significant error, because while the phantom may simulate the physical scatter and attenuation conditions for one neck, it is inadequate for another. Nevertheless, with the detector placed about 25 cm from the phantom, the percent error is acceptably small for meaningful clinical results, in which the normal range of uptake may vary from 6 to 30%—a fivefold variation.

The error caused by uncertainties due to different organ size and body habitus can be reduced by using pulse-height analysis to reduce the contribution due to scattered radiation. Another means of reducing error is to place the external detector at some distance from the organ of interest to reduce the error due to uncertainty of depth. For example, an error of 2 cm in depth at 10 cm from the detector produces a counting error of ±40%, while the same positional error at 20 cm distance from the crystal produces only about ±20% error.

To reproduce the scatter contributed by tissue surrounding and overlying the in vivo radioactive source, a variety of materials may be used that simulate the gamma-ray attenuation properties of soft tissue. These materials include water, presswood, lucite, and masonite. By carefully standardizing the counting geometry and instrument calibration, serial measurements in the same patient may be reproduced with a variability of about 10%. Variations between patients of different body habitus are much higher.

WHOLE BODY COUNTERS

The measurement of low levels of radioactivity, particularly when the radioactivity is widely distributed within the body, imposes special requirements on the construction and design of detectors. Whole body counters for measuring gamma-emitting radionuclides in the human body were originally conceived to measure radionuclide contaminations in radiation workers, but have since been used for a variety of clinical applications.[14,15]

Physical Characteristics

Whole body counters have two types of detectors, liquid and solid. The liquid scintillation whole body counter, developed by Anderson, consisted of a steel cylinder whose outer shell was filled with a mixture of toluene, p-terphenyl, and POPOP.[16] The design is shown in Fig. 3–18A. Various PM tubes are arranged around the cylinder, and the entire apparatus is enclosed in a shielded room to reduce background radiation. The advantage of the cylindric design is that it provides 4π geometry, so that sensitivity is largely independent of the spatial distribution of the radionuclide within the body.

Solid plastics in large volume have also

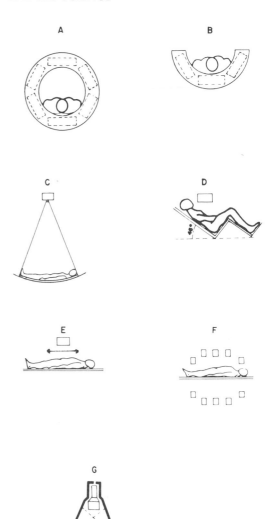

Fig. 3–18. Commonly used detector geometries in whole body counters. (From Kessler, W.V., et al.[17])

been used.[18,19] A common 2π configuration is shown in Figure 3–18B. While these counters have high sensitivity, the spectrometric resolution is quite poor, and their use must be largely restricted to counting previously identified radionuclides. The sensitivity of sodium iodide crystals is less because of smaller detector volumes, but they have much greater energy resolution, thus allowing radionuclide identification and quantitation by means of gamma-ray spectroscopy. Two basic characteristics of whole body counters that must be considered in all of their applications are (1) detector sensitivity and (2) uniformity of spatial response. Detector sensitivity depends essentially upon the efficiency of the detector and the level of background radiation. The uniformity of response depends upon the spatial relationship between the detector and the radiation source. Sensitivity can most easily be increased by enlarging the sensitive volume of the detector and/or reducing background radiation. To this end, the early trend of whole body counter construction was toward larger detector crystals and more elaborate shielding. The latter was necessary because, as the detector volume increases, the sensitivity to background radiation also increases. Best results are achieved by a judicious combination of detector size and shield mass, composition, and arrangement. By this means, it is possible to achieve a level of detectability in fractions of nanocuries sufficient to detect natural body burdens of K-40 and radium, which vary between 10^{-2} and 10^{-4} μCi.

Geometry

The detector geometry varies as functions of both the type of detector used and the position of the subject relative to the detector, but the system must always be designed to assure measurement reproducibility with changes in radionuclide distribution. Several detector arrangements are shown in Fig. 3–18.

The most commonly encountered systems make use of a stationary or moving couch geometry. The individual lies on a bed or couch viewed by one or more detectors (Fig. 3–18 E,F,G). In the case of a single detector, it may be fixed or moveable. Alternatively, the couch may move in relation to the detector.

An elaborate 54-detector system similar to that diagrammed in Fig. 3–18F has been constructed at Brookhaven National Lab-

oratories. It has a nearly invariant response to radionuclide distribution.[20] Other methods of improving uniformity include counting systems with rotational detectors and the substitution of Compton scatter for photopeak counting.[21]

Many shielding systems have been devised for the couch geometry. One of the simplest is the "shadow" shield (Fig. 3–18G).[22] In this counting system, the patient lies in a shielded trough. The detector overhead is also shielded, but open beneath. Either the trough or the detector moves longitudinally to scan the total length of the body. This system combines several desirable features, including favorable geometry, economy, and acceptable background levels for most counting problems.[23]

To avoid the high cost of these elaborate special-purpose counters, many laboratories have adapted more conventional instruments for whole body counting. Short et al. described the use of a scintillation camera which, without its collimator, has a high sensitivity and uniform response at some distance.[24] Rehani et al. have adopted a rectilinear scanner for the same purpose.[25]

Clinical Applications

Total Body Potassium

The fractional abundance of K-40 in natural potassium is *0.0118%*. From this relationship, it is possible to determine the total body potassium content by measuring the mass of K-40. With well-designed and carefully calibrated whole body counters, an accuracy of $\pm 5\%$ can be achieved, but the technique is not easy.[17,26,27,28,29] Because of the low abundance of K-40, its high-energy gamma emission (1.47 keV), and the ubiquity of potassium in the environment, elaborate detectors and shielding must be utilized. Organic scintillation detectors with 2π or 4π geometry have been used most often although the couch arrangement with multiple detectors (Fig. 3–18F) is also used.

The critical aspect in the direct measurement of K-40 is the calibration of the system. This calibration is generally performed by administration of K-42 to a group of normal subjects with various heights and weights or by constructing phantoms containing known amounts of potassium, which simulate the human distribution and approximate as closely as possible the geometry and gamma attenuation of the patient being counted. A range of normal individuals separated according to age and sex is measured and graphed according to height and weight.

Potassium is primarily an intracellular element and because relatively little exists in fat, potassium content is proportional to "lean body mass."

Lean Body Mass $\cong$
   Total Body Potassium (mEq)/68.1

Body Fat =
   Body Weight − Lean Body Mass

The measurement of total potassium is useful in studies of obesity and diets designed for weight loss without loss of lean body mass.[27] It is also an indicator of the fraction of intracellular water and in nutritional studies provides an index of global synthesis.

Total body potassium can be estimated with less sensitive counters by measuring total exchangeable potassium by the indicator dilution principle using K-42 (see vol. II, Chap. 22). The use of the whole body counter obviates collecting excreta and confining patients to metabolic units. Potassium-42 is usually administered intravenously, and the total body activity is determined. The retained fraction is determined again at 24 or 48 hr. This fraction plus the ratio of serum K-42 to cold serum potassium is used to calculate exchangeable potassium, which in turn is an estimate of total body potassium. Use of the whole body counter is somewhat more reproducible than the dilution technique,

which requires the determination of excreted K-42 to derive the retained dose.

Intestinal Absorption of Iron

Measurements of iron absorption are useful in several anemic and malabsorption diseases.[30,31,32] In the whole body counter technique, 0.5 to 5 μCi (~20–200 kBq) Fe-59 in the form of chloride, citrate, ascorbate, or hemoglobin-bound is administered orally. The absorbed fraction is determined by measuring total body activity 4 hr after ingestion and 14 days later. The advantage of whole body counting over other techniques is that measurements of excreta are avoided. It is especially useful for population studies in which it is important to avoid removing the patient from his normal habitat and routine.

Absorption of B_{12}

The technique of measuring B_{12} absorption is similar to that described for iron. B_{12} labeled with Co-58 or Co-60 is administered orally in doses of 0.5 to 1.0 μCi (~20–40 kBq). Total body activity is measured after administration and 7 to 10 days later. The normal absorbed fraction is between 45 and 80% of the administered dose. In patients with pernicious anemia, the absorbed fraction is 0 to 17%. This technique has been used by Belcher et al. and Reizenstein et al., among others.[33,34]

Strontium and Calcium

Calcium turnover studies using Ca-47 and Sr-85 have been helpful in understanding bone metabolism. Calcium-47 is used more often when measures of intestinal absorption and body retention are of interest. These studies are performed in a manner similar to that described for B_{12} absorption, counting 7 to 10 days after administration of the tracer.[35,36]

Strontium-85 has been used for studying bone metabolism in cases of osteoporosis, osteomalacia, and bone metastases.[37] The use of this tracer is valid because of the similar compartmental distribution and a longer useful physical half-life (64 days) than Ca-47.

REFERENCES

1. Anger, H.O.: Radioisotope cameras. *In* Instrumentation in Nuclear Medicine. Vol. 1. Edited by G.J. Hine. New York, Academic Press, 1967.
2. Zimmerman, R.E., Fahey, F.H., and Burns, R.E.: High pressure, multiwire proportional chamber for cardiac imaging. (Abst.) J. Nucl. Med., *21*:91, 1980.
3. Knoll, G.F.: Radiation Detection and Measurement. John Wiley & Sons, New York, 1979.
4. NCRP Report No. 50: Environmental Radiation Measurement. Washington, D.C., National Council on Radiation Protection, 1976.
5. Chung, V., Chak, K.C., Zacuto, P., and Hart, H.E.: Multiple photo coincidence tomography. Semin. Nucl. Med., *10*:345, 1980.
6. Sorenson, J.A.: Absorption-edge transmission technique using Ce-139 for measurement of stable iodine concentration. J. Nucl. Med., *20*:1286, 1979.
7. Bransome, E.D. (Ed.): The current Status of Liquid Scintillation Counting. New York, Grune and Stratton, 1970.
8. Crook, M.A., Johnson, P., and Scales, B. (Eds.): Liquid Scintillation Counting. Vols. 1 and 2. London, Heyden and Son, 1972.
9. Peng, C.T., Hanocks, D.L., and Alpen, E.L. (Eds.): Liquid Scintillation Counting. Vols. 1 and 2. New York, Academic Press, 1980.
10. Scales, B.: Questions regarding the occurrence of unwanted luminescence in liquid scintillation samples. *In* Liquid Scintillation Counting. Vols. 1 and 2. Edited by M.A. Crook, P. Johnson, and B. Scales. London, Heyden and Son, 1972.
11. Kobayashi, Y., and Mandsley, D.V.: Practical aspects of double isotope counting. *In* The Current Status of Liquid Scintillation Counting. Edited by E.D. Bransome. New York, Grune and Stratton, 1970.
12. Furlong, N.B.: Liquid scintillation counting of samples on solid supports. *In* The Current Status of Liquid Scintillation Counting. Edited by E.D. Bransome. New York, Grune and Stratton, 1970.
13. Ross, H.H.: Cerenkov radiations: photon yield application to (^{14}C) assay. *In* The Current Status of Liquid Scintillation Counting. Edited by E.D. Bransome. New York, Grune and Stratton, 1970.
14. Van Dilla, M.A.: Some applications of the Los Alamos human spectrometer. *In* Radioactivity in Man. Edited by G. Mennely. Springfield, Charles C Thomas, 1961.
15. Marinelli, L.D., et al.: Low-level gamma ray scintillation spectrometry: experimental requirements and biomedical applications. Adv. Biol. Med. Phys., *8*:81, 1962.
16. Anderson, E.C.: The Los Alamos human counter. Br. J. Radiol., *7*:27, 1957.
17. Kessler, W.V., et al.: A 4 liquid scintillation whole body counter. I-design operating characteristics and calibration. Int. J. Appl. Radiat. Isot., *19*:287, 1968.
18. Forbes, G.B.: A 4 plastic scintillation detector. Int. J. Appl. Radiat. Isot., *19*:535, 1968.
19. Delwaide, P.: A 4π plastifluor whole body counter for clinical use: calibration. Int. J. Appl. Radiat. Isot., *19*:535, 1968.
20. Cohn, S.H., Dombrowski, C.S., Pate, H.R., and Robertson, J.S.: A whole body counter with an invariant response to radionuclide distribution and body size. Phys. Med. Biol., *14*:645, 1969.
21. Cohn, S.H., and Palmer, H.E.: Recent advances in whole-body counting: a review. J. Nucl. Med. Biol., *1*:155, 1974.
22. Oliver, R., and Warner, G.T.: A clinical whole body counter using shadow field principle. Br. J. Radiol., *36*:806, 1966.
23. Kieffer, J.: Descricao, caracteristicas e desempenho de um prototipo de contador de corpo inteiro para uso clinico. *Tese* apresentada a Faculdade de Medicina da Universidade de Sao Paulo, 1970.
24. Short, M.D., Richards, A.R., and Glass, H.I.: The use of a gamma camera as a whole body counter. Br. J. Radiol., *45*:289, 1972.
25. Rehani, M.M. et al.: A simple and inexpensive clinical whole body counter. Nuklearmedizin, *15*:248, 1976.
26. Blahd, W.H., et al.: Electrolyte metabolism by whole-body counting techniques with particular reference to muscle disease and obesity in clinical uses of whole-body counting. Vienna, IAEA, *169*:186, 1966.
27. Woodward, K.T., et al.: Correlations of total body potassium with body water. Nature, *178*:97, 1956.
28. Forbes, G.B., Gallup, J., and Hursh, J.B.: Estimation of total body potassium-40 content. Science, *133*:101, 1961.
29. Forbes, G.B.: Methods for determining composition of the human body with a note on the effect of diet and body composition. Pediatrics, *29*:477, 1962.
30. Callender, S.T., et al.: The use of a single whole body counter for haematological investigations. Br. J. Haematol., *12*:276, 1966.
31. Deller, D.J.: Fe-59 absorption measurement by whole body counting: studies in alcoholic cirrhosis, hemochromatosis and pancreatitis. Am. J. Dig. Dis., *10*:249, 1956.
32. Pollack, S., Balcerzac, S.P., and Crosby, W.H.: Fe-59 absorption in human subjects using total body counting technique. Blood, *28*:94, 1966.
33. Belcher, E.H., Anderson, B.B., and Robinson, C.J.: The measurement of gastrointestinal absorption of Co-58 labeled vit. B_{12} by whole body counting. Nucl. Med. (Stuttg.), *3* :349, 1963.
34. Reizenstein, P.G., Conkite, E., and Cohn, S.H.: Measurement of absorption of vitamin B_{12} by whole body gamma spectrometry. Blood, *18*:95, 1961.
35. Caderquist, E.: Short term kinetic studies of ^{85}Sr and ^{47}Ca by whole body counting in malignant diseases of the skeleton. Acta Radiol., *2*:42, 1964.
36. Sargent, T., Linfoot, J.A., and Isaac, E.L.: Whole body counting of ^{47}Ca and ^{85}Sr in the study of bone diseases. *In* Clinical Uses of Whole Body Counting. Vienna, IAEA, 1966.
37. MacDonald, N.S.: Recent uses of total-body counter facility in metabolic research and clinical diagnosis with radionuclides. Whole Body Counting. Vienna, IAEA, 1962.

Chapter 4

STATISTICAL METHODS

SHELDON LEVIN

The subject of counting statistics is covered in many texts and monographs. This chapter attempts to simplify the usual statistical methodology as related to counting statistics through discussion of special characteristics of the Poisson distribution and their relationship to the Gaussian distribution.

GAUSSIAN DISTRIBUTION

The *Gaussian distribution function* is a mathematical statement describing in units of standard deviation the probability that an observation is greater than or equal to some fixed value. It is written as:

$$P(z \leq Z)$$
$$= \frac{1}{\sigma \sqrt{2\pi}} \int_{-\infty}^{Z} \exp \frac{-(x - \mu)^2}{2 \sigma^2} dx;$$

$$z = \frac{x - \mu}{\sigma} \qquad (1)$$

If the deviation $x - \mu$ is negative, then the probability is $1 - P(Z)$. The constants μ and σ are called *parameters* of the Gaussian distribution and are presumed to be known exactly. In practice, these parameters are not known and must be estimated from the data being analyzed; a caret (ˆ) is used to show that they are estimated. Thus the true population mean μ is estimated

by the sample average $\bar{x}$ and is calculated as:

$$\hat{\mu} = \bar{x} = \frac{\sum_{i=1}^{k} x_i}{k} \qquad (2)$$

where the values of x_i are the individually measured data points, k is the total number of points, and $\sum_{i=1}^{k} x_i$ is the sum of all observations. The other parameter of the Gaussian distribution, σ, is estimated by the sample standard deviation (s.d.) and is calculated as:

$$\hat{\sigma} = s.d. = \sqrt{\frac{\sum_{i=1}^{i=k} (x_i - \bar{x})^2}{k - 1}} \qquad (3)$$

Here again, k is the number of data points; however, the divisor is $k - 1$ because it yields a more accurate estimate of σ for small sample sizes. The standard deviation also is called the *root-mean-square* (rms) *error*. It provides a measure of the variability of observations on an individual basis and is expressed in the same units as the observations. The average and standard deviation are called *statistics* because they summarize the data. Rather than summing the deviations directly, the rms error is used, wherein the deviations from the mean $(x_i - \bar{x})$ are squared and the square root of their sum is then calculated. If this were not done, the deviations above and below the average would cancel, and the s.d. would always be zero.

POISSON DISTRIBUTION

The *Poisson distribution* differs from the Gaussian in many ways. It is a discrete rather than continuous distribution (i.e., it applies to discrete counts rather than to measured quantities), it has one parameter rather than two, and it is difficult to calculate and tabulate for large values of k because of its discreteness.

$$P(k) = \sum_{i=0}^{k} \frac{\mu^i}{i!} e^{-\mu}$$

which can be written as:

$$P(k) = e^{-\mu} \left(1 + \mu + \frac{\mu^2}{2!} + \frac{\mu^3}{3!} + \ldots + \frac{\mu^k}{k!} \right) \quad (4)$$

The symbol ! signifies *factorial* and is shorthand notation for the product of all digits up to the one factorialized. Thus 5! symbolizes the product $1 \times 2 \times 3 \times 4 \times 5 = 120$; 0! is defined as 1. The individual terms of the series give the probability of exactly k occurrences.

The sum of the terms of the series up to a given number k is the probability that up to k occurrences are observed, and 1 − P(k) is the probability of more than k occurrences. The parameter μ in the Poisson distribution represents the true mean number of events. Estimates of the population mean μ and the population standard deviation σ are particularly simple for the Poisson distribution:

$\hat{\mu} = N$, the observed number of events (e.g., counts) and
$\hat{\sigma} = \sqrt{N}$

There is a relationship between the Poisson and Gaussian distributions that

greatly simplifies their use.[1] For large numbers of counts, the Poisson distribution may be approximated accurately by the Gaussian distribution using $\mu = \mu$, $\sigma = \sqrt{\mu}$, and the estimates $\hat{\mu} = N$ and $\hat{\sigma} = \sqrt{N}$ (Fig. 4–1).

Poisson Distribution and Decay

In Chapter 3, the decay law was stated as:

$$dN/dt = -N\lambda$$

where λ is the decay constant expressing the probability that any particular atom will disintegrate in a unit of time. Multiplying by N, the number of atoms present, gives the rate of disintegration of the radioactive atoms per unit of time.

This equation can be rearranged and written in integral form to obtain:[2]

$$\int \frac{dN}{N} = -\int \lambda dt \quad (5)$$

which after integrating becomes:

$$\ln\left(\frac{N}{N_0}\right) = -\lambda t \quad (6)$$

Taking antilogs yields the familiar form:

$$N = N_0 e^{-\lambda t} \quad (7)$$

where N_0 is the number of atoms at time zero and N is the number remaining at time t. If μ is replaced by λt in the first

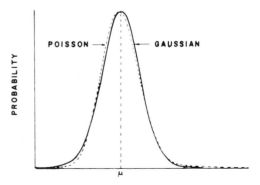

Fig. 4–1. Comparison of Poisson and Gaussian distributions for large values of N.

term of the Poisson series in equation (4), the following relationship may be stated:

$$P_0(t) = e^{-\lambda t}$$

which in terms of the Poisson distribution indicates the probability of observing exactly zero events when the true mean is λt. In terms of decay, it means the probability of no disintegrations or observed counts at time t. Alternately, the expression gives the probability that an atom survives t units of time.

If the above formula is multiplied by N_0, the number of atoms at time zero, it becomes:

$$N_0 P_0 (t) = N_0 e^{-\lambda t}$$

This indicates the expected number N of atoms that would survive t units of time given that the calculation begins with N_0. Thus:

$$N = N_0 e^{-\lambda t}$$

which is the same as the decay formula in equation (7).

The Poisson distribution, therefore, is appropriate in counting statistics because of its relation to the disintegration process.

RELATIVE STANDARD DEVIATION

The *relative standard deviation* (RSD), or *fractional error,* provides a measure of the variability as a fraction of the average value. It is defined as:

$$RSD = \frac{s.d.}{\bar{x}} \qquad (8)$$

and

$$\% \ RSD = \frac{100 \ s.d.}{\bar{x}}$$

For Poisson counting statistics, this simplifies to:

$$RSD = \frac{s.d.}{\bar{x}} = \frac{\sqrt{N}}{N} = \frac{1}{\sqrt{N}} \qquad (9)$$

and

$$\% \ RSD = \frac{100 \ s.d.}{\bar{x}} = \frac{100}{\sqrt{N}}$$

Table 4–1 shows how the RSD decreases as the number of counts increases.

Another use of the RSD, which is sometimes overlooked, is the estimation of the number of counts to achieve a given RSD. This is particularly useful in counting equipment that can be set for the total number of counts required. This method is valid only when the background is negligible, e.g., 1% of sample counts. If the formula

$$RSD = \frac{1}{\sqrt{N}}$$

simply is reversed, it becomes:

$$\sqrt{N} = \frac{1}{RSD}$$

Squaring it yields:

$$N = \frac{1}{(RSD)^2} \qquad (10)$$

Given, for example, that the RSD is required to be less than 0.05, or 5%, the following is calculated:

$$N = \frac{1}{(.05)^2} = \frac{1}{.0025} = 400$$

The result indicates that at least 400 counts, neglecting background, must be obtained to have the RSD no more than 0.05. Table 4–1 provides an insight into the required number of counts for a given % RSD.

TABLE 4–1. *Counts as a Function of RSD and % RSD*

Number of counts	RSD	% RSD
50	0.141	14.1
100	0.10	10.0
500	0.045	4.5
5000	0.014	1.4
50000	0.004	0.4

When the background count is not negligible, equation (10) may underestimate the required number of counts. A method that includes a term for background is therefore required. This method requires a preliminary estimate R_b of the ratio of the background counting rate to the sample counting rate. A rough estimate R_g of gross counting rates can often be obtained from previous similar data, and usually, the background counting rate is reasonably well known. Equation (10) becomes:

$$N = \frac{1 \; (1 + R_b/R_g)}{(RSD)^2 \; (1 - R_b/R_g)^2} \qquad (11)$$

which reduces to equation (10) when the value of R_b/R_g is small.

If it can be estimated, for example, that the sample, or gross, counting rate is ten times the background rate and a 5% maximum counting error is required, then the following can be estimated:

$$N = \frac{1 \; (1 + .1)}{(.05)^2 \; (1 - .1)^2}$$

$$= \frac{1}{.0025} \frac{1.1}{(.9)^2} = 543$$

In practice, this number is taken as a minimum. Estimates of N for several values of R_b/R_g with RSD = 5% are given in Table 4–2. Thus when the ratio of the background counting rate to the sample counting rate is 1/10 to 1/50, equation (11) is more accurate and should be used to estimate the sample counts.

TABLE 4–2. *Counts as a Function of R_b/R_g for 5% RSD*

R_b/R_g	N
1/10	543
1/20	465
1/50	424
1/100	412
1/500	402
1/10000	400

SUMS AND DIFFERENCES

It can be shown mathematically that sums and differences of observations of Gaussian distributed points are also Gaussian distributed.[1] This characteristic permits us to estimate the sum of a group of counts and the associated variability as well as the net (observed minus background) counts and the s.d. of the net count. If variables x_1 and x_2 are Gaussian distributed, then their sum $x = x_1 + x_2$ is Gaussian distributed with mean values:

$$\mu = \mu_1 + \mu_2$$
$$\sigma = \sqrt{(\sigma_1)^2 + (\sigma_2)^2}$$

and

$$\hat{\mu} = \bar{x}_1 + \bar{x}_2$$
$$\hat{\sigma} = s.d. = \sqrt{(s.d._1)^2 + (s.d._2)^2}$$

If x_1 and x_2 are counts N_1 and N_2, then the following is true:

$$\hat{\mu} = N = N_1 + N_2 \qquad (12)$$

and

$$s.d._{N_1+N_2} = \sqrt{(s.d._{N_1})^2 + (s.d._{N_2})^2}$$

This equation can be simplified for the Poisson distribution because $(s.d._{N_1})^2$ is simply N_1 and $(s.d._{N_2})^2$ is N_2. Thus:

$$s.d._{N_1+N_2} = \sqrt{N_1 + N_2} \qquad (13)$$

For the difference $X = X_1 - X_2$:

$$\mu = \mu_1 - \mu_2$$

but still

$$\sigma = \sqrt{(\sigma_1)^2 + (\sigma_2)^2}$$

COUNTING RATES

If counting rates are used instead of counts, then the counting rate R in cpm is:

$$R_{(cpm)} = \frac{N \; (counts)}{t \; (min)} \qquad (14)$$

and for the sum of two counting rates is:

$$R_{1+2} = R_1 + R_2 = \frac{N_1}{t_1} + \frac{N_2}{t_2} \qquad (15)$$

If the counting times are the same for the

two samples, i.e., if $t_1 = t_2 = t$, then $R_{1+2} = \frac{1}{t}(N_1 + N_2)$.

Time is assumed to be known exactly and is treated as a constant. Since the s.d. of a count N is $\sqrt{N}$, then for a counting rate:

$$\text{s.d.} = \frac{\sqrt{N}}{t} = \frac{\sqrt{Rt}}{t} = \sqrt{\frac{R}{t}} \quad (16)$$

The s.d. of the sum is:

$$\text{s.d.}_{1+2} = \sqrt{\frac{R_1}{t_1} + \frac{R_2}{t_2}} \quad (17)$$

This is called the *standard error* of the sum. If $t_1 = t_2 = t$, then

$$\text{s.d.}_{1+2} = \sqrt{\frac{R_1 + R_2}{t}}.$$

The average of several counts with equal counting times is:

$$\overline{N} = \frac{N_1 + N_2 + N_3 + N_4}{4}$$

and

$$\text{s.d.}_{\overline{N}} = \frac{1}{4}\sqrt{N_1 + N_2 + N_3 + N_4}$$

The average of several counting rates is:

$$\overline{R} = \frac{1}{4}(R_1 + R_2 + R_3 + R_4)$$

$$= \frac{1}{4}\left(\frac{N_1}{t_1} + \frac{N_2}{t_2} + \frac{N_3}{t_3} + \frac{N_4}{t_4}\right)$$

and

$$\text{s.d.}_{\overline{R}} = \frac{1}{4}\sqrt{\frac{R_1}{t_1} + \frac{R_2}{t_2} + \frac{R_3}{t_3} + \frac{R_4}{t_4}}$$

For equal counting times $t_1 = t_2 = t_3 = t_4 = t$:

$$\overline{R} = \frac{1}{4t}(N_1 + N_2 + N_3 + N_4)$$

and

$$\text{s.d.}_{\overline{R}} = \frac{1}{4}\sqrt{\frac{R_1 + R_2 + R_3 + R_4}{t}}$$

Nothing is to be gained from a set of repeated counts of the same sample other than to confirm that the Poisson process is correct.

If the difference between counting rates must be calculated, as in the case of background subtraction, the procedure is similar:

$$R_{1-2} = R_1 - R_2 = \frac{N_1}{t_1} - \frac{N_2}{t_2}$$

The s.d. of the difference is:

$$\text{s.d.}_{1-2} = \sqrt{\frac{R_1}{t_1} + \frac{R_2}{t_2}}$$

where $R = \frac{N}{t}$. For net counting rates:

$$R_{net} = R_g - R_b = \frac{N_g}{t_g} - \frac{N_b}{t_b} \quad (18)$$

and

$$\text{s.d.}_{net} = \sqrt{\frac{R_g}{t_g} + \frac{R_b}{t_b}} \quad (19)$$

OPTIMUM ALLOCATION OF BACKGROUND AND SAMPLE COUNTING TIMES

Jarett has shown that the most efficient allocation of time to minimize s.d.$_{net}$ occurs when:[3]

$$\frac{t_g}{t_b} = \sqrt{\frac{R_g}{R_b}} \quad (20)$$

This calculation is easier than may be imagined. The background counting rates and counting times are usually fairly well established. Also, some preliminary counts are often made on similar samples so that a crude estimate of the counting rate of the sample $R_g{}^*$ can be obtained. The optimum counting time for the sample can then be estimated:

$$t_g = t_b \sqrt{\frac{R_g{}^*}{R_b}}$$

This estimate is particularly helpful when the sample has a low counting rate, and counting times would be long.

Example 1. The background counting rate is usually 35 cpm and is counted for 10 min. The radionuclide in the sample to be counted is estimated at 500 cpm, based on the researcher's experience with similar material. What is the optimum counting time for the new sample?

$$t_g = 10 \sqrt{\frac{500}{35}} = 38 \text{ min}$$

If there were no "standard" background counting time, then the ratio of the sample to the background time could be determined as follows:

$$\frac{t_g}{t_b} = \sqrt{\frac{500}{35}} = 3.8 \text{ or approximately } 4$$

That is, the sample should be counted 4 times as long as the background for optimum allocation of time. Figure 4–2 gives the most efficient distribution of counting times as a function of gross and background counting rate ratios.

CONFIDENCE LIMITS

With estimates of the mean and standard deviation of a distribution that is assumed to be Gaussian, it is possible to compute with a prescribed degree of certainty the values (limits) within which the true mean is expected to fall. The values obtained for the estimated mean and s.d. will differ for repeated determinations of the same sample. The longer the counting process, the closer the estimate will be, so the next step is to bracket the true mean.

Estimates of the mean counting rate $\hat{\mu}$ and of the standard deviation $\hat{\sigma}$ can be used to determine confidence limits. The Gaussian distribution is such that 68% of the observations are expected to fall within one s.d. of the mean, and 95% of the observations are expected to fall within approximately two s.d.'s of the mean (actually 1.958). Figure 4–3 shows the area encompassed by ± 1, ± 2, and ± 3 s.d.'s.

Example 2. A 10-min determination of

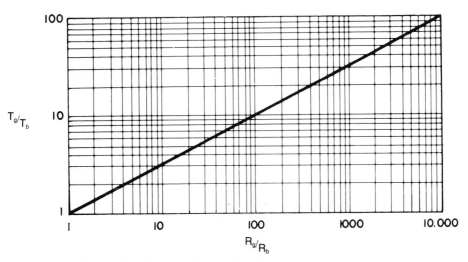

Fig. 4–2. Most efficient distribution of counting times.

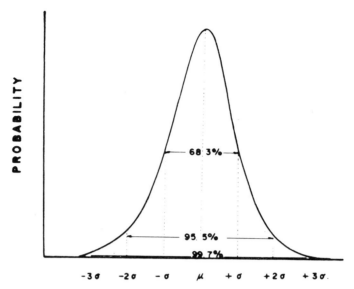

Fig. 4–3. Probability distribution of a Gaussian or normal curve showing the percentage of area defined by $\pm 1\sigma$, $\pm 2\sigma$, and $\pm 3\sigma$.

a sample yields 5480 counts. The background is 140 counts in 5 min. This yields:

$$R_{net} = R_g - R_b = \frac{N_g}{t_g} - \frac{N_b}{t_b}$$

$$= \frac{5480}{10} - \frac{140}{5} = 520 \text{ cpm}$$

$$\text{s.d.}_{net} = \sqrt{\frac{R_g}{t_g} + \frac{R_b}{t_b}} = \sqrt{\frac{548}{10} + \frac{28}{5}}$$

$$= 8 \text{ cpm}$$

For a Gaussian distribution, the true mean will lie within $\pm 1\sigma$ in 68% of observations; in this case, the mean $\pm 1\sigma$ is 520 $\pm$ 8 cpm, or 512 to 528. It may be stated with 95% confidence that the true counting rate lies between N $\pm$ 1.95 σ, in this case between 504 and 536, and so forth.

If the counting time were doubled, obtaining N_g = 10,975 for 20 min, and the same background of N_b = 140 counts in 5 min were used, then:

$$R_{net} = \frac{10975}{20} - \frac{140}{5} = 521 \text{ cpm}$$

and

$$\text{s.d.}_{net} = \sqrt{\frac{548.8}{20} + \frac{28}{5}} = 6 \text{ cpm}$$

This yields $\mu \pm 1\sigma$ limits of 521 $\pm$ 6: hence, the interval is 515 to 527 with 68% confidence. The $\mu \pm 1.95$ confidence limits are 509 to 533 cpm.

CHI-SQUARE DISTRIBUTION

The *chi-square distribution function* describes the distribution of the squares of independently distributed Gaussian quantities. If the variables x_i were Gaussian distributed, then the quantity:

$$X^2 = \sum_{i=1}^{k} \left(\frac{x_i - \mu}{\sigma} \right)^2 = \sum_{i=1}^{k} \frac{(x_i - \mu)^2}{\sigma^2} \quad (21)$$

would be distributed as X^2.

For the Poisson distribution, the number of counts N is Gaussian distributed for large values of N and the average $\overline{N}$ of a series of counts $N_i \ldots N_n$ is an estimate of the true mean. The σ is estimated by $\sqrt{N}$ for a single count, and the average $\overline{N}$ can be used to estimate σ^2 of the population. Cramer has shown that the following approximation holds:[1]

$$\sum_{i=1}^{k} \frac{(N_i - \overline{N})^2}{\overline{N}} = X^2 \qquad (22)$$

with k-1 degrees of freedom. The value of k should be 5 or larger.

If a series of counting determinations is made (whether from repeat measurements on the same sample or, e.g., from a series of samples of aliquots of the same radionuclide sample), determination of the homogeneity or lack of homogeneity of the counted values is possible.

Example 3. A particular sample was counted during ten random periods in a particular day. Are the readings homogeneous, or were there systematic changes during the day (e.g., voltage drops or calibration drift) that caused greater variability than could be expected from just "counting error"?

$$N_i$$
(Observed counts in each sample)

15970
17846
16157
16989
17534
16843
17235
16120
16756
17436

$\overline{N} = \Sigma N_i/k = 16{,}888$
s.d. $= \sqrt{\overline{N}} = 130$

To determine whether the value $\sqrt{\overline{N}}$ is consistent with Poisson variability, the X^2 is calculated. Applying formula (22):

$$X^2 = \Sigma \frac{(N_i - \overline{N})^2}{\overline{N}} = \frac{3{,}752{,}356}{16{,}888} = 222$$

By calculating the differences $N_i - \overline{N}$, the departures from expectation are examined individually, i.e., the true value of

the number of counts is estimated by the average count $\overline{N}$. To avoid negative values, the deviations are calculated, squared and then summed. Finally, the quantity $\Sigma (N_i - \overline{N})^2$ is divided by the estimate of the standard deviation squared, which in this case is $\hat{\sigma}^2 = \overline{N}$. The degrees of freedom here are the number of observations reduced by one, because the mean is also used in the calculation; $k - 1$ therefore becomes $10 - 1 = 9$ d.f.

An interesting characteristic of the theoretical X^2 distribution is that its expected value is the number of degrees of freedom; thus a computed value much greater than the number of degrees of freedom is expected to be significant. In example 3, the computed value of X^2 is 222, which is much greater than the expected value of 9. Table 4–3 gives the value of X^2 that must be exceeded for the sample to differ from expectation to give 90%, 95%, or 99% certainty. In other words, if the calculated value exceeds the tabled value for the appropriate number of degrees of freedom, then the probability of such an occurrence due to chance alone is said to be 1 in 10, 1 in 20, or 1 in 100. The value in Table 4–3 for 9 d.f. and probability of 0.01 (two-tailed) is $X^2 = 21.7$. The computed value 222 far exceeds that theoretical X^2, so something in addition to Poisson variability of counting error was operating, and the cause must be determined.

Chi-Square Distribution for Discrete Events

The chi-square distribution can also be used to compare the effectiveness of different diagnostic or therapeutic techniques. The quantity:

$$\Sigma \frac{(f_o - f_e)^2}{f_e} \qquad (23)$$

where f_o is an observed frequency of a discrete event and f_e is the expected frequency of the event, is distributed approximately as X^2. (The sum is taken over all categories.) The most common use of this test is in a 2×2 table where the ex-

TABLE 4–3. *Critical Values of the X^2 Distribution*

	Level of significance for one-tailed test					
	.10	.05	.025	.01	.005	.0005
Degrees of freedom	Level of significance for two-tailed test					
	.20	.10	.05	.02	.01	.001
1	1.64	2.71	3.84	5.41	6.64	10.83
2	3.22	4.60	5.99	7.82	9.21	13.82
3	4.64	6.25	7.82	8.84	11.34	16.27
4	5.99	7.78	9.49	11.67	13.28	18.46
5	7.29	9.24	11.07	13.39	15.09	20.52
6	8.56	10.64	12.59	15.03	16.81	22.46
7	9.80	12.02	14.07	16.62	18.48	24.32
8	11.03	13.36	15.51	18.17	20.09	26.12
9	12.24	14.68	16.92	19.68	21.67	27.88
10	13.44	15.99	18.31	21.16	23.21	29.59
11	14.63	17.28	19.68	22.62	24.72	31.26
12	15.81	18.55	21.03	24.05	26.22	32.91
13	16.98	19.81	22.36	25.47	27.69	34.53
14	18.15	21.06	23.68	26.87	29.14	36.12
15	19.31	22.31	25.00	28.26	30.58	37.70
16	20.46	23.54	26.30	29.63	32.00	39.25
17	21.62	24.77	27.59	31.00	33.41	40.79
18	22.76	25.99	28.87	32.35	34.80	42.31
19	23.90	27.20	30.14	33.69	36.19	43.82
20	25.04	28.41	31.41	35.02	37.57	45.32
21	26.17	29.62	32.67	36.34	38.93	46.80
22	27.30	30.81	33.92	37.66	40.29	48.27
23	28.43	32.01	35.17	38.97	41.64	49.73
24	29.55	33.20	36.42	40.27	42.98	51.18
25	30.68	34.38	37.65	41.57	44.31	52.62
26	31.80	35.56	38.88	42.86	45.64	54.05
27	32.91	36.74	40.11	44.14	46.96	55.48
28	34.03	37.92	41.34	45.42	48.28	56.89
29	35.14	39.09	42.56	46.69	49.59	58.30
30	36.25	40.26	43.77	47.96	50.89	59.70

pected frequency is computed from the same data set.

Example 4. In an experiment, 40 rats are irradiated at a dose expected to produce mortality within 30 days in 50% of them, which is the $LD_{50/30}$. Half of the animals are treated with a radioprotectant, which is expected to reduce mortality.

	LIVE	DIE	TOTAL
Treated	16	4	20
Not Treated	9	11	20
Total	25	15	40

Is the drug effective?
The table is given symbolically as follows:

	LIVE	DIE	TOTAL
Treated	a	b	a + b
Not Treated	c	d	c + d
Total	a + c	b + d	a + b + c + d = k

The expected frequencies can be computed from the marginal totals. Thus a, b, c, and d are the observed frequencies for the four conditions, and a + b + c + d = k.

$$a_e = \frac{a + c}{k} \times (a + b) \quad \text{is the expected frequency for a.}$$

$$a_e = \frac{25 \times 20}{40} = 12.5$$

$$c_e = \frac{a + c}{k} \times (c + d) \quad \text{is the expected frequency for c.}$$

$$c_e = \frac{25 \times 20}{40} = 12.5$$

$$b_e = \frac{b + d}{k} \times (a + b) \quad \text{is the expected frequency for b.}$$

$$b_e = \frac{15 \times 20}{40} = 7.5$$

$$d_e = \frac{b + d}{k} \times (c + d) \quad \text{is the expected frequency for d.}$$

$$d_e = \frac{15 \times 20}{40} = 7.5$$

X^2 can now be evaluated using the form:

$$X^2 = \Sigma \frac{(f_o - f_e)^2}{f_e}$$

thus

$$X^2 = \frac{(a - a_e)^2}{a_e} + \frac{(b - b_e)^2}{b_e} + \frac{(c - c_e)^2}{c_e} + \frac{(d - d_e)^2}{d_e}$$

By substituting the observed values from the first table in this example and estimates of the calculated expected values just given, the following is obtained:

$$X^2 = \frac{(16 - 12.5)^2}{12.5} + \frac{(4 - 7.5)^2}{7.5}$$
$$+ \frac{(9 - 12.5)^2}{12.5} + \frac{(11 - 7.5)^2}{7.5}$$
$$= \frac{3.5^2}{12.5} + \frac{(-3.5)^2}{12.5} + \frac{(-3.5)^2}{7.5} + \frac{3.5^2}{7.5}$$
$$= 0.98 + 0.98 + 1.63 + 1.63 = 5.23$$

There is always 1 d.f. for a 2 × 2 table.

The X^2 value for 1 d.f. is 2.71 for $P \le 0.05$ and 5.23 for $P \le 0.01$. In this case, the direction of the expected difference between the fractions was known *a priori*. This is called a *one-tailed test*; one- versus two-tailed tests are discussed more fully in the section "t Test for Two Independent Samples." For the one-tailed test, the probabilities in Table 4–3 are half of those for the two-tailed test. Thus, for the preceding example, if either the $P \le 0.05$ or $P \le 0.01$ significance level were chosen, the hypothesis of equality, i.e., that the treatment is not effective, would have to be rejected, because the computed value of X^2 is greater than the critical value of X^2, 2.71, for one degree of freedom. If the fraction expected to be larger were not known *a priori*, then the values given for the two-tailed test should be used.

Simplified Calculation for 2 × 2 Tables

Calculations can be simplified considerably for the 2 × 2 tables. Algebraic reduction leads to the formula:

$$X^2 = \frac{k \,(|ad - bc| - k/2)^2}{(a + b)\,(a + c)\,(b + d)\,(c + d)} \quad (24)$$

The vertical bars within the parentheses signify absolute value, i.e., the difference $|ad - bc|$ is always considered positive regardless of whether the algebraic sign is + or −. The quantity k/2 within the parentheses is subtracted as a correction for continuity, which brings the approximation closer to the actual values. The X^2 is only an approximation when used with discrete frequencies. It should be used with $k \geq 20$ and with five or more observations in each cell. Fisher's exact test (described later) should be used when these conditions are not met.

Without the correction for continuity, the simplified formula would yield the identical value for X^2 computed by the long method. Using the correction for continuity, the following is obtained:

$$X^2 = \frac{40 \, (|16 \times 11 - 4 \times 9| - 40/2)^2}{20 \times 25 \times 15 \times 20}$$

$$= \frac{40 \, (140 - 20)^2}{153600} = 3.84$$

which is smaller than the uncorrected X^2 and, of course, is still significant ($P \leq 0.05$) because it exceeds the tabled value of 2.71. By this method, however, it is not significant at $P \leq 0.01$.

This calculation indicates that the proportion of animals that have received the treatment and lived (16/20) is greater than the proportion of animals that have not received the treatment and lived (9/20), and that the difference is statistically significant at the $P \leq 0.05$ level. That is, in only 1 trial in 20 would the observed results occur by chance, so the claim that the drug is effective is accepted.

Fisher's Exact Test for 2 × 2 Tables

Fisher's exact test, an alternate procedure, is a bit more difficult to calculate but does not require reference to tables. It is most appropriate for small numbers of observations ($k < 20$) for which calculation is relatively easy and the X^2 approximation is least accurate. It belongs to a class of statistical techniques called *randomization tests.* In this test, rather than a value being calculated and the probability looked up in a table, the probability is calculated directly by taking all possible combinations of "favorable" results and dividing by all possible outcomes. This is similar to calculating the probability of a pair of 5's on the roll of dice, or rather, the

probability of a 10 or higher (i.e., a 10 or 11 or 12) on the roll of dice.

With the a, b, c, d notation of the X^2 tables given previously, the probability of obtaining the specific set of values in the 2 × 2 table due to chance may be computed as follows:

$$P = \frac{(a+b)! \, (c+d)! \, (a+c)! \, (b+d)!}{k! \, a! \, b! \, c! \, d!} \quad (25)$$

The probability of obtaining the observed result and all others that are less likely to occur is actually required. This probability is obtained by calculating the sum of the probabilities of all possible events, using equation (25) for each. For the numerator, equation (25) takes the product of the factorials of each of the four marginal totals, $a+b$, $c+d$, $a+c$, and $b+d$; for the denominator, the equation takes the product of the four factorials of the terms a, b, c, and d multiplied by the factorial of the total k. Factorial is explained after equation (4). Most programmable pocket calculators can be programmed to compute the quantity P fairly easily. A separate P calculation is made for each condition, and finally, the P's are summed. This can be done systematically by placing the smallest frequency in the upper left corner (the "a" position), renaming the categories, keeping the marginal totals constant, and computing the probabilities, as shown in example 5.

Example 5. A pilot experiment on a different radioprotectant, using a total of 20 experimental animals, produced the following 30-day surviving fractions: nontreated 4/10, treated 7/10. Is the drug effective? Form the 2 × 2 table.

	LIVE	DIE	TOTAL
Treated	$^a7$	$^b3$	$^{a+b}10$
Nontreated	$^c4$	$^d6$	$^{c+d}10$
Total	$^{a+c}11$	$^{b+d}9$	$^k20$

Place the smallest frequency, 3, in the "a" position.

a = 3	LIVE	DIE	TOTAL
Treated	[a]3	[b]7	10
Nontreated	[c]6	[d]4	10
Total	9	11	[k]20

a = 2	LIVE	DIE	TOTAL
Treated	2	8	10
Nontreated	7	3	10
Total	9	11	20

Keeping the marginal totals the same, form a series of tables, and make "a" successively 0, 1, 2, and 3. If the numbers from the preceding table are substituted into equation (25), the value for P_3 associated with a = 3 is calculated as follows:

$$P_3 = \frac{10!\ 10!\ 9!\ 11!}{3!\ 7!\ 6!\ 4!\ 20!}$$
$$= \frac{1.9074 \times 10^{26}}{1.2713 \times 10^{27}} = 0.150$$

The values for a at 0, 1, and 2 are calculated similarly:

a = 0	LIVE	DIE	TOTAL
Treated	0	10	10
Nontreated	9	1	10
Total	9	11	20

$$P_0 = \frac{10!\ 10!\ 9!\ 11!}{0!\ 10!\ 9!\ 1!\ 20!}$$
$$= \frac{1.9074 \times 10^{26}}{3.2037 \times 10^{30}} = 5.95 \times 10^{-5}$$

a = 1	LIVE	DIE	TOTAL
Treated	1	9	10
Nontreated	8	2	10
Total	9	11	20

$$P_1 = \frac{10!\ 10!\ 9!\ 11!}{1!\ 9!\ 8!\ 2!\ 20!}$$
$$= \frac{1.9074 \times 10^{26}}{7.1193 \times 10^{28}} = 2.679 \times 10^{-3}$$

$$P_2 = \frac{10!\ 10!\ 9!\ 11!}{2!\ 8!\ 7!\ 3!\ 20!}$$
$$= \frac{1.9074 \times 10^{26}}{5.9328 \times 10^{27}} = .0322$$

Thus $P = P_0 + P_1 + P_2 + P_3 = 0.0000595 + 0.00269 + 0.0322 + 0.150 = 0.184$

This computation gives the probability that, in the experiment described, the data obtained or a less likely set of data would occur approximately 18% of the time, or approximately one in five, due to chance alone. This method calculated the one-tailed probability for Fisher's exact test, which is required in this case, and it cannot be concluded that the radioprotective drug is effective. If a two-tailed test had been required, the computed probability of 0.184 would have had to be doubled. Examination of the four tables reveals that the three cases wherein a equals 0, 1, and 2 are worse than the one obtained (a = 3). Each has a probability of less than 0.05, which means that if an array with 2 in the "a" position had been obtained, the results would have been statistically significant.

For comparison, the X^2 test with the correction for continuity may be applied to these data with the realization that while n is 20, two of the cells have values of less than 5.

$$X^2 = \frac{k\ (|ad - bc|) - k/2)^2}{(a+b)\ (a+c)\ (b+d)\ (c+d)}$$
$$= \frac{20\ (|3 \times 4 - 6 \times 7| - 20/2)^2}{10 \times 9 \times 11 \times 10}$$
$$= 0.81$$

The actual probability of the X^2 distribution function for 1 d.f. and of a computed X^2 of 0.81 is $P = 0.368$ for the two-tailed test, or 0.181 for the one-tailed test, which means that the probability from the

X^2 method is very similar to that obtained from Fisher's exact test. The results are not significant in either method, i.e., the treatment has not been demonstrated to be effective.

McNemar's Test

Another use for the X^2 distribution is in testing for equality of proportions when the same individuals are measured on two separate occasions, or in comparing two methods used on the same individuals, with results stated in terms of a discrete observation.[4,5] An example might be the comparison of two imaging techniques in detecting a lesion.

	Analog Image		
Digital Image	− SCAN	+ SCAN	TOTAL
− Scan	a	b	a + b
+ Scan	c	d	c + d
Total	a + c	b + d	k

Each cell in the table contains the number of cases that either possess or do not possess the desired characteristic. The proportions of interest are those diagnosed as having a positive scan by method one ($P_1 = (c + d)/k$) and those diagnosed as having a positive scan by method two ($P_2 = (b + d)/k$). The difference between these proportions is:

$$P_2 - P_1 = \frac{c + d}{k} - \frac{b + d}{k} = \frac{c - b}{k}$$

Notice that the quantities a and d do not appear in the comparison. If c and b were equal, their average $(b + c)/2$ would be used as the expected value to form:

$$X^2 = \frac{(f_{o_1} - f_e)^2}{f_e} + \frac{(f_{o_2} - f_e)^2}{f_e}$$
$$= \frac{[c - (b + c)/2]^2}{\frac{b + c}{2}} + \frac{[d - (b + c)/2]^2}{\frac{b + c}{2}}$$

The notations f_{o_1} and f_{o_2} are the observed

frequencies, and f_e is the expected frequency. This reduces to:

$$X^2 = \frac{(c - b)^2}{c + b}$$

When a correction for continuity is introduced,[6] this becomes:

$$X^2 = \frac{(|c - b| - 1)^2}{c + b}$$

The vertical bars mean absolute values, i.e., the difference $|c - b|$ is considered positive regardless of the sign. This value of X^2 is then compared to the tabled X^2 distribution value with one degree of freedom.

Example 6. Seventy-five patients were studied using both conventional scintillation camera analog images and digitally enhanced images. The results were as follows:

	Analog Image		
Digital Image	− SCAN	+ SCAN	TOTAL
− Scan	20	5	25
+ Scan	10	40	50
Total	30	45	75

Are the results of the two methods comparable? The proportions of positive scans by each method are:

$$\frac{c + d}{k} = \frac{50}{75} \text{ for digital images}$$

and

$$\frac{b + d}{k} = \frac{45}{75} \text{ for analog images.}$$

The test compares the cases of disagreement:

$$X^2 = \frac{(|10 - 5| - 1)^2}{10 + 5} = 1.07$$

with 1 degree of freedom.

The tabled 0.05 significance level for X^2 with one degree of freedom is 3.84. In this case, a two-tailed test can be used because the only concern is whether or not the methods give the same results. The computed value does not exceed the tabled value; hence a difference between the two techniques cannot be asserted. Tested at the 0.05 significance level, then, the difference observed is not statistically significant.

COMPARISON OF TWO SETS OF CONTINUOUS MEASUREMENTS

t Test for Two Independent Samples

The determination of differences in thyroid uptake between two different isotopes of iodine in normal animals requires far greater differences in counts from animal to animal than would be due merely to "counting error." The counts, because they are reasonably high, can be considered a continuous variable. If the distribution of counts from animal to animal can be assumed to follow, more or less, a Gaussian distribution, then comparison of uptakes using the t test is appropriate. The t distribution contains the assumption that the underlying distribution is Gaussian but that the standard deviation is estimated from the data. The t distribution is almost identical to the Gaussian distribution for large sample sizes ($k \geq 200$ observations), and theoretically, it describes the behavior of the quantity:

$$t = \frac{\overline{x}}{s.d./\sqrt{k}} = \frac{\overline{x}}{SE_{\overline{x}}} \qquad (26)$$

The statistic $SE_{\overline{x}}$ is called the *standard error of the mean*. It is a measure of the variability of the sample mean whereas the standard deviation is a measure of the variability of individual observations. The more observations there are, the smaller the $SE_{\overline{x}}$ becomes. This rule is consistent with the principle that the larger the sample, the better the estimate of mean.

To compare two means, the following quantity is used:

$$t = \frac{\overline{x}_1 - \overline{x}_2}{SE_{\overline{x}_1 - \overline{x}_2}} \qquad (27)$$

where

$$SE_{\overline{x}_1 - \overline{x}_2} = \qquad (28)$$

$$\sqrt{\frac{(k_1 - 1)s.d._1^2 + (k_2 - 1)s.d._2^2}{k_1 + k_2 - 2} \times \frac{k_1 + k_2}{k_1 k_2}}$$

for small samples. If k_1 and k_2 are each over 30, the $SE_{\overline{x}_1 - \overline{x}_2}$ is approximated by:

$$\sqrt{\frac{s.d._1^2}{k_1} + \frac{s.d._2^2}{k_2}}$$

and if $k_1 = k_2 = k$ then:

$$SE_{\overline{x}_1 - \overline{x}_2} = \sqrt{\frac{s.d._1^2 + s.d._2^2}{k}} \qquad (29)$$

The quantity t is compared to the tabled theoretical value using $k_1 + k_2 - 2$ degrees of freedom (Table 4–4).

Example 7. The following series of net counts were taken one per animal.

Radionuclide 1	Radionuclide 2
10586	9842
9856	8312
10128	9468
12642	10840
8744	7259
9425	8870
7932	8226
10973	9620
$\overline{x}_1 = 10036$	$\overline{x}_2 = 9055$
$\sqrt{\overline{x}_1} = 100$	$\sqrt{\overline{x}_2} = 95$
$s.d._1 = 1438$	$s.d._2 = 1121$
$SE_{\overline{x}_1} = 569$	$SE_{\overline{x}_2} = 396$
$k_1 = 8$	$k_2 = 8$

Examination of each set of observations determines whether the biological variability dominates, i.e., whether the variability exceeds what would be expected from Poisson variability. Treating the observations as a series of counts allows the following to be computed:

$$X^2 = \sum_{i=1}^{k} \frac{(N_i - \overline{N})^2}{\overline{N}} = \frac{(k - 1)\,\sigma\overline{N}^2}{\overline{N}}$$

where k is the number of subjects in the sample.

Radionuclide 1   *Radionuclide 2*

$$X^2 = \frac{(8-1)(1438)^2}{10036} \qquad X^2 = \frac{(8-1)(1121)^2}{9055}$$

$$= 1442 \qquad\qquad = 971$$

The degrees of freedom for each is $k - 1 = 8 - 1 = 7$ because there are eight Poisson observations in each. X^2 for 7 d.f. at the 5% significance level (two-tailed) is 14.1, a value many times exceeded by the computed values. Hence the s.d. computed as $\sqrt{\Sigma(N_i - \overline{N})^2/k - 1}$ (the conventional method of computing $\hat{\sigma}$) is compared in this way to the Poisson estimate of variability provided by $\sqrt{\overline{N}}$. Thus 1438 has been compared effectively to the Poisson estimate of 100 counts for radionuclide 1, and 1121 has been similarly compared, in a sense, to 95 counts for radionuclide 2. The X^2 test has verified that the Poisson variability is small compared to the observed individual-to-individual variability. This step is usually not necessary but has been included as an example of the methodology.

The t test now can be applied to the data to determine whether the two groups are different. If there is reason to believe from previous work that one group tends to be larger than the other, the differences observed can be studied to determine whether they are consistent with that hypothesis.

For the data given earlier in which $k_1 = k_2 = k = 8$, the following is computed:

$$SE_{\overline{x}_1 - \overline{x}_2} = \sqrt{\frac{(s.d._1)^2 + (s.d._2)^2}{k}}$$

$$= \sqrt{\frac{(1438)^2 + (1121)^2}{8}}$$

$$= 645$$

The quantity t then becomes:

$$t = \frac{\overline{x}_1 - \overline{x}_2}{SE_{\overline{x}_1 - \overline{x}_2}} = \frac{10036 - 9055}{645} = 1.52$$

The value for degrees of freedom is $k_1 + k_2 - 2 = 14$. This computed value is compared with the critical value for 14 degrees of freedom in Table 4–4. At this time, it must be determined whether a "one-tailed" or a "two-tailed" test is required. If it is known *a priori* that the difference between the averages observed could have been either negative or positive (i.e., that $\overline{x}_1$ could have been either larger or smaller than $\overline{x}_2$), then the test is considered two-tailed. This is because a large negative value of t would be associated with a value in the left tail, while a large positive value of t would be associated with a value in the right tail. If it cannot be decided *a priori* which way the difference must go, a significance test that assumes half the values in the left tail and half in the right tail must be used. On the other hand, if it is known *a priori* that one of the two groups will be larger, then the difference $\overline{x}_1 - \overline{x}_2$ must always be in a particular direction. In this case, the "one-tailed" test is used.

In example 7, if the second group is assumed *a priori* to be smaller, and if $P < 0.05$ is selected, a value $t = 1.761$ is found in Table 4–4, using the heading marked "one-tailed" for 14 d.f. The tabled value is larger than the computed value of $t = 1.52$, so the hypothesis of equality cannot be rejected and it cannot be asserted that the true mean μ_1 is greater than μ_2. When a value of t that is close to significance is obtained, the experiment may be repeated using a larger sample size; if the averages and the s.d.'s then remained about the same, the $SE_{\overline{x}_1 - \overline{x}_2}$ would become smaller because k would be larger, as indicated in equation (29), and the computed value of t would be larger, as indicated in equation (26).

t Test for Paired Comparisons

Whenever a test is administered to a series of animals or patients and then either the same test is repeated under a different condition or a different test is adminis-

TABLE 4–4. *Critical Values of the t Distribution*

	Level of significance for one-tailed test				
	.05	.025	.01	.005	.0005
	Level of significance for two-tailed test				
df	0.1	.05	.02	.01	.001
1	6.3138	12.7062	31.8205	63.6567	636.6193
2	2.9200	4.3027	6.9646	9.9248	31.5991
3	2.3534	3.1824	4.5407	5.8409	12.9240
4	2.1318	2.7764	3.7470	4.6041	8.6103
5	2.0150	2.5706	3.3649	4.0322	6.8688
6	1.9432	2.4469	3.1427	3.7074	5.9588
7	1.8946	2.3646	2.9980	3.4995	5.4079
8	1.8595	2.3060	2.8965	3.3554	5.0413
9	1.8331	2.2622	2.8214	3.2498	4.7809
10	1.8125	2.2281	2.7638	3.1693	4.5869
11	1.7959	2.2010	2.7181	3.1058	4.4370
12	1.7823	2.1788	2.6810	3.0545	4.3178
13	1.7709	2.1604	2.6503	3.0123	4.2208
14	1.7613	2.1448	2.6245	2.9768	4.1405
15	1.7531	2.1315	2.6025	2.9467	4.0728
16	1.7459	2.1199	2.5835	2.9208	4.0150
17	1.7396	2.1098	2.5669	2.8982	3.9651
18	1.7341	2.1009	2.5524	2.8784	3.9217
19	1.7291	2.0930	2.5395	2.8609	3.8834
20	1.7247	2.0860	2.5280	2.8453	3.8495
21	1.7207	2.0796	2.5176	2.8314	3.8193
22	1.7171	2.0739	2.5083	2.8188	3.7921
23	1.7139	2.0687	2.4999	2.8073	3.7676
24	1.7109	2.0639	2.4922	2.7969	3.7454
25	1.7081	2.0595	2.4851	2.7874	3.7252
26	1.7056	2.0555	2.4786	2.7787	3.7066
27	1.7033	2.0518	2.4727	2.7707	3.6896
28	1.7011	2.0484	2.4671	2.7633	3.6739
29	1.6991	2.0452	2.4620	2.7564	3.6594
30	1.6973	2.0423	2.4573	2.7500	3.6460
40	1.6839	2.0211	2.4233	2.7045	3.5510
50	1.6759	2.0086	2.4033	2.6778	3.4960
100	1.6602	1.9840	2.3642	2.6259	3.3905
200	1.6525	1.9719	2.3451	2.6006	3.3398
∞ (z:)	1.6449	1.9600	2.3263	2.5758	3.2905

Compiled by W.E. Jackson, AFRRI, Bethesda, MD.

tered to the same individuals, the two sets of measurements are likely to be correlated. The reason for such correlation is that if the tests are designed to measure the same characteristic, an individual's high response on one test most likely would be high on the second test, and vice versa. If the results are correlated, then the t test for two independent samples is not applicable because the samples are not independent. The *paired t test* is designed for this purpose.

The simplest calculations for this test involve forming the differences between the individuals in the two sets of measurements, computing $\bar{x}$ s.d., and $SE_{\bar{x}}$ for the differences, and computing the value t.

Example 8. Suppose now that the two sets of data from example 7 were obtained from the same eight animals.

Subject	Radio-nuclide 1	Radio-nuclide 2	$\Delta = x_1 - x_2$
1	10586	9842	744
2	9856	8312	1544
3	10128	9468	660
4	12642	10840	1802
5	8744	7259	1485
6	9425	8870	555
7	7932	8226	−294
8	10973	9620	1353

$$\bar{\Delta} = 981$$
$$\text{s.d.} = 692$$
$$SE_{\bar{\Delta}} = 245$$

If results from the two radionuclides are the same, the average of the differences is expected to be zero. If that average is significantly different from zero, then the two tests are considered different.

$$t = \frac{\bar{\Delta}}{SE_{\bar{\Delta}}} = \frac{981}{692/\sqrt{8}} = 4.00$$

In this case, the degrees of freedom are $k - 1 = 7$, one less than the number of pairs of observations. For a one-tailed test with 7 degrees of freedom, Table 4–4 shows the tests to be significantly different at $P \le 0.005$.

Using the appropriate test can have an important effect on interpretation of the data in cases of paired observation. In example 7, the two groups were assumed to be independent, and the difference was not statistically significant. In example 8, however, the appropriate test for paired comparisons was used, and the difference was statistically significant at $P \le 0.005$.

NONPARAMETRIC TESTS

A class of tests that can be substituted for the conventional statistical tests, which usually rely on the fact that the observations follow a Gaussian distribution, are nonparametric, or distribution-free, tests. Two such tests that replace the independent and paired t tests are presented here. These are particularly useful with data that are quite variable, that have suspected outliers, or that are suspected of departing markedly from the Gaussian distribution—e.g., data from a possible mixture of two strains (old/young, sick/well, etc.) that cannot be separated and might cause a bimodal response. If subjects used for the two experimental treatments were chosen randomly, then the bimodality should affect both groups similarly. Although the averages might not be representative of a clean population, the observed changes due to treatment could be valid. If the sample sizes are large (at least 30 in each), the usual t test might yield valid results. Because of the large variance, smaller samples most likely would not show real differences, and conclusions would be suspect because of the departure from the Gaussian distribution.

Paired Observations—Wilcoxon Signed Rank Test

The Wilcoxon test is applicable under the same conditions as the paired t test.[5,7,8] In fact, the test is up to 95% as efficient in its use of the data. It is preferred by many researchers, particularly when linearity of scaling is an issue, such as when physicians are asked to assign a number to the degree of a test's abnormality. Although the scaling results can be ranked in such a case, averaged values have little meaning.

In the Wilcoxon test, data are arranged as they were in the t test for paired comparisons, but their differences are ranked, the sign of the difference is ignored, and the sign is appended afterward. The ranks of the positive values are summed to obtain T_+, and the negative values are summed separately to obtain T_-. A differ-ence of zero is excluded from the ranking, and the sample size is reduced by 1. The test statistic chosen is the smaller of the two values, T_- or T_+ and is compared to the appropriate value in Table 4–5 where k is the number of pairs. If the computed value is less than or equal to the tabled value, conclude that the two groups are different.

Example 9. Data from the previous example, with minor changes, and a ninth pair of observations are used:

Subject	Nuclide 1	Nuclide 2	Δ	Absolute Rank	Sign of Rank
1	10586	9842	744	(4)	+
2	10132	8312	1820	(9)	+
3	10128	9468	660	(3)	+
4	12642	10840	1802	(8)	+
5	8744	7259	1485	(6)	+
6	9425	9110	315	(2)	+
7	7932	8226	− 294	(1)	−
8	10973	9620	1353	(5)	+
9	12051	13846	− 1795	(7)	−
	$\bar{x}_1 = 10290$	$\bar{x}_2 = 9614$	$\bar{\Delta} = 677$		
	$s.d._1 = 1497$	$s.d._2 = 1901$	$SE_{\bar{\Delta}} = 388$		$T_- = 8$
			$t = \dfrac{\bar{\Delta}}{SE_{\bar{\Delta}}} = 1.74$		$T_+ = 37$

(one tail) $t_{.05}$, 8 d.f. $= 1.859$

For this example, the sum of the positive ranks is $T_+ = 37$, and the sum of the negative ranks is $T_- = 8$. The T_- is the smaller value and should be compared to the tabled value. For a one-tailed test, the tabled value for k = 9 and for $P \leq 0.05$ of the Wilcoxon test is T = 8 from Table 4–5. If the computed T_- quantity is less than or equal to the tabled value, the hypothesis of equality is rejected. In this example, the computed value equals the tabled value, and it must be concluded that the set of values for the first radionuclide was significantly higher than that for the second. A two-tailed test doubles the probability and requires use of the appropriate column headings in the table.

Using the previously described paired comparison t test on the same data yields a computed t = 1.74 and a tabled (Table 4–4) one-tailed value for 8 d.f. at the $P \leq 0.05$ of 1.859, which is not significant; therefore, the uptake of radionuclide 1 could not be considered significantly greater. On the other hand, the Wilcoxon procedure indicates that the two groups are different. The most reasonable explanation for the difference between the two outcomes is that because of the single observation on radionuclide 2 for the ninth subject, which was inconsistent with the others, the t test is the wrong test to use.

Mann-Whitney Test for Two Independent Samples

A nonparametric test developed by Mann and Whitney that is a valid substitute for the independent-samples t test is appropriate for the same conditions as the Wilcoxon test (i.e., non-Gaussian, large variability, and occasional outliers), but it is applicable for two independent samples rather than related measurements.[9]

The critical value U in the Mann-Whitney test is calculated as follows: Assemble observations from the two samples and rank them from the lowest to the highest value, disregarding which sample the value came from. At the same time, retain the identity of each sample, e.g., write the values from sample 1 in red and those for sample 2 in blue, or offset the values as shown in example 10. Assign the rank (1) to the smallest value and assign the rank $(k_1 + k_2)$ to the largest. Then sum the ranks of Sample 1 separately from those in Sample 2. If the data from one of the two sam-

ples is clearly larger than the other, its rank sum should be much larger than the sum of the ranks for the other sample. S_1 and S_2 are the sums of the ranks of the first and second samples, respectively.

The test statistic is $T_1 = S_1 - k_1(k_1 + 1)/2$ where k_1 is the number of observations in Sample 1, or $T_2 = S_2 - k_2(k_2 + 1)/2$. The smaller of the computed values T_1 or T_2 is then compared to the tabled value for the appropriate sample size. Degrees of freedom are not used in either of these tests; the k refers to the number of observations in a sample. If $k_1 = k_2$ (i.e., if the sample sizes are equal), then the smaller sum of ranks is used.

Example 10. Data from example 9 are used assuming that the two samples are independent and ranked as described above.

This quantity can be compared with the tabled value of T (sometimes designated U) that is available in most nonparametric statistical texts,[5,10] and in many standard statistical texts.[11] For experiments in which each of the samples consists of eight or more observations, a simple approximation is available in place of using the extensive Mann-Whitney tables. Computing T for this quantity is not necessary; instead, the value S is used to compute a new statistic Z:

$$Z = \frac{2S - k_1 k_2}{\sqrt{\dfrac{k_1 k_2 (k_1 + k_2 + 1)}{3}}} \qquad (30)$$

The quantity Z is approximately Gaussian distributed, with the approximation improving with increasing sample size. For this example, the following is obtained:

$$Z = \frac{2(73) - 9 \times 9}{\sqrt{\dfrac{9 \times 9 \ (9 + 9 + 1)}{3}}} = 2.87$$

The values in the t table for ∞ degrees of freedom are actually the Gaussian distribution values of Z (Table 4–4). For a

Counts		*Ranks*	
Sample 1		*Sample 1*	
	Sample 2		*Sample 2*
	7259		(1)
7932		(2)	
	8226		(3)
	8312		(4)
8744		(5)	
	9110		(6)
9425		(7)	
	9468		(8)
	9620		(9)
	9842		(10)
10128		(11)	
10132		(12)	
10586		(13)	
	10840		(14)
10973		(15)	
12051		(16)	
12642		(17)	
	13846		(18)
S = Σ Ranks		$S_1 = 98$ $S_2 = 73$	

$$T_2 = S_2 - \frac{k_2(k_2 + 1)}{2}$$

$$= 73 - \frac{9 \times 10}{2} = 28$$

TABLE 4–5. *Table of Critical Values of T in the Wilcoxon Matched-Pairs Signed-Ranks Test*

	Level of significance for one-tailed test			
	.05	.025	.01	.005
	Level of significance for two-tailed test			
k	.10	.05	.02	.01
6	2	0	—	—
7	4	2	0	—
8	6	4	2	0
9	8	6	3	2
10	11	8	5	3
11	14	11	7	5
12	17	14	10	7
13	21	17	13	10
14	26	21	16	13
15	30	25	20	16
16	36	30	24	19
17	41	35	28	23
18	47	40	33	28
19	54	46	38	32
20	60	52	43	37
21	68	59	49	43
22	75	66	56	49
23	83	73	62	55
24	92	81	69	61
25	101	90	77	68
26	110	98	85	76
27	120	107	93	84
28	130	117	102	92
29	141	127	111	100
30	152	137	120	109

From Wilcoxon, F., and Wilcox, R.A.[8] Reproduced with the permission of the American Cyanamid Company.

one-tailed test with $P \leq 0.05$, the computed value Z must exceed the tabled value of $Z = 1.645$. A two-tailed test requires a value of $Z = 1.96$. Clearly, the Mann-Whitney test shows the two groups to be unequal.

Reference to the table of the Gaussian distribution is necessary, but the test procedure is based on rankings. Although the data contain what appears to be a maver-

ick, the test shows the groups to be significantly different ($P \leq 0.01$). The conventional t test for independent samples gives:

$$t = \frac{\overline{x}_1 - \overline{x}_2}{\sqrt{\dfrac{(s.d._1)^2 + (s.d._2)^2}{k}}} = \frac{677}{806} = 0.84$$

This value is clearly not significant because the one-tailed $t_{.05} = 1.746$ for 16 degrees of freedom; however, use of the nonparametric test that is not sensitive to outliers shows that the groups are significantly different. It is the appropriate test to use.

TREATMENT OF SPURIOUS OBSERVATIONS

When data are collected, whether in connection with a complex experiment or a routine isotope-counting series, one or more observations appear occasionally that seem inconsistent with the other data. An experienced technician usually will go to the measuring device, examine it carefully, and repeat the counts, or perhaps will have a pathologist do a postmortem examination (in the case of animal experiments) in an attempt to assign a cause to the maverick data point. If none can be found, the researcher is in a quandary: Should he include the observation in statistical computations and distort both the average and standard deviation if the observation is spurious? Or should the data point be discarded, possibly making the s.d. smaller than it really is and shifting the average away from the direction of the outliers?

Many times, an investigator may feel justified in discarding a data point, particularly if it is only one of a large set of similar observations and if the point is, for example, 5 or 10 times the size of the remainder of the group of observations. At other times, even the most experienced investigator has difficulty in deciding how to treat the apparent outlier.

Two approaches can be taken: (1) use of a statistically valid method for the rejection of outliers, and (2) use of nonparametric statistical methods that are not affected by outliers (the approach preferred by many statisticians). The Wilcoxon and the Mann-Whitney tests presented earlier are two methods that compare groups of data and are not sensitive to outliers. Other methods are presented in Siegel and in Conover.[5,10]

Rejection of Outliers

To consider rejection of outliers, one must be confident that systematic errors (e.g., calibration drift) have not affected the data, that the observations are homogeneous (e.g., animals are from a single shipment, reagents from a single batch, injection by a single individual), and that subjects have had a single treatment or treatment combination. Furthermore, all of the rejection methods require the observations to be from a Gaussian distribution, with the exception of the suspected outliers. Examples of data that should not be routinely purged of suspected outliers are (a) an entire day's output of a radioisotope-counting lab, because it includes a mixture with too great a variety of determinations and biologic samples; (b) the data from an experiment wherein several treatments are examined with only a few data at each treatment; and (c) retrospective data, e.g., from hospital records in which conditions, technicians, or treatment conditions have changed.

Data that might lend themselves to purging of suspected outliers are a large calibration run or observations from a single treatment in which previous experience has shown data to be consistent with the Gaussian distribution.

Despite the fact that statisticians universally discard Chauvenet's criterion because it rejects data at a probability level that changes as a function of sample size,

it is still recommended by some authors.[12] The subject is ignored in almost all statistical texts because there is no universal test for outliers and almost every case requires a different technique. Excellent summaries of rejection procedures are given by Grubbs and by Anscombe.[13,14]

The method presented here was suggested by Pearson and Chandra Sekar and was based on work by W.R. Thompson.[15,16] It is valid for a series of observations in which one observation is suspect. Some have applied it a second time, realizing that because the procedure was applied twice, the probability will be greater than that selected.

In the Thompson method, the average ($\bar{x}$) and the standard deviation (s.d.) are calculated by the usual methods. Then the suspect data point is selected, which will be the largest observation $x_{(n)}$ or the smallest observation $x_{(1)}$. Either of the following quantities is calculated:

$$T_{(n)} = \frac{x_{(n)} - \bar{x}}{s.d.} \text{ or } T_{(1)} = \frac{\bar{x} - x_{(1)}}{s.d.}$$

Note that the denominator is s.d. and not S.E. as in many other statistical tests. This quantity is compared to the appropriate value in Table 4–6. If the calculated T exceeds the tabled value, then the data point is rejected. In using the significance level 1% or 5% a one-tailed test is assumed, i.e., the experimenter knows in advance of examining the data whether outliers will be too large or too small.

Table 4–6 gives the distribution in percentage points of the deviation of the largest observation from the sample mean; the individual observations are assumed to be Gaussian distributed.[13]

Example 11. Data from example 9 (p. 87) for the Wilcoxon signed rank test allows a determination of whether the last observation from Nuclide 2 data, subject 9, is

TABLE 4–6. *Thompson Criterion for Rejection of Single Outlier*

Table of Critical Values for T (One-sided Test) When Standard Deviation is Calculated from the Same Sample

Number of Observations n	5% Significance Level	2.5% Significance Level	1% Significance Level
3	1.15	1.15	1.15
4	1.46	1.48	1.49
5	1.67	1.71	1.75
6	1.82	1.89	1.94
7	1.94	2.02	2.10
8	2.03	2.13	2.22
9	2.11	2.21	2.32
10	2.18	2.29	2.41
11	2.23	2.36	2.48
12	2.29	2.41	2.55
13	2.33	2.46	2.61
14	2.37	2.51	2.66
15	2.41	2.55	2.71
16	2.44	2.59	2.75
17	2.47	2.62	2.79
18	2.50	2.65	2.82
19	2.53	2.68	2.85
20	2.56	2.71	2.88
21	2.58	2.73	2.91
22	2.60	2.76	2.94
23	2.62	2.78	2.96
24	2.64	2.80	2.99
25	2.66	2.82	3.01
30	2.75	2.91	
35	2.82	2.98	
40	2.87	3.04	
45	2.92	3.09	
50	2.96	3.13	
60	3.03	3.20	
70	3.09	3.26	
80	3.14	3.31	
90	3.18	3.35	
100	3.21	3.38	

From Grubbs, F.E.[13] With permission of Technometrics.

an outlier. For these data, $\bar{x}_2 = 9614$, s.d.$_2$ = 1901, and the largest observation, $x_{(9)}$ – 13846. The following is computed:

$$T_{(9)} = \frac{x_{(9)} - \bar{x}_2}{\text{s.d.}_2} = \frac{13846 - 9614}{1901} = 2.23$$

The tabled value for $P \leq 0.05$ for T with 9 observations is 2.11. A rejection of $x_{(9)}$ because T exceeds the tabled T value is therefore justified.

REFERENCES

1. Cramer, H.: Mathematical Methods of Statistics. Princeton, NJ, Princeton University Press, 1946.
2. Evans, R.D.: The Atomic Nucleus. New York, McGraw-Hill, 1955.
3. Jarett, A.A.: Statistical Methods used in the Measurement of Radioactivity with Some Useful Graphs and Nomographs. Oak Ridge National Laboratory Report AECU-232, June 1946.
4. McNemar, Q.: Note on the sampling error of the difference between correlated proportions or percentages. Psychometrica, *12*:153, 1947.
5. Siegel, S.: Nonparametric Statistics for the Behavioral Sciences. New York, McGraw-Hill, 1956.
6. Edwards, A.L.: Note on the correction for continuity in testing the significance of the difference between correlated proportions. Psychometrica, *13*:185, 1948.
7. Wilcoxon, F.: Individual comparisons by ranking methods. Biometrics Bulletin, *1*:80, 1945.
8. Wilcoxon, F., and Wilcox, R.A.: Some Rapid Approximate Statistical Procedures. Princeton, American Cyanamid Co., 1964.
9. Mann, H.B., and Whitney, D.R.: On a test of whether one of two random variables is stochastically larger than the other. Ann. Math. Statist., *18*:50, 1947.
10. Conover, W.J.: Practical Nonparametric Statistics. New York, John Wiley & Sons, 1971.
11. Brown, B.W., and Hollander, M.: Statistics, A Biomedical Introduction. New York, John Wiley & Sons, 1971.
12. Chauvenet, W.: A Manual of Spherical and Practical Astronomy. Vol. 2. Philadelphia, J.B. Lippincott, 1863. Appendix 558–566.
13. Grubbs, F.E.: Procedures for detecting outlying observations in samples. Technometrics, *11*:1, 1969.
14. Anscombe, F.J.: Rejection of outliers. Technometrics, *2*:123, 1960.
15. Pearson, E.S., and Chandra Sekar, C.: The efficiency of statistical tools and a criterion for the rejection of outlying observations. Biometrika, *XXVIII*:308, 1936.
16. Thompson, W.R.: On a criterion for the rejection of observations and the deviation to the sample standard deviation. Ann. Math. Statist., *6*:214, 1935.

Chapter 5

COMPARTMENTAL ANALYSIS

PAULO ROBERTO LEME

Living organisms exist fundamentally by a complex of interrelated dynamic processes. A continuous interchange of substances occurs between the organism and its environment, and numerous interdependent physicochemical phenomena are related to absorption, distribution, utilization, metabolism, and excretion of biologic substances. Of particular interest to the study of biologic compartments is a quantitative understanding of the temporal, spatial, and structural transitions that these substances undergo within the organism. These transitions are referred to as kinetics.

RADIOACTIVE TRACERS AND INDICATORS

Relatively little information can be obtained about the kinetics of a substance within the organism in its normal state of functioning. An acceptable means of studying kinetics in a biologic system is to introduce into the system a perturbation or stimulus and observe the response to this stimulus. Such a perturbation must be sufficiently gentle so as not to alter the behavior of the system, yet active enough to be measurable. Radioactive tracers provide an ideal means of accomplishing this end because:

1. They possess the same relevant physical, chemical, and biologic properties as the substance being traced.
2. They are easily measured, either in vivo or in vitro, by their emitted radiations.
3. They can be used in such small quantities that they do not alter the system into which they are introduced.

Small differences in biochemical behavior between a radioactive tracer and the nonradioactive substance can occur owing to the difference in mass numbers between the stable and the radioactive isotopes, which is called the *isotopic effect*. Such differences, however, are rarely significant.

A difference does exist between radioactive *tracers* and radioactive *indicators*. The former has the same chemical structure as the substance being studied. Examples are I-131, used to study the behavior of stable I-127, and Fe-59, used to trace Fe-56. A radioactive indicator has a different chemical structure from the substance traced, and it may or may not be an integral part of the biologic system. It has some biologically similar property, however, such as distribution space or metabolism. Typical examples of radioactive indicators are radiostrontium, used to study the kinetics of calcium, or radioiodinated albumin, used to study plasma protein metabolism. Radioactive indicators generally possess more significant kinetic differences than do tracers.

BIOLOGIC COMPARTMENTS

A substance within a living organism generally is manifested in various discrete states. Each state can be characterized by its *distribution* (in a body fluid, or within an organ parenchyma), by some *chemical form* (protein bound, free state, or by-product), or by a combination of the two (such as a substance bound to an enzyme in the circulation). Each discrete state is called a *biologic compartment.* The total of all of these discrete states is called the *pool* of the substance.

Within a compartment, all particles or elements of the substance are indistinguishable from one another. Particles can be transferred from one compartment to another by crossing some chemical or physical barrier, such as a membrane, or by chemical transformation. Within any compartment, all particles must have the same probability of transfer from one compartment to another.

Particles of a substance may combine with one another in the transformation to a second compartment. When particles of two states, A and B, couple to form a particle of a third state C, the process is called a *second-order transition* and can be represented mathematically by:

$$\frac{dC}{dt} = k{\cdot}A{\cdot}B \qquad (1)$$

where $\frac{dC}{dt}$ is the rate of transition and k is a proportionality constant. When a transition involves n different particles, the process is termed *nth order.* All enzymatic reactions are second-order processes or greater.

When the transition of a particle of state

A to state C does not require any other substance, the process is termed *linear,* or *first-order,* kinetics and may be defined by:

$$\frac{dC}{dt} = k{\cdot}A \qquad (2)$$

In this case, the rate of reaction is directly proportional to the quantity of particles present in state A.

If the rate of transition, or turnover rate, is independent of the number of particles present, the process is *zero order*:

$$\frac{dC}{dt} = k \qquad (3)$$

In a zero-order process, the mechanism of transition frequently is saturated, so that only a fixed number of particles can undergo this transition. A zero-order process is also linear. It can be proved that *the response of any system, even nonlinear (second order or greater), to a radioactive tracer is always linear or first order.*[1]

COMPARTMENTAL MODEL

A compartmental model that represents the biologic system and its kinetic behavior with regard to the substance being studied can usually be constructed. A model is composed of a finite number of compartments with defined probabilities of transition, or transfer of substances, between them. In Figure 5–1, the compartments are represented by numbered circles of the same size, neglecting the volumes and masses of distribution. Transitions are represented by arrows and can be *reversible,* as between compartments 1 and 2 and between 2 and 3, or *irreversible,* as between compartments 1 and 3, between compartments 3 and 4, and between compartment 1 and the external environment. The starred arrow indicates a compartment into which a radioactive tracer was introduced to study the system.

A compartmental model can be de-

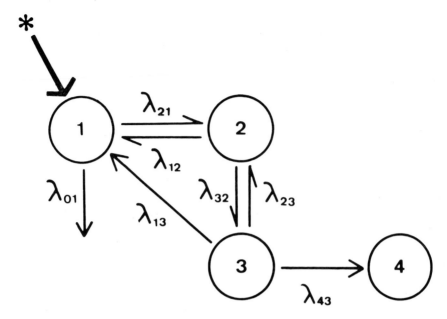

Fig. 5–1. Schematic representation of a compartmental model in which the compartments are represented by circles and transitions of the substance traced between compartments are represented by arrows. The starred arrow represents the introduction of a tracer.

scribed mathematically by a group of ordinary differential equations. Each equation describes the rate of variation of particles in a particular compartment as a function of time. In the example of Figure 5–1, the following system of differential equations appears:

$$\frac{df_1}{dt} = -\lambda_{01}f_1 - \lambda_{21}f_1 + \lambda_{12}f_2 + \lambda_{13}f_3 \qquad (4)$$

$$\frac{df_2}{dt} = \lambda_{21}f_1 - \lambda_{12}f_2 - \lambda_{32}f_2 + \lambda_{23}f_3 \qquad (5)$$

$$\frac{df_3}{dt} = \lambda_{32}f_2 - \lambda_{13}f_3 - \lambda_{23}f_3 - \lambda_{43}f_3 \qquad (6)$$

$$\frac{df_4}{dt} = \lambda_{43}f_3 \qquad (7)$$

where:

f_i (i = 1, 2, 3, ...) represents the quantity of tracer in compartment i as a function of time $f_i(t)$, usually

expressed as a fraction of the quantity of tracer introduced.

λ_{ij} is the fractional rate of transfer, which represents the fraction of tracer that is transferred to compartment i from compartment j in unit time and is expressed in units of $time^{-1}$.

λ_{oj} is the fractional rate of transfer outside the system.

Thus each product $\lambda_{ij}f_j$ represents the quantity of tracer being transferred from compartment j to compartment i at any time t. (Observe that f_j varies with time.)

This system of differential equations can be represented generically by:

$$\frac{df_i}{dt} = \lambda_{i1}f_1 + \lambda_{i2}f_2 + \ldots - \lambda_{1i}f_i \ldots$$
$$(i = 1, 2, \ldots n) \qquad (8)$$

A system is said to be in *dynamic equilibrium*, or in a *steady state*, when the quantity of substance traced in each compartment and the rates of transfer remain constant with time. A system in dynamic equilibrium is *open* when a substance is eliminated by the system, and this elimination is compensated exactly by introducing a substance from which it is synthesized. In this circumstance, the coefficients λ_{ij} are constant.

Such a system of equations, along with the initial conditions $f_i(0)$, i.e., the quantity of tracer in each compartment at time zero, defines the kinetic behavior of the radioactive tracer in the model. In the example of Figure 5–1, the initial conditions are $f_1(0) = 1$ and $f_2(0) = f_3(0) = f_4(0) = 0$, since at this instant, all of the tracer introduced is still in compartment 1.

The solution of this group of differential equations consists of finding a group of algebraic equations for $f_1(t)$, $f_2(t)$, ... $f_n(t)$ that define the quantity of tracer in each compartment as a function of time.

In the case of linear kinetics, the solution consists of a group of equations that are a sum of n exponential terms:

$$
\begin{aligned}
f_1 &= A_{11}e^{-\lambda_1 t} + A_{12}\,e^{-\lambda_2 t} + \ldots + A_{1n}\,e^{-\lambda_n t} \\
f_2 &= A_{21}\,e^{\lambda_1 t} + A_{22}\,e^{-\lambda_2 t} + \ldots + A_{2n}\,e^{-\lambda_n t} \quad (9) \\
f_n &= A_{n1}\,e^{+\lambda_1 t} + A_{n2}\,e^{-\lambda_2 t} + \ldots + A_{nn}\,e^{-\lambda_n t}
\end{aligned}
$$

These equations constitute a transient solution, which is to say that they refer to the radioactive tracer A. The solution of the dynamic equilibrium consists of determining the mass M_j of the substance traced as well as the turnover rates ρ_{ij} between the various compartments and between these compartments and the outside environment. The turnover rate ρ_{ij} is the mass of the substance traced that is transferred to compartment i from compartment j in unit time and is determined by the product of the mass transferred and the fractional coefficient of transfer:

$$\rho_{ij} = \lambda_{ij}M_j \quad (10)$$

In dealing with an open system, one must consider the mass of substance traced that enters the system in unit time from some external source, for example, the diet. This mass may be represented by U_i. Both ρ_{ij}

and U_i are expressed in units of mass per unit of time, e.g., mg/day.

From these considerations, the dynamic equilibrium of the example in Figure 5–1 may be defined by the following group of algebraic equations:

$$
\begin{aligned}
U_1 + \lambda_{12}M_2 + \lambda_{13}M_3 - \lambda_{21}M_1 - \lambda_{01}M_1 &= 0 \\
U_2 + \lambda_{21}M_1 + \lambda_{23}M_3 - \lambda_{12}M_2 - \lambda_{32}M_2 &= 0 \quad (11) \\
U_3 + \lambda_{32}M_2 - \lambda_{23}M_3 - \lambda_{13}M_3 - \lambda_{43}M_3 &= 0
\end{aligned}
$$

This system of equations can be generalized:

$$U_i + \lambda_{i1}M_1 + \lambda_{i2}M_2 + \ldots - \lambda_{1i}M_i - \ldots = 0 \quad (12)$$
$$(i = 1, 2, \ldots, n)$$

FORMULATION OF MODELS AND COMPARTMENTAL ANALYSIS

The process of model formation is the inverse of the preceding description. When experimental observations have been made, the next step is to determine the nature of the system responsible for these observations.

After the introduction of a radioactive tracer into the system, serial samples are taken from the greatest possible number of sources. A typical case might involve intravenously injecting a tracer, followed by taking samples of whole blood plasma, urine, and feces at varying times after introduction of the tracer. Both the radioactivity and the concentration of the substance traced are then determined. External measures of radioactivity over such relevant areas of the body as liver, kidneys, precordium, and even the total body may also be utilized.

The experimental data thus obtained can be expressed in various units. In general, it is preferable to express the radioactivity measured as *fraction of the dose injected per milligram of traced substance* (specific activity), as *fraction of the dose per milliliter of the sample taken* (radioactive concentration), or simply as *fraction of the dose* (activity).

From the experimental data, a family of

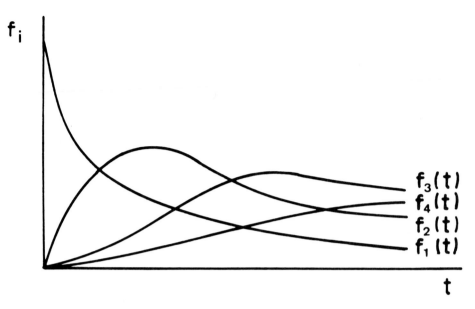

Fig. 5–2. Family of curves describing the evolution of tracer in each compartment. The curves constitute transient solutions to the system of differential equations $f_i(t)$.

curves can be constructed to reflect the evolution of the tracer as a function of time (Fig. 5–2). The process of model formulation then involves various steps: (1) postulating a model, (2) adjusting the parameters of the model to the experimental data, (3) testing the model, and (4) elaborating new experiments.

DETERMINING THE NUMBER OF COMPARTMENTS

Each of the experimental curves can be expressed mathematically by one or more exponentials, i.e., an algebraic sum of exponential terms such as those in equation (9). The first step in compartmental analysis is to determine the number of compartments of the model. It can be proven that with linear kinetics, *the number of compartments with reversible changes necessary to reproduce the experimental data is at least equal to the number of exponential terms of the experimental curves.*[2]

Analysis of the curves can be made graphically or with the use of a computer.

The graphic procedure can be illustrated by successive subtractions called *curve stripping,* or *peeling.* In Figure 5–3, the solid dots represent an experimental curve of the variation of a tracer in a compartment into which it was introduced, expressed in fractions of dose injected, and represented on a semilogarithmic scale. The final portion of the curve is linear. Because the scale is logarithmic, this portion can be represented by the exponential term $A_1 e^{-\lambda_1 t}$. When this linear portion is extrapolated to time zero, the value A_1 is found at the intercept of the ordinant axis, or 0.1. The fractional coefficient of transfer λ_1 can be determined from the slope of the extrapolated line and the relation:

$$\lambda_1 = \frac{\ln 2}{T_{1/2,1}} \qquad (13)$$

where $T_{1/2,1}$ is the half-time of the first exponential, i.e., the interval of time necessary for the value of the exponential to be reduced to half its initial value, or $A_1/2 = 0.05$. From the graph, this is found to be 5 days.

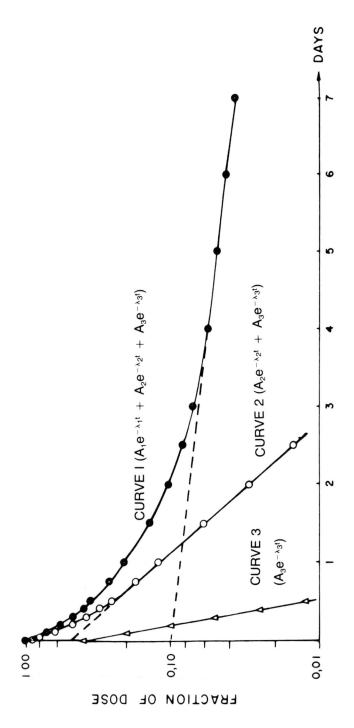

Fig. 5–3. Deconvolution of experimental curve 1 (Fig. 5–2) into three exponential terms by the method of successive subtractions.

Therefore:

$$\lambda_1 = \frac{0.693}{5.0} = 0.139 \text{ days}^{-1}$$

Then, from each point of experimental curve 1 is subtracted the corresponding value of the extrapolated line. These differences are plotted on the same graph to yield curve 2. If curve 2 is a straight line, the original curve would represent two exponential terms. In Figure 5–3, only the last part of curve 2 is linear. The process, therefore, is repeated and the extrapolation of curve 2 to zero time yields the second exponential term $A_2 e^{-\lambda_2 t}$. Analogous to what was done for the first exponential term, A_2 is found from the intercept and λ_2 from the relation $\lambda_2 = \dfrac{\ln 2}{T_{1/2,2}}$ and are 0.5 and 1.39 days^{-1} respectively.

The process is repeated to obtain curve 3, which in this case is a straight line. The values $A_3 = 0.4$ and $\lambda_3 = 6.93$ days^{-1} are found in a similar manner. Curve 1 of Figure 5–3 can now be expressed mathematically as the sum of three exponential terms:

$$f_t = 0.1 \, e^{-0.139t} + 0.5 \, e^{-1.39t}$$
$$+ \, 0.4 \, e^{-6.93t}$$

Thus the simplest model capable of accounting for the data in Figure 5–3 must contain at least three compartments of reversible changes.

Minimum numbers of compartments are spoken of because, in the initial stages of analysis, a model is in general a simplification of the system. This is due principally to the limitations of the available data and to the inherent fluctuations of the data. These limitations relate to the capacity of resolution for each group of data: rapid processes cannot be resolved and processes with close rates of variation cannot be distinguished. Thus in Figure 5–3, a process resulting in a fourth, rapid exponential could have occurred (e.g., with a $T_{1/2,4} = 0.001$ day^{-1}), so that at the time of the first sample (at $t = 0.1$ day), the process would have already reached equilibrium. Again, it could be that the first exponential term might in reality be a consequence of two processes whose $T_{1/2}$ do not differ by more than 10% and thus reflect only a single exponential. The fact that the experimental curves, which reflect the kinetics of the radioactive tracer, can be expressed in identical exponential terms as the solution of the system of differential equations that define the model attests to the adequacy of this type of model in representing the kinetics of the tracer. In determining the minimum number of compartments in the model, it is not necessary, although it may be desirable, to have more than one experimental curve.

DEFINING THE MODEL

Once the number of compartments has been determined, it is necessary to determine the number of parameters of the model or, in other words, to describe the model properly. The most general model with three compartments, compatible with the data in Figure 5–3, is represented by Figure 5–4A, although models B and C also satisfy these data. Only more information about the system can orient the selection of a particular model. Such information might come from experimental data from other compartments, from the elimination of the tracer from the system, or from certain physiologic or biochemical restrictions known about the system that provide more structure to the model.

In the absence of sufficient information about the selection, a model with the least number of interconnections or transitions can be chosen. A series (catenary) or a parallel (mamillary) model is usually preferred (Fig. 5–4B and 5–4C). Afterwards, an arbitrary choice must be made.

The general criterion used in formulating a model is simplicity: always start with the simplest model compatible with the data while observing the physiologic, bio-

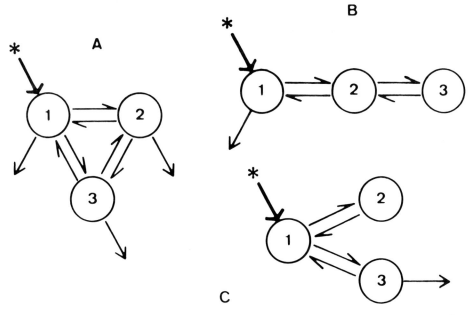

Fig. 5–4. Three 3-compartment models compatible with the data of Fig. 5–3. *A.* The most general model. *B.* Series or catenary model. *C.* Parallel or mamillary model.

chemical, and physicochemical restrictions known about the system. At a later stage, additional experiments are undertaken to test the model further; changes in the model are made as new information necessitates a change in the original concept.

DETERMINING THE PARAMETER VALUES

Once the model has been chosen, the next step is to determine the *values of the parameters* that will reproduce the experimental data. There are two general methods of solution: the *deterministic* (algebraic or analytic) process and the *stochastic* (or probabilistic) process.

Deterministic Process

In this process, the coefficients ij are determined from their mathematical relations with the coefficients of the exponential terms A_{ij} and λ_j. Such relations are obtained with the solution of the system of differential equations that characterize the model.

To illustrate this process, consider the compartmental model proposed for tri-iodothyronine (T_3) kinetics in humans.[3,4] After the intravenous injection of 120 μCi of T_3 labeled with I-125, the plasma concentration curve $C_1(t)$, expressed as fraction of administered dose per liter, can be represented mathematically by:

$$C_1(t) = 0.080\ e^{-10.2t}$$
$$+\ 0.020\ e^{-0.57t} \quad (14)$$

where t is expressed in days.

The distribution volume V_1 of the compartment into which the tracer is introduced can be determined by the relation:

$$C_1(0) = \frac{f_1(0)}{V_1} \quad (15)$$

where $C_1(0)$ is the concentration at zero time and $f_1(0)$ is the quantity of tracer at that time, expressed as fraction of administered dose and therefore equal to 1.

Making t = 0 in equation (14) and substituting in equation (15) produces:

$$V_1 = \frac{1}{0.10} = 10.0 \text{ liters}$$

The fact that V_1 is greater than the plasma volume indicates that the T_3 is distributed outside the vascular space.

The two exponential terms of $C_1(t)$ justify the two-compartment model shown in Figure 5–5. The differential equations that describe the tracer kinetics in the model are:

$$\frac{df_1}{dt} = -(\lambda_{01} + \lambda_{21})f_1 + \lambda_{12}f_2 \quad (16)$$

$$\frac{df_2}{dt} = \lambda_{21}f_1 - \lambda_{12}f_2 \quad (17)$$

$$\frac{df_0}{dt} = \lambda_{01}f_1 \quad (18)$$

where equation (18) describes the cumulative loss of tracer from the system. The solution of this group of differential equations yields:

$$f_1(t) = A_{11} e^{-\lambda_2 t} + A_{12} e^{-\lambda_2 t} \quad (19)$$

$$f_2(t) = A_{21} e^{-\lambda_1 t} + A_{22} e^{-\lambda_2 t} \quad (20)$$

The value for $f_1(t)$ can be obtained from equation (14) multiplied by the distribu-

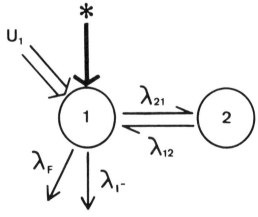

Fig. 5–5. Two-compartment model used to describe T_3 kinetics. Compartment 1 is the plasma space and compartment 2 the intracellular space. U_1 is the rate of T_3 synthesis; λ_{I^-} and λ_F represent deiodination and fecal loss respectively. (From Koutras, D.A., et al.[3])

tion volume V_1 from equation (15), which yields:

$$f_1(t) = 0.80\ e^{-10.2t} + 0.20\ e^{-0.57t} \quad (21)$$

In the process of solving equations (16), (17), and (18), the following relationships between the various values for λ_{ij}, which are to be determined, and the terms A_{ij} and λ_j arise:

$$\lambda_{01} = \frac{1}{\dfrac{A_{11}}{\lambda_1} + \dfrac{A_{12}}{\lambda_2}} \quad (22)$$

$$\lambda_{21} = A_{11}\lambda_1 + A_{12}\lambda_2 - \lambda_{01} \quad (23)$$

$$\lambda_{12} = A_{12}\lambda_1 + A_{11}\lambda_2 \quad (24)$$

From the preceding equations, the following values of the parameters are obtained: $\lambda_{01} = 2.33$ days^{-1}; $\lambda_{21} = 5.94$ days^{-1}; and $\lambda_{12} = 2.50$ days^{-1}.

A determination of free radioiodine in the plasma provides a value of 95.5%, which permits the parameter λ_{01} to be separated into two parts, λ_{I^-} and λ_f, representing deiodination of the T_3 and fecal loss respectively. They are expressed numerically as follows:

$$\lambda_{I^-} = 0.955 \times 2.33 = 2.23\ \text{days}^{-1}$$

$$\lambda_F = 0.10\ \text{day}^{-1}$$

A measure of the plasma T_3 concentration permits the determination of mass M_1 by the relation:

$$C_1 = \frac{M_1}{V_1} \quad (25)$$

In the example, $C_1 = 1.0\ \mu g/l$. Therefore $M_1 = 10.0\ \mu g$. M_2 can be determined by the conditions of the dynamic equilibrium:

$$U_I + \lambda_{12}M_2 - \lambda_{21}M_1 - \lambda_{01}M_1 = 0 \quad (26)$$

$$\lambda_{21}M_1 - \lambda_{12}M_2 = 0 \quad (27)$$

Equation (27) yields $M_2 = 23.8\ \mu g$ and equation (26) yields $U_1 = 23.2\ \mu g/day$

where U_1 represents the rate of T_3 synthesis by the thyroid.

The turnover rates of T_3 determined by the product $\lambda_{ij}M_j$ are expressed in g/day: $\rho_{21} = \rho_{12} = 59.4$; $\rho_I^- = 22.3$; and $\rho_F = 1.0$.

The volume V_2 is determined in terms of *plasma equivalent space,* defined as the hypothetical volume that the substance traced would occupy if it were distributed with a uniform concentration equal to that in the plasma.[5] This is expressed mathematically as:

$$\frac{M_1}{V_1} = \frac{M_2}{V_2} \qquad (28)$$

Therefore $V_2 = 23.8$ liters. Such a large space suggests a high intracellular concentration of T_3.

This type of analysis, while interesting, suffers several limitations:

1. It requires an understanding of relatively complex mathematical operations for the solution of the differential equations.
2. Small alterations in the formulated model may require repeating all calculations.
3. Small imprecisions in the values of the constants of the exponential terms are amplified in the intermediate calculations, which results in large errors in the derived parameters.
4. A statistical treatment of the data becomes impractical.

Stochastic Process: Using the Analog Computer

This method consists of gradually adjusting by trial and error the values of the model parameters until they reproduce the experimental data. Because it is a time-consuming process, it requires the aid of a digital or analog computer.

Functionally, an analog computer is an electronic system used to simulate a real system. Its name derives from the *analogy* between the variables of a real system, such as biologic compartment, and the elements of an electronic circuitry. For example, the quantities of tracer in various biologic compartments may be represented by voltages that are proportional to them. This analogy results from the fact that the differential equations that describe the evolution of a tracer as a function of time are identical to the differential equations that describe variations of voltage as a function of time.

In the example of the two-compartment model of Figure 5–5, equations (16), (17), and (18) can be simulated by the circuit shown in Figure 5–6. Voltages representing the terms that form $\dfrac{df_1}{dt}$, $\dfrac{df_2}{dt}$, and $\dfrac{df_0}{dt}$ are introduced into amplifier integrators represented by the symbol $-\!\!\rhd\!-$; the impulses leaving these amplifiers then represent $-f_1$, $-f_2$ and $-f_0$. (The signal is inverted when passing through an amplifier.) To

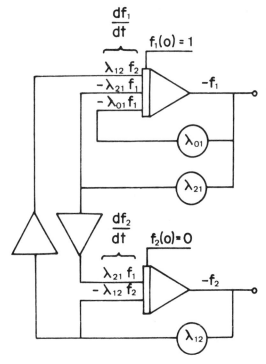

Fig. 5–6. Analog computer program to resolve differential equations (16) and (17) relative to the model of T_3 in Fig. 5–5.

multiply f_1 and f_2 by the corresponding constants λ_{ij}, potentiometers represented by the symbol $-\bigcirc-$ are used. The symbol $-\triangleright-$ represents amplifiers whose function is only to invert the signal. The initial values of f_1, f_2, and f_0 at zero time are introduced into the amplifiers. Scale factors are utilized to avoid very high or very low voltages. The output from the integrators is maintained at the initial values $f_1(0)$ and $f_2(0)$ until a key operation is called up, after which the output varies with time according to equations (16), (17), and (18).

The solutions to the differential equations, i.e., the curves $f_1(t)$, $f_2(t)$, and $f_0(t)$, can be traced on paper with an X-Y plotter or can be observed on an oscilloscope screen. These curves are then compared with the experimental curves, and the values of the potentiometers representing the various values of λ_{ij} are varied until the desired fit is obtained.

Analog computers are particularly valuable, as they permit adjustments in a relatively short time and are inexpensive to operate. On the other hand, their precision leaves something to be desired, and they do not permit statistical treatments. The values of the parameters λ_{ij} obtained with an analog computer provide excellent initial estimates for subsequent analysis by a digital computer.

Stochastic Process: Using the Digital Computer

Because of their great versatility, operational capacity, rapid calculations, and precise results, digital computers are practically indispensable in model development and in compartmental analysis. Over a period of several years, Berman, Shahn, and Weiss developed an integrated methodology of general use, which was programmed for digital computers in a way that allowed the researcher to use it without understanding the sophisticated machinery or the complex mathematics.[6,7] The program, called SAAM (Simulation, Analysis And Modeling), has been contin-

ually improved, the final version being SAAM 25.[8]

The data entered into the SAAM program are the experimental measurements and their corresponding times. The measurement error, i.e., the standard deviation or coefficient of variation, must also be entered for each point. To each group of data corresponding to measurements q_i from the same locale—plasma, red cells, feces, urine, external counts, etc.—is designated a component i (i = 1,,2,3, . . .).

Once the group of data is entered, a numerical solution to the system of differential equations that define the model is calculated, and the calculated and observed values are compared. This phase is known as *simulation.* The initial estimates of the system parameters are then adjusted by an iterative process until a least squares fit of the observed values q_i is obtained. The final results include values of the adjusted parameters with their respective standard deviations; a solution of the dynamic equilibrium, i.e., M_i and ρ_{ij}; a list of all the values $q_i(t)$, both experimental and calculated; and a graph of these values on either a linear or logarithmic scale.

Programs like the SAAM are useful because:

1. They do not require a detailed understanding of the mathematics.
2. Alterations in the model formulated are easily executed.
3. They do not require intermediate manipulations of the data.
4. They permit statistical treatment sufficiently elaborate to provide for each parameter of the model, as well as for each calculated data point and estimated statistical error.

One disadvantage of this method is the difficulty (which decreases with practice) of providing initial estimates of the parameter values. It is worth pointing out, however, that the SAAM program permits analysis of models in which the parameters λ_{ij} vary with time, resolves nonlinear differential equations, permits the adjustment of linear combinations of exponentials, performs spectral analysis, and has many other useful functions. Perhaps one of the most powerful characteristics of the program is the possibility of analyzing the kinetics of substances when perturbations are introduced into the system, such as a drug that alters the kinetics of the substance studied.

TESTING THE MODEL

Finally, it is necessary to judge whether the adjusted model chosen is consistent and unique. When systematic deviations between the calculated and observed values occur (which can easily be verified by visual inspection of the resulting curves), the model is considered inconsistent and requires modification. Such deviations may occur when the model lacks sufficient freedom to adjust the data. In this case, inconsistencies can be reduced by increasing the degree of freedom, whether by the modification of fixed parameter values to adjustable values or by the addition of new parameters.

When systematic deviations do not occur but large standard deviations in the calculated parameter values are observed, the model is not unique, and is badly chosen. This situation may occur when the quantity of information contained in the experimental data is inadequate to define the model chosen. Often additional physiologic or biochemical information about the system can orient the choice of a more appropriate model. When the parameter values can be determined with reasonable precision, the model is considered consistent, unique, and acceptable.

CONCLUSION

Compartmental models are valuable instruments in the study of unknown systems. They represent formally the investigator's conceptualization of a system at the experimental level. A model is rarely equal to the actual system. In the process of evolution of a model, the first of the series is generally an oversimplification of the system; however, as the number of experiments increase and the models are successively modified, the discrepancies between the model and the system disappear.

Besides the extensive investigations on iodine metabolism, recent years have seen an intensive application of compartmental models in the kinetics of such substances as calcium,[9,10,11,12] iodine,[4,13] magnesium,[14,15] sodium and potassium,[16,17] citrate,[18] albumin,[19] triglycerides and fatty acids,[20,21,22] glucose,[23,24,25,26] insulin,[27,28] aldosterone,[29,30] collagen,[31] rose bengal,[32] and methotrexate.[33]

REFERENCES

1. Berman, M., et al.: The application of multicompartmental analysis to problems of clinical medicine. Ann. Intern. Med., *68*:423, 1968.
2. Berman, M., and Schoenfeld, R.: Invariants in experimental data on linear kinetics and the formulation of models. J. Appl. Physiol., *27*:1361, 1956.
3. Koutras, D.A., et al.: Endemic goiter in Greece: thyroid hormone kinetics. J. Clin. Endocrinol. Metab., *30*:479, 1970.
4. Berman, M.: Iodine kinetics. *In* Methods of Investigative and Diagnostic Endocrinology. Edited by J.E. Rall and I.J. Kopin. Amsterdam, North-Holland, 1972.
5. Brownell, G., Berman, M., and Robertson, J.: Nomenclature for tracer kinetics. Int. J. Appl. Radiat. Isot., *19*:249, 1968.
6. Berman, M., Shahn, E., and Weiss, M.F.: The routine fitting of kinetic data to models: a mathematical formalism for digital computers. Biophys. J., *2*:275, 1962.
7. Berman, M.: Compartmental analysis in kinetics. *In* Computers in Biomedical Research. Vol. 2. Edited by R. Stagey and B. Waxman. New York, Academic Press, 1965.
8. Berman, M., and Weiss, M.F.: SAAM Manual. U.S. Public Health Service Publication No. 1703. Washington, D.C., U.S. Government Printing Office, 1967.
9. Neer, R., et al.: Multicompartmental analysis of calcium kinetics in normal adult males. J. Clin. Invest., *46*:1364, 1967.
10. Birge, S.J., et al.: Study of calcium absorption in man: a kinetic analysis and physiologic model. J. Clin. Invest., *48*:1705, 1969.
11. Phang, J.M., et al.: Dietary perturbation of cal-

cium metabolism in man: compartmental analysis. J. Clin. Invest., 48:67, 1969.

12. Ramberg, C.F., Jr., et al.: Calcium kinetics in cows during late pregnancy, parturition and early lactation. Am. J. Physiol., 219:1166, 1970.

13. Ermans, A., et al.: Metabolism of intrathyroidal iodine in normal men. J. Clin. Endocrinol. Metab., 28:169, 1968.

14. Avioli, L.V., and Berman, M.: Mg^{28} kinetics in man. J. Appl. Physiol., 21:1688, 1966.

15. Avioli, L.V., and Berman, M.: Role of magnesium metabolism and the effects of fluoride therapy in Paget's disease of bone. J. Clin. Endocrinol. Metab., 28:700, 1968.

16. Burg, M.B., Grollman, E.F., and Orloff, J.: Sodium and potassium flux of separated renal tubules. Am. J. Physiol., 206:483, 1964.

17. Chandler, W.K., and Maves, H.: Sodium and potassium currents in squid axons perfused with fluoride solutions. J. Physiol., 211:623, 1970.

18. Tashjian, A.H., and Whedon, G.D.: Kinetics of human citrate metabolism: studies in normal subjects and in patients with bone disease. J. Clin. Endocrinol. Metab, 23:1029, 1963.

19. Gill, J.R., Jr., Waldmann, T.A., and Bartter, F.C.: Idiopathic edema. I. The occurrence of hypoalbuminemia and abnormal metabolism in women with unexplained edema. Am. J. Med., 52:444, 1972.

20. Eaton, R.P., Berman, M., and Steinberg, D.: Kinetic studies of plasma free fatty acid and triglyceride metabolism in man. J. Clin. Invest., 48:1560, 1969.

21. Shames, D.M., et al.: Transport of plasma free fatty acids and triglycerides in man: theoretical analysis. J. Clin. Invest., 49:2298, 1970.

22. Quarfordt, S.H., et al.: Very low density lipoprotein triglyceride transport in type IV hyperlipoproteinemia and the effects of carbohydraterich diets. J. Clin. Invest., 49:2289, 1970.

23. Segal, S., Berman, M., and Blair, A.: The metabolism of variously C^{14} labeled glucose in man and an estimation of the extent of glucose metabolism by the hexose monophosphate pathway. J. Clin. Invest., 40:1263, 1961.

24. Atkinson, A.J., Jr., and Weiss, M.F.: Kinetics of blood-cerebrospinal fluid glucose transfer in the normal dog. Am. J. Physiol., 216:1120, 1969.

25. Kronfeld, D.S., Ramberg, C.F., Jr., and Shames, D.M.: Multicompartmental analysis of glucose kinetics in normal and hypoglycemic cows. Am. J. Physiol., 220:886, 1971.

26. Shames, D.M., Berman, M., and Segal, S.: Effects of thyroid disease on glucose oxidative metabolism in man. A compartmental model analysis. J. Clin. Invest., 50:627, 1971.

27. Sherwin, R.S., et al.: A model of the kinetics of insulin in man. J. Clin. Invest., 53:1481, 1974.

28. Insel, P.A., et al.: Modeling the insulin-glucose system in man. Fed. Proc., 33:1865, 1974.

29. Ayers, C., et al.: The effect of chronic hepatic venous congestion on the metabolism of D,L-aldosterone and D-aldosterone. J. Clin. Invest., 41:884, 1962.

30. Davis, J.O., et al.: Metabolism of aldosterone in several experimental situations with altered aldosterone secretion. J. Clin. Invest., 44:1433, 1965.

31. Phang, J.M., et al.: Compartmental analysis of collagen synthesis in fetal rat calvaria. I. Perturbations of proline transport. Biochem. Biophys. Acta, 230:146, 1971.

32. Turco, G.L., et al.: The kinetics of I^{131} rose bengal in normal and cirrhotic subjects studied by compartmental analysis and a digital computer. J. Lab. Clin. Med., 67:983, 1966.

33. Leme, P.R., et al.: Kinetic model for the disposition and metabolism of moderate and high-dose methotrexate (NSC-740) in man. Cancer Chemother. Rep., 59:811, 1975.

Chapter 6

IMAGING SYSTEMS

Jon Erickson

A large part of the practice of nuclear medicine is the production of images that display the distribution of a radioactively labeled pharmaceutical. This chapter examines the various methods and equipment used to produce these diagnostic images. Although the rectilinear scanner is becoming rare in the practice of nuclear medicine, it is included in this chapter because of its importance in the development of imaging techniques. Detailed discussions of collimation and modulation transfer function are presented in the section "Scintillation Cameras."

RECTILINEAR SCANNERS

Practical radionuclide imaging in humans began in 1951 with Benedict Cassen's development of an automatic scanning device. This instrument was fitted with a collimated calcium tungstate crystal capable of graphically registering radionuclide distributions within body organs. In fact, the first commercial systems contained calcium tungstate crystals and single-bore collimators similar to those of Cassen's original instrument. Because of the small bore of the collimator, a reasonable resolution was achieved for small organs. This device presented few obstacles

since the only organ then scanned was the thyroid.

With the development of NaI(Tl) crystals, much larger detector sizes were possible. To take advantage of the greater area exposed to the photon flux, Newell constructed a collimator with multiple holes, all converging to a *focal point* in space (Fig. 6–1).[2] There is a plane at the focal point for which the system has the greatest resolution; objects above and below this plane are less resolved. The resulting image therefore is likened to an x-ray tomograph. The collimated detector, which contains a NaI(Tl) crystal usually 3, 5, or 8 in. in diameter and 2 in. thick, sweeps back and forth over the organ distribution in an X-Y raster. The detector is connected to a recorder system through either a rigid mechanical arm or electronic encoding devices. The recorder registers the activity detected in some appropriate display format. The image may be a 1:1 representation or a reduction by a predetermined minification factor.

Collimators

The fundamental purpose of the collimator is to exclude all photons arising from the radioactive source except those within the field of interest.

Collimators are of many types. Selection

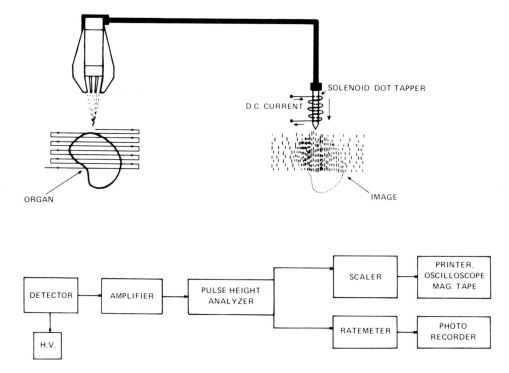

Fig. 6–1. Rectilinear scanner fitted with a focused collimator and solenoid dot tapper to register the image on paper.

of a collimator depends upon (1) the energy of the photons emitted by the isotope being scanned, (2) the resolution required (and therefore the organ imaged), (3) the sensitivity required for adequate count density, and (4) the depth below the collimator face to be scanned.

Collimators generally are made of lead, which is inexpensive and easy to mill and mold. They are described according to their number of holes: single bore or multihole; their relative sensitivity: fine, medium, and coarse; their relative resolution: high, medium, and low; the energy for which they are intended: high, medium, and low; and their depth of focus: usually between 3 in. and 5 in. Collimator holes may be round, hexagonal (*honeycomb*), or quadrilateral. Hexagonal holes generally have the best characteristics because of the uniform septal thickness between them and their optimum arrangement for a circular crystal. The thickness of the septa

depends upon the energy of the gamma ray to be collimated. Very thin septa are possible with low-energy nuclides such as I-125, Hg-197, and Tc-99m. The angle that the septal walls make with the crystal face largely determines the focal length.

The number and length of holes and thickness of the septa determine the collimator's sensitivity and resolution. Figure 6–2 shows three types of collimators with varying sensitivities and resolution. The single-hole collimator in Fig. 6–2a (also called a *straight bore collimator)* has high sensitivity but low resolution because the field of view is broad. The collimator in Figure 6–2b has higher resolution but low sensitivity. The focused, multichannel collimator in Figure 6–2c is a reasonable compromise between sensitivity and resolution.

Resolution is the power of the system to differentiate two points on a plane. Probably the most common method of com-

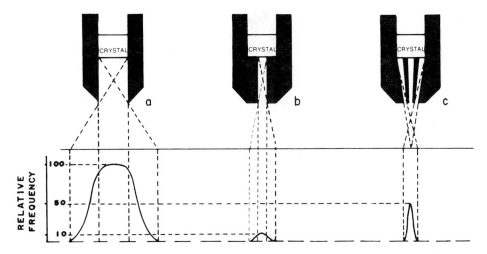

Fig. 6–2. Three collimators with different resolution and sensitivities. Collimator *a* has high sensitivity but low resolution. Collimator *b* has high resolution but low sensitivity. Collimator *c* has high resolution and intermediate sensitivity.

paring collimators in a clinical setting is to fill a phantom that has known variations of structure with a solution of the radionuclide to be used, scan it with two collimators, and visually compare the results. This means of evaluation, however, is quite subjective and may fail to distinguish small differences in collimator performance.

Another simple means of evaluating resolution is to plot the isoresponse curves in air by constructing a paper plane parallel to and bisecting the collimator holes. A point source is then placed at the focal point, where the highest counting rate is recorded. The small area around which this peak activity does not vary is the 100% isoresponse curve (Fig. 6–3). A family of curves is then drawn for decreasing percentages of the peak activity.[3] One estimate of the collimator resolving power is given by the distance in centimeters between the focal point and the 50% isoresponse curve, perpendicular to the collimator axis. The smaller this distance, the higher the collimator resolution. The collimator sensitivity may be judged by the counts/min/µCi measured from a point source at the focal point.

Not only is this method laborious, but it is difficult to find the exact plane bisecting the collimator. For many years, collimator resolution was expressed in terms of its response to scanning a point source at the collimator focal distance (Fig. 6–4). The full width of this response curve at half its maximum height (FWHM) is approximately the separation at which two point sources may be distinguished. Scanning the point source at only the focal distance, however, does not fully describe the collimator response. For example, the FWHM as a single value does not fully define the collimator response to the two isotopes shown in Figure 6–4. The flaring of the tails of the I-131 curve is due primarily to septal penetration by the higher-energy I-131 gamma rays.

A more rigorous method of determining resolution is by scanning a line source, wherein the difficulty of precisely aligning the collimator and the point source is avoided. By passing a line source across the collimator's field of view at different distances Z from the collimator, a series of *line spread functions* is generated (Fig. 6–5). The curve at the focal distance is identical to the *point spread function*

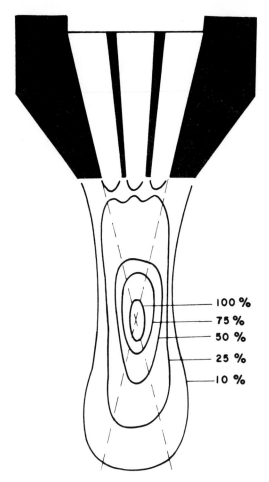

Fig. 6–3. Isoresponse curves of a focused collimator.

shown in Figure 6–4. The resolution at various distances from the collimator is thus defined.

Scanner Adjustments

The signal coming from the detector is much like that of any other scintillation detector and must be processed before being displayed. Several factors have important effects on the outcome of the final image.

Pulse-Height Analyzer

The purpose of the pulse-height analyzer is to exclude scattered radiation, which degrades the image, and to exclude higher-energy photons in the cases of dual tracer studies or radionuclides with multiple gamma emissions. The analyzer is adjusted so that the window encloses the photopeak of interest. The appropriate settings for each radionuclide must be determined for each instrument by plotting the pulse-height spectrum. In scanners equipped with multichannel analyzers, this procedure is easy. With single- or dual-channel analyzers, the procedure described in Chapter 2 must be performed. With such higher-energy radionuclides as I-131 and In-113m, a symmetric window 15 to 20% of the photopeak energy in width is usually employed. For lower-energy radionuclides, an asymmetric window usually is preferred to reduce the contribution of photons scattered through small angles, since lower-energy gamma photons lose less energy in scattering than do higher-energy gamma photons. With this technique, the lower discriminator is set closer to the photopeak.

The use of two or more spectrometers is of value in scanning In-111, Ga-67, Se-75, and Yb-169, which have more than one photopeak. Better resolution and image contrast are obtained by eliminating scattered photons between the peaks.

Speed and Line Spacing

Scanner speed is determined by a control that governs the *motor speed,* or the rate with which the detector passes over the organ. *Line spacing* is the distance indexed in the y direction after each scan pass. Both of these factors determine the *information density* in the image. They are related by:

$$\text{Information density} = \frac{\text{counts}}{\text{area}}$$

$$= \frac{\text{maximum count rate}}{\text{scan speed} \times \text{line spacing}}$$

Schultz et al. have suggested that 1000 to 1500 counts/cm² are required for the detection of "cold" lesions.[4] Hot lesions require somewhat lesser densities.

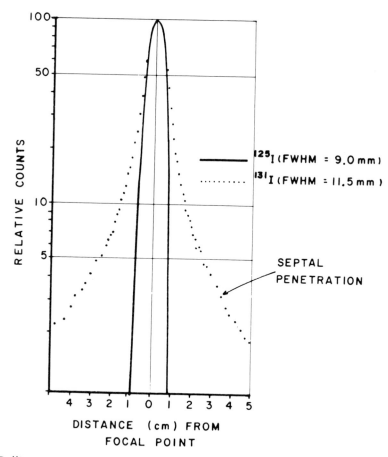

Fig. 6–4. Collimator response characteristics (point spread functions) for two photon energies as a function of the distance of the point source from the focal point in the focal plane.

The line spacing must also be matched to the recording parameters. For optimum appearance, rows of dots must not have large spaces between them. For both dot scans and photoscans, the bottom of the dot should just touch the top of the dots below. A smoother image often can be obtained by overlapping the lines (half-spacing), although this practice increases scanning time and generally does not increase lesion detectability.

In photorecorders, the light pipe determines dot size. For high-density scans, such as thyroid scans, a small-aperture light pipe is used. This light pipe requires narrower line spacing, usually 0.2 cm. Larger light pipes are used for brain and liver scans so that wider line spacing, 0.35 cm to 0.40 cm, can be achieved.

Time Constant

The *time constant* determines the ratemeter response and is essentially a smoothing device. Once the information has been received, this device largely determines how fast it is displayed on either the dot scan or the photoscan. A ratemeter has an exponential buildup and decay. Therefore, it imposes a delay between the time of photon detection and the time of imaging recording. To be effective, the time constant must be matched to the scanner speed and the rate of information received. If the time constant is too long, the slow ratemeter decay "drags" information from areas of high counting rate into areas of lower counting rate, which produces a *scalloping* effect at the image

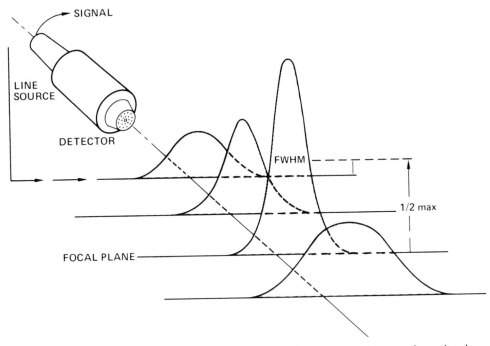

Fig. 6–5. Collimator response to a line source scanned at various distances from the detector. These curves define the line spread functions.

margins that obscures small variations in the radionuclide distribution. If the time constant is too short, a mottled scan appearance results. In general, shorter time constants are used for high counting rates, and longer time constants for low counting rates.

Digital ratemeters also may be used with rectilinear scanners. These buffered scalers accept and store pulses as the detector moves over the organ. At the end of a preset scanning distance, they generate a pulse equal to the counts stored. The photorecord thus produces a dot of intensity proportional to the counts detected in that distance. The ratemeter then is reset and begins again.

Image Display

A variety of image display modes are possible with all scanning devices. The paper dot display is the oldest (Fig. 6–1). Three formats of paper records are encountered. The dot tapper uses a solenoid-powered tapper to make a black mark on plain paper. Teledeltos paper is heat sensitive and blackens when the hot stylus is applied. Color scans combine the tapper arrangement with a multicolor ribbon. The ribbon color is controlled by the ratemeter through a *range differential,* so that both color and dot density indicate the range of activity.

In general, two settings control the dot record. The *dot factor* is a buffering function that determines how many impulses must be received before a dot is recorded. This function is controlled by a selector designated 2, 4, 8, 16, 32, and 64. The dot factor is determined by the maximum counting rate:

$$\text{Dot factor} = \frac{\text{maximum counts/min}}{\text{scan speed} \times 10}$$

If the dot factor is set too low, the solenoid will jam at high counting rates. Also, there will be loss of contrast resolution in the higher counting rate regions because of the limited intensity range of the dot tapper paper display. If the dot factor is too high, valuable detail will be lost over areas of lower counting rates.

Usually, *a background erase* adjustment (also called *background suppression* or *background cutoff)* is available. With this rate-limiting function, counting rates below a preselected minimum are not recorded (Fig. 6–6). This feature is useful in increasing *contrast,* especially where blood background is high.[6] Injudicious use of this setting, however, also results in loss of detail or in distortion of the true image size.

Photoscans

In photorecording, a light source replaces the tapper, and photographic film replaces the paper. The major advantage is that film density (gray scale) combines with dot density to produce an added range of information density difference. The light source may be a small incandescent bulb or a photocathode tube. With both, the light intensity is varied in proportion to counting rate either by modulating the light output or by varying the duration of exposure.

Incandescent bulbs use a focusing lens to project the point of the filament onto the film. A shaped aperture may be used to produce square or round dots on the film. Some clinicians prefer to use a Gaussian light spot of varying size by defocusing the filament image slightly to give a dark center with a lighter penumbra. This action smooths the image and reduces the appearance of the dot mosaic.

Contrast enhancement in photorecording operates analogously to the range differential in color dot scans. When enhancement is increased, the slope of optical density is increased with increasing counting rates (see "Contrast," Chap. 23). Background cutoff operates in the same way as the dot record. As with dot records, care must always be taken to avoid losing information in the modification process.

The *density* of the photorecording is usually controlled by the power to the light source. This adjustment must be determined for each type of film used and also must be adjusted according to the information density and scanner speed. In many scanners, this adjustment is set automatically as a function of other controls, but a manual adjustment always exists as well. The problems of underexposure and overexposure are universal in photo-

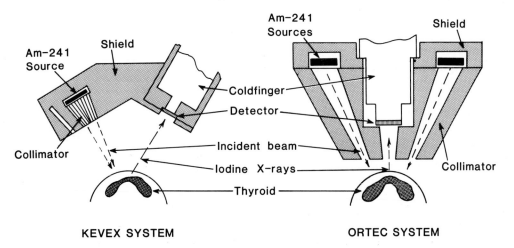

KEVEX SYSTEM   **ORTEC SYSTEM**

Fig. 6–6. Two source-detector configurations for fluorescent scanning of the stable iodine content of the thyroid. (Adapted from Patton, J.A.[5])

graphic processes; they always cause a loss of detail.

Variable Persistence Oscilloscope

On most modern rectilinear scanners, persistence oscilloscopes provide the technician with a continuously developing visible record of the scan's progress. As the scan proceeds, the electron beam in the oscilloscope is positioned by controls on the scanning mechanism. The beam is turned on and off as the detector system encounters activity in its field of view. Special construction of the cathode-ray tube (CRT) allows the images to remain displayed until intentionally erased by the operator. This corresponds to the use of the persistence oscilloscope on scintillation cameras. This device is enormously useful in determining whether the proper scanning limits have been set, the proper area is being scanned, or the patient has moved; it eliminates having to wait until the scan has been completed and the "hard copy" film developed.

Fluorescent Scanning

A form of rectilinear scanning that does not involve the injection of radioactive material has been implemented in a few locations.[5] Fluorescent scanning makes use of the fact that atoms, when irradiated by X-rays or gamma rays of the appropriate energy, in turn emit radiation characteristic of the irradiated isotope. The most commonly imaged element in fluorescent scanning is iodine. If iodine is irradiated by photons greater than 33.2 keV, there is a finite probability that a K-shell electron will be removed from the atom by photoelectric absorption. When this takes place, the vacancy is filled promptly by an electron from the L shell. Excess energy is carried off by either an Auger electron or a characteristic x-ray. For iodine, the K-characteristic x-ray energy is 28.5 keV. From a physical standpoint, the most efficient energy for production of the characteristic x-ray is only slightly greater than the 33.2-keV ionization energy of the K-shell electron. Radiation of this low energy, however, would be attenuated severely by the tissue before reaching the iodine. Higher-energy radiation is less efficient but provides greater penetration and hence a reduced dose of radiation. Two types of radiation sources have been used: Americium-241 (half-life 450 years, 60-keV gamma rays) and specially filtered x-ray tubes.[7]

Fluorescent scanning is used primarily in imaging the stable iodine content of the thyroid. This method was first developed by Hoffer.[8] Two systems are currently available for fluorescent thyroid scanning. Both use the Am-241 sources for excitation and are available as adaptations to standard rectilinear scanners (see Fig. 6–6). The Kevex system uses a single Am-241 source mounted to the side of the lithium-drifted silicon (Si(Li)) solid-state detector. The Ortec system, on the other hand, uses a series of Am-241 sources mounted concentrically around the detector. In both systems, the sources are collimated to localize the irradiation to the area being viewed by the detector and to minimize the amount of scattered photons. Source strengths of 10 to 20 Ci of Am-241 are used in these systems.

Compared to conventional imaging procedures, fluorescent scanning provides several benefits: (1) No substance, whether stable or radioactive, needs to be injected into the patient. (2) The radiation dose of 15 to 60 mrads to the thyroid, which is limited to the neck region, is low compared to the 200 to 250 mrads for Tc-99m pertechnetate and 2 to 20 rads for I-131 sodium iodide scans. Patients with iodine pools saturated from contrast media or those taking thyroid suppressants can be studied. A method for quantifying thyroid iodine content has been reported by Patton et al.[9]

SCINTILLATION CAMERAS

In contrast to scanners, which collect information about the radioactivity distribution in sequence, *scintillation cameras* collect data in parallel. Cameras are sensitive within their entire field of view at all times and therefore are capable of recording dynamic processes as well as static distributions; scanners are limited to the latter.

Of the several designs described in the literature, only a few have been produced commercially, primarily owing to considerations of cost, reliability, and clinical usefulness. This chapter presents only those systems that are widely used or have clinical promise. Of the camera designs currently available, the Anger single-crystal system is by far the most widely used.

Anger Scintillation Camera

The scintillation camera is a stationary device that images distributions of radioactive material by a combination of collimation and electronic positioning circuitry. Although significant system improvements have occurred in recent years, the camera concept has remained basically unchanged since it was proposed by H.O. Anger in 1957.[10]

The scintillation camera, as shown in Figure 6–7, consists of several distinct components, including collimator, radiation detector, position circuitry, and image display. Each is discussed separately. The collimation system has been reserved for last because it varies with the special configurations in which the camera is used.

Radiation Detector and Position Determination

The radiation detector on present-day scintillation cameras consists of a large-diameter (28-cm to 41-cm) NaI(Tl) single crystal 0.64 cm to 1.25 cm thick. This crystal is viewed by several *photomultiplier* (PM) tubes, which sense the light produced by photon absorption in the crystal. If the energy of an absorbed photon is assumed to be deposited at a single point in the crystal and the light is assumed to radiate from this point, then the amount of light sensed by any individual PM tube is directly related to its proximity to the point of absorption.

There were 19 PM tubes in the early scintillation cameras.[11] Present-day cameras utilize from 37 to 91 tubes. To determine the position and energy of the interaction in the crystal accurately, it is important that the amount of light collected from the crystal be high. Maintaining this level is accomplished in most cases by use of a specially designed plastic light pipe. The ability of the light pipe to collect light maximally from each scintil-

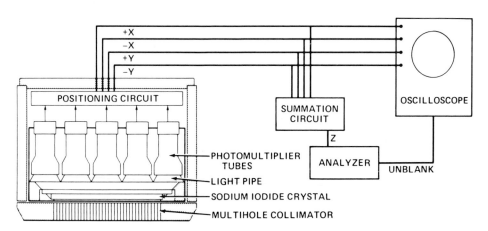

Fig. 6–7. Block diagram of the Anger scintillation camera showing the major parts of the image-forming system.

lation and to distribute it correctly to the PM tubes determines the spatial resolution, linearity, and uniformity of the camera. A thin light pipe provides better resolution, whereas a thick one provides better uniformity.

The PM tubes are connected to an electronic network, which has been designed so that each tube contributes a fixed portion of its output signal to the generation of a set of four position signals. Figure 6–8 is a schematic representation of this electronic network. Each PM tube is connected through capacitors to four output leads called $X+$, $X-$, $Y+$, and $Y-$. The amount of signal that each tube contributes to these four leads is directly proportional to the capacitance values shown in the diagram. Thus tube 7 contributes an equal

amount to each of the four coordinate signals, while tube 1 contributes three times as much to $X-$ as it does to $X+$. In this manner, the position of an interaction in the crystal can be determined by examining the relative magnitude of the four output signals. In addition, the four signals are fed into a summation circuit, which determines the total amount of light produced and hence the total amount of energy deposited in the crystal. The output of the summation circuit, the *Z pulse*, is used for energy discrimination by the pulse-height analyzer.

The selection of the energy window to be used for a particular imaging study has been simplified in the scintillation camera by virtue of two characteristics of modern cameras: the display oscilloscope and the

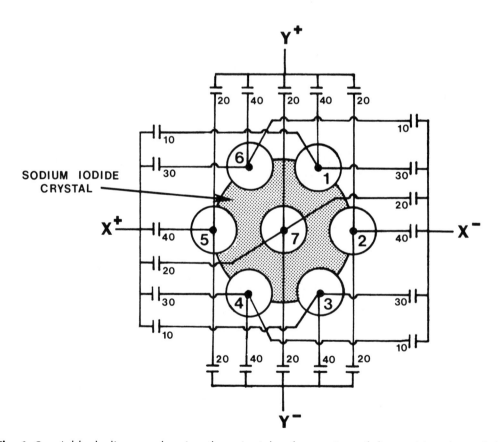

Fig. 6–8. A block diagram showing the principle of operation of the position-determining circuitry of the scintillation camera.

stability of solid-state electronics. The display oscilloscope provides a visual display of pulse heights and window position to aid the operator in making adjustments. Two types of pulse-height display are commonly available (Fig. 6–9), though not both on all cameras.

The long-term stability of modern solid-state electronics makes it possible to provide the camera user with preadjusted energy windows, which are set up to the customer's specifications when the manufacturer delivers the camera. These energy selections are then available simply by depressing the appropriate push-button control.

Modern scintillation cameras have up to three single-channel analyzers (SCAs), which may be used singly for single-peak radionuclides or in conjunction with one another in the case of an isotope that has several useful photons (e.g., Ga-67, with peaks at 93, 184, 296, and 388 keV).

Image Display

If the Z pulse meets the window requirements, the X and Y position signals are applied to the deflection plates of a cathode-ray oscilloscope. Accepted pulses from the analyzer are used to unblank the oscilloscope, which results in a flash of light on the screen at a position directly related to the position of the interaction in the detector. When a photographic film is exposed to the light flashes from the display oscilloscope, a picture that represents the distribution of activity being imaged is obtained, with the more exposed areas of film representing areas of greater radioactivity. The basic scintillation camera has a display scope that may be photographed with positive or negative film. A multiformat device, available from most manufacturers, usually contains a larger cathode-ray display tube with an x-ray film cassette holder and is capable of positioning the individual images at several locations on the film as determined by the technologist. The several images on a single piece of film may be either multiple views of a single static study or the sequential images of a dynamic study. Figure 6–10 shows a part of a radionuclide cer-

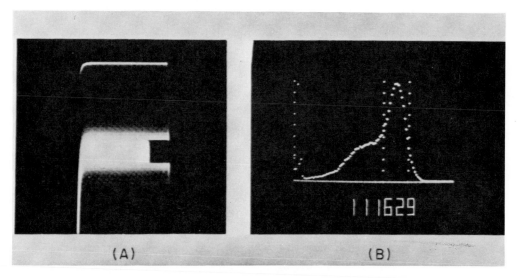

Fig. 6–9. Two methods for selecting the pulse-height interval of a scintillation camera. (A) Energy window appears as a dark rectangle within the stretched pulse spectrum on the cathode-ray tube of the Searle camera. A 20% window centered on the photopeak is shown. (B) Energy window is defined by two vertical lines set on the spectral display of the hundred-channel analyzer of the Picker camera. The digits indicate the counts between the two vertical lines. (From Hine, G.J., and Erickson, J.J.[13])

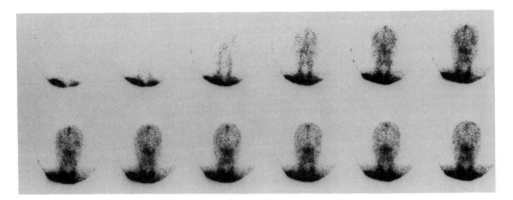

Fig. 6–10. Multiformat images showing the movement of activity during a dynamic brain blood-flow study.

ebral angiogram in which the change in activity distribution is recorded as the bolus moves through the circulatory system of the head.

Collimation

In the preceding discussion of the image production mechanism, the exposed areas of the image on the film were stated to represent areas of radionuclide concentration. More accurately, however, they represent only the distribution of gamma rays absorbed by the detector crystal. The re-

lationship to the actual radioactivity distribution is determined by the collimator in front of the crystal. The collimator most commonly used with the scintillation camera is the parallel multihole collimator, shown schematically in Figure 6–11. This collimator consists of an array of lead channels perpendicular to the face of the crystal. Each channel accepts gamma rays only from the activity directly in front of it and prevents (within physical limits) photons from other areas from entering the detector. The spatial resolution is best

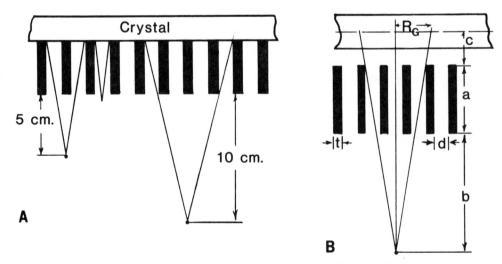

Fig. 6–11. Orientation of lead septa to the crystal in a parallel-hole collimator. *A.* Uncertainty in source position increases with distance from collimator. *B.* Geometric resolution R_G may be calculated as discussed in text.

nearest to the collimator and is degraded with increasing distance. The sensitivity, on the other hand, decreases only slightly with distance because as the distance increases, the spatial concentration of photons decreases by the inverse square of the distance, but the total area of crystal exposed to the source increases by the square of the distance. This explanation is true only in the absence of any scattering material, which tends to attenuate the number of photons exponentially as distance increases. As with all collimators, the performance of the parallel multihole collimator is determined by the number of holes, hole diameter, length of hole, septum thickness, and collimator material. Constructing a more efficient collimator for low-energy gamma rays is possible because the septa can be thinner and more holes of smaller diameter can be used. Camera manufacturers normally supply several different parallel multihole collimators, each with special attributes that render them suitable for various clinical studies.

The choice of which collimator to use for a clinical study is determined by the spatial resolution and sensitivity required as well as the energy of the gamma ray emitted by the isotope to be mapped. Some tomographic or special-purpose imaging also requires specification of the hole shape or orientation, as with the seven-pinhole or slant-hole collimators discussed in the section "Tomography" in this chapter.

The geometric resolution R_G of a parallel-hole collimator (Fig. 6–11) is given by the equation:

$$R_G = d(a_e + b + c)/a_e$$

where a_e is the effective length of the collimator septa and is related to the actual septal length by the equation:

$$a_e = a - 2\mu^{-1}$$

where μ is the linear attenuation coefficient for the collimator material.[14] This re-

lationship provides for penetration of the corners of the septa by the gamma rays being imaged. Similarly, the geometric efficiency can be described by the equation:

$$G = \{Kd^2/a_e(d + t)\}^2$$

Note that this geometric efficiency is independent of source depth provided that there is no attenutation in the material between the source and the collimator. The value K in this equation is a function of both the shape of the collimator hole and of the distribution pattern of holes in the collimator.

Several other points should also be noted. These equations indicate that resolution is a function of the first power of the hole diameter while sensitivity is a function of the square of the diameter. Sensitivity is inversely proportional to the square of the collimator thickness, but dependence of the geometric resolution on collimator thickness is less than linear. This means that collimator length affects sensitivity much more strongly than it affects the resolution. Septal thickness affects sensitivity by reducing the area available for radiation to reach the crystal. In general, the septal thickness should be sufficient to stop 95% of the incident radiation along the path of minimum attenuation. One difficulty with using high-resolution imaging devices to image high-energy gamma emitters is that the required thickness of the collimator septa often causes the shadows of the septa to be visible in the image.

Several collimators have been designed to make the effective field of view either smaller or larger than the crystal diameter. These devices include diverging, converging, and pinhole collimators. The diverging collimator was designed to increase the effective field of view of the camera. In this case, the holes, instead of being parallel, are constructed so that they diverge at the face of the collimator (Fig. 6–12). Thus the image size is strongly dependent upon the object's distance from

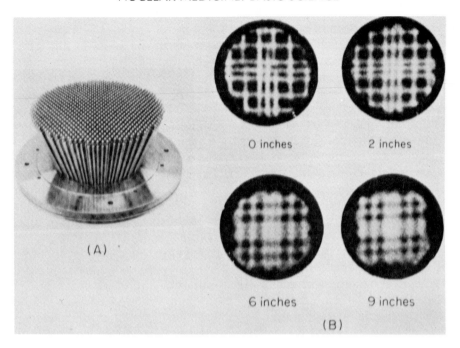

O inches   2 inches

6 inches   9 inches

(A)

(B)

Fig. 6–12. Diverging collimator for scintillation cameras. (A) The pins employed for casting the collimator show increasing divergence of holes from center of collimator toward its edge. (Courtesy of Searle.) (B) Images at 0, 2, 6, and 9 in. from face of diverging collimator show reduction of image size and deterioration of resolution with increasing distance. Line sources are 1 and 2 in. apart. (From Hine, G.J., and Erickson, J.J.[13])

the collimator. The image produced by a source distribution close to the collimator is larger than that produced by the same distribution at a greater distance. This characteristic introduces a distortion in the images of such thick organs as the liver, because the images of the distribution of radioactivity at all depths of the organ are superimposed. This problem is not serious for simple imaging procedures and does allow large organs, such as both lungs or large livers, to be imaged in a single view.

In such instances as brain imaging of small infants a magnified image of the isotope distribution is desirable. Such a device is the reverse of the diverging collimator in that the holes converge to a focal point at a distance in front of the camera face to produce images that increase in size as distance increases. These collimators produce the same type of image

distortion as do the diverging collimators, but they do not interfere severely with routine imaging procedures, especially for thin, high-contrast organs.

The popularity of these two special-purpose collimators and the fact that they are usually used with low-energy gamma emitters has given rise to the *reversible collimator,* in which a central core is made so that it can be removed from the supporting structure, reversed, and replaced to produce the complementary collimation characteristics.

The pinhole collimator, shown in Figure 6–13, operates on the principle of the old-fashioned box camera. Consisting of a small opening at the end of a conical lead shield, it projects an inverted radiation image onto the crystal detector. The resolution and sensitivity of this collimator are functions of the pinhole diameter. As the pinhole diameter increases, the solid

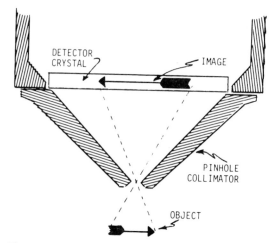

Fig. 6–13. Pinhole collimator showing inverted image of the radioactive object as projected on the crystal.

angle of radiation accepted by the collimator for each point of the source increases, thereby increasing its apparent size on the detector face. This aspect reduces the collimator resolution but increases its sensitivity. The image size depends highly on the source-to-aperture distance. When the source-to-aperture distance is equal to the aperture-to-detector distance, the radiation image projected on the detector is equal in size to the source. Reducing the source-to-aperture distance magnifies the image, while increasing the distance reduces the image size. Because of this strong dependence upon source distance, the pinhole collimator is best suited for high resolution imaging of such small thin organs as the thyroid.[15]

Performance and Evaluation

Field Uniformity and Resolution

Two properties of a scintillation camera are especially important in clinical diagnostic studies: the ability to produce the same counting rate from a point source placed at different points in the field of view, and the ability to determine the position of photon interaction accurately.

Early scintillation cameras, when irradiated with a uniform or "flood" field of

activity, produced images that displayed definite areas of increased activity. This variation of count density would seem at first to be simply a result of nonuniform sensitivity in the crystal. The major contribution, however, results from positioning distortions.[16] For example, a positioning distortion in both the X and the Y directions toward tube centers, which represents less than 0.5% integral nonlinearity, results in a compression of the count or dot density. If the distortion is effective over 20 mm, a 20-mm square in the object area is compressed to an 18-mm square in the image. The count density is then increased by approximately 20% over a corresponding undistorted area.

In a well-tuned camera, the counting efficiency varies by less than ±2% if the photopeak is centered in a 20% window. Variations in count densities caused by variations in counting efficiency as a function of position become a problem only if the camera is detuned. In general, the variation in counting efficiency is responsible for only a small part of the count-density variation. Early scintillation cameras exhibited counting rate variations of ±15% when well tuned. This amount of variation is easily discernible to the eye and could contribute to faulty interpretation of clinical studies. With the introduction of better light pipes, more PM tubes, and better tuning procedures, this variation has dropped to less than ±10%.

Thin-Crystal Technology

Early scintillation cameras were constructed with a crystal thickness of 12.5 mm (½ in.). This thickness was a worthwhile compromise, for it provided a clinically useful tool that could be constructed economically with known technology. In recent years, the drive to increase intrinsic spatial resolution of camera systems has caused manufacturers to construct cameras with thinner crystals and reduced lightpipe thicknesses. The thickness of the crystal affects spatial resolution by the following process. When a gamma ray is absorbed in the crystal, the light emitted radiates out from the point of interaction. Between the time of emission and its detection by the photomultiplier, the light may be partially absorbed by the crystal itself or may undergo multiple scatterings within the crystal. Both processes reduce the accuracy with which the positioning circuitry determines the source of the light and therefore the point of interaction in the crystal. For low-energy gamma rays of Tl-201 (70 keV) and Tc-99m (140 keV), the majority of interactions in the crystal take place near the entry side of the crystal. For Tl-201, 97% of the gamma rays are absorbed in the first 2 mm of crystal while for Tc-99m, 80% of the gamma rays are absorbed in the first 5 mm. Thus, for these most commonly used isotopes, the second half of the 12.5-mm crystal simply contributes to reduced spatial resolution without adding significantly to the sensitivity.

At the present time, many cameras with small fields of view, which are designed primarily for cardiac studies utilizing Tc-99m and Tl-201, have been constructed with crystal thicknesses of 6.25 mm (¼ in.). This improves the intrinsic Tc-99m resolution from 5.5 mm to 3.8 mm while leaving the sensitivity for Tl-201 unchanged and reducing the sensitivity of Tc-99m by only 15%. For cameras with large fields of view, which are used with all isotopes—including I-131 (361 keV), the crystal thickness has been reduced on many designs to 9.4 mm (⅜ in.). This results in a Tc-99m spatial resolution of 4.4 mm and only a 6% loss in sensitivity. For I-131, this design provides a resolution of 3.3 mm and a sensitivity reduction of only 23%.[17]

Concurrent with the change in crystal thickness have been changes in designs of the light pipe and of photomultiplier tubes. The use of round photomultiplier tubes requires some mechanical method of collecting the light that would normally

pass out of the crystal and into the small spaces between the tubes. In most cases, the light pipe is constructed to collect this light by placing reflectored surfaces in the interstices between the photomultipliers. These reflect light back to the appropriate photomultiplier for processing, thus increasing the efficiency of light collection. In some cases, the face of the light pipe is painted to control the angles and directions from which light can be collected. This process tends to reduce somewhat the completeness of light collection, but it increases the uniformity of the flood image. At least one manufacturer (Picker) has replaced the round tubes with hexagonal-shaped tubes and completely eliminated the light pipe.[12]

Energy Window Selection

The value of eliminating scattered radiation has been emphasized by a number of authors. Beck et al. determined that the optimum window setting for 140-keV gamma rays is a lower level of 126 keV and an upper level high enough to include all photopeak events.[18] The expected improvements in performance have been confirmed clinically with a scintillation camera by Sanders et al.[19] Using an offset window, however, brings the scintillation camera to the edge of unstable operation. As long as the photopeak is centered, a small shift in gain of a PM tube shifts the energy peak for that phototube, so that some counts are lost and others are gained, which results in only a small change in counting efficiency. If the energy selection window is not centered, any small shift in the energy peak can cause significant and often objectionable variations in counting efficiency.[16] Although offsetting the energy peak in the window eliminates some scattered radiation and improves spatial resolution, it may have a deleterious effect on field uniformity. Several manufacturers now offer a feature that allows the technician to position the energy selection window accurately on the photopeak.

These automatic centering circuits, when activated, operate by shifting the gain of the energy amplifier until the output of the analyzer is maximum. This amplifier setting is then maintained for the rest of the study. When utilizing any method that allows precise and accurate adjustment, one restriction must be kept in mind. If a small point source is used in front of a collimated camera, the isotopic spectrum produced is predominately that resulting from the single PM *directly* over the source. To obtain an accurate window setting for the entire crystal surface, either an uncollimated detector or an extended source must be used.

Deadtime

While the camera processes the positional and energy information from each pulse, it is unable to begin processing a second pulse, so some interaction events are lost. This deadtime can be as short as 3 μsec or as long as 75 μsec, depending on the specific instrument and the data processing that is applied to the detected events. A second source of count loss is pulse pair pileup.

In some dynamic studies, 15 to 20 mCi of activity may enter the field of view of the camera. With a high-efficiency collimator, counting rates as high as 300,000 cps into the single-channel analyzer are encountered.[20] Several authors have shown that the deadtime of an Anger scintillation camera is a combination of *paralyzable* and *nonparalyzable* components.[21,22] The elements of the camera system up to and including the SCA constitute the paralyzable component while all data processing beyond the SCA is nonparalyzable. It is important to exercise care when comparing scintillation cameras on the basis of deadtime. Several factors that are often not mentioned when deadtimes are stated can have significant effects on the measured deadtimes, e.g., SCA window setting, nuclide used, scatter conditions, positions of internal timing controls, and the deadtime of data processing hardware. Muehllehner et al. state that the observed losses for events falling within a certain window depend on the number of events falling both inside and outside the analyzer window.[22] As a result, as the ratio of "window" to "non-window" events decreases, the percentage of "window" events lost increases, thereby exhibiting an apparently longer deadtime. The decrease in "window" to "non-window" counting rate may result from a narrowing of the SCA window, introduction of scattering material, or the use of a nuclide with a smaller photopeak to nonphotopeak ratio, e.g., I-131 instead of Tc-99m.

Modern scintillation cameras incorporate several electronic innovations that allow them to process counting rates on the order of 300,000 to 400,000 cps.[20] These electronic features include:

1. Circuitry to analyze the rise time of energy pulses, which thereby permits a priori processing for rapid rejection of very high or very low energy pulses that would not be accepted by the SCA. This processing reduces the deadtime for scattered events.

2. Analog buffers for temporary storage of events that accept input pulses while the slower data processing sections are handling prior events.

3. Circuitry to reject pulse pair pileup and eliminate coincidence events. Piled-up events result in prolonged scintillation pulses, which can be detected because they do not meet specific decay criteria.

4. Replacing the analog position circuitry with digital electronics to reduce the time required to obtain position information (see "All-Digital Camera" in this chapter).

Spatial Resolution and Modulation Transfer Function

The spatial resolution of an imaging system is the measure of its ability to distinguish variations in a distribution of radio-activity. In the past, several methods of characterizing spatial resolution have been proposed. One method is to express spatial resolution as the minimum dis-tance by which two point sources can be separated and still be resolved in the image as two separate sources. While this is a rough estimate of resolution, it is im-precise and depends strongly on the cri-teria used to define separation.

A more sophisticated method of defin-ing collimator response as well as the per-formance of every component within the detector system is by the *modulation transfer function* (MTF).[23] Consider a de-tector passing over a series of line sources, as in Figure 6–14. The sources each con-tain some activity S_{max}, between which there is no activity, S_{min}. Because the re-sponse of the system is not perfect, the detector traces a pattern of maximum and minimum counting rates, as illustrated in

Figure 6–14. The modulation of the source distribution is defined as:

$$M_s = \frac{S_{max} - S_{min}}{S_{max} + S_{min}}$$

and that of the detection instrument out-put is defined as:

$$M_I = \frac{C_{max} - C_{min}}{C_{max} + C_{min}}$$

If the lines are far enough apart so that the counting rate falls to zero between the line sources, and if $S_{max} = C_{max}$ and $S_{min} = C_{min}$, then $M_s = M_I = 1$ and the *modu-lation transfer* = 1. This means that one can completely distinguish the lines as separated. As the lines are placed more closely together, however, the valleys fill in, and C_{min} increases. Ultimately, the lines are spaced so close together that no modulation in the detector response occurs and MT = O.

The MTF defines the accuracy with

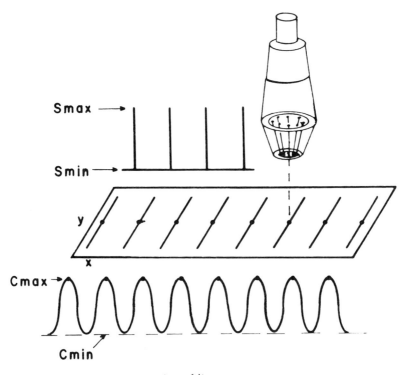

Fig. 6–14. Detector response to a series of line sources.

which variations (modulation) in the source are transferred to an observed counting rate (or image contrast) that is:

$$MTF = \frac{M_I}{M_s}$$

If one plots the modulation transfer versus spatial frequency (lines/cm), curves such as those shown in Figure 6–15 result. Curve A represents a system in which there is relatively little scatter or septal penetration; curve B represents a system with greater septal penetration or sensitivity to scattered radiation.

One method of determining the MTF of a camera system is to scan a radioactive equivalent of the star phantom of optics. With this fan-shaped source, the cross section at any radius is a sinusoid. The modulation is then measured at each radius. The primary problem with this method is the difficulty of obtaining quantitative values for higher spatial frequencies.

A second method of measuring MTF is a more indirect method based on a technique often used to test electronic amplifiers. In this method, the input to the system is a narrow pulse signal. If the pulse approximates a delta function, the Fourier transform of the input signal indicates that it contains all frequencies with an equal weight of 1. Even if the input signal is not a true delta function, the only restriction is that it must contain frequencies above those to which the instrument can respond. The Fourier transform of the output signal directly represents the MTF. In the case of an imaging system, the pulse input is obtained by using a narrow line source. The Fourier transform at a given spatial frequency v obtained from a scan of a line source is given by the equation:

$MTF(v_i)$

$$= \frac{\int_{-\infty}^{+\infty} L(x)\cos 2\pi v x \, dx + i \int_{-\infty}^{+\infty} L(x)\sin 2\pi v x \, dx}{\int_{-\infty}^{+\infty} L(x) \, dx}$$

where $L(x)$ is the amplitude of the line

source response as a function of position x along the scan line.

If the scan of a line source is digitized by collecting the output of the SCA and correlating it with the source position to obtain a digitized image of the source, it is possible to calculate the MTF for the device. If the line source image is obtained at sufficiently small increments, the foregoing equation may be approximated by:

$$MTF(v_i) = \frac{\sum_{j=n}^{m} L(x_j)\cos(2\pi v_i x_i) + i \sum_{j=n}^{m} L(x_j)\sin(2\pi v_i x_i)}{\sum_{j=n}^{m} L(x_j)}$$

$$= cosMTF + sinMTF$$

where x_n and x_m are positions on each side of the peak beyond which the line spread is effectively zero. The absolute value is determined by:

$$|MTF| = \left((cosMTF)^2 + (sinMTF)^2 \right)^{1/2}$$

In the process of imaging a distribution, the primary source of information degradation is the collimator—for three reasons. First, to provide a reasonable number of counts to produce an image, the collimator must have holes of finite dimension. Second, scattered radiation can enter the holes of the collimator and pass into the detector; thus, the collimator has a scatter response that is directly related to the hole size. Third, the collimator, even though constructed of dense material, cannot prevent all septal penetration. Even at low energies the primary and scattered radiation has a finite probability of passing unattenuated through the collimator body.

The line spread and its Fourier transform, the MTF, are capable of demonstrating the degree to which each factor affects the response of the camera system. If the camera response is symmetric and septal penetration and scatter are minimal, the response curve or line source response approximates a Gaussian curve, as shown in Figure 6–5. Increasing septal penetration causes the line source response to broaden

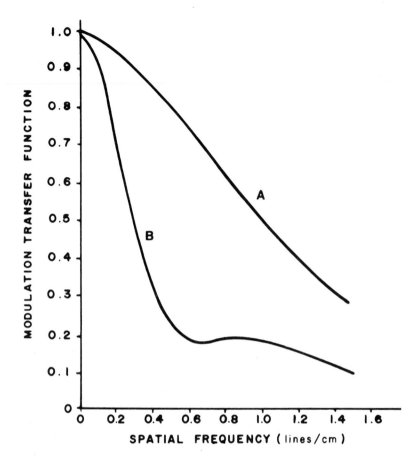

Fig. 6–15. Modulation transfer function of a scintillation camera to: *A,* I-125 source, and *B,* I-131 source.

at the base. It would be expected that the system whose MTF is curve A in Figure 6–15 would better resolve fine detail. The introduction of scatter to the line spread has essentially the same effect as septal penetration, and in a practical imaging situation, the two are difficult to distinguish. The response of the collimated detector system is always a function of the distance between the source and the collimator, the photon energy, and the scattering media present. As a result, the complete MTF description of an imaging system must include the effects of these variables. For the scintillation camera, the resolution must be assessed over a wide field of view, i.e., the entire crystal area.

Uniformity Correction Devices

Reducing crystal thickness, as discussed earlier, improves spatial resolution at the expense of greater nonuniformity in the flood field. The latter results from more efficient light collection by the photomultipliers and decreased light scatter, since light scatter tends to even out the response. For most thin-crystal cameras, it is no longer possible to adjust the gain of the photomultiplier circuits manually to improve field uniformity. For this reason, all commercial manufacturers have designed automatic uniformity correction circuitry that adjusts the detector response to correct for inherent nonuniformities. These devices stem from four separate design concepts, some of which are used in combination to produce the desired correction.

In the ideal camera, the spectral response of the detection system would be such that a gamma ray of a given energy interacting in the crystal would produce the same size signal independent of the position of the interaction. In fact, the response of the detector system varies over the face of the crystal owing to variations in the efficiency of the scintillator, the photomultiplier gains, coupling of PM tubes to the crystal, and other uncontrollable factors. The result is illustrated in Figure 6–16. The photopeaks of the spectra collected at various points in the crystal do not coincide exactly, and when the individual spectra are summed to form the overall spectrum from the camera, the distribution about the photopeak is necessarily broader than that from individual PM tubes. Thus an energy window wide enough to encompass the entire photo-

peak of the summed spectra is wider than necessary in almost every subregion of the detector. Those areas in which the window is too wide on the low-energy side collect more scatter than those areas in which the window is too wide on the high-energy side.

This problem is corrected by dividing the detector area into several subregions (usually 64 × 64) and collecting a spectrum for each. The location of the photopeak in each subregion is determined during calibration collection and stored in a microprocessor memory. During subsequent imaging procedures, the position of each interaction is determined by the positioning electronics and by the calibration factor obtained from the memory for that region of the detector. The calibration factor is used to adjust automatically the electronics that determine if the interaction represents a gamma ray of acceptable energy. This mechanism produces a camera with 4096 individually adjusted single-channel analyzers rather than a single averaged analyzer. When properly implemented, deadtime is not increased because the memory and associated electronics are sufficiently fast to process the signals in real time.

This method allows a narrower window to be used without degrading uniformity. Use of the narrower window and the more accurate positioning of the photopeak in the window result in a more uniform field and in improved spatial linearity. The actual implementation of this correction procedure varies with different manufacturers. Some systems require the user to collect a calibration image periodically, while in other systems, the calibration factors are written into a *read only memory* (ROM) during manufacturing and are not changed thereafter. Both methods of implementation appear to produce satisfactory results.

The second method of uniformity correction is a version of the original attempts at uniformity correction. This method as-

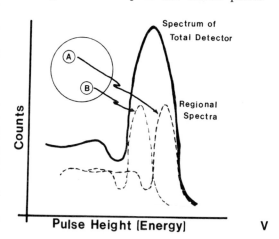

Fig. 6–16. Pulse-height spectrum of total detector is the sum of the individual regional spectra.

sumes that nonuniformity is simply a result of variations in sensitivity over the face of the detector. This correction procedure follows the procedure described for energy correction. The detector area is subdivided into a number of regions (again usually 64 × 64). During calibration, the number of counts obtained in each subregion from a flood source is determined. A correction factor for each region is then stored in a corresponding memory location. During imaging procedures, the total counts in each subregion are adjusted to provide an apparently uniform sensitivity. This is done by either adding or subtracting counts from each region based on the correction factor stored in the corresponding memory location. In some systems, this correction is accomplished solely by subtracting or suppressing counts in the more sensitive regions so that the overall sensitivity is reduced to that of the least sensitive region. Other systems add counts to areas of low sensitivity to make them appear more sensitive. At least one system uses a compromise and adds counts to the areas of low sensitivity and suppresses counts in the areas of high sensitivity. This last method is the only one in which the overall count is not changed. The subtraction, or *count skimming,* method results in a decrease in the overall sensitivity while the additive, or *count injection,* method provides an apparent increase in sensitivity. The primary problem with this type of sensitivity correction is that it compromises the usefulness of the image data in quantitative studies in which the actual true counting rates in regions of the image must be obtained, and yet it fails to address the true source of the image nonuniformity. Also, the effect of the correction procedure on the system sensitivity depends strongly on the type of nonuniformity. For example, a count skimming system is affected much more strongly by the presence of a single cold spot than by the presence of a single hot spot. In the former case, counts must be suppressed

from the majority of the detector, while in the latter case, counts are suppressed only from the hot spot. Systems that utilize this correction technique have a sensitivity 10 to 15% higher or lower when enabled than when the camera is operated without correction. The direction of the change depends, of course, on whether the counts are skimmed or added. This method is seldom used as the sole method for correction in modern imaging systems; it is usually combined with one or more of the other techniques.

Two cameras currently marketed employ a uniformity correction based on the standpoint that nonuniformity arises from misplaced events. In this technique, the ability of the positioning electronics to indicate the location of an accepted interaction correctly over the face of the detector is quantitatively determined. Correction factors are calculated and stored in a read only memory. During imaging, the location of the interaction is determined as accurately as possible by the standard camera electronics. This position is then used to determine which memory location is addressed to provide the correction factors. Both X and Y corrections are performed. The correction factors represent small adjustments that are combined with the basic position determination to provide an accurate final event location.

This technique, commonly referred to as *dot shifting,* is difficult to calibrate, and as a result, the calibration is performed in the factory during manufacturing. To perform the calibration a rectangular array of points is obtained by imaging a shadow mask consisting of a lead sheet with the corresponding array of holes. The image is collected in a computer system and examined by software to determine the actual location of the centroid of the peak from each hole. A correction factor then is calculated, which if applied to the image, would shift the peak to the location specified by the geometry of the lead mask. The correction factors for both the X and Y coordinates then are written into a ROM for use during the collection procedures.

A fourth calibration system is not directed strictly at the problem of nonuniformity but rather at the problem of drifts in the detector photomultipliers and associated electronics. Even in cameras that are optimally adjusted to maximize uniformity, there still remains the problem of how to deal with electronic drift that results in a detuned system. Two manufacturers have addressed this problem by installing light-emitting diodes (LEDs) in the detector assembly so that, when they are activated, the light emitted is detected by the PM tubes. By prior calibration, the expected photomultiplier output is known. Any shift from the expected value represents a change in electronic gain. The LEDs are activated periodically, and the resultant electronic gain determinations are used to modify the contents of an energy calibration matrix, such as is produced by the first method described.

As stated previously, most present camera systems use a combination of these calibration methods. At the present time, the ZLC system from Siemens performs an energy correction in parallel with a dot-shifting correction. The Picker Corporation Micro-Z performs an energy correction followed by dot skimming to increase uniformity. The Elscint Dymax camera systems perform a series of corrections consisting of an energy correction, a dot shift, and a combination of count rejection and injection. The General Electric 400A camera system with Autotune uses a combination of the LED phototube balancing, energy correction, and dot shifting.

The use of these correction and calibration techniques has resulted in the production of reliable imaging instruments, with spatial resolution approximately 3.5 mm FWHM, spatial linearity approximately 1% or better over the entire field of view, and a field uniformity of 4 to 5%.

Energy resolution for the Tc-99m photopeak is commonly 11 to 13%.

Mobile Camera

The increase in nuclear cardiac procedures has given rise to the design of small field of view, low-energy, mobile scintillation cameras. Evaluation of cardiac function involves the use of Tl-201 and Tc-99m with gamma-ray energies of 70 keV and 140 keV respectively. Because of these low energies, the camera detector head can be constructed with thinner shielding. The reduced weight has made possible the construction of mobile cameras that can be taken to critical care areas in the hospital.

All-Digital Camera

Genna et al. have described an experimental digital imaging system in which the positional information is obtained by use of a calibration, or "lookup," table.[24] The system is calibrated initially by scanning a point source over the imaging array and measuring the PM response to the radiation from the source as a function of position. The position of an interaction in the detector of a gamma ray from an unknown distribution of activity is then determined by comparing the light output of the photomultiplier array with corresponding values in the lookup table for which the exact position is known.

This method of determining the positional information, as opposed to using weighting resistors or capacitors in an analog computer arrangement, does not depend heavily on the uniformity of the crystal and photomultiplier response. In the analog camera, the combination circuits and position determination matrices are designed with the assumption that the crystal, light pipe, and optical coupling are all perfectly uniform and identical. Since this is not the case, however, adjustments are included to allow the serviceman to compensate for nonuniformities in response as well as for unequal PM tube response.

In the digital camera, no assumptions are made regarding field uniformity because all positional information is obtained for the calibration procedure. A commercial version of the digital camera has been introduced by the Elscint Company. In this camera, the electronic signals produced by the photomultiplier tubes are processed immediately by an ADC. The resultant digital signals are then passed through X and Y positional analysis circuits which have been constructed from values obtained during the calibration process. The use of dual ADCs on each of the PM tubes allows extremely high counting rate capability by allowing the PM tubes to process succeeding counts while the positioning circuitry and thresholding system continues to analyze and process prior counts. The commercial camera has a specified counting rate capability in excess of 200,000 cps at a 10% loss level.

The use of digital circuitry directly at the PM tube allows computers to perform a much wider range of quality-control procedures. This in turn should lead to a more reliable and easily repaired camera system. The increased complexity in the detector system, however, has made the camera more expensive. Also, the manufacturer's computer must be purchased with the camera in order to derive all of the benefits from the digital system.

Microprocessor-Controlled Camera

The Siemens Scintiview system represents an attempt to gain the advantages of a digital system without actually converting to a completely digital imaging head. In this system, a microprocessor computer system replaces the control console of the normal camera. The user of the camera enters the control operations through a pushbutton system in response to options displayed on a CRT display. The software to drive the microprocessor is contained in

read only memory in the processor electronics.

The Scintiview is a combination camera and computer and as such is capable of not only data collection but also rather sophisticated data reduction. The present model is capable of routine static imaging but is also able to perform dynamic studies and multigated cardiac imaging procedures. The system contains its own ECG system for gated procedures. Data can be stored and retrieved via a floppy disk. Image interaction for region-of-interest choices in the analysis of cardiac function studies is provided by a lightpen.

This camera provides all normal camera operations as well as several that would be impossible with an external computer system. The use of the CRT provides a great deal of flexibility in operator interaction. The choice of position for the energy window is facilitated by precalibrated windows and automatic adjustment of the window during use. Display of the energy spectrum through the window indicated on the CRT allows the operator to verify that the system is functioning correctly. The indication of the amount of correction required to center the window over the peak of interest while the system is operating is a useful quality control procedure.

Image Intensifier Camera

The Anger scintillation camera is limited in its overall resolution because of its poor intrinsic resolution, particularly at low gamma-ray energies. Many groups have made a substantial effort to develop cameras with a high intrinsic resolution. The image intensifier, as used in radiology for amplification of dim radiographic images, has become the object of much of these efforts because it is an extremely sensitive light amplifier with high resolution. An isotopic imaging camera must also possess a number of other properties, however, such as high detection efficiency, uniform field response, pulse-height discrimination to eliminate scattered events, high counting rate capability, and a large field of view.

The most obvious approach to the use of the image intensifier as a scintillation camera is to replace the PM tubes and pulse positioning electronics.[25] In this system, the light generated by the scintillation crystal is focused onto the input photocathode of the image intensifier by a large, high-efficiency lens. Pulse-height analysis can be accomplished by collecting a fraction of the light either at the edge of the crystal or near the lens. The intensifier is turned on only if an acceptable event has occurred. Because of the extremely small size of the light sample used for analysis, the discrimination is poor. This design allows the use of large-diameter flat crystals with high detection efficiency and achieves high resolution (~2 mm) with a deadtime of about 1 μsec.

In an attempt to remove the lens, which causes considerable light loss, an array of CsI(Tl) crystals has been mounted directly on the face of a large-diameter image intensifier.[26] Again, pulse-height discrimination is achieved by sampling the light. As in the first system, the pulse-height discrimination is marginal, and spatial resolution is limited to approximately 5 mm by the finite crystal size (3 mm wide × 16 mm long). The deadtime of this system is approximately 1 μsec.

Alternatively, a thin crystal can be placed either inside the first image intensifier stage or directly on the outside face of the intensifier.[27,28] The crystal used was CsI(Tl) or CsI(Na), bent to fit the curvature of the intensifier input window. Whereas Kellershohn gated a second stage of intensification to achieve pulse-height discrimination, Ter-Pogossian recorded the output of the first stage using a sensitive TV camera. Some pulse-height discrimination was achieved in the latter system by placing a lower and upper discriminator on the scan signal from the TV camera. This latter method allowed simultaneous processing of events occurring at different points in the crystal, with a potential for high counting rate capability while still maintaining pulse-height discrimination.

An image intensifier camera that appears to combine the high intrinsic spatial resolution of the image intensifier with the better energy resolution of the Anger scintillation camera has been described by Mulder and Pauwels and is shown schematically in Figure 6–17.[29] Their system consists of an array of small scintillation crystals, either 5000 individual crystals or 300 blocks of 25 crystals each, mounted on the face of a large image intensifier tube (30 cm or 36 cm in diameter). Coupled to the large tube is a series of three smaller tubes connected together by fiber optics. The light output of the last amplifier tube is collected by four PM tubes. The signals from the PM tubes are used to determine both the pulse amplitude and the X and Y coordinates of the gamma event. If the pulse amplitude falls in the selected energy window, the scintillation is displayed on an oscilloscope just as for an Anger camera. With this design, Mulder and Pauwels succeeded in obtaining an energy resolution of 20%. Because the detector consists of an array of individual crystals 4 mm × 4 mm, this design can be altered to accommodate higher energies by simply lengthening the crystals from the current thickness of 1 cm to as much as 2.5 cm. Contrary to its effect in Anger cameras, this change should not affect the spatial resolution but can substantially improve the efficiency.

The light emitted by an individual detector crystal is distributed in the output of the last image intensifier tube in a Gaussian distribution of light intensity. While the four PM tubes theoretically determine the center of the light distribution, some statistical uncertainty does exist. If the detector is irradiated by a uniform radioactive source, the image produced is an array of spots (one for each crystal), each with

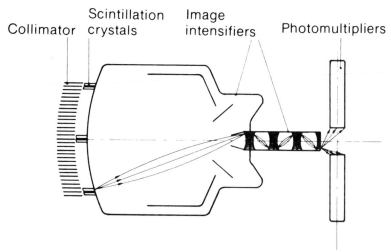

Fig. 6–17. Schematic of image intensifier scintillation camera using multiple crystals, with position and energy determined by four PM tubes (only two shown) viewing output phosphor. (From Mulder, H., and Pauwels, E.K.J.[29])

a full width at half maximum of 0.25 cm at 140 keV.

To eliminate these spots and smooth out the image, the entire detector assembly is moved in a circular path 7.5 cm in radius, while at the same time, the display for this detector motion is electronically compensated. The FWHM of the line spread function for the total imaging system is 4 mm.

Computerized Multicrystal Gamma Camera

In 1963, Bender and Blau introduced a design for a computerized multicrystal gamma camera. This instrument consisted of an array of 294 sodium iodide crystals arranged in 14 rows of 21 detectors each.[30]

Each row and column of the detector grid is optically coupled to separate PM tubes. Pulses that occur simultaneously in any pair of orthogonal phototubes uniquely identify the crystal in which the interaction has taken place. The principle of generation is illustrated in Figure 6–18 by a simplified 2 × 2 crystal array. When a gamma ray is absorbed in one of the crystals, the light produced is divided between the two PM tubes to which that particular detector is connected. The outputs from these two PM tubes are summed and analyzed in the camera's pulse-height analyzer.

This camera is inherently a digital imaging device in that each event produces an X (row) and a Y (column) address. By using this address to drive a digital computer memory, information is generated that can then be displayed or processed.

The detector head of the multicrystal gamma camera consists of 294 crystals, each of which is viewed individually and has a square cross section that is 0.8 cm to a side and 3.8 cm long. The energy resolution of this camera is degraded by the long light pipes used to couple the crystals to the PM tubes. Because only about 20% of the light presented to the light pipe by the crystal actually reaches the PM tube, the energy resolution is decreased by a factor of approximately two compared to conventional gamma-ray spectroscopy. Thus the clinical images have decreased contrast because of difficulty in discriminating against small-angle scatter at gamma-ray energies below 200 keV.

One reason for designing a multicrystal gamma camera was to achieve high counting rates. Removal of the analog position-

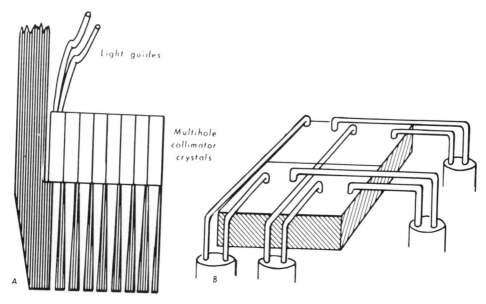

Light guides

Multihole collimator crystals

A   B

Fig. 6–18. Simplified drawing illustrating principle of multicrystal gamma camera in which each of the four detector crystals is optically coupled by light pipes to two PM tubes whose output is used to generate position and energy information. *A*, Cross-section through the collimator. *B*. Four-crystal schematic. (From Kuhl, D.E.[15])

ing electronics as used in the Anger cameras allowed extremely fast data processing from this camera. As with the Anger camera, this camera has both a paralyzable and nonparalyzable component to its deadtime. Up to approximately 180,000 cps, the deadtime is relatively constant at 2.25 μsec but increases to 2.9 μsec at 230,000 cps, at which time the paralyzing component begins to cause a serious distortion in the counting rate response. The coarse spatial resolution, however, makes the basic camera unsuitable for high-resolution static imaging. To provide this capability, the detector is equipped with a high-resolution collimator and a computer-controlled multiposition bed.

The 294-crystal array can be regarded as an assembly of 294 rectilinear scanners fixed in space with respect to each other. Because the detectors are spaced 1.1 cm apart, it is necessary for each detector to scan only a 1.1 cm × 1.1 cm area to cover the entire field of view, as all other detectors scan a corresponding area simultaneously. The scan could be performed by a continuous motion over the 1.1 cm × 1.1 cm area just as with a rectilinear scanner. In practice, however, the array is displaced in discrete steps in both the X and the Y directions. The displacement for each step is equal to one fourth of the 1.1 cm distance to be scanned, and a total of 16 equal steps covers the 1.1 cm × 1.1 cm area for each of the 294 detectors. Instead of moving the camera, the patient containing the radioactivity is displaced by the movable bed, which is under computer program control.

This system produces an image of an area 24 cm × 16 cm. For larger areas, the bed is indexed the width of the array, and a second set of measurements is taken.

The multicrystal camera is provided with three parallel hole collimators of 2.5-cm, 3.8-cm, and 6.4-cm thickness. The 6.4-cm collimator provides high-resolution collimation with a FWHM ranging from 3 mm at the collimator face to 10 mm at 10 cm. The medium and coarse resolution collimators of 2.5-cm and 3.8-cm thickness represent reasonable compromises to achieve higher efficiency with lower but still sufficient spatial resolution.

Rotating Laminar Camera

To overcome some of the inherent disadvantages of using sodium iodide for stationary cameras, designs for the use of solid-state detectors for imaging systems have been investigated. One such example is the rotating laminar camera constructed with a germanium crystal (ROLEC). The camera described by Urie et al. consists of a single germanium slab 45 mm on a side, with grooves cut into the slab to form the detector channels as shown in Figure 6–19.[31] Mounted in front of the detector are tungsten plate collimators that serve to restrict the field of view of the individual detector elements to the area directly in front of the respective element. In the experimental configuration, the detector is divided into 30 channels, each 1.47 mm wide. The tungsten plates are 0.18 mm thick, 35 mm high, and aligned with the segmenting grooves. During data collection, the detector is rotated in equally spaced increments through 180° about an axis perpendicular to the face of the detector slab. At each incremental location,

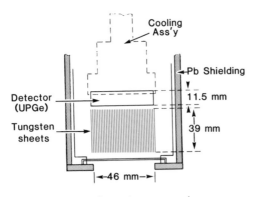

Fig. 6–19. High-purity germanium camera system with tungsten collimator sheets mounted for rotation inside lead-shield container.

the data are collected from the 30 elemental detectors transferred to a large computer for reconstruction by a filtered back-projection technique similar to that used for transmission CT images. The images are displayed as a 30 × 30 matrix with 16 gray levels.

Because of the size of the detector, objects to be imaged are limited to a maximum length of 4.5 cm. The spatial resolution at the face of the collimator is 3 mm, which decreases to 6 mm at a depth of 10 cm. Because of the better energy resolution of the germanium detector, the camera maintains a high resolution at depth. Specification of sensitivity for a rotating laminar camera is a complex problem because of the mathematical reconstructions involved in the production of the image. Although the germanium detector is somewhat less efficient for absorption of technetium gamma rays than is sodium iodide, this problem is partially offset by the unique collimator design. The laminar collimator exposes nearly 25% more of the detector area than do Anger-camera collimators. The lack of collimator septa along the length of the individual detector elements allows photons to be accepted from a much larger solid angle, thereby increasing detection efficiency. The reconstruction technique is particularly sensitive to low counting statistics. Theoretical calculations based upon the characteristics of the sodium iodide scintillation camera and the laminar emission camera indicate that acquisition times for the latter have to be increased over that for the Anger detector.[32] Because the image production does involve mathematical reconstruction techniques, the imaging time for a given signal-to-noise ratio increases with increasing detector size. The use of a high-resolution germanium detector, however, augments the image resolution at depth.

Tomography

In planar imaging with the scintillation camera, the radiation emitted by all overlying structures in front of the camera is superimposed onto the image. This makes it impossible to determine from any one view the relative distance of various structures from the face of the camera. This was less of a problem when rectilinear scanners with focused collimators were used, because some ability to discriminate between overlying structures was provided by the operator's choice of scanner-to-patient distance. With scintillation cameras, the problem of depth discrimination has been solved by several techniques for tomographic mapping, some with greater clinical success than others.

Tomographic slices are denominated *transaxial* if they are oriented perpendicular to the long axis of the body and *longitudinal* if they are oriented parallel to the long axis of the body. Tomographic techniques are also based on the type of isotopic decay used for imaging, i.e., single-photon emissions computed tomography (SPECT) and positron emission transaxial tomography (PETT).

Single-Photon Longitudinal Tomography

Three forms of longitudinal tomography based on single-photon imaging techniques have proved sufficiently useful to be produced commercially. These are the scanning camera (PHO/CON), the seven-pinhole collimator, and the slant-hole collimator. Several other techniques are of interest but for one reason or another have not attained commercial status and remain research techniques.

The oldest of the current commercial techniques is the scanning camera system, which was first discussed by Anger in 1966 and was commercially produced by Siemens Corporation under the name PHO/CON. In its current version, the scanner consists of two opposed probes mounted on a full-body scanning table. The probes are standard Anger cameras with 10-in. NaI(Tl) crystals fitted with focused collimators. Current versions of the instrument have 19 PM tubes. The elec-

tronics used to drive the cameras are those developed for the large field of view camera by Siemens and are capable of high counting rates with pulse pileup rejection.

The tomographic images are produced by special electronic circuitry during the rectilinear scan. Each probe is capable of producing six individual images that represent six equally spaced planes in the patient's body. Thus the complete scanning process produces 12 complete images.

Figure 6–20 illustrates the principle of operation of the tomographic scanner. Consider a point source at level A in front of the collimator. As the source moves from position 1 to position 5, its image moves across the detector in the same direction as shown in the lower part of Figure 6–20. At level B, the field of view is narrower, so the source produces an image in the detector only at positions 7, 8, and 9. At level C, the focal plane, the source is imaged only at position 13. Beyond the focal plane at levels D and E, the relationship between the source and its image is reversed so that the image moves in a direction opposite to that of the source.

In the original instrument, images representing the distributions of radioactivity at the various levels were produced by utilizing a special lens arrangement for each level desired. The lens arrangement for each level was designed to compensate for the motion of the image so that the activity at that level was imaged in focus while activity at other levels was smeared out and acted simply as increased background.

This lens system has been replaced in recent instruments by an electronic multiformat display in which six separate images are generated on the face of a large CRT display. Each of the individual images is electronically compensated to produce the image of the desired plane.

The overall resolution (R_0) for sources on any plane in the subject is given by the equation:

$$R_0 = (R_c^2 + R_p^2 + R_e^2)^{1/2}$$

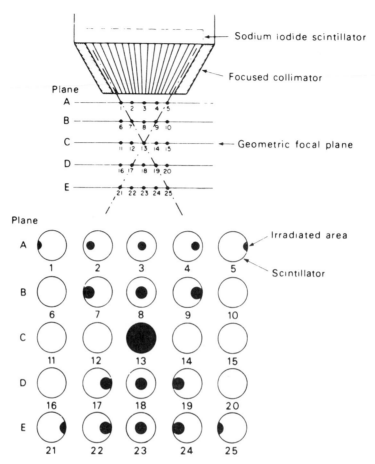

Fig. 6–20. Operation of the multiplane longitudinal scanning camera. Images of activity at different levels in front of the focused collimator move at different rates across the detector. Compensation for these differences in motion for each level results in an in-focus image of the activity on each plane of interest. (From Anger, H.O.[33])

where the resolution of the collimator central hole, collimator parallax, and the scintillator-phototube combination are given by R_c, R_p, and R_e respectively.[11] When spatial resolution is plotted as a function of depth for several planes, it is seen to be a combination of the response of a scintillation camera with a parallel-hole collimator combined with the response of a focused collimator adjusted for each of the readout planes. The resolution as a function of depth is relatively uniform, decreasing only slightly with increasing depths. Passing downward through each focal plane, the resolution increases

slightly and the interplane resolution decreases slightly. Because the collimator contributes two of the three factors in the resolution equation, it has more effect on the resolution than does the scintillator-phototube portion of the system.

Anger has shown that for 140-keV photons, resolution is good at depths of up to 10 cm. Resolution is theoretically highest with photons in the range of 0.2 to 0.5 MeV because absorption of the higher-energy gamma rays by large amounts of overlying tissue is appreciably less and because a larger fraction of scattered gamma rays is removed by pulse-height discrimination.[11]

The clinical utility of the multiplane tomographic scanning camera has been investigated by McRae and Anger.[34] They state that the tomoscanner does provide better images in thick organs than do conventional scintillation cameras. The tomographic scintigrams provide an excellent guide to the depth of lesions in small organs.

The tomographic scanner does not remove counts produced by activity that lies outside the chosen focal plane. The counts persist as random background that can obscure faint structures even when the structures of interest lie in the focal plane of the given tomogram.[33] Attempts have been made to remove interference by processing the data with a computer following completion of the scan. The technique that appears most successful is an iterative one that uses initially constructed slices to estimate the amount of extraneous information, i.e., counts from outside the plane of interest.[35] The images then are processed for removal of the estimated extraneous activity to produce more exact representations of the tomographic planes. This processing requires a significant amount of computational hardware and time. Regardless, the unprocessed images from present instruments are quite good.

Seven-Pinhole Tomography

Seven-pinhole tomographic techniques as introduced by Vogel et al. in 1978 represent another method of obtaining longitudinal tomographic images with the scintillation camera.[36] In this case, the parallel-hole collimator normally used for imaging is replaced by a specially designed collimator containing seven individual pinholes. When a distribution of activity is viewed with this collimator, seven separate images are formed on the crystal face. Each image represents a view of the activity from a slightly different angle. If properly combined by shifting and scaling,

three-dimensional information about the activity distribution can be reconstructed from these images.

Figure 6–21 illustrates the collimator and the imaging system. Because the nature of the image processing required to produce the tomographic slices is complex, and because the camera and collimator must be calibrated to correct for deficiencies in linearity and uniformity, reconstruction requires use of a digital computer. In the reconstruction, the images are combined to produce one or more images representing selected places in the organ imaged. The amount of image shifting and scaling prior to combining the individual pinhole images depends on the depth of the plane.

The seven-pinhole technique has the advantage of producing tomographic images without requiring a complicated mechanical scanning system. On the other hand, only a relatively small volume can be imaged. In fact, the size of the distribution is limited to the field of view of the individual pinholes. The presence of large amounts of activity outside the field of

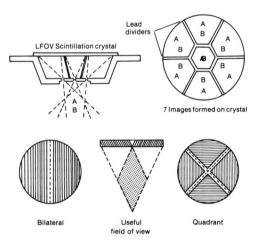

Fig. 6–21. Tomographic collimators. Top) Seven-pinhole collimator, showing position of sources A and B on scintillation camera detector. Bottom) Slant hole collimators, showing limited field of view of both bilateral and quadrant hole designs.

view produces artifacts in the reconstructed images because the various pinholes are not all viewing the same distribution.

The seven-pinhole collimator system suffers from other disadvantages, which compromise its clinical usefulness. The method suffers from the decreased sensitivity common to all pinhole imaging techniques. In addition, the reconstruction technique is sensitive to counting statistic noise. These limitations require extended data collection for high-quality clinical images. The extended time involved provides an opportunity for patient motion as well as for redistribution of the labeled pharmaceutical, both of which tend to degrade the image quality. Because of the relatively narrow viewing angle between the individual pinholes, the tomographic capability is strongly depth-dependent. That is, structures closer to the collimator are better separated than those farther away.

The most successful application of the seven-pinhole collimator has been myocardial imaging using Tl-201.[37] Imaging of other organs has not been universally successful. The technique appears to be quite sensitive to the technologist's skill and to the care with which the data are collected. The positioning of the patient also has an effect on the images produced. The use of cardiac gating to eliminate the effects of cardiac motion is also possible with this technique since the images are collected with a stationary camera. This allows cardiac synchronized tomographic images without significant additional hardware.

Rotating Slant-Hole Collimator

An attempt to overcome the sensitivity and depth-dependence characteristics of the seven-pinhole collimator has resulted in the design of the quadrant slant-hole collimator (QSH). This is a variation of the rotating slant-hole collimator introduced in 1970 by Muehllehner. The QSH has a collimator core composed of four 90° pie-shaped segments (Figure 6–21). Each segment is constructed of parallel holes slanted at a 25° angle, which produce a diamond-shaped field of view with a clinically effective range of 7.5 cm to 18 cm from the collimator. In normal use, tomograms can be produced from two four-view images taken with a 45° rotation of the collimator between image collections.

Because this collimator is essentially a parallel-hole collimator, it shares the same advantages. That is, the resolution and sensitivity are weak functions of distance from the collimator face, and the sensitivity is much greater than that of the pinhole collimator. The segmental images produced by this collimator do not undergo the minification process that takes place with the pinhole collimator, and the uniformity of sensitivity over the fields of view of the individual collimator segments is much improved over the seven-pinhole collimator.

This tomographic technique has not gained wide acceptance. Because there is a need for two images, the technique cannot be used easily for gated imaging and cannot be used at all for tomographic imaging of dynamic processes. It is commercially available, however, as an imaging option from several manufacturers. The spatial resolution of the QSH technique is approximately 7 mm FWHM at 7.5 cm, increasing to 12 mm at 15 cm.

Stochastic Coded Aperture

There are several imaging methods that produce longitudinal tomographic images. They have not had as widespread acceptance as the three techniques already discussed. Of special interest are the Fresnel zone plate and the stochastic coded aperture.

The stochastic coded aperture is an attempt to make better use of the detector area of the scintillation camera (Fig. 6–22). The seven-pinhole collimator requires that the individual images do not overlap on the face of the detector. This

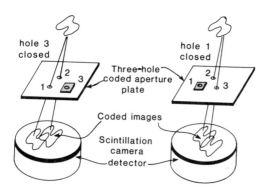

Fig. 6–22. With stochastic coded apertures, the images may overlap on the detector and are decoded by using several images with various holes closed. (Adapted from Rogers, W.L.[38])

limits both the amount of magnification and the size of the field of view. The stochastic coded aperture system allows images to overlap on the detector face and decodes the overlap by using images recorded with different combinations of pinholes. The overlapped images are in a sense decoded by imaging the distribution of activity through several hole configurations and then applying an iterative arithmetic reconstruction technique.

A system based on this design has been described by Rogers.[38] This system uses an aperture plate with 73 pinholes. The data are collected by shielding the aperture plate so that nine holes are open at any one time. Successive nine-hole combinations are collected and then processed to produce the tomographic images. This operation is equivalent to solving 73 simultaneous equations for 73 unknowns. In this application, each unknown is represented by a single pinhole image.

The tomography results from each pinhole viewing the source from a slightly different angle. By combining individual pinhole images appropriately, tomographic planes are reconstructed.

Use of this system to image the thyroid and facial bones has been described by Keyes.[39] As with the seven-pinhole collimator, the depth resolution is strongly dependent on the field of view and therefore on the imaging angles involved. The increase in image contrast due to this geometry also is useful for situations in which there is little contrast between normal and abnormal tissue. This renders the thyroid an appropriate organ for which to use this system.

The two greatest disadvantages of this system are the limited angles from which images are obtained and the time required for computer processing. The system described by Rogers and Keyes requires approximately two hours to produce four tomographic slices. Dedicated processors, however, can probably reduce this to an acceptable time and preliminary clinical data indicate a need for further investigation.

Fresnel Zone Plate

The Fresnel zone plate consists of a single shadow plate constructed according to a mathematical formula (Fig. 6–23). The aperture in the plate consists of a series of concentric rings whose widths and densities are calculated from the Fourier transform of the image of a point source obtained with a single-pinhole collimator. Tomographic images can be obtained from

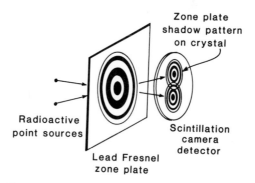

Fig. 6–23. The Fresnel zone plate is constructed by using a mathematical formula for the transparent ring dimensions so that the image can be decoded by a well defined mathematical manipulation. (Adapted from Rogers, W.L., et al.[40])

the coded aperture image by a mathematical manipulation based on Fourier transform theory.[41]

Data from planes outside the plane of interest interfere with the high-quality reproduction of the tomographic image by increasing the average background of the reconstructed plane. This is the same effect as is present in all other limited-angle techniques and can be partially corrected by iterative image-processing techniques and background subtraction. The advantage of the Fresnel zone plate over the time-coded stochastic aperture is that only one image is required to obtain all of the tomographic information.

Longitudinal tomographic imaging systems are mechanically simple to construct, but they suffer from several disadvantages that limit their clinical usefulness. There are listed by Budinger as follows:[43]

1. Statistical noise is increased during image reconstruction.
2. Attenuation correction is difficult and further increases noise.
3. Systems requiring complex decoding require significant amounts of computer time.
4. Pinhole systems that possess geometric distortion cause image distortion.
5. Pinhole systems have a nonuniform sensitivity.
6. There is limited angle sampling in all systems.

The presence of statistical noise makes it difficult to perform extensive processing without seriously degrading the images. The lack of attenuation correction limits the ability of the longitudinal tomography to produce quantitative results. The extensive computation time required for such techniques as the stochastic coded aperture and the Fresnel zone plate renders their application in routine clinical imaging doubtful. Because of the distortions and nonuniformities of the pinhole systems, successful application depends on calibration procedures and technical expertise.

The list of disadvantages is not intended to imply that longitudinal tomography is not useful. The scanning camera, seven-pinhole collimator, and the slant-hole collimator have proved clinically useful for qualitative imaging. Such coded aperture forms as the seven-pinhole collimator are useful for dynamic and gated studies.

Transverse Tomography

Transverse tomographic imaging systems using single-photon emitters (SPET) fall primarily into two groups. In the first, the equipment is designed specifically for tomographic imaging and is limited entirely to this procedure or to some restricted extension of it. The second class of instruments includes versions of the scintillation camera. The latter group has gained the most widespread clinical use. There are several reasons for this, one of which is that the technology is familiar to both user and manufacturer, which thereby eliminates the problems and expense of new manufacturing technologies and re-education of the user. Equally important, the rotating camera systems can be used for classic imaging procedures as well as tomography.

As stated earlier, one of the primary restrictions of longitudinal tomographic techniques is the limited viewing angles used to collect the data. The obvious method of overcoming this limitation is to move the camera so that the effective viewing angle is increased. This solves the problem of viewing angle but introduces other reconstruction problems.

The rotating camera system is shown schematically in Figure 6–24. A photograph of a commercial version of the scanner is shown in Figure 6–25. In this system, the patient lies on a pallet under the camera heads while data are collected from multiple angles around the patient. Some commercial versions use a single

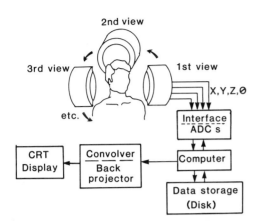

Fig. 6–24. Schematic of rotating camera tomography showing three positions of the camera head about the subject.

camera head. In an alternate version, the camera remains stationary and the patient is rotated.[43] This produces the same image relationships but is less satisfactory because it requires more patient cooperation.

The basic imaging procedures are the same for both the single and the dual-headed systems. The dual-headed scanner, however, does have an advantage in that it is possible to reduce the time required to collect a sufficient number of images for adequate tomographic reconstruction. Also, addition of the second camera head provides an opportunity to apply some attenuation correction.

Two methods of data collection are used for clinical procedures. They differ only in the motion of the detector heads. In the *step and shoot* method, the camera head is stepped between imaging positions and allowed to remain stationary while the image is collected. In the second method, the image data are collected during continuous camera rotation. The step and shoot method is perhaps easier to discuss in explaining the tomographic reconstruction process.

The most common method of tomographic image reconstruction is *filtered backprojection* which is based on a technique similar to that used for x-ray trans-

mission CT.[44] If a simple square distribution of activity, as shown in Figure 6–26A, is viewed by a detector placed parallel to the Y axis, a distribution of counts as shown on the Y axis is detected. Similarly, a detector parallel to the X axis produces the *count profile,* or *projection* P, as shown in the figure. The aim of tomographic reconstruction is to produce a two-dimensional representation of the original activity distribution from these and similar sets of projections taken at many angles about the source distribution.

The simplest method of reconstructing the source distribution from observed counts is to reverse the collection process and place the counts from an individual location in a given projection back out along the line perpendicular to the face of the detector (i.e., to "backproject" the data). There is no evidence that some areas of the reconstructed source should receive more counts than others during backprojection of data from any given projection. For this reason, the counts from a given point in a profile are distributed uniformly throughout the field of view for the detector at that point. This process is represented by the lines emanating from the X and Y axes in Figure 6–26B. When this operation is performed, the simple source distribution is roughly reconstructed as shown by the dark square in the center of Figure 6–26B. Also present, however, are areas of lower, but still significant, activity in the areas outside the main source. These "arms" on the reconstructed source image tend to reduce the contrast between the actual source distribution and the background. Actual reconstruction of a real distribution involves the use of many more sets of projection data, but the reduced contrast effect is present no matter how many projections are used.

Correction of the reduced contrast effect of the simple backprojection reconstruction is accomplished by modifying (i.e., *filtering*) the counting data before the backprojection is performed. The original

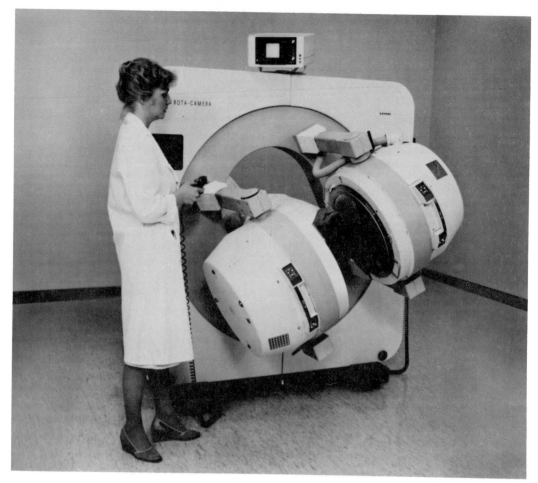

Fig. 6–25. A commercial single-photon emission tomographic scanner using two scintillation camera detector heads. (Photo courtesy of Siemens Gammasonics.)

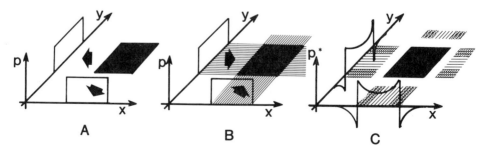

Fig. 6–26. Simple backprojection of data obtained (*A*) results in artificially high background (*B*). Reprocessing (i.e., filtering) prior to backprojection produces a high contrast image (*C*).

projections P are obtained as shown in Figure 6–26A and then are mathematically modified (P*) to the shape illustrated in Figure 6–26C, so that there are negative components. These negative components from one view (e.g., along the Y axis) cancel some of the positive components from other views (e.g., along the X axis). As shown in Figure 6–26C, this results in a reproduction of the original source distribution as in the simple backprojection example but with a much reduced background activity. Including data from views in other positions around the source increases the definition of the activity distribution without increasing the apparent background activity.

The choice of the exact mathematical form of the filter to be used for reconstruction depends on a large number of factors and is not appropriate for discussion in this text. These factors include, however, considerations of the expected source distribution, the characteristics of the data-collection device, the spatial resolution, and the amount of statistical noise permitted in the final image.

In general, the reconstruction of transaxial images from single-photon emitters is not quite as easy as it is for transverse tomography. The most serious problem inherent in single-photon tomography is attenuation of photons in the material between the point of emission and the detector. Photons emitted close to the surface of the patient's body have a much higher probability of reaching the detector than do those emitted from deep internal organs. This means that two identical sources at different distances from the detector appear to have different activities. This is an effect not taken into account during the simple filtered backprojection reconstruction, and it can result in serious artifacts if ignored.

Three methods of attenuation correction have been described. Budinger describes a method that requires data collected from opposing views of the organ being imaged.[45] It is a modification of the use of the geometric mean of the counts from opposing detectors to reduce the effects of tissue thickness. In this case, the geometric mean (i.e., the square root of the product of the two values) of corresponding opposed views is formed. This value is then modified to take into account the thickness and the average activity distribution. A complex multiplicative factor is combined with each of the projection values. This is an effective correction method but does depend on finding the correct thickness of the object.

The second method ignores attenuation effects in the first reconstruction but follows an iterative correction based on the estimated attenuation coefficients of the tissue surrounding each image pixel. After construction of the first uncorrected image, a second image is produced in which each pixel is obtained by multiplying the corresponding pixel in the first image by a factor that is a function of the distance of the pixel from the detector and of an estimated attenuation coefficient. The difference between this second image and the first is used as a correction array for producing a final image.

The third method involves modifying the data in the projection measurements before they are used to construct an image.[46,47] In this case, each data value in each projection is multiplied by a factor $e^{+\mu d_k}$, where μ is the attenuation coefficient and d_k is the distance from a line through the center of the circle of reconstruction and parallel to the projection array to the edge of the object. The modified data are then backprojected into the image following multiplication by a filter factor which depends on the distance of the pixel from the line through the center of reconstruction.

In general, corrections for attenuation in which the attenuation coefficients are used to perform the corrections appear to work best.

Single-Photon Tomography

There are primarily two types of scanning systems for single-photon tomography.[42,45] The first system is basically the same as those in first-generation transmission CT machines (i.e., a linear scanning motion combined with a rotating gantry). The second system is a more complex combination of rectilinear scanning and rotation.

Kuhl and Edwards described the first SPET system, which was used with the MARK I scanner.[48] In this system, the planar views of the isotopic distribution were collected by performing normal rectilinear scans at several angular orientations about the patient. These scans were then reprocessed to produce tomographic views. While this system was somewhat successful, it was never developed commercially.

The Tomogscanner II manufactured by J & P Engineering Limited in England is similar in design to the tomographic systems of Kuhl and Edwards.[49] It consists of two opposed 4-in. detectors mounted on a U-shaped arm that straddles the patient. The mounting is such that the detectors are able to move perpendicular to the long axis of the patient and perform a single transverse scan. After each pass, the U-shaped arm is rotated 6 degrees. A total of 30 transverse scans are collected and stored for later reconstruction.

Data from this device are reconstructed into the tomographic images by the previously discussed method of filtered backprojection. The diameter of the tomographic slice can be either 27 cm for head images or 49 cm for body images. The scanning times for this instrument represent one of its most severe disadvantages. Dworkin reported scanning times ranging from 90 min for six slices of the liver to 45 min for three images of the heart.[50] This extended scanning time requires preliminary imaging with a conventional camera to optimize patient positioning so that lesions are not missed by the relatively thin tomographic slice.

The addition of more detectors reduces the scanning time but not enough to eliminate the need for the preliminary camera imaging. The physical characteristics of the Tomogscanner depend on the detector separation, which varies from 20 cm to 76 cm.[49] The FWHM at the center of the tomographic slice with a 30-cm separation is 15.5 mm. This increases to 26.5 mm with a 64-cm detector separation. The off-center resolution varies from 19 mm to 24.5 mm at 10 cm from the center. In tissue-equivalent material, the resolution is more constant, ranging from 19.5 mm to 22 mm FWHM.

The disadvantages of the Tomogscanner, which are shared by many ECT systems, are difficulty in positioning, reduced counting rate due to low sensitivity of the detector system, longer imaging times, necessity of screening patients for positioning information. The advantages, however, are an ability to provide quantitative information about isotope distribution, an ability to see behind areas of high activity, and for some selected cases, increased sensitivity and specificity.

A more complex scanning motion is performed by the Union Carbide 710 Brain Imager.[51] In this system, the scanner consists of twelve detectors mounted at 30°-increments around the patient (Fig. 6–27). The individual detectors execute a rectilinear scan in the plane of the tomographic slice as each index of the rectilinear scan moves the detector in or out from the patient. The direction of motion depends on the detector's angular position, with alternate detectors moving in and the others moving out. The effect of this scanning motion is to move the focal point of the focused collimators over the area covered by the tomographic slice.

This scanning motion obviates the need for the rotational motion required of other systems. Scanning times from 2 min to 5 min may be selected by the operator. The

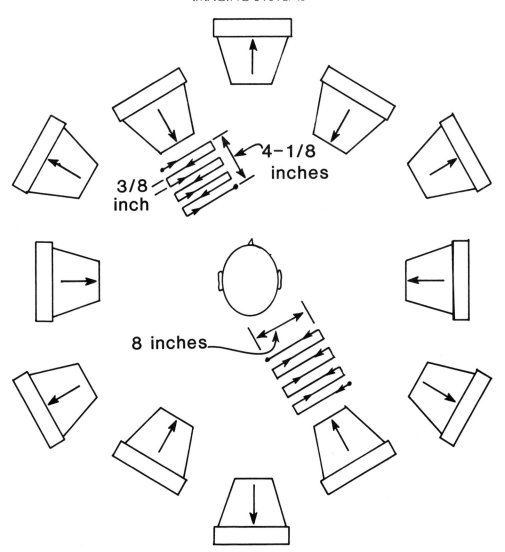

4–1/8 inches

3/8 inch

8 inches

Fig. 6–27. The Union Carbide 710 Brain Imager consists of twelve detectors that simultaneously execute the small rectilinear scan. Depth information for the tomographic slice is provided by focused collimators on each detector. (Adapted from Williams, L.E., et al.[51])

scanning area is a circle 20 cm in diameter, useful only in scanning heads. The detector shielding is sufficient for gamma-ray energies of up to 300 keV. The images are reconstructed by filtered backprojection following completion of the scan. After the first scan is completed image formation occurs simultaneously with collection of data for the second slice. Reconstruction time is 3 min. The images are displayed in a 128 × 128 format with a 16-level gray scale.

The spatial resolution of this system varies only 2% over the area of the tomographic slice and averages 9 mm for the image, and less processing is needed to reduce statistical noise to 11.5 mm. The correlation between pixel counts and the specific activity in the field of view is excellent and shows a sensitivity of approximately 200 counts/min/μCi.

Positron Tomography

When a positron is emitted from the nucleus of an atom, it travels only a short distance before combining with a free negative electron. This action produces two 511-keV annihilation photons, which move away from the point of annihilation in opposite directions at the speed of light. By placing two detectors on opposite sides of a positron-emitting source, the annihilation radiation can be detected as essentially simultaneous absorption of the gamma photons in the two detectors. If these detectors are scintillation cameras, it is possible to define a plane between them upon which the positron source must lie (Fig. 6–28).

Collecting many thousands of these coincidence events makes it possible to reconstruct images of the source distribution in the space between the detectors. Reconstructing these images is accomplished by selecting a plane of interest and assuming that a point source of activity lies on that plane at the point where the two an-

nihilation photons pass through it. Figure 6–28 shows the source distributions that would result by reconstructing planes at points A and B from the three annihilation events shown. The resulting image would show a single, denser point in plane A while the image would appear diffuse in plane B. Reconstruction of several serial planes permits reconstruction of the radionuclide distribution in these dimensions. One of the principal advantages of positron imaging is that the sensitivity of the imaging system is essentially independent of the position of the source in the space between the two detectors. This statement is true because as the source moves away from one of the detectors, it moves closer to the other. A second advantage of positron systems is that theoretically no physical collimation of the detectors is required to obtain the spatial resolution; thus high sensitivity is permitted. In prac-

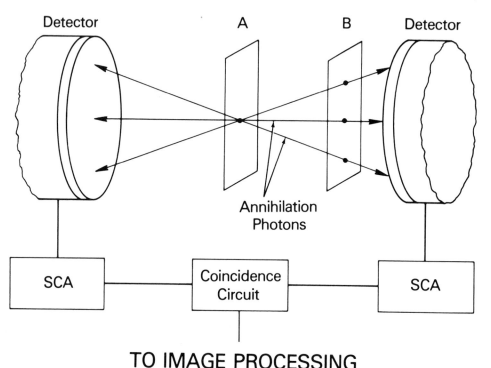

Fig. 6–28. A schematic representation of positron imaging by coincidence detection of the 511-keV annihilation gamma rays, showing the source distribution on two planes that could produce the detected events.

tice, however, some collimation is required to restrict the detection of non-coincidence events by either detector. These events result from several sources, including the scattering of one of the 511-keV gamma rays out of the field of view, the scatter within either detector crystal, and the cascade gamma rays emitted by the positron source. Noncoincidence events degrade the system response by increasing the deadtime of the system so that fewer of the coincidence gamma rays can be processed. They may also introduce spurious or pseudo-coincidence events. Spurious coincidence can be reduced further by pulse-height analysis, but only at the expense of increased deadtime.

Figure 6–29 illustrates some of the various detector configurations that have been devised for positron tomographic imaging.[53,54] The most straightforward design utilizes a low-resolution "focal detector" opposite the primary collimated scintillation camera.[55] This system provides adequate images on planes close to the primary imaging detector, but because of the lower resolution of the second detector, images of deeper planes within the patient suffer from degraded resolution. This design also suffers in that it is a serial system, that is, an event anywhere in the detector disables the system for the length of time it takes to process the event. Thus small amounts of activity, may overload the system. Furthermore, a 1-cm thick detector crystal in the primary imaging detector is only about 17% efficient for 511-keV photons.

Because of these limitations, other multidetector systems have been designed. Two of these, the hybrid positron scanner and the multicrystal-array positron camera, were designed and constructed at Massachusetts General Hospital by Brownell and his associates.[56] The hybrid positron scanner consisted of a total of 18 NaI(Tl) detectors arranged in two equal columns. Each of the nine crystals was paired with its direct opposite as well as

the two detectors on either side of its opposing detector. The entire detector assembly made four passes to form a 36-line rectilinear image of a 20 cm × 25 cm area.

To scan a larger area with short imaging times, a multidetector camera system was designed with two opposed arrays of 127 NaI(Tl) crystals each (Fig. 6–29B). Each crystal in this array is paired with its direct opposite and its 24 nearest neighbors for coincidence detection—a possibility of 2549 crystal pairs. This instrument has a resolution of 1 cm (FWHM) with a detector separation of 50 cm. The sensitivity of the system has been measured at 1000 counts/min/μCi. The positron imaging capabilities of the multicrystal-array positron camera have been clinically useful in imaging $^{13}NH_3$ and Ga-68 ATP distributions in the brain.[57]

To obtain transaxial images, the detectors of both the single-crystal and the multicrystal detector systems must be rotated. Because both of these detectors are two-dimensional imaging devices, introduction of more complicated motions into the imaging systems is unncessary.

The two detector configurations shown in parts C and D of Figure 6–29 were developed to increase sensitivity. The hexagonal ring configuration of Figure 6–29C is typical of the *positron emission transaxial tomographs* (PETT) series of positron scanners. This configuration was designed initially by Phelps, Ter-Pogossian, and Hoffman.[58] Each bank of detectors consists of 44 to 70 NaI(Tl) detectors that range from 7.5 cm to 17 cm in length in the axial direction with a 5-cm cross section, depending on the design of the individual system.

In collecting positron decay information, each detector in a given bank is coupled in coincidence with several detectors in the opposite detector bank. In this way, the spatial sampling resolution at any given detector position is increased. Because of the finite size of the individual detectors and therefore the limited num-

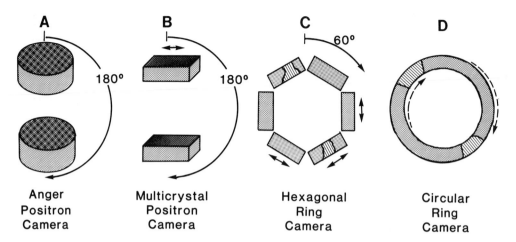

Fig. 6–29. Four detector configurations for positron emission tomography. (Adapted from Phelps, M.E., et al.[52])

ber of spatial samples obtainable, it is necessary to provide a small linear scanning motion to move the individual detector to slightly different positions throughout the imaging procedure. At the end of a short traverse (4 cm to 5 cm), the entire hexagonal gantry is rotated through an angle of 3 degrees, and the linear scan is repeated.

Images from the PETT scanners are produced by convolution processing similar to the transmission CT scanners and displayed on a CRT display (see Vol. II, Chap. 6). Spatial resolutions on the order of 0.9 cm to 2.5 cm FWHM are possible with this scanner design. A design similar to the PETT series is the ECAT scanner sold by Ortec. New scanners are continually being produced; the primary differences lie in changes in detector size, electronic design, and shielding for collimation. The one significant limitation that this "scan and increment" design has is the long imaging times, which make it difficult to perform serial scans when an isotope with a short half-life is used. Scanning times typically are in the range of several minutes. Attempts to overcome this handicap have led to the design of scanners with several rows of detectors in each bank. Thus it is possible to construct a scanner that contains four rows of detectors in each bank capable of producing up to seven separate transaxial slices simultaneously.

The fourth detector design is one in which a complete circle of detectors is used to define the image plane (Fig. 6–29D). The initial design contained 32 NaI(Tl) detectors in a circular array.[59] This system could acquire sufficient data for construction of a tomographic image of the brain in only 5 sec using Ga-68 EDTA. Since development of this first instrument, several others have been constructed along the same lines. Brooks described a system containing 128 bismuth germanate (BGO) detectors mounted in four rings and having an inside diameter of 38 cm.[60] This system can provide seven transaxial slices with a data acquisition time of only 1 sec and has a maximum counting rate capability of 1.5×10^6 cps.

As with the hexagonal ring detector array, the size of the detectors and the limitations on the associated electronics that can be supported by the circular ring design require the detector assembly to execute an auxiliary motion to increase the sampling resolution. This usually takes the form of a small oscillation of the detectors but can be accompanied by a short rotation of the entire ring.[61]

In general, positron imaging systems

suffer from a serious lack of information containing photons. The signal-to-noise ratio for clinical images can be increased somewhat by imaginative programming of the reconstruction algorithm, but such an increase is limited. Ter-Pogossian has described a data collection and reconstruction technique that includes the time-of-flight information about the photons in the production of the image.[62] When a positron undergoes annihilation, the two photons leave the point of annihilation in opposite directions. If the annihilation site is not precisely at the halfway point of the line separating the two detectors, one photon will take a slightly longer time to reach the farthest detector. With present-day electronics, time differences in detected events can be measured at subnanosecond (10^{-9}) levels. This enables the system to determine the source of an annihilation event to within 15 cm of the line midway between the two detectors. When this time-of-flight information is combined with the filtered backprojection reconstruction, the signal-to-noise ratio in the resultant images can be increased by a factor of approximately four.

QUALITY ASSURANCE OF IMAGING INSTRUMENTS

Both the correct functioning and the correct usage of instrumentation are important in considering quality assurance. This section examines some critical factors regarding the use of imaging equipment in the clinical laboratory as well as methods of measuring the equipment's physical characteristics.

Collimator Selection

All of the imaging devices described in this chapter, with the possible exception of some positron tomography systems, require the use of physical collimation to produce images. High-quality images depend on correct selection and use of collimation. The choice of collimator for rec-

tilinear scanners depends on the photon energy of the radionuclide used, the depth of the organ being imaged (i.e., the focal depth), and the spatial resolution desired. The choice of collimator for scintillation cameras depends on the gamma-ray energy, the resolution (or sensitivity) desired, and the organ size. The organ size may determine whether or not a converging or diverging collimator, or perhaps a pinhole collimator is selected.

As discussed earlier in this chapter, inherent in all collimators is an inverse relationship between spatial resolution and sensitivity. In theory, obtaining clinical images with the highest spatial resolution would be ideal. For statistical reliability, however, it is also important to have a sufficient number of photons. If it is impossible for the patient to remain stationary for the extended length of time required by a high-resolution collimator, some compromise must be made. Choosing appropriate collimation on the basis of resolution versus sensitivity is determined by clinical realities, and most likely there will be different decisions made for different laboratories and even for different patients undergoing the same examination.

Collimator choice based on photon energy seems more straightforward, except in the case of radionuclides that emit photons of more than one energy. This is not a problem if the photon of interest is the one with the highest energy. For example, Xe-133 emits photons of several energies, but only the highest-energy (81-keV) photon is used for organ imaging. The lower-energy photons in this case do not significantly affect the image, although they may limit the maximum counting rate because of coincidence losses. In the case of I-131, in which the 364-keV (82%) photon is of clinical interest, the 610-keV ($\sim$ 7%) photon must be considered in the design of the collimator. Failure to consider this photon results in significant degradation of organ images, because of septal penetration by the high-energy photons. Similarly, when Ga-67 is used, the presence of the photons at 300 keV (16%) and 394 keV (4%) must be recognized as possibly contributing to background, as a result of both septal penetration and scatter into lower-energy windows.

The overall spatial resolution R_o of the imaging system is given by the equation:

$$R_o = \sqrt{R_i^2 + R_s^2 + R_g^2}$$

where R_i is the intrinsic detector resolution, R_s is the scatter resolution, and R_g is the geometric resolution.[63]

For rectilinear scanners, the intrinsic resolution is effectively zero because the detector itself has no means of positioning a detected photon. The scintillation camera, however, has positioning circuitry, and the intrinsic resolution is directly related to photon energy. Geometric resolution tends to decrease with increasing gamma energy because of the additional lead required for collimation. In general, the higher the energy, the better the intrinsic resolution. From the preceding equation, it is apparent that there is a limit beyond which spatial resolution cannot be improved by physical collimation.

One aspect of collimator choice that has become important with the development of newer, thin-crystal cameras designed to maximize the resolution of Tc-99m is that these cameras may have significantly thinner shielding around the detector head. This is especially true of mobile cameras for which total instrument weight is a design consideration. The thinner detector shielding renders the use of the higher-energy isotopes more difficult. The high-energy photons of I-131 and Ga-67 penetrate the side of the detector head and contribute to the overall background. This problem cannot be controlled by the orientation of the head. With thicker shielding, the presence of other patients in the imaging area can be tolerated by appropriately positioning the patient being imaged so that the other activity sources are excluded from the field of view. This is not as effective with thinner shielding because the penetration is not a function of the collimator construction or position.

Energy-Window Selection

The choice of window setting is a trade-off of sensitivity to the primary photons versus the ability to discriminate against scattered photons. If a relatively wide energy window is used to increase sensitivity, then a proportionately larger number of scattered photons are accepted as valid events. Table 3–1 shows the scattering angle required to reduce the photon energy by 10%. This table indicates that for the most commonly used isotope, Tc-99m, photons scattered through an angle of up to 40° yield a photon of sufficient energy to fall within an energy window whose width is 20% of the photopeak energy of 140 keV. When the energy window is opened to increase the counting rate, much of the increase may come from the inclusion of scattered photons, which decreases resolution. While this trade-off would be advantageous for a first-pass cardiac study, it would not be appropriate for bone scanning.

One method of increasing sensitivity without a corresponding increase in scattered photons is to use an asymmetric energy window, adjusted so that its center is above the photopeak. Obviously, the amount of improved sensitivity is limited. Once the window includes all of the photopeak, no further increase in detection efficiency occurs with raising the upper-level discriminator. Asymmetric windows are effective for simple counting systems and for rectilinear scanners but less successful with scintillation cameras.[64] As shown in Figure 6–16, the energy spectrum produced by the scintillation camera is a composite of the individual spectra generated by each PM tube. Because it is difficult to align the PM tubes perfectly, an asymmetric energy window may exclude significant portions of the photopeaks from some tubes in the camera. This can result in a serious degradation in field uniformity.[65]

There is no question that the image contrast is increased by using an asymmetric window to exclude scatter, but the possibilities for image degradation are sufficiently great to prevent its becoming standard practice.

Deadtime

In most systems, the total amount of information lost because of instrument deadtime is a function of the counting rate. The amount of information lost because of deadtime should be negligible over the range of counting rates encountered in clinical studies.

Depending on their electronic configuration, counting systems are either nonparalyzable or paralyzable. In a nonparalyzable system the instrument is unable to respond for a fixed period of time following a detected event. At the termination of the processing time, the instrument becomes live and is able to process further interactions. The length of time for which the detector system is dead is independent of any events that may occur in the detector during the deadtime. In a paralyzable system, the length of time for which the system is dead depends on the number of events that occur during the processing time. The two types of systems are illustrated in Figures 3–6 and 3–7. These figures demonstrate that a paralyzable system can remain permanently unable to process data if the counting rate is sufficiently high.

Both the scintillation camera and the rectilinear scanner contain components with both types of deadtime characteristics.[21] This makes it difficult to characterize the response of these systems completely by measuring a single deadtime value at a single counting rate. For the sake of standardization and the ability to make comparisons between systems, however, the concept of a single deadtime value has become widely used. This problem is addressed further in the section "Scintillation Cameras."

With rectilinear scanners, if the system is operated at or near its counting rate limit, it becomes difficult to detect variations in the distribution of activity in the organ being imaged. In terms of a liver scan, for example, this effect could prevent the detection of low-contrast cold lesions in the liver. For this reason, it is inappropriate simply to increase the amount of activity given the patient to increase counting rate and reduce the imaging time. It is important to know the counting rate capability of the detector and to recognize its limitations in terms of expected increased counting rate with increased dose given to the patient.

Deadtime in camera systems causes fewer problems in static imaging, although the situation is the same as that for the rectilinear scanner, i.e., low-contrast cold lesions can be obscured by a counting rate that approaches instrument saturation. Another more serious problem, however, occurs when the scintillation camera is used for quantitative dynamic flow studies. Since the percentage of events that are lost depends on the counting rate, a larger percentage is lost at high than at low counting rates.[66] At high counting rates, the peak of the activity curve is distorted, even with the relatively modest deadtime. If the area under the curve is used for quantitative determinations, the deadtime strongly influences the results. In many instances, complete compensation for this limited response is impossible. Because of this, it is important to know the relationship between true and observed counts over the entire range of system operation.

Several innovative approaches to the reduction of deadtime have been introduced by various manufacturers. The multicrystal gamma camera originally devised by Bender and Blau was intended to increase sensitivity to medium- and high-energy gamma rays, e.g., those from I-131 and Ba-

137m.[30] The unique advantage of a multidetector system from the standpoint of deadtime is that the detector array is essentially a parallel detector system whereby only the single crystal in which an interaction takes place is affected. All other detectors remain in their unperturbed states and are able to accept and process photons. This causes a detector system to be limited by the electronics, not by the recovery time of the scintillation crystal as in the case of the Anger scintillation camera. The deadtime for the detector array is approximately 0.5 μsec.[67] Adding electronic processing and computer memory, however, increases the deadtime to approximately 2.25 μsec.

Several electronic innovations have been introduced by manufacturers of single-crystal scintillation cameras to reduce deadtime. In the normal operation of the camera, the summed output of the PM tubes is measured by the pulse-height analyzer, which determines the amount of energy deposited in the crystal. This determination is made under the assumption that the light output from the crystal was zero just prior to the interaction and that all the light resulting from each interaction is collected and processed. As the counting rate increases, this assumption may not remain valid. If the light in the detector does not decay to zero before the next event, pulse pileup results, with the consequent rejection of valid photons (see "Instrument Deadtime," Chap. 3). Baseline shift occurs when a second pulse falls on the "tail" of the preceding pulse. If the pulse height is insufficient to fall within the analyzer window, it is rejected.

Two common techniques to overcome these drawbacks of standard pulse-height analysis are (1) the use of a floating baseline for the pulse from the PM tubes and (2) a "leading-edge" technique that makes an early estimate of the pulse height based on an early determination of the rising slope of the pulse. These two techniques often are combined to decrease the effective deadtime of the single-crystal camera. In the floating baseline technique, the value of the electronic signal just prior to the initiation of a new pulse is remembered, and the determination of energy is made by the SCA based on this non-zero baseline. This technique allows the camera to process interactions that occur closer together than the decay time of the crystal/PM tube system and can significantly shorten the time required for a new interaction to be processed. In the leading-edge method of energy estimation, the initial slope of the pulse from the PM tubes is examined, and a decision is made on the likelihood of the pulse falling within the energy window. If the slope is too flat, the pulse is likely to fall below the window and if it is too steep, the pulse is likely to fall above the window. In either case, further processing of the pulse is discontinued, thus freeing the electronics to process the next pulse more quickly.

These two techniques are not without problems. Using the floating baseline makes it more difficult to determine accurately from the light output the position of the interaction because there is a practical limit to the ability to determine the beginning threshold light value precisely. Also, because the threshold is changing constantly throughout the pulse integration process, some assumptions are required regarding the characteristics of the decaying first pulse. Both of these effects reduce the spatial resolution of the camera operating in this mode. The problem with the slope-detection method of decreasing deadtime is that it makes it possible for valid counts to be discarded when the initial slope is relatively far from that expected. Fortunately, at the high counting rates encountered during use of these techniques, the percentage of counts lost because of misestimates of the predicted peak value is small compared to the increase in processed counts resulting from the decreased deadtime.

One major limiting factor in processing

counts to produce clinical images is the time required to move the electron beam of the display oscilloscope into the correct position. In older cameras, this required approximately 4 to 6 μsec. In some systems with large-display multiformat imaging devices, this time may reach 10 to 15 μsec. Since the determination of correct energy and position may require one μsec or less, any decrease in the display time will have an important effect on overall deadtime. One approach to correcting this problem is to provide analog buffers that can store several sets of coordinates in the order in which they occurred, so that if the display system is busy, subsequent events are remembered and displayed when the system becomes available again.

Instrumentation Quality-Control Procedures

There are numerous tests that can be performed on both rectilinear scanners and scintillation cameras to provide assurance of proper instrument operation. Because of the complexity of both of these devices, a single "best" testing procedure does not exist. Nor does any one test evaluate all aspects of instrument function. Several tests are described, all of which the operator should understand.

Rectilinear Scanners

Since the rectilinear scanner obtains it positional information by a combination of collimation and a comparatively simple mechanical motion, the routine quality-assurance tests deal primarily with the electronics that process the counting information. There are only a few routine tests that should be performed daily.[68] These tests provide the operator with a quantitative indication of the counting function. They are quantitative, however, only in the sense that they provide a numerical value that can be compared with similar values obtained over the previous days and weeks. None of the tests, by themselves, can be used to imply that the instrument is functioning according to factory specifications.

All nuclear counting equipment, scanners included, have a means of generating a simulated counting signal that can be used to test the timing and scaler operation. This "60-cycle" test signal generates at 60 cps simulated counting rate. The test can be performed each morning to check for correct operation of the scaler system. If the results deviate from the expected value, the scaler, timer, or signal source should be suspected of faulty functioning and must be checked.

Measurement of the peak-to-scatter or peak-to-total counts provides a determination of the correct operation of the crystal, PM tube, amplifier, and SCA. This value is determined by measuring the number of counts detected in a standard SCA window relative to the number detected by the system when the window is either disabled or opened as wide as possible. This measurement gives the operator an indication of the amount of scatter or nonphotopeak counts relative to the number of photopeak counts. Any gross change in the crystal, PM tube, amplifier, or SCA window changes the value of this ratio. This simple test can be easily performed every day with either a standard Cs-137 source or a small amount of the isotope being imaged. This value can be used only as an indication of change in the operational characteristics, not as an absolute indication of correct instrument operation.

Another test that should be performed every day is a standard scan of a stepwedge phantom, designed to produce counting rates at the photoplotter that range from zero to some maximum value. A scan of this phantom will indicate correct operation of the photodisplay or the device used for the production of the clinical images.

An alternative to daily testing is the use of a total-performance phantom that stresses the imaging abilities of the scanner. This phantom usually has the shape of a human organ, e.g., the brain or liver. Within the phantom are placed lesions of known size and position. These phantoms are available from a variety of sources, but the ones most commonly used are designed by the College of American Pathologists (CAP). The brain phantom designed by this group is a plastic construction containing 2-cm round lesions at depths ranging from 2.5 cm to 11.5 cm from the top surface. Use of the total-performance phantom to evaluate the scanner tests the machine's ability to make clinical images but does not provide quantitative measurements. Changes in any of the functions tested by the peak-to-total measurement and by the scan of the step wedges also produce changes in the image of the phantoms. Consequently, lesion-to-background contrast and the spatial resolution change, which changes the appearance of the marginally detectable lesions.

Note that both of the tests suggested for daily operational checks of the scanner involve the production of images, which must be processed by whatever method is used for routine clinical images. This is intentional since it is important to test operation of the entire image production system rather than merely some of its aspects.

Scintillation Cameras

Quality assurance for scintillation cameras is more complex than for rectilinear scanners. Not only must the nuclear counting electronics be evaluated, but the electronic positioning circuitry must also be tested. Determination of the position of photon interaction in the scintillation camera crystal is complex and is prone to error. Most errors made by the positioning electronics result in observable artifacts in the clinical image; these can be assessed by the routine quality-assurance tests. The artifacts generally fall into two categories: those that appear as mispositioned interactions and those that cause the detector to appear to have nonuniform sensitivity.

These image defects are present in all cameras to some degree. Currently, construction of a camera with perfectly uniform sensitivity and zero image distortion is impossible. Other such artifacts as those resulting from defects in the crystal or collimators usually can be detected without special testing or by the use of special phantoms.

Radiation Sources

All quality-assurance tests for scintillation cameras involve use of radioactive sources. Since a uniform response throughout the crystal area is essential, tests of detector uniformity must provide uniform irradiation. Several methods provide uniform irradiation of the detector. In most cases, there are no practical differences in results of tests performed with different sources if they are properly used.

Many institutions prefer to perform uniformity tests with the collimator in place to protect the crystal. In this case, an extended source distribution must be used. Two types of extended sources are available.[69] Commercial plastic sources loaded with Co-57 are easy to use because they do not have to be recharged every day, and the 122-keV photon of Co-57 is close enough to the 140 keV of Tc-99m to test for proper operation of the system. The operator should realize that Co-57 is reactor-produced and may be contaminated by Co-56 and Co-58, which emit 810-keV and 511-keV photons. If the images produced by one of these sources have defects otherwise unexplainable, the source should be examined carefully for uniformity and contamination.

The second distributed source is a water-filled disc to which is added 0.5 to 10 mCi of Tc-99m. The advantage of this source is that the amount of activity can be adjusted to individual situations. Since the total volume of the source may be as much as 2 l, there is no restriction regarding the specific activity of the added Tc-99m. The only restriction on such activity is that it should not be in the form of macroaggregated albumin, which tends to plate out onto the plastic in an irregular distribution. Obviously, care must also be taken to mix any added activity completely.

If the uncollimated detector is to be irradiated, a single point source can be used.[70] This may be either a small sealed vial or a syringe held in a special holder to allow it to be repositioned accurately after each use. Whenever the uncollimated detector is exposed, it must be protected to prevent physical damage to the crystal or contamination by radioactivity. Care must also be exercised to limit the technician's exposure to these sources.

Transmission Phantoms

Several transmission phantoms have been devised to assess camera operation (Figure 6–30).[70] They consist of regular arrays of lead absorbers, which are supported by Lucite plates and can be affixed to the detector face. These phantoms can be irradiated by any of the sources described, because they are thin and do not require an extended source when used with the uncollimated camera.

The four-quadrant bar phantom consists of four sets of lead bars with different spacings. The bar width is equal to the space between bars, and each set is perpendicular to the adjacent sets. The specific bar widths vary with manufacturers but range from 0.2 cm to 1.5 cm. This phantom was one of the first designed to measure the spatial resolution of scintillation cameras. Ideally, the phantom should have at least one set of bars that are marginally separable by the camera being evaluated. The fact that the bars extend only halfway across the detector limits this phantom's usefulness in examining the linearity of the camera.

The Hine-Duley phantom was designed to overcome the disadvantages of the quadrant phantom. This phantom consists of a series of parallel bars extending completely across the detector. It has five sets of bars with three different spacings. As with the quadrant phantom, the width of the bars and the separation vary according to manufacturer. The primary problem with this phantom is that the bars with minimal separation, which best test spatial resolution, cover only a small portion of the detector. On the other hand, spatial linearity is well evaluated, even though two images are required to examine both directions.

The parallel-line-equal-space (PLES) phantom was designed to evaluate spatial resolution over the entire detector area. This phantom consists of a single set of lead bars of equal width and spacing that cover the entire detector area. To evaluate cameras of different resolving capabilities, this phantom is sold in several line separations. The phantom must be imaged in two orientations to evaluate the detector capabilities completely, and it provides no variation in bar spacing.

Orthogonal-hole phantoms were designed to evaluate both resolution and linearity. The original design consists of an

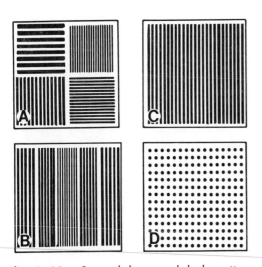

Fig. 6–30. Several bar- and hole-pattern phantoms used to evaluate gamma cameras. *A.* Quadrant. *B.* Hine-Duley. *C.* PLES. *D.* Orthogonal hole.

array of equal-sized round holes drilled in a lead sheet, which in turn is supported by a plastic sheet. The phantom is available in three hole sizes and separations. This phantom provides a solution to the problem of having to image bar phantoms in two directions to test both axes of the camera. The holes in the phantom are close enough together to allow the eye to estimate linearity from the row pattern. The symmetry of the array allows both axes to be evaluated simultaneously. This phantom suffers the same disadvantages, however, as the PLES phantom in that the size and separation of the holes must be chosen with the resolution of the camera in mind, since to test resolution adequately, the holes should be just barely detectable. Because of this disadvantage, a single laboratory may require two or more such phantoms if cameras with differing resolutions are to be tested.

A solution to this requirement is the Bureau of Radiological Health (BRH) phantom.[71] The structure of this phantom is similar to that of the Hine-Duley phantom. It consists of groups of holes 2.5 mm in diameter with the horizontal spacing varying between the groups. The vertical spacing is fixed at 5 mm center to center (2.5 mm edge to edge), while the horizontal spacing ranges from 4 mm center to center (1.5 mm edge to edge) in the center group of holes to 9.5 mm center to center (7.0 mm edge to edge) in the outer groups. Again, the difficulty with this phantom is that the finest resolution capability is tested in only a small region of the crystal.

Total-Performance Phantoms. There are three "total-performance" phantoms designed to evaluate global function of the scintillation camera. These phantoms permit subjective evaluations, not quantitative evaluations, and are best used for intercomparisons of imaging systems. The CAP phantom, the total-performance phantom discussed earlier, can also be used to evaluate scintillation cameras.[72] These are transmission phantoms into

which absorbers have been placed to simulate lesions. These phantoms eliminate the need for loading and handling a phantom with radioactivity; only a source is required. The Rollo phantom is an arrangement of spherical voids with varying amounts of surrounding radioactivity, which results in a known range of lesion sizes with a known object-to-background ratio. The range of lesion size and contrast ratios allows an estimate of effectiveness of an imaging device in the presence of realistic scatter conditions. Even though it is intended for evaluation of new devices and imaging techniques, the Rollo phantom can be used for routine camera evaluations less frequently than daily. It can be used beneficially on a semiannual or annual basis for a global test of the camera system.

The Mould liver phantom is a plastic model of the human liver that contains lesions of known size and position.[73] It is filled with radioactivity and may be placed in a large water bath to simulate scattering conditions in the patient. It is useful for monitoring camera operation in terms of image quality and scatter rejection.

Deadtime

As discussed earlier, scintillation cameras possess both paralyzable and nonparalyzable components, which prevent the use of a single deadtime value to describe the camera response completely. The protocol prescribed by the American Association of Physicists in Medicine (AAPM), however, permits a reasonable estimation of the camera response in patient studies as well as comparisons of camera operation with manufacturer specifications.[74]

Since the purpose of deadtime measurements is to obtain a parameter that has clinical significance, use of a source configuration that simulates clinical scatter conditions is important. The two-source method defined by the AAPM utilizes a special plastic source holder that simulates the scatter configuration encountered in cardiac studies. Two Tc-99m sources, R_1 and R_2, which individually produce counting rates of approximately 20,000 cps, are counted individually and combined (R_{12}). The background corrected counting rates are then used in the following formula:

$$\tau = \frac{2R_{12}}{(R_1 + R_2)^2} \cdot \ln \left[\frac{(R_1 + R_2)}{R_{12}} \right]$$

A counting rate at which a 25% loss in counts occurs can be calculated from the following equation:

$$R = \frac{.75}{\tau} \cdot \ln \left(\frac{100}{75} \right) = \frac{0.216}{\tau}$$

This value is important because at this rate a 2% increase in administered activity produces only a 1% increase in observed counting rate.

The peak counting rate attainable with the camera also depends on correct camera operation. This is measured by placing a source of approximately 500 μCi (18.5 MBq) of Tc-99m in front of the uncollimated detector. Starting with the source at some distance from the camera, the operator brings the source incrementally closer to the crystal. At each step, the counting rate is determined. The counting rate rises to a maximum and then falls as the source continues to be brought closer to the detector.

Sensitivity

Sensitivity is the ratio of counts recorded to the photons reaching the detector crystal. Sensitivity is a function of photon energy, crystal thickness, energy window setting, deadtime, and collimation. Most parameters that affect sensitivity are the camera's physical characteristics, which have been fixed during manufacturing. Deadtime, however, is one parameter that can change as the system ages or is modified. The sensitivity of the

camera should be measured at installation and periodically thereafter, e.g., at semiannual or annual intervals. The relative sensitivity of all collimators should be measured at installation. A method for measuring relative collimator sensitivity has been published by the AAPM.[74] This method consists of placing a calibrated source of radioactivity on the face of the collimated detector and measuring the counting rate obtained with each collimator. To avoid interference from the collimator septa, a distributed source configuration such as a flat bottom flask or Petri dish should be used. The total amount of radioactivity should be such that an insignificant number of counts are lost due to deadtime with the most sensitive collimator. The results of the measurements are expressed in counts/sec/μCi.

Uniformity and Linearity

Field uniformity and linearity measurements are routine quality-assurance tests that should be performed daily. In general, these tests are subjective, consisting of visual inspection of a high-quality image of the *flooded* detector with and without a transmission phantom. Both images can be collected by using either an extended source with the collimator in place or a point source of activity with the collimator removed (Fig. 6–31). The only requirement is that the tests be peformed in the same manner each day.

The presence of the field uniformity correction devices on modern cameras adds another aspect to the routine testing of uniformity and linearity. In some cameras, these devices can be disabled for testing, while in others, they cannot. One problem created by the presence of these correction devices is that they may hide a defect in the camera until it is so severe that the correction mechanism no longer compensates for it. If the correction device can be disabled, the flood should be examined at least weekly or biweekly with the device bypassed. This uncorrected image will

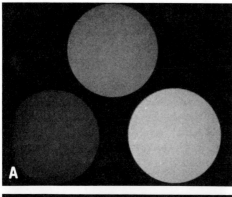

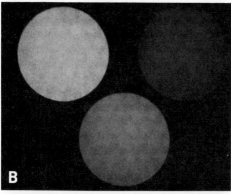

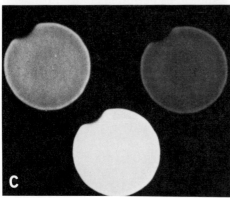

Fig. 6–31. Flood images showing a uniform field (A), inadequate gain adjustment resulting in accentuation of the PM tubes (B), and defect due to nonfunctioning PM tube (C).

monitor slow changes in detector response that are hidden by the correction device.

Linearity tends to change slowly with time and usually does not need monitoring on a daily basis. Any gross changes in linearity also affect uniformity and there-

fore do not go undetected. Weekly or biweekly tests of linearity are generally adequate for routine clinical operation. As cameras become used more intensely for single-photon emission tomography, the intervals between testing may need to be shortened because nonlinearities smaller than those that interfere with diagnoses from simple planar views cause artifacts in the reconstructed tomographic images.

Window Adjustment and Width

The calibration of the SCA window usually is not monitored except at installation or after a major repair of the nuclear counting circuitry. Accurate calibration requires the use of a multichannel analyzer.[74] Daily quality assurance, however, should include monitoring the SCA window setting to ensure that it is set to the appropriate position. It is possible for the preset windows on many newer cameras to drift slightly with time. When this occurs, service personnel should be notified.

Computer Assistance in Quality Control

Early applications of dedicated computers to quality assurance dealt primarily with nonuniformity in detector response. The initial approach consisted of applying correction functions to the clinical images. These functions were obtained by collecting a flood image and calculating a correction matrix to make the detector response uniform.[75,76] This method was not widely used in clinical practice, however, because nonuniformities were soon understood to arise primarily from mispositioning of photon interactions and only minimally from nonuniform sensitivity. Most modern uniformity correction is applied internally by altering the X and Y outputs from each PM tube.

The many parameters required to describe scintillation cameras completely make it difficult to characterize the daily quality-control test results by a single, or even two or three, numerical values. Several investigators have described computer processing techniques aimed at producing useful indicators of camera response.[77,78,79]

A more complete computerized program has been described by Hasegawa et al.[80] Sensitivity, spatial resolution, and spatial linearity all are determined from a single image of a specially constructed orthogonal-hole phantom. The algorithm searches the image to locate the counting peaks corresponding to the holes in the orthogonal phantom. Once the peaks are located, the computer calculates the FWHM to provide a measure of resolution. The variation of the detected peak locations from theoretical intersections of a perfect grid is used as an indication of linearity. Point-source sensitivity is provided by the amplitude of the individual peaks. All values generated by analysis of the test image are displayed in numerical and graphic form. The total evaluation time required is approximately 20 min.

REFERENCES

1. Cassen, B., et al.: Instrumentation for ^{131}I use in medical studies. Nucleonics, 9:46, 1951.
2. Newell, R.R., Saunders, W., and Miller, E.: Multichannel collimators for gamma-ray scanning with scintillation counters. Nucleonics, 10:36, 1952.
3. Harris, C.C., et al.: Collimators for radioisotope scanning. In Progress in Medical Radioisotope Scanning. Oak Ridge, TN, ORINS, 1962, p. 25.
4. Schultz, A.G., Knowles, L.G., Kohlenstein, L.C., et al.: Quantitative assessment of scanning-system parameters. J. Nucl. Med., 11:61, 1970.
5. Patton, J.A.: X-ray fluorescence imaging. In Imaging for Medicine. Vol. 1. Edited by S. Nudelman and D.D. Patton. New York, Plenum Press, 1980.
6. Cederlund, J.: Information theory and radioisotope scanning. In Medical Radioisotope Scanning. Vol. 1. Vienna, IAEA. 1964.
7. Johnson, P.M., Esser, P.D., and Lister, D.B.: Fluorescent thyroid imaging: Clinical evaluation of an alternative instrument. Radiology, 130:219, 1979.
8. Hoffer, P.B., Jones, W.B., Crawford, R.B., et al.: Fluorescent thyroid scanning: A new method of imaging the thyroid. Radiology, 90:342, 1968.
9. Patton, J.A., Hollifield, J.W., Brill, A.B., et al.: Differentiation between malignant and benign solitary thyroid nodules by fluorescent scanning. J. Nuc. Med., 17:17, 1976.
10. Anger, H.O.: A New Instrument for Mapping Gamma-Ray Emitters. Biology and Medicine Quarterly Report UCRL-3653. Washington, D.C., 1957.
11. Anger, H.O.: Radioisotope cameras. In Instrumentation in Nuclear Medicine. Edited by G.J. Hine. New York, Academic Press, 1967.
12. Patton, J.A., Rollo, F.D., and Brill, A.B.: Recent advances in nuclear medicine instrumentation. IEEE Trans. Nucl. Sci., NS-27:1066, 1980.
13. Hine, G.J., and Erickson, J.J.: Advances in scintigraphic instruments. In Instrumentation in Nuclear Medicine. Edited by G.J. Hine and J.A. Sorenson. New York, Academic Press, 1974.
14. Tinkel, J.B., and Barbiere, J.C.: Collimators: Theory and practice. Picker J. Nucl. Med., 2:6, 1981.
15. Kuhl, D.E.: Physical principles of radionuclide scanning. In Principles of Nuclear Medicine. Edited by H.H. Wagner, Jr. Philadelphia, W.B. Saunders, 1968.
16. Wolff, J.R.: Calibration methods for scintillation camera systems. In Quantitative Organ Visualization in Nuclear Medicine. Edited by P.J. Kenny and E.M. Smith. Coral Gables, FL, University of Miami Press, 1971.
17. Sano, R.M., and Tinkel, J.B.: Consequences of crystal thickness reduction on gamma camera resolution and sensitivity. J. Nucl. Med., 19:712, 1978.
18. Beck, R.N., et al.: Effects of scattered radiation on scintillation detector response. In Medical Radioisotope Scintigraphy. Vol. 1. Vienna, IAEA, 1969.
19. Sanders, T.P., Sanders, T.D., and Kuhl, D.E.: Optimizing the window of an Anger camera for [99m]Tc. J. Nucl. Med., 12:703, 1971.
20. Murphy, P., Arseneau, R., Maxon, E., Thompson, W.: Clinical significance of scintillation camera electronics capable of high processing rates. J. Nucl. Med., 18:175, 1977.
21. Sorenson, J.A.: Deadtime characteristics of Anger cameras. J. Nucl. Med., 16:284, 1975.
22. Muehllehner, G., Jaszcyak, R.J., and Beck, R.M.: The reduction of coincidence loss of radionuclide imaging cameras through the use of composite filters. Phys. Med. Biol., 19:504, 1974.
23. Beck, R.N.: A theory of radioisotope scanning systems. In Medical Radioisotope Scanning. Vol. 1. Vienna, IAEA, 1964.
24. Genna, S., Pang, S., and Smith, A.: Digital scintigraphy: Principles, design, and performance. J. Nucl. Med., 22:365, 1981.
25. Mallard, J.R., and Wilks, R.J.: The Aber-gammascope. An image intensifier gamma camera. In Medical Radioisotope Scintigraphy. Vol. 1. Vienna, IAEA, 1969.
26. Moody, N.G., Paul, W., and Joy, M.K.G.: A Survey of Medical Gamma-Ray Cameras. Proc. IEEE, 58:217, 1970.
27. Ter-Pogossian, M.M., et al.: An image tube scintillation camera for use with radioactive isotopes emitting low-energy photons. Radiology, 69:463, 1966.
28. Kellershohn, C., Degrez, A., and Lansiart, A.J.: Deux nouveau types de detecteurs pour camera

a rayons X ou γ. *In* Medical Radioisotope Scanning. Vol. 1, Vienna, IAEA, 1964.

29. Mulder, H., and Pauwels, E.K.J.: A new nuclear medicine scintillation camera based on image-intensifier tubes. J. Nucl. Med., *17*:1008, 1976.
30. Bender, M.A., and Blau, M.: The autofluoroscope. Nucleonics, *21*:52, 1963.
31. Urie, M.M., Mauderli, W., Fitzgerald, L.T., and Williams, C.M.: Rotating laminar emission camera with GE detector: Experimental results. Med. Phys., *8*:865, 1981.
32. Mauderli, W., Fitzgerald, L.T., and Urie, M.M.: Rotating laminar emission camera with GE detector: An analysis. Med. Phys., *8*:871, 1981.
33. Anger, H.O.: Tomographic techniques. *In* Instrumentation in Nuclear Medicine. Edited by G.J. Hine and J.A. Sorenson. New York, Academic Press, 1974.
34. McRae, J., and Anger, H.O.: Clinical results from the multiplane tomographic scanner. *In* Tomographic Imaging in Nuclear Medicine. Edited by G.S. Freedman, New York, Society of Nuclear Medicine, 1973.
35. Chang, L.T., MacDonald, B., and Perez-Mendez, V.: Axial tomography and three dimensional image reconstruction. IEEE Trans. Nucl. Sci., NS-*23*:568, 1976.
36. Vogel, R.A., Kirch, D., LeFree, M., et al.: A new method of multiplanar emission tomography using a seven pinhole collimator and an Anger scintillation camera. J. Nucl. Med., *19*:648, 1978.
37. Rollo, F.D., and Patton, J.A.: Perspective on seven pinhole tomography. J. Nucl. Med., *21*:888, 1980.
38. Rogers, W.L.: The pseudorandom time modulated aperture. An algebraic description. *In* Emission Computed Tomography: The Single Photon Approach. HHS publication. FDA 81-8177, 1981, p. 133.
39. Keyes, J.W.: Tomographic applications: Thyroid and facial bones. *In* Emission Computed Tomography: The Single Photon Approach. HHS publication. FDA 81-8177, 1981, p. 141.
40. Rogers, W.L., Han, K.S., Jones, L.W., and Bierwalter, W.H.: Use of Fresnel zone plate for gamma imaging. J. Nucl. Med., *13*:612, 1972.
41. Budinger, T.F., and MacDonald, B.: Reconstruction of the Fresnel-coded gamma camera images by digital computer. J. Nucl. Med., *16*:309, 1975.
42. Budinger, T.F.: Physical attributes of single photon tomography. *In* Emission Computed Tomography: The Single Photon Approach. HHS Publication. FDA 81-8177, 1981, p. 6.
43. Budinger, T.F., Derenzo, S.E., Gullberg, G.T., et al.: Emission computed axial tomography. J. Comp. Assist. Tomog., *1*:31, 1977.
44. Brooks, R.A., and DiChiro, G.: Image reconstruction in computed tomography. Radiology, *117*:561, 1975.
45. Budinger, T.F.: Physical attributes of single-photon tomography. J. Nucl. Med., *21*:579, 1980.
46. Gulberg, G.T., and Budinger, T.F.: The use of filtering methods to compensate for constant attenuation in single photon emission computed tomography. IEEE Trans. Biom. Eng., BME-*28*:142, 1981.
47. Tertiak, O.J., and Metz, C.: The exponential radon transform. SIAM. J. Appl. Math., *39*:2, 1981.
48. Kuhl, D.E., and Edwards, R.Q.: Image separation radioisotope scanning. Radiology, *30*:653, 1963.
49. Elliott, A.T., Hanson, M.E., and Britton, K.E.: Tomogscanner 2S technical evaluation. *In* Emission Computed Tomography: The Single Photon Approach. HHS publication. FDA 81-8171, 1981, p. 211.
50. Dworkin, H.J.: Initial impressions of whole body tomographic scanning. *In* Emission Computed Tomography: The Single Photon Approach. HHS Publication. FDA 81-8177, 1981, p. 199.
51. Williams, L.E., Loken, M.K., Cook, A.M., et al.: Physical characteristics of the Union Carbide 710 brain imager. *In* Emission Computed Tomography: The Single Photon Approach. HHS publication. FDA 81-8177, 1981, p. 245.
52. Phelps, M.E., Hoffman, E.J., Huang, S.C., and Kuhl, D.E.: IEEE Trans. Nucl. Sci., NS-*26*:2746, 1979.
53. Phelps, M.E.: Emission computed tomography. Semin. Nucl. Med., *7*:337, 1977.
54. Brownell, G.L., Correia, J.A., and Zamenhof, R.G.: Positron instrumentation. Rec. Ad. Nucl. Med., *1*:1, 1978.
55. Aronow, S.: Positron scanning. *In* Instrumentation in Nuclear Medicine. Edited by G.J. Hine. New York, Academic Press, 1967.
56. Brownell, G.L., and Burnham, C.H.: Recent developments in positron scintigraphy. *In* Instrumentation in Nuclear Medicine. Edited by G.J. Hine and J.A. Sorenson. New York, Academic Press, 1974.
57. Hoop, B., et al.: Techniques for positron scintigraphy of the brain. J. Nucl. Med., *17*:473, 1976.
58. Phelps, M.E., Hoffman, E.J., Mullani, N.A., et al.: Transaxial emission reconstruction tomography: Coincidence detection of positron-emitting radionuclides. *In* Non-Invasive Brain Imaging Computed Tomography and Radionuclides. Edited by H. DeBlanc and J.A. Sorensen. New York, Society of Nuclear Medicine, 1975.
59. Robertson, J.S., Marr, R.B., Rosenblum, B., et al.: Thirty-two crystal positron transverse section detector. *In* Tomographic Imaging in Nuclear Medicine. Edited by G.S. Freedman. New York, Society of Nuclear Medicine, 1973.
60. Brooks, R.A., Sank, U.J., DiChiro, G., et al.: Design of a high resolution positron emission tomograph. The neuro-PET. J. Comp. Assist. Tomog., *4*:5, 1980.
61. Kanno. I., Uenrura, K., Muira, S., and Muira, Y.: HEADTOME: A hybrid emission tomograph for single photon and positron emission imaging of the brain. J. Comp. Assist. Tomog., *5*:216, 1981.
62. Ter-Pogossian, M.M., Mullani, N.A., Ficke, D.C., et al.: Photon time-of-flight assisted positron emission tomography: J. Comp. Assist. Tomog., *5*:227, 1981.
63. Beck, R.N.: The scanning system as a whole: General considerations. *In* Fundamental Problems in

Scanning. Edited by A. Gottschalk and R.N. Beck. Springfield, IL, Charles C. Thomas, 1968.

64. Rollo, F.D., and Schulz, A.G.: Effect of pulse height selection on lesion detection performance. J. Nucl. Med., *12*:690, 1971.

65. Rollo, F.D., and Harris, C.C.: Factors affecting image formation. *In* Nuclear Medicine Physics, Instrumentation and Agents. Edited by F.D. Rollo. St. Louis, C.V. Mosby, 1977.

66. Budinger, T.F.: Clinical and research quantitative nuclear medicine system. *In* Medical Radioisotope Scintigraphy. Vienna, IAEA, 1972.

67. Grenier, R.P., Bender, M.A., and Jones, R.H.: A computerized multi-crystal scintillation gamma camera. *In* Instrumentation in Nuclear Medicine. Edited by G.J. Hine and J.A. Sorenson. New York, Academic Press, 1974.

68. MacIntyre, W.J., Flynn, M.J., and Wegst, A.V.: Quality assurance of testing of rectilinear scanners. *In* Quality Control in Nuclear Medicine. Edited by B.A. Rhodes. St. Louis, C.V. Mosby, 1977.

69. Paras, P., VanTuinen, R.J., and Hamilton, D.R.: Quality control for scintillation cameras. *In* Quality Control in Nuclear Medicine. Edited by B.A. Rhodes. St. Louis, C.V. Mosby, 1977.

70. Rollo, F.D.: Quality assurance in nuclear medicine. *In* Nuclear Medicine Physics, Instrumentation and Agents. Edited by F.D. Rollo. St. Louis, C.V. Mosby, 1977.

71. Paras, P., Hine, G.J., and Adams, R.: BRH Test pattern for the evaluation of gamma-camera performance. J. Nucl. Med., *22*:468, 1981.

72. Hermann, G.A.: Imaging quality control program. J. Nucl. Med., *16*:957, 1975.

73. Mould, R.F.: A liver phantom for evaluating camera and scanning performance in clinical practice. Br. J. Radiol., *44*:810, 1971.

74. American Association of Physicists in Medicine Report No. 6: Scintillation Camera Acceptance Testing and Performance Evaluation. New York, American Institute of Physics, 1980.

75. Morrison, L.M., Bruno, F.P., and Mauderli, W.: Sources of gamma-camera image inequalities. J. Nucl. Med., *12*:785, 1971.

76. Bruno, F.P., Morrison, L.M., Mauderli, W., et al.: Computer-generated correction of non-uniform detector response of a gamma camera. J. Nucl. Med., *11*:623, 1970.

77. Hattner, R.S., and Kaufman, L.: An algorithm for mapping and quantitating the uniformity of a radionuclide distribution using a scintillation camera and a small digital computer. J. Nucl. Med., *15*:534, 1975.

78. Cox, N.J., and Diffey, B.L.: A numerical index of gamma-camera uniformity. Br. J. Radiol., *49*:734, 1976.

79. Cohen, G., and Keriakas, J.G., Padikal, I.N., et al.: Quantitative assessment of field uniformity for gamma cameras. Radiology, *118*:197, 1976.

80. Hasegawa, B.H., Kirch, D.L., DeFree, M.T., et al.: Quality control of scintillation cameras using a minicomputer. J. Nucl. Med., *22*:1075, 1981.

Chapter 7

COMPUTER SYSTEMS

STEPHEN BACHARACH AND
MICHAEL LINCOLN

Computers used in medicine perform a wide range of operations, from the control of simple instruments to reconstruction of tomographic images from complex physical data. In many instruments, the computer's existence is unknown or transparent to the user, and properly so, for devices should be designed so that the user can operate them correctly without knowing the details of their inner workings. The operation of computers that control most instruments needs to be understood no more than the principles of solid-state electronics need to be understood to play a transistor radio. Such underlying principles can be ignored, however, only when use of the instrument is well defined. This condition is not met by the computers used to collect and process images in nuclear medicine. As yet, there are no standard methods for processing and analyzing computer-acquired studies. Nor are there standard methods for acquiring data. It is not yet known how to make full use of the information contained in the digitized images of nuclear medicine.

In nuclear medicine, computers are used to acquire and manipulate data (images), which ultimately are assessed in a subjective way by clinicians. Several methods can be used to acquire and ma-

nipulate images. A good computer system allows considerable flexibility in the acquisition, processing, and display of images. Such flexibility in turn requires the user to understand how these different functions affect the data.

In the first section of this chapter, use of the computer as an instrument is discussed, and attention is given to the associated devices (*hardware)* essential to its operation. The remaining sections discuss *software*—that is, the programs used to acquire and process data.

OVERVIEW

The nuclear medicine computer system is made up of several major components, each of which may be considered independently (Fig. 7–1). Although not all systems contain every peripheral device shown in Figure 7–1, every system must contain the five basic elements shown: a module for *data acquisition*, a module for *mass storage,* a module for *image display,* a *computer,* and a *keyboard terminal.* The three modules are connected to the computer, which the user controls through the keyboard terminal.

Data produced by an imaging system (usually an Anger scintillation camera)

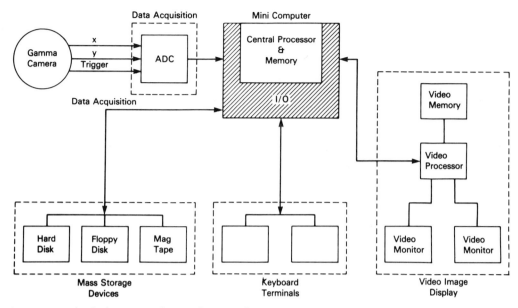

Fig. 7–1. Block diagram of a nuclear medicine computer system.

must first be digitized, i.e., converted to numbers, before being passed to the computer. This conversion is performed by the analog-to-digital converter (ADC) shown in Figure 7–1. The converted data are accepted by the input/output (I/O) circuitry of the computer. The *central processor unit* (CPU) of the computer then decides (under the user's direction) what to do with the data. The data can be stored temporarily in the computer memory, processed further by the CPU, transferred to disks or magnetic tape for long-term storage, or passed to the video processor for display on a television monitor. The components necessary to perform each of these tasks are discussed in detail in the following sections.

CAMERA-COMPUTER INTERFACE[1,10]

Digital computers operate only on numeric data. Therefore, the first step in acquiring a nuclear medicine image is to convert the image into a pattern of numbers. This process is referred to as *digitizing* the image and is performed by the ADC.

The elements of a nuclear image that determine the design and operation of the ADC should be considered first. An analog nuclear medicine image consists of a two-dimensional array of dots, similar to those in newsprint images. The dot density is proportional to the regional concentration of the radionuclide within the organ scanned (Fig. 7–2). The computer organizes these data into a digital image, which is divided into a square grid or matrix in the camera field of view. Each square in the grid is called a *picture element,* or *pixel.* For each gamma ray detected within the detector, the corresponding pixel value is incremented by one digit. This process is illustrated in Figure 7–2, in which the gamma camera field is divided into an array of 8 × 8 pixels. For a variety of reasons (e.g., limitations in computer memory size, computing speed, the resolution of the camera), typical matrix sizes range from 32 × 32 to 128 × 128.

Data produced by the Anger camera consist of two analog signals X and Y, and a third logic signal called the *trigger pulse.* The X and Y signals are *analog signals* because their amplitudes are the analog of

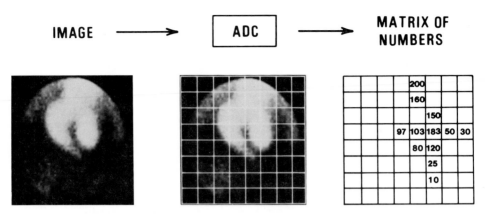

Fig. 7–2. Digitization of an image. The field of view of the scintillation camera is divided into a matrix, here illustrated 8 × 8 for simplification.

(i.e., proportional to) the X and Y coordinates of the location of the detected gamma ray. The trigger signal is the output of the energy window of the gamma camera. It is a *logic signal* rather than an analog signal because its amplitude carries no information; it is simply generated (if a gamma ray is within the selected energy window) or not generated (if the gamma ray's energy is outside the window).

Each gamma ray striking the detector produces these three signals if its energy is within the selected window. These signals are directed to the ADC. Whenever the ADC senses a trigger pulse, it converts (digitizes) the accompanying X and Y signals into a pair of numbers that are the X and Y coordinates of the pixel in the digital image. Usually, two ADCs are used: one for X and one for Y.

Several techniques can be employed to perform the digital conversion. These techniques must be rapid enough to convert one signal pair before the next signal pair arrives from the camera. If a second signal pair arrives while the ADCs are still converting a previous signal, the second signal pair may be missed, which contributes to the system deadtime. Ideally, ADC deadtime should be shorter than the most closely spaced pulses that the gamma camera is capable of producing (typically a few microseconds). One fast method for per-

forming the conversion is called the *successive approximation* method. A basic form of this method is illustrated in Figure 7–3. An analog *comparator* circuit is used to compare the X or Y signal to a list of voltages generated by a resistor network. In the figure, the signal voltage is compared to a voltage selected from a set of 256 voltages (typically the middle value—the 128th voltage in the example of Figure 7–3). Thus the value 128 serves as the first approximation of the digital value of the signal. If the comparator circuit discovers that the signal voltage is greater than the selected voltage, a new value is selected from the list. This new estimate would be halfway between the first estimate (128) and the maximum (256). This series of approximations is repeated eight times, and each time, the new value selected from the table approximates the true value more closely.

THE COMPUTER[1,2,4,5,9,10]

The computer in most nuclear medicine systems is composed of three basic sections: the I/O circuit, the memory, and the CPU (Fig. 7–1). The I/O module transfers information to and from various peripheral devices (the ADC, disks, terminals, etc.). The computer memory is divided up into discrete locations for storing num-

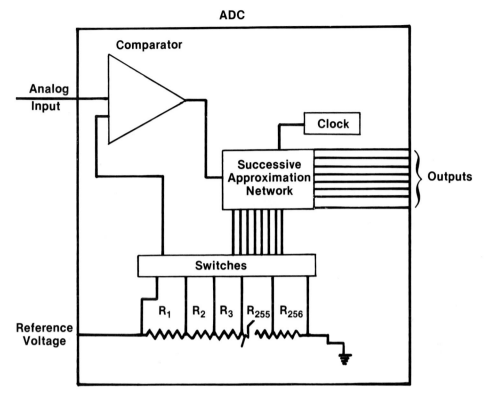

Fig. 7–3. Analog-to-digital converter. The analog voltage is compared to a series of voltages from the reference resistor network, using a binary search algorithm. The output is a binary number proportional to the input voltage amplitude.

bers. Each storage location is called a *word* of computer memory. The memory can be used to store any numeric data of interest. For example, each of the numbers comprising the pixels of a digitized image may be stored temporarily in a separate word of memory. Computer memory is also used to store *programs,* that is, lists of instructions (each represented by a number) that the user wishes the computer to carry out.

Cost and design constraints limit the number of words of memory in a computer. The size, i.e., the largest numeric value, of each word is also limited. The need for a size limit becomes obvious if the problem of storing numbers on a pad of paper is considered. If each number falls in the range of 0 to 99, only two digits are required to "store" each number by writing it on the paper. If the numbers are

allowed to be as large as 9999, four digits are required, which uses more storage space (room on the paper) than if only two digits are allowed. By virtue of the binary system in which the computer stores numbers, the largest number that can be stored in a word of the computer's memory is usually 65,535, or $(2^{16}-1)$. Therefore, the largest number of counts that can occur at a single pixel is limited to 65,535. Usually, this limitation does not cause any difficulty, except perhaps when imaging small objects containing high concentrations of radioactivity (e.g., a "hot" syringe), which result in many counts within a small number of pixels.

Because the number of words in the computer memory is limited, storage of not one number but two numbers in each word is frequently desirable. Each half-word of memory is called a *byte* of memory and can store a number only as large as 255 (2^8–1). At first, it might seem that a half-word should be able to store a number half as large as a full word. That this is not so can be understood from the previous example of writing a number on paper. With a word capable of holding four digits, a number as large as 9999 can be stored, while with a half-word capable of holding only two digits, a number only as large as 99 can be stored.

This example differs from computer words, however, in that the computer uses not a decimal numbering system, but a binary numbering system. The digits of the binary system (called *bits,* for *bi*nary dig*its)* are not powers of 10 but powers of 2. If the pixels of an image are stored in bytes, only half as much memory is needed, allowing, for example, twice as many images to be stored in the computer memory at once. The 255 count maximum of each byte may pose problems, however. Consider the image of a 2 million count flood field. When this field is digitized as a 128 × 128 matrix (16,384 pixels), each pixel contains approximately:

$$\frac{2,000,000 \text{ counts}}{16,384 \text{ pixels}} = 122 \text{ counts per pixel}$$

This number of counts can indeed be stored in 1 byte. If a 64 × 64 matrix is used instead, the same 2 × 10^6 count flood produces approximately 488 counts in each pixel, a number too large to store as a byte. In this case, a full word of storage must be used for each pixel.

The third computer component is the CPU. The CPU can be thought of as the "brains" of the computer. It is used to control all I/O operations, to manage the use of the memory, and to perform arithmetic (addition, multiplication, etc.) and logic operations (e.g., comparisons for equality) on data stored in memory. These arithmetic and logic tasks usually can be performed on the order of 10^6 operations per sec. Such data manipulations as tomo-

graphic reconstructions and certain image enhancing techniques require even greater computation speed than the CPU can provide. In these special instances, incorporation of hardware modules that speed computations may be desirable. Two devices commonly used for this purpose are the *floating point processor,* which greatly speeds the performance of noninteger arithmetic calculations, and the *array processor,* which allows image filtering (used for tomographic reconstruction) to be performed at high speed.

Mass Storage Devices[9,10]

Usually, digitized images, programs, and other useful data are stored temporarily in memory, in either byte or word mode. Because memory size is limited (and expensive), and because the memory is erased when the power is turned off, it is unsuitable for long-term data storage. The most common device for storage of images is a magnetic disk. There are two kinds of magnetic disks: *hard* and *flexible* (or *floppy*). A disk storage system consists of two parts: the disk itself (similar in shape to a phonograph record), on which data is stored, and the disk drive (analogous to a phonograph player), which is the device used to read from or record onto the disk.

Hard disks are available in many capacities. Popular storage sizes range from ten megabytes to hundreds of megabytes. The number of images that can be stored on a disk can be determined from the matrix size of each image and from the disk capacity. For example:

10 megabyte disk = 5 × 10^6 words
If image size = 64 × 64 (word mode)
= 4096 words/image

Then the image capacity is:

$$= \frac{5,000,000 \text{ words}}{4096 \text{ words/image}}$$

≈ 1220 (64 × 64) word mode images

This value is an upper limit, because

frequently the disk is also used to store data other than images. Another important consideration is the length of time required to retrieve data, once stored. Images stored on hard disks typically require tens of milliseconds to retrieve.

Hard disks, then, allow rapid access to a large volume of data stored in a reasonably small space. The disk and disk drive are quite fragile; they are sensitive to shocks (mechanical and thermal) and to the presence of dust and particulate matter (e.g., smoke). For this reason, the disk itself is most commonly an integral part of a protective plastic container, called a *disk pack*, the whole of which may be inserted into the disk drive.

There are two kinds of hard disks: fixed and removable. In removable disks, the disk pack can be removed from the disk drive. When a disk pack has been filled with images, it is removed from the disk drive and stored on a shelf, and a new disk pack is inserted. This is expensive, as each 10-megabyte disk pack may cost from $50 to $100; a larger-capacity disk pack costs much more. On the other hand, a fixed disk (sometimes called a *Winchester disk*) does not separate from the drive. It is, however, less expensive to manufacture, and since the unit (disk pack and drive) can be sealed in an airtight and dust-tight enclosure, it is less prone to environmental damage.

Floppy Disks

The floppy disk units also consist of two parts: a disk drive and the "diskette" on which the data is actually stored. Diskettes are removable and can store one-half to one million bytes of information. Floppy disks are much slower than hard disks; it may take the computer some seconds to read an image from them. Both floppy disk drives and diskettes are considerably less expensive than hard disks. Floppy disks are much less subject to environmental and mechanical damage. They are typically stored not in a bulky case, as are hard disks, but in a plastic jacket. On a "per word" basis, floppy disks cost roughly the same as fixed disks. Their small size (both physically and in terms of storage capacity) makes them convenient for storing patient images. A series of gated cardiac images obtained from one subject are easily stored on a single floppy disk.

Video Display[1,6,10,11]

The video display device is specialized in the nuclear medicine computer. Usually, the display is controlled by a separate microcomputer with its own memory (the video memory) and limited processing capabilities. For example, the ability to vary the background and brightness scales continuously without affecting the stored, raw data is desirable. Furthermore, the ability to display cyclic images in an endless loop or "movie" format is important and is best accomplished without having to access the disk memory repeatedly. Color displays are often incorporated to highlight certain features of an image (see Chapter 23).

Hardware Considerations and Digital Resolution

When digitizing a gamma camera image with an ADC, the user must first select an appropriate "digital resolution," i.e., the size matrix into which the camera field of view is divided. Digital resolution usually is expressed in units of pixels per centimeter in both the horizontal and vertical directions. Digital resolution can also be expressed as a *pixel density,* or the number of pixels spread over the field of view divided by the field area. In this case, the units of resolution are pixels per square centimeter.

Sometimes, the digital resolution is stated misleadingly as simply the size matrix into which the image is divided, for example, a "64 × 64" resolution. Usually, this means that the field of view is divided into a matrix of 64 pixels × 64 pixels (4096 in all). The corresponding digital resolution is ambiguous unless the camera field of view is known. A 64 × 64 image represents different resolutions for large and standard field of view cameras (Table 7–1).

After the ADC digitizes the image into a matrix, the computer must store the array of numbers in its memory. From Table 7–1, a 32 × 32 image uses 4 times less memory than a 64 × 64 image, since the former contains 4 times fewer pixels as the latter. Because computer memory is limited, the digital resolution (and hence the matrix size) is chosen with care.

How does the user determine the proper digital resolution for a particular study? The answer, as often happens in nuclear medicine, involves a trade-off between good spatial resolution and high counting statistics. For a given total number of counts, the higher the digital resolution, the smaller the number of counts at each pixel. If counting statistics are not the limiting factor, a good rule of thumb is to estimate first the resolution expected from the camera and collimator (including the effects of scatter and finite patient-to-collimator distance). This resolution distance then should be spanned by about 3 to 5 pixels so that further resolution is not lost by the digitization process. Thus a camera and collimator capable of 1-cm resolution would require a digital resolution of 3 to 5 pixels per cm to avoid loss of resolution from digitization. A resolution much higher than this provides little further information, uses much more computer memory, and results in poorer statistics at each pixel. A digital resolution significantly lower than this may fail to reproduce adequately the information present in the original image. The "gamma camera resolution" referred to here is not the "intrinsic camera resolution" but rather some more realistic estimate of the camera's actual ability to distinguish objects under the conditions of scatter, limited counts, and background present in the image under consideration. For most gated cardiac blood pool images, this resolution would be worse than 1 cm.

Analog Zoom

Frequently, the matrix sizes listed in Table 7–1 do not permit optimal digital resolution. For example, a gated cardiac image may require a matrix larger than 64 × 64 to avoid a scalloped ventricular wall. Computer memory, however, may be insufficient to accomodate a fourfold larger 128 × 128 matrix. In such cases, the *analog zoom* feature on most computers is used to magnify a small part of the image (e.g., the cardiac chambers) and to digitize only selected areas of the image rather than the entire field of view. This feature increases digital resolution without changing matrix size. The price paid is a reduction in the camera's apparent field

TABLE 7–1. *Matrix Characteristics for 16-bit Memory*

Matrix size	No. pixels	Max. counts per pixel	Memory required (words)	Resolution (pixels/cm)	
				37 cm LFOV	25 cm FOV
32 × 32	1024	255 (byte mode)	512	0.86	1.3
		65535 (word mode)	1024		
64 × 64	4096	255	2048	1.7	2.6
		65535	4096		
128 × 128	16,384	255	8192	3.5	5.1
		65535	16384		
256 × 256	65,536	255	32768	6.9	10.2
		65535	65536		

of view, an acceptable price if the organ of interest is small.

The analog zoom is usually specified as a factor by which each axis of the image is magnified. For example, assume at no zoom (zoom factor of 1.0) a 64×64 matrix just encompasses the 25-cm field of view of the camera (Fig. 7–4A). The digital resolution is 64 pixels/25 cm = 2.6 pixels/cm. At a zoom factor of 1.5, the X and Y axes of the image are each magnified by a factor of 1.5 (Fig. 7–4B). The new digital resolution is $1.5 \times 64/25$ cm = 3.8 pixels/cm. The digital resolution is 50% higher and is equivalent to digitizing the camera field of view with a 96×96 matrix. Similarly, a 64×64 matrix at a zoom factor of 2.0 is equivalent to the digital resolution of a 128×128 matrix but requires only one fourth of the memory, because only the central field of the camera image is digitized and stored.

SOFTWARE[4,8]

In modern computers, the cost of writing and developing software (programs) is a major fraction of the system cost because of the great amount of time required to write and test ("debug") programs. There are several languages in which computer programs can be written. Each has different functions, and each has its strengths and weaknesses. These languages include (1) machine language, (2) assembly language, (3) high-level languages (e.g., Fortran or Basic), and (4) command languages.

Machine Language

The CPU of every computer has a relatively small repertoire of instructions that it can carry out (often 100 or fewer). Usually, these instructions are simple, for example, "Add one to the value stored in a specific memory location," or "Skip the next instruction if the number stored in a specified memory location is zero." Each elementary instruction recognized by the CPU is represented by a number. These numbers are the *language* of the CPU (the *machine language)*. To perform complex tasks, hundreds or thousands of such simple instructions must be executed in the proper sequence by the computer. Such a sequence of instructions is tedious to write, because it consists simply of a long list of numbers.

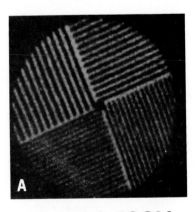

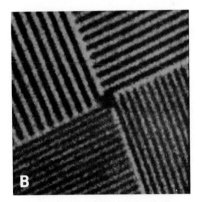

ANALOG ZOOM = 1.0

ANALOG ZOOM = 1.5

Fig. 7–4. Analog zoom. *A.* Bar phantom with analog zoom = 1. *B.* Bar phantom with analog zoom = 1.5. The zoomed image not only is enlarged but has a larger number of pixels per cm^2 of image area.

Assembly Language

Assembly language was devised to make machine language programming easier and faster. In assembly language programs, numeric coding has been replaced by a series of mnemonics, which is easier to use. A special program called an *assembler* translates the mnemonics into the machine language, which the CPU understands.

High-Level Languages

Such high-level languages as Fortran and Basic are used widely in computers. These languages allow the programmer to give instructions to the computer in a more human-oriented manner, using a mixture of English and algebra—for example, "Let AREA = 3.1416 × R^2." A special program then is used to translate each of these "human" language instructions into the many machine language instructions that the CPU understands. In the case of the AREA example, this translation might result in dozens of machine language instructions.

There are two major types of high-level languages: interpreted languages and languages that must be compiled. Interpreted languages are translated line by line (by a program called an *interpreter*). That is, if the program consists of ten lines of instructions, the interpreter translates the first line, executes the requested task, translates the second line, executes the second task, and so on. Whenever the program is used, it is retranslated and re-executed line by line. Languages that must be compiled, such as Fortran, are treated differently. A compiler program is used first to translate all lines of the program; the program is then executed. If the program is used again, it need not be retranslated.

When a computer runs a program written in an interpreted language, the process is much slower than when it runs an equivalent program written in a compiled language. In the former case, the CPU must spend much of its time interpreting program lines, often several times in the case of loops, whereas in languages such as Fortran, the compiler has already interpreted the program into machine language prior to execution. Thus, at run time, the CPU only needs to execute the precoded program. This not only is faster than an interpreted program but also saves memory, because the compiler itself does not need to be in memory at run time. Nonetheless, there are disadvantages to using compilers. Compiled programs are difficult to modify and require programming skill to specify all parameters fully prior to execution.

To choose among high-level languages, a detailed knowledge of the application and its limitations is necessary. Fortunately, this is not usually necessary with nuclear medicine computers, as they are supplied with software to perform most operations required. Most computers use Fortran or a combination of interpreted Basic and compiled Basic (for improved speed). Modification of existing programs for specific applications generally requires support from the system supplier.

Command Languages[7,12]

To enable individuals not expert in programming to make minor modifications in acquisition and processing software, most nuclear medicine systems are supplied with a *command language* or "macro-language." A command language allows the stringing together of commands and predefined variables so that complex processing and acquisition protocols can be used with only one or a few keystrokes. Sophisticated computer systems may have command languages that permit loops and branching, which can be useful for increasing efficiency and speed.

Some examples of the software supplied with nuclear medicine computers serve to illustrate the indispensable functions they have come to perform, even in routine imaging procedures.

Static Frame Mode Acquisition

Variations of the image with time are considered unimportant in static scans. The user first selects the proper digital resolution (hence the appropriate matrix size and zoom factor). The computer then sets aside room in memory for this matrix. When the acquisition is begun, the ADC digitizes the X and Y coordinates of each count processed by the gamma camera. This pair of coordinates determines the location of the corresponding pixel, whose numeric value is then incremented by one. In this way, a record is kept of the number of counts occurring at each pixel. Usually, a second counter that accumulates total counts is incremented also. The computer or the scintillation camera can stop acquisition, based on either time or total counts. Upon terminating acquisition, the matrix is stored on either a floppy or a hard disk. This process of sorting the gamma camera data into an image, or frame, is referred to as *framing* the data.

In many nuclear medicine studies, it is desirable to follow the changing organ distribution of a radionuclide as a function of time. This requires a sequence of images over time. There are two basic methods by which this process may be accomplished, and there are advantages and disadvantages of each.

Dynamic Frame Mode Acquisition[1,3,9,10]

One method for following changing patterns of activity is to acquire the data in *dynamic frame mode.* In this mode, the user first specifies (1) the matrix size desired, (2) either the duration of each image or the number of images to be acquired each second, and (3) the total duration of the study. Specification of the number of images per sec is usually referred to as the *framing rate.* For example, if the study duration is 60 sec at a framing rate of 2 frames per sec, 120 images will be created. Few nuclear medicine computers are large enough to hold this many images in memory. Almost always, the images must be stored on disk after they are created. In dynamic acquisition, for example, each image could be acquired as described for a static acquisition and then transferred to disk, and the next image could be acquired. The second image, however, could not be created until the first had been written to disk and its matrix in memory reset to zero. This process (especially the disk transfers) takes time—time during which data would normally be lost.

To illustrate the general method by which this problem is circumvented, consider a 64 × 64 (word mode) matrix size at a framing rate of 4 images per second (0.25 seconds per image). The computer sets aside space in memory for *two* 64 × 64 matrices. For the first 0.25 second, data would be stored (framed) into the first matrix in memory. During the second 0.25 sec, data would be stored in the second matrix. Simultaneously, the computer would transfer the first matrix from memory to disk and reset each element of the first matrix to zero. At the end of the second 0.25-sec interval, data would be transferred to the first matrix again, while the second was being written to disk.

Several practical considerations are apparent. First, the computer must have sufficient memory to hold *two* images in memory at the same time. This often sets an upper limit on the matrix size allowable for dynamic acquisition. Second, images cannot be acquired any more rapidly than they can be written to disk, which usually sets an upper limit on the possible framing rate. Since a 64 × 64 image contains only one fourth as many pixels of data as does a 128 × 128 image, the former can be written to disk four times faster than a 128 × 128 image can, and usually, the maximum framing rate is about four times faster. Likewise, byte mode images can support twice the framing rate as word mode images. Finally, because hard disks can record data at a much faster rate than can floppy disks, dynamic frame mode acquisitions can be performed at a higher frame rate on hard disks. Typical dynamic framing rates achievable by modern computers, using hard disks are shown in Table 7–2.

Dynamic frame mode studies can be acquired in byte mode rather than word mode when the framing interval is short enough, that is, when the chance of exceeding 255 counts in any pixel is small.

Usually, dynamic frame mode acquisitions are the simplest, most straightforward solution to the problem of dynamic acquisition. Several factors must be considered, however, when dynamic frame mode acquisitions are performed:

1. A large number of images are often required for high framing rate studies (e.g., first-transit cardiac ventricular function studies).
2. The temporal resolution (framing rate) required must be determined in advance.
3. The framing rate is limited by the disk writing speed, especially for large matrix sizes.
4. In some circumstances, much more data must be stored on the disk than are actually used in analyzing the image.

In most clinical studies, these factors are inconsequential. In a few special cases, however, they become serious limitations, especially when the required framing rate can be determined only from the data itself. In such cases, list mode acquisition may be preferable.

TABLE 7–2. *Typical Framing Rates Using a Hard Disk*

Matrix size (bytes)	Maximum frame rate (images/sec)
32 × 32	200
64 × 64	50
128 × 128	15
256 × 256	Static only

List Mode Acquisition[1,3,10]

In *list mode* acquisition, the computer simply records in sequence the position (X,Y) of each photon detected by the camera. Later, when the study is complete, this sequential "list" of data is sorted into frames whose matrix size and rate are then determined. To retain timing information, the list also contains timing marks so that the time of each photon occurrence may be determined. Typically, these are recorded every msec.

Two potential disadvantages of list mode acquisition are apparent. First, the list must be stored on disk. If a one-million count study is to be acquired, one million words (plus 1000 words per sec for timing marks) must be stored. Second, at the conclusion of the study, the data are not yet ready for visual inspection but must be framed into images. This sorting proceeds exactly as in a dynamic frame mode acquisition except that the data comes from the disk instead of from the gamma camera. The necessity for retrospective framing adds a few extra minutes of processing to the study. The patient need not be present during this time, however, and neither the framing rate nor matrix size is limited except by the time resolution inherent in the timing marks. If the initial framing rate and matrix size selected are inappropriate, the study need not be repeated. Instead, the data are simply reframed from the disk at the newly selected temporal or spatial resolution. The list mode data can then be discarded and that space on the disk reused.

Dynamic frame mode acquisitions usually require less disk space than list mode acquisitions. High counting rate studies in particular are usually handled more efficiently in frame mode. Under certain conditions, however, the reverse is true. For example, consider a first-pass cardiac dynamic study of 20 sec duration with a peak counting rate of 60,000 cps, a 64 × 64 matrix size, and a framing rate of 25 per sec. List mode acquisition would require a disk space for $20 \times 61{,}000$ words per sec (including timing marks) $= 1.22 \times 10^6$ words. The disk space required is independent of matrix size or framing rate. For dynamic frame mode acquisition, the disk space consumed critically depends on framing rate and matrix size. For the above example:

$$20 \text{ sec} \times 25 \text{ frames/sec}$$
$$\times 4096 \text{ words/frame} = 2.0 \times 10^6 \text{ words}$$

In this case then, using a list mode acquisition conserves disk space. It is also more flexible, because framing rate and matrix size can be altered after the study.

Table 7–3 summarizes the advantages and disadvantages of frame and list mode acquisition. Note that in list mode acquisition the maximum counting rate must be less than the maximum speed at which the disk is capable of storing data (typically 100,000 to 200,000 words per sec). Dynamic frame mode is not limited by counting rate, but instead, the product of framing rate and matrix size must not exceed the maximum rate at which data can be written to disk.

Gated Acquisitions[1,9,15]

Many physiologic events occur too quickly to allow adequate counting statistics with sufficient temporal resolution. If an event is cyclic, *gated studies* can be performed. In a gated study, some physiologic parameter is used to demark the cycle. For example, in framing the cardiac cycle the electrocardiographic R wave is used as a gate to demark the cycle. Gated studies can be acquired in either frame or list mode.

In cardiac gated studies, the heart cycle is defined as an R-R interval. This cycle then is divided into as many frames as are necessary to provide the desired temporal resolution. For example, 16 images are usually adequate for recording cardiac wall motion. If the average R-R interval is 800 msec, then 16 images correspond to a framing rate of 50 msec/frame or 20 frames per sec. The computer then establishes in its memory 16 separate matrices of the desired spatial resolution (e.g., 64×64), into which counts are sorted sequentially. At each R wave, which marks the beginning of a new cycle, data are sorted into the first matrix. After 50 msec have elapsed, data are acquired into the second matrix in memory, and so on, until the next R wave. At each R wave, data are sorted into the first matrix again. Usually, several hundred cycles are required to obtain adequate statistics in the composite, 16-image cycle. Following acquisition, the frames can be displayed sequentially and looped, giving the cine effect of a beating heart. Many parameters are measured from such studies (see Vol. II, Chap. 17).

Implicit in the method of gating is the assumption that all cycles are equivalent. The composite gated image sequence may not reflect reality, however, in patients in whom the R-R interval is highly variable. Nonetheless, gated cardiac imaging has proved to be of great value and is widely used. Other cyclic phenomena (e.g., the respiratory cycle) have also been studied using the concept of "gating" but have

TABLE 7–3. *A Comparison of List and Frame Mode Acquisition*

	List mode	Dynamic frame mode
Disk usage	Equals total counts	Independent of total counts
	Independent of matrix size	Increases with increasing matrix size
	Independent of framing rate	Increases with increasing framing rate
Matrix size	Unlimited	Limited by maximum disk writing speed
Frame rate	Unlimited	Limited by maximum disk writing speed
Maximum counting rate	Limited by disk writing speed	Unlimited (except by system deadtime)

proven less useful than gated cardiac studies.

IMAGE PROCESSING[3,7,11,12]

Digital images frequently require further processing (1) to improve visual appearance, which enhances clinical interpretation, and (2) to derive quantitative information from the images. In addition, further processing can be used to rearrange images for easier disk storage and retrieval.

Altering Visual Perception

Commercial nuclear medicine computer systems provide many methods of altering image appearance. Some common procedures and their effects are discussed here.

Contrast. When digital images are displayed, there is a predefined relationship between image intensity and counts. For example, with a linear relationship, the displayed brightness of each pixel is directly proportional to the number of counts stored at that pixel, and the "hottest" pixel is displayed with the brightest intensity. *High display contrast* implies a large change in brightness for a given fractional change in counts, and *low display contrast* implies a small change in brightness for the same fractional change in counts.

Thresholding. An image is *thresholded* by setting to zero counts all pixels with counts below a certain selected value, called the *lower-level threshold,* or *limit.* Notice in Figure 7–5B that the appearance of image pixels above the threshold is not altered; the contrast of the image is not changed. Thresholding can be used to focus the observer's attention on a particular portion of the image above the thresh-

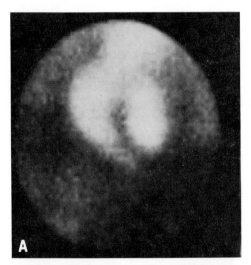

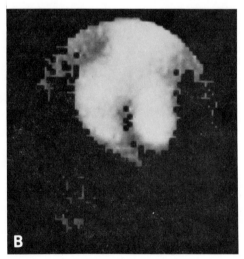

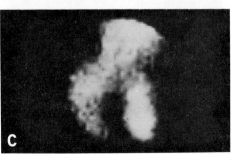

Fig. 7–5. Thresholding versus background subtraction. *A.* Original image of heart. *B.* Same image as in A, but all pixels with counts less than 100 have been set to zero brightness. Note creation of artificial edges. *C.* Same image with 100 counts subtracted from each pixel. Image rescaled so that highest count pixel is brightest. Note increased contrast.

old. It is also possible to set upper-and lower-level thresholds so that pixels exceeding the upper level and those below the lower level are set to zero. This is called *windowing* the image.

Often an image of an organ that has been (lower-level) thresholded gives the appearance of having a well-defined edge, the location of which depends upon the value selected for the threshold. While a fixed-threshold method of edge detection may be of use occasionally, it can also produce misleading edges (see "Contrast," Chap. 23).

Background Subtraction. When an image of an organ is viewed, the elimination or reduction of counts from surrounding tissue is sometimes desirable. In a xenon lung ventilation image, for example, background activity from the muscle and fat tissues of the surrounding chest wall is detected. A commonly employed, but simplistic, scheme for compensating for this background activity uses the assumption that the background is constant everywhere within the image; thus this value is subtracted from each pixel in the image. This method is illustrated in Figure 7–5C for a gated blood pool image.

Unlike thresholding, background subtraction does alter the image contrast—by increasing it. To see that this is so, consider the following example. Imagine a lung image with a background activity averaging 50 counts per pixel. Assume that under these conditions the hottest pixel in the lung contains 150 counts and the coldest pixel contains 50 counts. Contrast of the image can be expressed as the change in brightness per fractional change in counts, with a value of zero representing minimum brightness and a value of 1.0 representing maximum brightness. If the hottest pixel (150 counts) in the lungs were displayed at the maximum brightness of 1.0 then the coldest pixel in the lung (50 counts) should be displayed at a brightness of 0.33. The display contrast of the image then is:

Display Contrast

$$= (1.0 - 0.33)/100 \text{ counts}$$

$$= 0.67 \text{ per 100 counts}$$

If 50 counts then are subtracted from each pixel, and the image again is displayed so that the hottest pixel (now $150 - 50 = 100$ counts) is displayed at maximum brightness (1.0), then the coldest spot is displayed at zero counts and therefore at zero brightness. The new contrast is:

Display Contrast $= (1.0)/100$ counts
$$= 1.0 \text{ per 100 counts}$$

Thus background subtraction has increased the display contrast by about 50%. Often, this change in contrast enhances the clinician's ability to observe small changes in activity (perfusion or ventilation) within the lungs. Background subtraction increases image contrast by spreading a smaller range of counts over the full range of available brightness.

Logarithmic Images. Occasionally, an image has regions of high counts containing clinical structure (i.e., meaningful changes in counts) as well as regions of low counts containing clinical structure. If this image is displayed in the usual manner (brightness proportional to counts), it is possible for detail to be missed from one or both of these regions. Contrast in the bright region could be enhanced by background subtraction but at the expense of losing the low count density region. Logarithmic imaging offers a solution to this dilemma. By calculating the logarithm of the counts in each pixel, detail in both regions can be visualized simultaneously. Suppose an image contains one region with approximately 100 counts per pixel plus a "hot spot" of 140 counts per pixel. Suppose a second region of the image has an average count per pixel of 10,000 with a hot spot of 14,000. Although the 40% change in counts from 14,000 to 10,000 might be easily visible when the image is displayed in a linear manner, the same

40% count change from 140 to 100 would be imperceptible. These transformations are illustrated in Table 7–4.

When brightness is directly proportional to counts, the 40% count density change in the high region of the image produces a brightness change 100 times greater than that of the 40% change in the cold region. When the logarithm of counts at each pixel is displayed, the 40% change in the hot region results in exactly the same brightness difference as does the 40% change in the cold region. This equalization is obtained at a cost of (1) nonlinearity between absolute counts and brightness and (2) reduction in contrast at the high count density region of the image.

Other forms of contrast manipulation are possible. Brightness can be made proportional to the exponential value of counts, which emphasizes the high count area of the image. Many computers allow a graphic transformation of counts to brightness in which the user enters a counts-brightness curve with a lightpen or joystick. Thus an image can have a linear representation of counts to brightness in one range but a logarithmic representation in another. Logarithmic and graphic transformation are illustrated in Figure 7–6 from a gated blood pool scan. The clinician can use these techniques to emphasize subtle changes in tracer concentration.

Smoothing. All images have statistical fluctuations owing to limited counts. If the fluctuations are large, the ability of the clinician to interpret the image is impaired. The best means for improving such an image is to collect more counts. When this is not practical, however, several mathematical operations are available that may improve the appearance of the image. These operations are generally called *smoothing* operations and they have both advantageous and deleterious effects on the perceived image quality. A common method of smoothing an image is illustrated in Figure 7–7. This method involves averaging the counts from a group of neighboring pixels and replacing the center pixel in the smoothed image with this average value. The averaging can be performed either by counting all values equally or by counting pixels far from the center pixel less heavily in the average than the closer pixels (called *weighted smoothing*). The number of pixels used in the average may vary. In Figure 7–7, nine points have been used, and the weighting factors are shown. This technique therefore is referred to as *nine-point weighted smoothing*.

Smoothing reduces statistical noise by averaging. The averaging process, however, results in loss of resolution—edges become blurred. Several factors are important when deciding whether or not to smooth an image. First, smoothing by averaging should be applied only for visual purposes (to aid in qualitative image interpretation or in drawing a region of interest). Usually, computations are performed best on the original data. Second, spatial smoothing by averaging should be applied only when counting fluctuations are the principal factor affecting visual perception. Applying this type of smoothing operation to an image that has high counts per pixel does not significantly improve

TABLE 7–4. *Linear and Logarithmic Transformations of Pixel Counts to Image Brightness*

Linear		Logarithmic	
Counts	Brightness	Log counts	Brightness
14,000	1.0	4.15	1.0
10,000	0.7	4.0	0.96
140	0.01	2.15	0.52
100	0.007	2.0	0.48

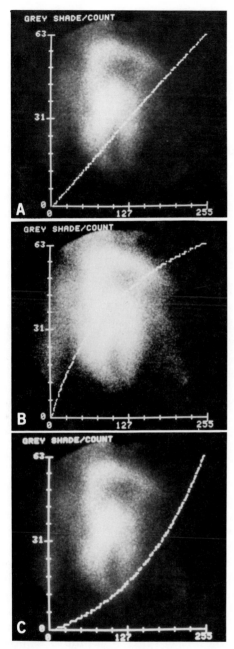

Fig. 7–6. Image manipulation. *A.* Original image of the heart. Display brightness (gray shade) is graphed linearly against counts. *B.* Logarithmic transformation. Note increased visualization of such low-count density structures as the aorta. *C.* Exponential transformation. High count areas are emphasized, primarily right and left ventricular outflow tracts.

visual "smoothness" but does decrease resolution (e.g., blurring true changes in such counts as those occurring at organ edges or at borders between hot and cold regions).

Some spatial smoothing operations are attempts to avoid the problem of blurring true edges by adjusting the "amount" of smoothing at different regions within the image—smoothing heavily where statistics are the principal cause of the observed counting fluctuations, smoothing less heavily in regions where changes in counts are not explainable on a statistical basis. Such smoothing operations are called *nonstationary* because the degree of smoothing varies over the image. Again, quantitative information present in the image generally is not preserved following application of nonstationary smoothing procedures, which are used primarily to improve visual perception.

The aforementioned smoothing procedures are all *spatial* in nature, i.e., the averaging procedures are performed in the X and Y directions of a single image. When smoothing is performed in dynamic studies, time is an extra dimension to be considered. *Temporal* smoothing (often combined with spatial smoothing) is used frequently in processing cardiac wall-motion images prior to cinematic display or definition of left ventricular regions of interest (ROIs). The same techniques used for spatial smoothing apply to temporal smoothing, except that only one dimension, time, is used.

To understand five-point temporal smoothing, consider the tenth image in a series of 24 dynamically acquired gated cardiac images. The five-point temporally smoothed value of the nth pixel in this image is created by averaging its counts with the nth pixel counts in images 8 and 9 and in images 11 and 12. This averaging procedure may be weighted or not, and may be stationary or nonstationary in time, just as with spatial imaging. If temporal imaging is combined with spatial

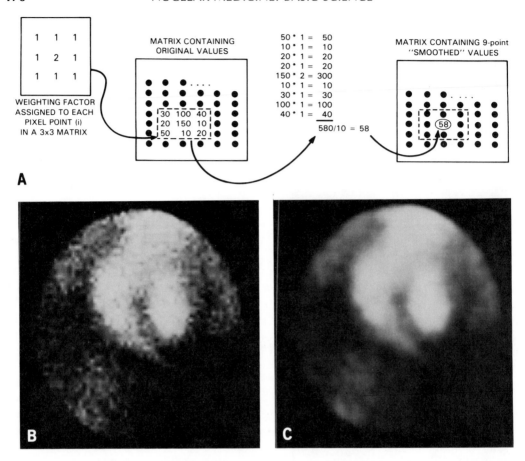

Fig. 7–7. Smoothing. *A.* Smoothing technique for 9-point weighted smooth. *B.* Original image. *C.* Nine-point weighted smoothed image.

imaging, the two spatial dimensions of smoothing (e.g., 9 points—3 pixels in X and 3 pixels in Y) are combined with the temporal smoothing (e.g., 5 points in time). In this case, the resulting pixel value is influenced by the content in 45 temporally and spatially neighboring pixels.

Quantifying Images[7,11–16,18,19]

Many images already are in a form that allows quantification of useful clinical parameters with minimal processing. For example, in a lung perfusion image the counts at any pixel need only be divided by the total counts to calculate fractional blood flow to the lung region corresponding to that pixel. The displayed result is a *functional image* because the value at each pixel represents not counts, but rather the value of a functional parameter, in this case fractional blood flow.

Care is needed in performing the division operation. Many nuclear medicine computers allow only integer numbers (0,1,2,...) to be stored at each pixel. Fractional numbers are rounded off to the next lower integer value. Since the total counts in a perfusion image is large compared to the value at any pixel, it is possible for each pixel value to be "rounded-off" to zero following the division, which results in a blank image. This is avoided by first scaling the image by a suitable factor so that the resulting counts at each pixel lie, for example, between 0 and 100. For such numeric manipulations, word mode data often are more convenient than byte mode data.

Occasionally, a single image does not contain the quantitative information sought. This occurs most frequently in dynamic imaging, in which the images vary with time. Often in such a case, the images can be combined into a single functional image to display the quantitative information. Consider an end diastolic image and an end systolic image, both obtained from a gated cardiac blood pool scan. To evaluate the volume of blood ejected from each region within the ventricles (the *regional stroke volume),* a functional image can be created by subtracting the end systolic image from the end diastolic image. Each pixel in this image, then represents the regional stroke volume. A bright pixel represents a region with a high stroke volume (a large difference between end systole and end diastole), and a dark pixel a region with a low stroke volume (Fig. 7–8). Subtraction of images requires an understanding of how the computer is programmed to deal with negative numbers. Usually, negative numbers can be avoided by thresholding the resulting image with a lower-level threshold of zero, which sets all negatives to zero.

Time-Activity Curves. In most dynamic studies, quantitative clinical information is obtained by observing the changing counts in a given region over time. Figure 7–9 illustrates a Hippuran renogram in which the regional concentration of radiohippuran is followed within the ROI through the uptake (rising curve) and excretion phase (*washout).* Such a curve is referred to as a *time-activity curve* (TAC). The ROIs can be regular or irregular in contour and can be determined either by keyboard insertion of X-Y coordinates or by drawing directly on the video display with a lightpen or "joystick."

The ROI identifies for the computer which pixels are to be used in creating the TAC. TACs are created by plotting on the Y axis the number of counts within each ROI of each image versus the frame number on the X axis, each of which represents a selected time interval. TACs themselves can be analyzed further either subjectively by visual inspection, or objectively by quantifying some parameter of interest from the TAC. All arithmetic processing techniques used with images, such as background subtraction and smoothing, also are useful for TACs.

Occasionally, determining the function of each region of the organ is useful. If information from a large number of different regions are sought, the generation of individual TACs becomes quite cumbersome. To overcome this problem, TACs are created for each pixel of an image and then processed to produce some *index of function.* Each numeric index is assigned a proportionate intensity, and the matrix is displayed as a functional image.

In practice, this functional image is often interpreted more easily than are several hundred TACs. Consider the following example. During a radioxenon ventilation study, the patient continuously breathes a xenon-oxygen mixture until equilibrium between the gas and plasma concentrations is reached. Then, dynamic frame mode acquisition is begun as the patient is switched to room air. The ensuing sequential images record the washout of xenon as a measure of regional airflow.

The TAC produced from each pixel within the lung can give a numeric indication of the relative airflow to the region corresponding to that pixel. A functional image is produced, with a TAC created for each pixel, but instead of being stored, it is background subtracted, and the washout slope is calculated. This index is then stored in a 64 × 64 matrix, creating a new image in which the value at each pixel is proportional to regional airflow. The clinician then is able to evaluate the 4069 TACs and regional airflow values easily, by simply observing the single functional image.

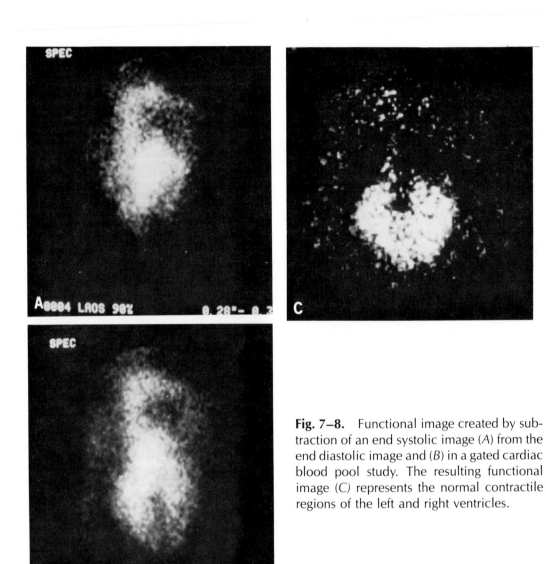

Fig. 7–8. Functional image created by subtraction of an end systolic image (A) from the end diastolic image and (B) in a gated cardiac blood pool study. The resulting functional image (C) represents the normal contractile regions of the left and right ventricles.

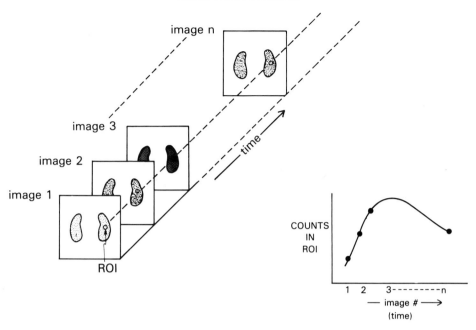

Fig. 7–9. Creation of a time activity curve from a region of interest within the kidney after injection of I-131 Hippuran.

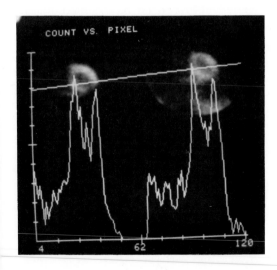

Fig. 7–10. Activity profile: exercise (left) and redistribution (right) Thallium images in the 45-degree LAO projection. The profile line is 3 pixels wide.

Activity Profiles. Slices of a two-dimensional image can be taken in any orientation within the image plane to create an activity profile. The profile may consist of a line one pixel wide or up to the entire width of the image. The profile then is displayed as a graph of counts per pixel (averaged for the line width) on one axis and pixel number on the other axis. This technique is useful for showing small differences in counts between nonadjacent areas or in the same area at different times. For example, consider the exercise and redistribution Thallium heart images in Figure 7–10. The similarity of the profiles suggests that regional perfusion to the tissues lying in this plane varied uniformly.

Volumetric Display. Two-dimensional images can be displayed as a three-dimensional representation using the count density for the third dimension. In such images, peaks represent regions of high counts, and valleys low counts. These images are of limited usefulness, owing to the difficulty of displaying a three-dimensional image on a CRT. Volumetric display is most valuable when the brightness scale of the CRT is limited.

Image Orientation. Orientation of images can be changed to obtain better comparisons between similar images. Orientation parameters include both rotation of 90°, 180°, or 270° within the plane of the original image and rotation about a vertical or horizontal axis. Sophisticated computer programs can also rotate or translate images in lesser multiples, although doing so may affect the original data by cutting off the corners of the image. Images can also be superimposed or laid side by side, with the same degree of magnification for enhanced comparison and analysis.

Deadtime Correction. The gamma camera and the computer system require a finite amount of time to detect, process, digitize, and store each scintillation event. This usually requires approximately 1 to 10 μsec. During this deadtime, all or part of the system is unable to accept new scintillation events. As discussed in Chapter 3, correction for nonparalyzable deadtime can be approximated by the equation:

$$R = \frac{r}{1 - r\tau}$$

where R is the true counting rate, r is the observed rate, and τ is the deadtime. This factor is applied to each pixel of the image. Valid correction is much more complicated, however, because the deadtime is caused by all radiations that reach the detector, both photopeak and scattered radiation. Because the amount of scattered and attenuated radiation is a factor of the radionuclide, patient, collimator, and camera, deadtime calculations should be made for each imaging system, under typical acquisition conditions.

Uniformity Correction. Anger cameras do not produce a uniform image when exposed to a uniform source (flood) of radiation. This nonuniform response is due to three effects: (1) The nonuniform energy response of the detector, (2) spatial nonlinearities and (3) nonuniformities in the sensitivity of the detector and collimator. The last of these three errors is easily corrected by the computer. First, a flood image is acquired and digitized using the same matrix size as will be used in the clinical image. After suitable normalization, the clinical image to be corrected is divided by the flood image. Regions of low sensitivity, which produce cold areas on the clinical image, are therefore increased by dividing by a small number, while hot areas are reduced by dividing by a large number. The flood field uniformity correction *does not* correct for the effects of spatial nonlinearities or energy nonuniformities. In fact, if these sources of error are not corrected prior to making the flood correction, artifacts may be produced in the clinical image.

Special dedicated computers are available that can make the required linearity and energy corrections "on-the-fly" (i.e., in real time on an event-by-event basis). Recently, such computer systems have been incorporated as an integral part of the gamma camera, significantly improving the quality of clinical images.

Fourier Analysis of Cyclic Data. Any cyclic curve can be represented mathematically by a sum of sinusoid and cosinusoid curves of various amplitudes and frequencies, known as a *Fourier series.* The principles are familiar in music: Any complex tone (e.g., a note played on a piano) can be identically reproduced by adding together the proper number of pure tones (called harmonics) of varying pitch (frequency) and intensity (amplitude).

Fourier series are useful in analyzing the cyclic data produced from gated cardiac studies. As an example, consider a TAC produced from a left ventricular ROI. This TAC is a cyclic function of time and can be written as a Fourier series:

$$TAC = A_1 \sin (f_t) + A_2 \sin (2\ f_t) + A_3 \sin (3\ f_t) + ...$$
$$+ B_1 \cos (f_t) + B_2 \cos (2\ f_t) + B_3 \cos (3\ f_t) + ...$$
$$= \sum_{n=1}^{\infty} A_n \sin (n\ f_t) + B_n \cos (n\ f_t)$$

where A_n and B_n are the amplitudes, or intensities, of each frequency (called a *harmonic*). The *fundamental frequency f*, or first harmonic, is given by $2\pi/p$ where p is the period of the cardiac cycle in sec. Note that ∞ in the summation implies that, in principle, an infinite number of harmonics is required to reproduce a curve exactly.

In practice, because the left ventricular TAC often closely resembles a cosine wave, fewer terms (harmonics) are needed to describe the TAC. In Figure 7–11A, a left ventricular TAC is shown. In Figure 7–11B is the Fourier series that describes this TAC if all harmonics except the first are omitted. Curve B has the same general shape as the TAC but is missing much detail (e.g., the rapid filling, the diastasis period, atrial contraction, etc.). In Figures 7–11C, 7–11D, and 7–11E, two, three, and four harmonics are added, producing a curve successively closer to the original. If the number of harmonics were increased still further, the Fourier series would eventually reproduce the original identically (including the statistical fluctuations). By omitting the high-frequency harmonics (e.g., using only the first four harmonics, as in Figure 7–11E), a much smoother curve is produced. This is a principal use of Fourier series—to smooth, or *Fourier filter*, TACs by omitting high-frequency harmonics.

Fourier series are also used in cardiac *phase analysis*, in which the TAC is assumed to be described adequately by one harmonic. An examination of Figures 7–11A and 7–11B reveals that B is only a crude approximation of A. *Phase* is defined as the degree to which the single harmonic curve is asymmetric. For example, in Figure 7–11B, there are seven more points to the right of end systole than to the left. Each point in this figure represents 20 msec, therefore the "phase" of this TAC is said to be 7 points × 20 msec = 140 msec shifted to the right. Phase is usually expressed in units of degrees rather than msec. By convention, 360° is equal to the entire TAC (52 points in this example). Therefore, the 7-point shift of Figure 7–11B equals $\left(\dfrac{7}{52}\right) \times 360° = 48°$ shift to the right.

Phase shift can also be calculated directly from the first harmonic amplitudes in the Fourier series (phase = $\tan^{-1}(A_1/B_1)$). This method is used by most computer programs. Phase is nothing more than a measure of asymmetry. It is not a measure of any specific physiologic function although TAC asymmetry is influenced by many physiologic factors.

Fourier analysis can be applied to gated

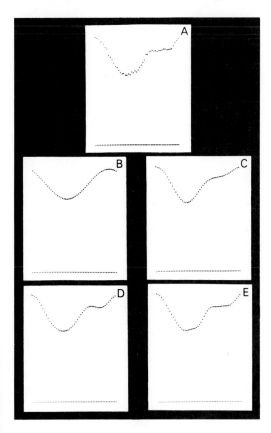

Fig. 7–11. Fourier analysis of TACs. *A*. TAC derived from left ventricle. *B*. One-harmonic representation of TAC. *C*. Two-harmonic representation. *D*. Three-harmonic representation. *E*. Four-harmonic representation.

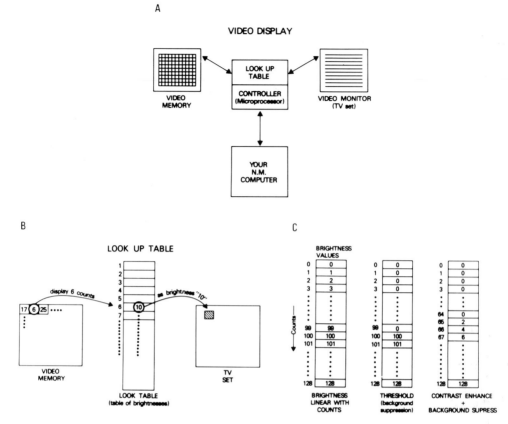

Fig. 7–12. Video display. *A.* Components of video display. *B.* Use of look-up table to convert counts to brightness. *C.* Use of look-up table to alter image through thresholding and contrast enhancements.

image sequences as well as to the TACs derived from them. By calculation of a Fourier series for each single-pixel TAC in the image sequence and omission of all high harmonics, effective temporally smoothed images are obtained. Also, the principles of functional mapping can be applied to the phase calculated at each pixel, yielding a functional map of Fourier phase.

IMAGE DISPLAY[6,11]

One of the most clinically important functions of a nuclear medicine computer system is to enhance images. Unlike non-computerized imaging, the computer permits a high degree of flexibility in image

display. This flexibility is both advantageous and potentially troublesome. It is advantageous because each image can be optimally displayed for perception of structure. The clinician can select the relationship between counts and brightness so as to view each image at all desired contrasts and brightnesses. A disadvantage of this flexibility is that the computer then is able to produce many images from one set of data, which makes interpretation more complex by requiring real understanding of the computer's image-manipulation software.

On most modern computer systems, images are presented on a video display. The video display consists of three major elements: the display memory, in which dig-

A

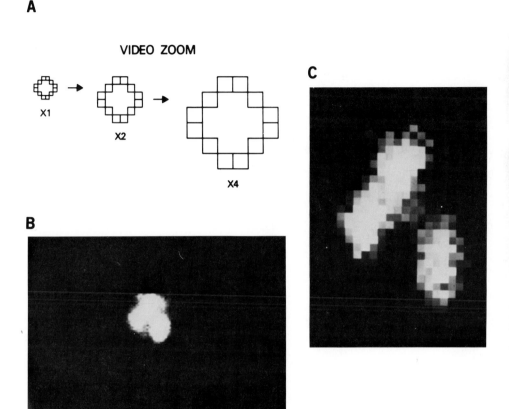

Fig. 7–13. Video zoom. *A*. Zoom × 1, × 2, and × 4. *B*. Gated cardiac image: zoom = 1. *C*. Gated cardiac image: zoom = 4.

itized information can be stored; a monitor on which the image actually appears (usually a standard commercial TV set); and the video processor, a small computer that controls the display. For example, the video processor can sequentially display images stored in the video memory, thus creating a cinematic display of a dynamic image sequence.

An important task of the video processor is to translate the numeric values of the image matrix into various intensities of light on the display. This translation from digitized image to display brightness is determined by a *look-up table,* used to control the display's visual aspects that affect perception. Figure 7–12 illustrates a video display system and its look-up table. The look-up table can be thought of as a table

of brightness values, often called *gray scale* values. The first brightness value corresponds to zero counts. Subsequent brightness values, which may vary linearly, exponentially, logarithmically, or arbitrarily, correspond to progressively increasing counts. By altering the look-up table, as in Figures 7–12B and 7–12C, the visual effects of thresholding and background subtraction can be achieved without altering the data.

Most display systems can be used to alter the size of the image by a feature known as *video zoom,* illustrated in Figure 7–13. Note that in these figures, unlike analog zoom discussed earlier, video zoom increases only the size of the image—not the resolution. The principal use of video zoom is to adjust the image size to the

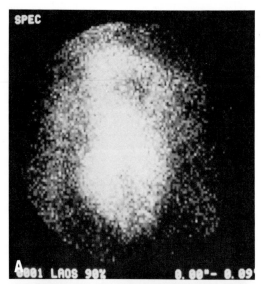

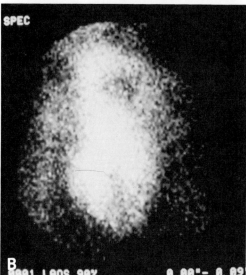

Fig. 7–14. Interpolation. *A.* Uninterpolated gated cardiac image. *B.* Same image after interpolation.

viewing distance. Increasing the zoom, however, increases pixel edge effects. This can be offset partially by *interpolation,* which creates more pixels in video display than are actually present in the computer matrix by averaging adjacent pixels to "make up" intermediate pixels (Fig. 7–14). Although this may improve the image cosmetically, it cannot substitute

for a proper combination of viewing distance and image size.

Color Displays

Video display systems also can be used to display different count ranges as different colors. To do so, not one, but three look-up tables are used, one for each of the three primary colors of the color TV monitor—red, green, and blue. The disadvantage of color is that it is unnatural, that is, a particular color does not have any natural relevance or widely accepted meaning related to imaging (Is green "hot" or "cold"? Is yellow a defect, or is red?). Also, the borders between regions of different colors stand out as edges to the eye, edges as arbitrary as values in the look-up table used to produce them (see Chapter 23).

One worthwhile use of color might be to display functional images, in which many easily distinguishable colors could be used to represent the various functional values of the parameter of interest. Another potential use of color displays is based on the fact that there are two attributes to a particular color (e.g., red): its intensity and its frequency (i.e., its "redness"). Theoretically, several quantities could then be represented in a single image. The value of one quantity might be represented by the intensity of a color, while a second quantity might be represented by the frequency (i.e., the particular color). Unfortunately, the human eye's perception of intensity is itself a function of color.

The ability to alter and enhance images and to extract maximum information from imaging procedures has rendered computers indispensible to most imaging laboratories. With picture archiving systems on the horizon, all or most imaging studies may soon be digitized, stored, and viewed from video consoles rather than from emulsion-based film. Some "all-digital" departments already exist.

REFERENCES

1. Bacharach, S.L., Green, M.V., Ostrow, H.G., et al.: Instrumentation and data processing in cardiovascular nuclear medicine: Evaluation of ventricular function. IEEE Trans. Nucl. Sci., NS-27, 1980, p. 1095.
2. Bell, C.G., Mudge, J.C., and McNamara, J.E.: Computer Engineering: A DEC View of Hardware Systems Design. Bedford, MA, Digital Press, 1978.
3. Hine, G.J., and Sorenson, J.A. (Eds.): Instrumentation in Nuclear Medicine. Vol. 2. New York, Academic Press, 1981.
4. Mano, M.N.: Computer System Architecture. Englewood Cliffs, NJ, Prentice Hall, 1976.
5. Rollo, E.D. (Ed.): Nuclear Medicine Physics: Instrumentation and Agents. St. Louis, C.V. Mosby, 1977.
6. Todd-Pokropek, A.E., and Pizer, S.M.: Displays in scintigraphy. *In* Medical Radionuclide Imaging. Vol. 1. Vienna, IAEA, 1977.
7. Proceedings of the Sixth Symposium on Sharing of Computer Programs and Technology in Nuclear Medicine. Atlanta, Society of Nuclear Medicine, 1976.
8. Shaw, A.C.: The logical design of operating systems. Englewood Cliffs, NJ, Prentice Hall, 1974.
9. Holman, B.L., and Parker, J.A.: Computer-Assisted Cardiac Nuclear Medicine. Boston, Little, Brown, 1981.
10. Lieberman, D.E. (Ed.): Computer Methods: The Fundamentals of Digital Nuclear Medicine. St. Louis, C.V. Mosby, 1977.
11. Information Processing in Medical Imaging. Proceedings of the Sixth International Conference. Paris, INSERM Vol. 88, 1979.
12. Medical Radionuclide Imaging. Proceedings of International Symposium—Heidelberg 1980. Vienna, IAEA, 1980.
13. Esser, P.D. (Ed.): Functional Mapping of Organ Systems and Other Computer Topics. New York, Society of Nuclear Medicine, 1981.
14. Maddox, D.E., Holman, B.L., Wynne, J., et al.: The ejection fraction image: A noninvasive index of regional left ventricular wall motion. Am. J. Cardiol., *41*:1230, 1978.
15. Hamilton, G.W., Williams, D.L., and Caldwell, J.H.: Frame rate requirements for recording time-activity curves by radionuclide angiography. *In* Nuclear Cardiology: Selected Computer Aspects. Edited by J.A. Sorenson. New York, Society of Nuclear Medicine, 1978.
16. Champeney, D.C.: Fourier Transforms and Their Physical Applications. New York, Academic Press, 1973.
17. Reference deleted.
18. Bacharach, S.L., deGraff, C.N., van Rijk, P., et al.: Fourier distribution map: Toward an understanding of what they mean. *In* Functional Mapping of Organ Systems and Other Computer Topics. Edited by P.D. Esser. New York, Society of Nuclear Medicine, 1981.
19. Links, J.M., Douglass, K.H., and Wagner, H.N.: Patterns of ventricular emptying by Fourier analysis of gated blood-pool studies. J. Nucl. Med., *21*:978, 1980.

Chapter 8

PRODUCTION OF RADIONUCLIDES

HOMER B. HUPF AND
JOHN HARBERT

Nearly all of the naturally occurring radionuclides that are found in sufficient abundance for use in tracer studies have long half-lives, which make them unsuitable for medical use. All medically important radionuclides are produced in nuclear reactors or particle accelerators of various types. This chapter examines the radionuclides most frequently used in nuclear medicine and identifies their modes of production and general details of processing.

REACTOR-PRODUCED RADIONUCLIDES

A nuclear reactor consists essentially of a tightly contained enclosure with a central core of fissionable fuel, usually U-238 and U-235, the latter enriched significantly above its natural abundance of 0.7%. Uranium-235 undergoes spontaneous fission ($T_{1/2} \sim 7 \times 10^8$y), which yields two smaller, more stable fission fragments and two or three neutrons per fission event. Some of these fission neutrons stimulate additional fission events. For example, if each nucleus undergoing fission produces two neutrons capable of stimulating two additional events, the sequence of the fission events would increase in geometric proportion, or

2:4:8:16:32:64:128. . . leading to a *chain reaction.* The relationship between the number of fissions in one generation and the number of fissions in the immediately preceding generation is called the *multiplication factor.* When this factor is greater than unity, the speed of the chain reaction increases and the reaction is called *supercritical.* When the factor is less than unity, the reaction eventually ceases and is said to be *subcritical.* The reaction is *sustained,* or *critical,* when the factor equals unity exactly.

The average number of neutrons produced per fission is approximately 2.4. To sustain criticality, an equilibrium must be established between the rate of neutron production and the rate of dissipation by either escape or absorption. The size, shape, and composition of the reactor core are all important in achieving and sustaining a chain reaction. If the U-235 is contained within a small sphere, most of the neutrons escape the system without producing a critical reaction. As the radius of the sphere increases, neutron escape increases as r^2, but absorption increases as r^3. Combining the appropriate radius with a sufficient quantity of fuel achieves a critical radius and critical mass. In the case of pure U-235, the critical radius is about

8.7 cm and the critical mass is about 5.2 kg.

In a nuclear reactor, the speed of the reaction is governed by control rods made of a material with a high *cross section* for neutrons, such as boron or cadmium; the rods are raised or lowered to speed or slow the nuclear reaction (Fig. 8–1). The *moderator* also slows the neutrons, thereby increasing the probability of neutron absorption by U-235 nuclei. The moderator is distributed throughout the fuel and consists of such light atoms as hydrogen, deuterium, or carbon. These nuclei have low cross sections for neutron absorption, but cause elastic collisions, which slow them to a *thermal neutron* state (about 0.3 eV). This energy state is most efficient in inducing fission. Some reactors, e.g., the "swimming pool" reactor, are moderated by water that circulates between the elements and serves as a coolant. Deuterium is an even more efficient moderator.

Usually, the target to be irradiated is inserted into the reactor core by a pneumatic conduction system, which is enclosed within a suitable container called a *thimble.* This system is best used to produce radionuclides of relatively short half-lives. Nuclides with longer half-lives may be extracted from fixed targets attached to the control rods or may be processed from spent fuel rods.

Principal Nuclear Reactions

Several nuclear reactions can occur in the course of neutron activation. The most common production mode is the (n, γ) reaction, known also as the *neutron capture* reaction:

$$^A_Z X \ (n, \ \gamma) \ ^{A+1}_Z X$$

In this reaction, the target nucleus $^A_Z X$ captures a neutron, forming an excited nucleus $^{A+1}_Z X^*$, which undergoes deexcitation by emission of a *prompt* gamma ray. The resulting nucleus is usually radioactive and most often decays by beta emission because of neutron excess (Figs. 1–1 to 1–4). Because the product is an isotope of the target atom, the product will not be carrier-free. Only a tiny fraction of the tar-

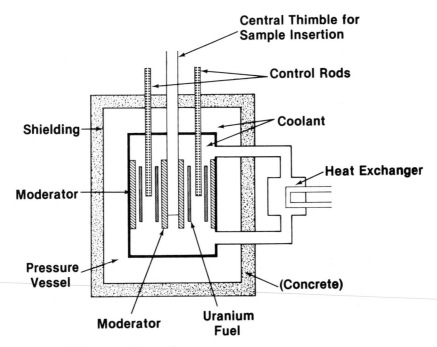

Fig. 8–1. Essential features of a nuclear reactor.

get nuclei are activated (1:10⁶ to 1:10⁹), so that specific activity is quite low. Szillard and Chalmers described a process to separate the formed radioisotope based on the fact that the recoil energy generated by nuclear emission of a photon after neutron capture is often sufficient to break the chemical bond in the target material.[1] An appreciable number of the activated nuclei then exist in a chemical form different from that of the target atoms, and this difference allows chemical separation. An example is the separation of trivalent Cr-51 after neutron bombardment of hexavalent potassium chromate. Specific activities of 30 mCi/mg are easily obtainable.

Carrier-free products result when the activated nucleus is a short-lived intermediate, as in the production of I-131 from Te-130:

$$^{130}_{52}\text{Te (n,}\gamma\text{) } ^{131}_{52}\text{Te (}\beta^-, T_{1/2} = 25 \text{ min) } ^{131}_{53}\text{I}$$

Both Tc-99m and In-113m are obtained from parent nuclides produced by (n,γ) reactions. The relatively long half-lives of the parents Mo-99 (66.6 hr) and Sn-113 (115 days) make these nuclides ideal for use in generator systems (see Chapter 9).

(n,p) and (n,α) Reactions

In these reactions, the incident neutrons have energies in the 2-MeV to 6-MeV range, resulting in the emission of charged particles. In (n,p) reactions, the atomic number of the product nuclide decreases by one while the mass remains the same:

$$^A_Z\text{X (n,p)}^A_{Z-1}\text{X}$$

For (n,α) reactions, the atomic number decreases by two and atomic mass decreases by three:

$$^A_Z\text{X (n,}\alpha\text{) }^{A-3}_{Z-2}\text{X}$$

The products in these cases are separated easily from the target by chemical means and are thus carrier-free radionuclides. Some examples of these reactions are listed in Table 8–1.

TABLE 8–1. *Some Reactor-Produced Radionuclides*

Radionuclide	Principle production	
	Decay modes	Reaction
¹⁴C	β⁻	¹⁴N (n,p) ¹⁴C
²⁴Na	β⁻,γ	²³Na (n,γ) ²⁴Na
³²P	β⁻	³¹P (n,γ) ³²P
		³²S (n,p) ³²P
		³⁴S (n,γ) ³⁵S
³⁵S	β⁻	³⁵Cl (n,p) ³⁵S
⁴²K	β⁻,γ	⁴¹K (n,γ) ⁴²K
⁴⁷Ca	β⁻,γ	⁴⁶Ca (n,γ) ⁴⁷Ca
⁵¹Cr	EC,γ	⁵⁰Cr (n,γ) ⁵¹Cr
⁵⁹Fe	β⁻,γ	⁵⁸Fe (n,γ) ⁵⁹Fe
⁷⁵Se	EC,γ	⁷⁴Se (n,γ) ⁷⁵Se
⁹⁹Mo	β⁻,γ	⁹⁸Mo (n,γ) ⁹⁹Mo
¹¹³Sn	EC,γ	¹¹²Sn (n,γ) ¹¹³Sn
¹²⁵I	EC,γ	¹²⁴Xe (n,γ) ¹²⁵Xe→¹²⁵I
¹³¹I	β⁻,γ	¹³⁰Te (n,γ) ¹³¹Te→¹³¹I

BUILDUP OF RADIOACTIVITY

The buildup of radioactivity produced in a thin target when irradiated by a source of particles is given by the equation:

$$dN/dt = n\phi\sigma - \lambda N$$

where N is the number of atoms undergoing the reaction, n is the number of target nuclei capable of undergoing the reaction, φ is the flux density of particles per cm² per sec, σ is the cross section for the particular reaction in barns, 10^{-24} cm² (10^{-28} m² in SI units), and λ is the decay constant of the radionuclide formed. In this equation, nφσ equals the number of transformations per sec, and −λN describes the radioactive decay occurring during irradiation. After irradiation continues for some finite time t, the number of radioactive nuclei N* formed is found by integration:

$$N_t^* = \frac{n\phi\sigma}{\lambda} (1 - e^{-\lambda t})$$

The amount of activity formed is calculated using the relations between mass in g; the atomic weight A; and Avogadro's number, 6.02×10^{23} atoms/mol:

$$\text{Activity} = \frac{6.02 \times 10^{23} \, \phi\sigma}{A} (1 - e^{\lambda t}) \text{dps/g}$$

$$(\text{or Bq/g})$$

Dividing by 3.7×10^{10} dps/Ci

$$\text{Activity} = \frac{1.62 \times 10^{13} \, \phi\sigma}{A} (1 - e^{-\lambda t}) \text{ Ci/g}$$

This equation gives the *specific activity* at any time t.

The buildup of activity is illustrated in Figure 8–2. The curve approaches a limit where the rate of production equals the rate of disintegration. The point at which activity reaches a maximum is known as the *saturation specific activity.* When t is *long* with respect to $T_{1/2}$:

$$\text{Maximum activity} = \frac{1.62 \times 10^{13} \, \phi\sigma}{A} \text{Ci/g}$$

Figure 8–2 shows that maximum activity is reached after approximately five half-lives. In fact, irradiation longer than 3 to 4 half-lives is inefficient. The rate of production is:

$$R = \frac{6.02 \times 10^{23} \, \phi\sigma}{A} \text{ activations/g sec}$$

$$= \frac{1.62 \times 10^{13} \, \phi\sigma}{A} \text{ Ci/g sec}$$

This equation assumes no attenuation of flux by the target. Of course, this does not hold for thick targets, nor for bombardment with charged particles, in which particle flux decreases as the particles pass through the target material of thickness X, i.e., $\Delta\phi/\Delta X$ is high. The activation cross section also decreases because of loss of particle energy. Lapp and Andrews discuss these considerations in more detail.[2]

The reaction cross sections noted in these equations are the *activation cross sections.* The cross section values listed in nuclide charts are the *isotopic cross sections* for specific reactions and specific nuclides. For example, consider the production of Sn-113 by the ^{112}Sn (n,γ) ^{113}Sn reaction. The cross section for this reaction is 0.9 barns,[3] and the isotopic abundance of metallic tin is 95%. In a 1-g tin target:

$$N = \frac{6.02 \times 10^{23} \times 0.95}{112}$$

In a flux of 10^{12} neutrons/cm^2/sec, the maximum activity produced per gram would be:

$$= \frac{N \, \phi\sigma}{A \, (3.7 \times 10^{10})}$$

$$= \frac{6.02 \times 10^{23} \times 0.95 \times 10^{12} \times 0.9 \times 10^{-24}}{112 \times 3.7 \times 10^{10}}$$

$$= 0.123 \text{ Ci}$$

$$= 4.55 \times 10^{9} \text{ Bq}$$

The maximum activity obtainable in these reactions is a linear function of the concentration of the nuclei undergoing reaction. Targets should be packed as densely as possible, and when the natural abundance of the reacting nuclide is low, isotopic enrichment may be necessary to increase specific activity. For example, the production of Ca-45 from the ^{44}Ca (n,γ) ^{45}Ca reaction is facilitated greatly by using Ca-44 that is enriched tenfold above its 2.06% natural abundance. Nevertheless, the final specific activity is low.

NUCLEAR FISSION

Fission of U-235 or Pu-239 gives rise to a great variety of nuclides, whose masses

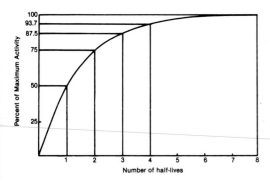

Fig. 8–2. Buildup of activity as a function of time (in half-lives) of bombardment.

range from 72 to 162, with the majority between 95 and 135. Some fission products useful to medicine are Sr-90, Mo-99, I-131, and Xe-133. While fission products may be recovered from spent fuel rods, the usual method is by processing targets of enriched U-235 inserted directly into the reactor core. The separation of radionuclides obtained by fission is difficult because many radionuclides are formed, and usually several isotopes of the same element are formed. Thus, separation of I-131 from stable I-127 and long-lived I-129 ($T_{1/2}$ = 1.6×10^7 yr) is nearly impossible. On the other hand, Mo-99 used in the preparation of ^{99}Mo- ^{99m}Tc generators can be recovered in high specific activities.

PARTICLE ACCELERATORS

Charged particle accelerators may be divided into two groups based on the acceleration path: linear and circular. Particle acceleration in both groups is accomplished by electrostatic attraction between the charged particle and an oppositely charged drift tube, separated by an electronically insulated gap. In a *linear accelerator,* or LINAC, segmented drift tubes of increasing length are aligned linearly, up to one mile in length in some cases (Fig. 8–3). High-frequency alternating current is applied to each tube segment, so that adjacent segments are oppositely charged. Charged particles injected into the tube are accelerated in the segment gaps, owing to the temporary opposite charge in the succeeding tube. The velocity, or kinetic energy, of the accelerated particle is directly related to the electrostatic charge applied and to the total length of the assembly. Energies of up to 800 MeV for protons and in the GeV range for electrons have been achieved at National Laboratory facilities. The type of particle accelerated and the energies generated are selected carefully according to the nuclear reaction desired and the target material used.

In a *circular accelerator,* or *cyclotron,* the accelerated particles are held in a tight spiral by the application of a magnetic field perpendicular to the particle's direction. Initially, charged particles to be accelerated are injected into the center of a space between two hollow D-shaped copper tanks (Fig. 8–4). Opposite alternating electric charges are placed on the "D's" and oscillated at frequencies of about 10^7 Hz.

The charged particle is accelerated into the oppositely charged "D," is bent by the magnetic field, and returns to the gap in time to be accelerated across the gap and into the other "D," which is now oppositely charged. The velocity, or energy, of the particle increases each time the particle passes through the gap, and the radius of the particle's path increases. Proton energies approaching 30 MeV are

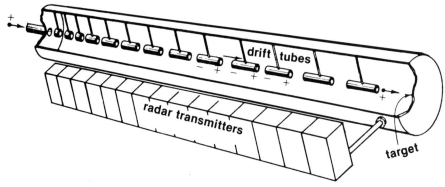

Fig. 8–3.   Schematic diagram of a linear accelerator.

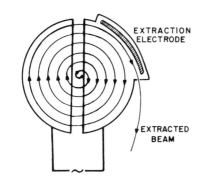

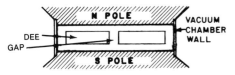

Fig. 8–4. Schematic diagram of a cyclotron.

achieved with an orbit radius of less than 40 cm.

Cyclotrons capable of accelerating protons, deuterons, alpha particles, and He-3 ions to energies between 8 MeV and 40 MeV are available commercially and are the principal machines used for radionuclide production.

PRINCIPAL NUCLEAR REACTIONS

Charged particle nuclear reactions change the number of protons in the nuclei of the target atoms and therefore change the element. For example, cyclotron production of Ga-67 from isotopically enriched Zn-68 utilizes the following nuclear reaction: ^{68}Zn (p,2n) ^{67}Ga. Occasionally, the product of the nuclear reaction is the radioactive parent of the desired nuclide. For example, Tl-201 ($T_{1/2}$ = 73.5 hr) is the daughter of Pb-201 ($T_{1/2}$ = 9.4 hr) formed by the $^{203}Tl(p,3n)$ ^{201}Pb reaction using isotopically enriched Tl-203 as the target. Just as chemical reactions either absorb energy (must be heated) or release energy (heat is released), nuclear reactions either absorb or release energy. This energy is expressed as a Q value and can be calculated from the differences in the sum of the masses of the reactants and products. For example:

$$^{68}Zn + p \rightarrow {}^{67}Ga + 2n + Q$$
$$67.9248 + 1.0073 = 66.9282 + 2.0173 - 0.0134$$
$$Q = -.0134 \text{ amu} \times 931.4 \text{ MeV/amu} = -12.48 \text{ MeV}$$

The energy Q must be supplied by the projectile causing the nuclear reaction. For a positively charged particle (p^+, d^+, $^3He^{++}$, $^4He^{++}$) to penetrate the nucleus of a target atom, sufficient energy must be supplied to overcome the potential barrier due to coulombic repulsion of like charges. Therefore, to effect a charged particle reaction, positively charged projectiles must be accelerated to energies sufficient to overcome the potential barrier of the positively charged nucleus even though the nuclear reaction itself may be exoergic. In general, (p,n) reactions are formed in the 10-MeV to 15-MeV range, (p,2n) in the 15-MeV to 25-MeV range, p,3n) in the 20-MeV to 35-MeV range, etc. To determine Q values experimentally, a stack of thin foils is placed in the charged particle beam and irradiated for a known time at known beam current. Following irradiation, each foil is assayed for the various radionuclides produced by the reactions (x,n), (x,2n), (x,3n), etc. All data from the foils are plotted for activity produced versus energy produced for the various reactions. The resulting curves for each reaction are called *excitation functions* and describe the production yield in μCi/μA-hr over an energy range.

The beam current can be determined accurately by integrating the current produced in an evacuated aluminum Faraday cup or from the radioactivity induced in high-purity metallic disks placed in the beam during the bombardment. The disks are made of such a metal as copper or silver, for which the excitation function (μCi/μA-hr) has been thoroughly studied and is well known.

For the production of any radionuclide, several nuclear reactions are possible. The best method is chosen by the energy and charged particles available, physical and chemical properties of the target material, competing nuclear reactions and the radionuclidic purity desired, total activity required (i.e., mCi or Ci), and economic considerations.[4] An example is the production of I-123 ($T_{1/2}$ = 13 hr), for which more than a dozen nuclear reactions are possible, each with its own set of problems and advantages. With few exceptions, the radiopharmaceutical industry uses proton reactions in the 15-MeV to 30-MeV range for production of radionuclides. Some typical reactions for accelerator-produced radionuclides are shown in Table 8–2.

PRODUCTION YIELDS

Production rates for charged particle nuclear reactions follow the same rules as described earlier in this chapter and can be calculated from reaction cross section values. The concept of flux, however, as presented for nuclear reactors is not practical for cyclotron production. Instead, the beam of charged particles generated per sec is measured as *beam current* in microamperes. The area over which the beam is spread depends upon the beam profile and target configuration. Radionuclide production is optimized by delivering as

TABLE 8–2. *Some Accelerator-Produced Radionuclides*

Radionuclide	Principal decay mode	Nuclear reaction
^{11}C	β^+	$^{11}B(p,n)^{11}C$ $^{10}B(d,n)^{11}C$ $^{14}N(p,\alpha)^{11}C$
^{13}N	β^+	$^{12}C(d,n)^{13}N$ $^{16}O(p,\alpha)^{13}N$
^{15}O	β^+	$^{14}N(d,n)^{15}O$ $^{16}O(p,pn)^{15}O$
^{18}F	β^+,EC	$^{16}O(\alpha,pn)^{18}F$ $^{20}Ne(d,\alpha)^{18}F$
^{43}K	β^-,γ	$^{40}Ar(\alpha,p)^{43}K$
^{52}Fe	β^+,EC	$^{50}Cr(\alpha,2n)^{52}Fe$
^{57}Co	EC	$^{56}Fe(p,\gamma)^{57}Co$
^{67}Ga	EC	$^{66}Zn(d,n)^{67}Ga$ $^{68}Zn(p,2n)^{67}Ga$
^{75}Br	β^+,EC	$^{74}Se(d,n)^{75}Br$ $^{74}Se(p,\gamma)^{75}Br$
^{81m}Kr	γ	$^{79}Br(\alpha,2n)^{81}Rb \xrightarrow[T_{1/2}=4.7\text{ hr}]{EC,\beta^+} {}^{81m}Kr$
^{111}In	EC	$^{111}Cd(p,n)^{111}In$ $^{112}Cd(p,2n)^{111}In$
^{123}I	EC	$^{122}Te(d,n)^{123}I$ $^{123}Te(p,n)^{123}I$ $^{124}Te(p,2n)^{123}I$ $^{127}I(p,5n)^{123}Xe \xrightarrow[T_{1/2}=2.1\text{ hr}]{EC,\beta^+} {}^{123}I$
^{201}Tl	EC	$^{200}Hg(d,n)^{201}Tl$ $^{201}Hg(d,2n)^{201}Tl$ $^{203}Tl(p,3n)^{201}Pb \xrightarrow[T_{1/2}=9.4\text{ hr}]{EC,\beta^+} {}^{201}Tl$

much beam current as the target can withstand at the optimum particle energy. The limiting factor is usually the rate at which heat can be removed from the target to prevent it from melting. The amount of heat generated in the target is the product of the particle energy and the beam current; therefore, as particle energy is increased, the beam current must be decreased to produce the same heat load.

Usually, production yields are reported as mCi/μA-hr (1 μA bombardment for 1 hr) at a given particle energy and target size and thickness.

CYCLOTRON TARGETS

A *cyclotron target* is a deposit of a chemical element on a target base or holder of high thermal conductivity. Ideally, the target material is a monoisotopic element having a low vapor pressure and high melting point. The target base is usually composed of copper, nickel, silver, or aluminum, with machined holes for water cooling. An internal target intercepts the beam inside the D-shaped tank and must be designed to dissipate large quantities of heat. These high-power targets are usually metallic elements electroplated or vapor-deposited on a copper base for high thermal conductivity.

The cyclotron beam may be deflected from its circular orbit inside the "Ds" and extracted into an evacuated beam tube external to the tank. Targets placed in this beam are called *external targets.* With external targets, space and configuration requirements are not severe, and greater flexibility is possible. Extracted beam currents generally are much lower than internal currents, and cooling requirements are less stringent. Foils, pressed powder, and gaseous targets, though not feasible as internal targets, are possible as external targets.

Because the radionuclide produced in charged particle reactions differs chemically from the target material, separation

yields a carrier-free product. High beam current internal targets are quite radioactive (i.e., often more than 1000 R/hr), owing in part to short-lived radionuclides induced in the target base, thus they must be chemically processed in a hot cell, or with other heavily shielded containment, using remote manipulation. Usually, the target material is an expensive isotopically enriched stable isotope and must be recovered chemically after separation of the desired product. The monetary investment of materials, equipment, and personnel required for target preparation, processing, and recovery coupled with generally lower yields results in higher costs for cyclotron-produced radionuclides than for reactor-produced products.

Examples

Gallium-67

Gallium-67 is commercially prepared using the ^{68}Zn (p,2n) ^{67}Ga reaction. Isotopically enriched Zn-68 is electroplated on a copper internal target base. Naturally occurring zinc (18.5% Zn-68) can be used; however, the Ga-67 yield is reduced accordingly, and the content of 9.5-hr Ga-66 is increased. The target is bombarded at an incident proton energy of 26 MeV for 10 to 20 hr, producing several curies of Ga-67.

Iodine-123

Several nuclear reactions are capable of forming I-123. Unfortunately, all of them have some disadvantages that translate to high cost: low-yield, poor radionuclidic purity or high energy requirements. The ^{127}I (p,5n) ^{123}Xe $\rightarrow$ ^{123}I reaction produces large quantities of relatively pure I-123, with varying, but generally low, percentages of I-125 as radionuclidic impurity. This reaction requires 60 MeV to 70 MeV protons, and cyclotrons having this energy are few and expensive to build. A good compromise is the ^{124}Te(p,2n) ^{123}I reaction, currently used to produce commercially I-123. Isotopically enriched Te-124 is pressed into an external cup target and bombarded with 20 MeV to 25 MeV protons for several hours, producing 100 mCi to 200 mCi per hr. The principal impurity is 4 to 5% I-124 at the time of clinical use.

Fluorine-18

Fluorine-18 is one of several relatively short-lived positron-emitting radionuclides that are produced from gaseous external targets. Other such radionuclides include O-15, N-13, and C-11.

The most useful nuclear reaction for production of F-18 is $^{20}Ne(d,\alpha)^{18}F$, which uses naturally occurring neon gas with 0.1% fluorine carrier contained in an external gas target. Deuterons between 2 and 14 MeV used to bombard the target produce approximately 350 mCi in one hr. At the end of bombardment, the gas in the target is released and conducted through a suitable system of tubing and valves to a reaction vessel for subsequent chemical processing.

In the preparation of F-18-2-deoxy-2-fluoro-D-glucose (F-18 FDG), the anhydrous F-18 as F_2 is bubbled through a cooled solution of 3,4,6 tri-O-acetyl D-glucal in freon-11 to form glycopyranosyl fluoride.[5] After the freon evaporates, the residue is dissolved in petroleum ether and passed over a silica gel column to remove impurities. The mixture is evaporated to dryness, suspended in dilute hydrochloric acid, and refluxed to hydrolyze the product to F-18 FDG.

Similar on-line systems have been developed for processing O-15, N-13, and C-11.

REFERENCES

1. Szillard, L., and Chalmers, T.A.: Chemical separation of radioactive element from its bombarded isotope in the Fermi effect. Nature, *134*:462, 1934.
2. Lapp, R.E., and Andrews, H.L.: Nuclear Radiation Physics. 4th ed. Englewood Cliffs, NJ, Prentice Hall, 1934.
3. Lederer, C.M., Shirly, V.S., et al.: Table of Isotopes. 7th ed. New York, John Wiley & Sons, 1978.
4. Tilbury, R.S., and Laughlin, J.S.: Cyclotron production of radioactive isotopes for medical uses. Semin. Nucl. Med., *4*:245, 1974.
5. Barrio, J.R., et al.: Remote, semiautomated production of F-18-Labeled 2-deoxy-2-fluoro-D-glucose. J. Nucl. Med., *22*:372, 1981.

Chapter 9

RADIONUCLIDE GENERATOR SYSTEMS

LELIO G. COLOMBETTI

Modern imaging systems demand high photon fluxes to achieve well-resolved static images and statistically meaningful measurements. The use of short-lived and ultrashort-lived radionuclides to maintain acceptably small absorbed doses of radiation is becoming increasingly popular. Radionuclide generators provide an ideal means of eliminating the two major impediments to the use of short-lived nuclides, namely, cost of production and uncertainty of transportation. The long-lived parent is shipped to the nuclear facility in a suitable separation system from which the short-lived daughter can be extracted as needed over the functional life of the system.

The evolution of radionuclide generators can be traced back to the early twenties, when Failla separated Rn-222 from Ra-226.[1] During World War II, Ba-140 was used as a source of the shorter-lived daughter, La-140.[2] The idea caught on, and many investigators developed new generator systems, among them Tc-99m, Ga-68, Sr-87m, In-113m, and I-132.[2,3,4,5,6,7,8,9,10]

To be useful, a generator system must have certain basic properties:

1. It must yield a daughter with high radiochemical and radionuclidic purity.

2. It must be safe and simple to operate.
3. It must be sterile and pyrogen-free.
4. The product must be convenient for the preparation of radiopharmaceuticals.
5. It must be capable of multiple separations.
6. The daughter's half-life should be less than 24 hr. Otherwise, the radionuclide is better obtained directly from a commercial source.

RADIOACTIVE EQUILIBRIA

In a generator system, the parent-daughter relationship can be described by:

$$\frac{dN_1}{dt} = -N_1\lambda_1 \tag{1}$$

and

$$\frac{dN_2}{dt} = N_1\lambda_1 - N_2\lambda_2 \tag{2}$$

where:

N_1 = the number of atoms of the parent isotope.

N_2 = the number of atoms of the daughter isotope.

λ_1 = the disintegration constant of the parent isotope.

195

λ_2 = the disintegration constant of the daughter isotope.

$N_1\lambda_1$ represents the rate at which daughter atoms are formed, and $N_2\lambda_2$ represents the rate of their disappearance. Upon integration:

$$N_1 = N_1^0 e^{-\lambda_1 t} \qquad (3)$$

and

$$N_2 = \frac{k\lambda_1}{\lambda_2 - \lambda_1} N_1^0 (e^{-\lambda_1 t} - e^{-\lambda_2 t})$$

$$+ N_2^0 e^{-\lambda_2 t} \qquad (4)$$

where:

N_1^0 = initial number of parent atoms.
N_2^0 = initial number of daughter atoms.
k = the fraction of parent atoms decaying to the daughter isotope.

Equation (4) describes the growth of the daughter nuclide and determines its activity at any time t. If at t = 0 the quantity of daughter is zero, equation (4) becomes simply:

$$N_2 = \frac{k\lambda_1}{\lambda_2 - \lambda_1} N_1^0 (e^{-\lambda_1 t} - e^{-\lambda_2 t}) \qquad (5)$$

In some generator systems, the daughter decays in turn to a third stable isotope:

$$\frac{dN_3}{dt} = \lambda_2 N_2 \qquad (6)$$

and

$$N_3 = N_1^0 \left(1 + \frac{k\lambda_1}{\lambda_2 - \lambda_1} e^{-\lambda_2 t} \right.$$

$$\left. - \frac{k\lambda_2}{\lambda_2 - \lambda_1} e^{-\lambda_1 t} \right) \qquad (7)$$

Using the relationship between activity A (in dps) and the number of radioactive atoms N:

$$N = \frac{A}{\lambda} = \frac{AT_{1/2}}{0.693} = 1.44\, AT_{1/2}$$

and substituting A for N in equation (4):

$$A_2 = \frac{k\lambda_2}{\lambda_2 - \lambda_1} A_1^0 (e^{-\lambda_1 t} - e^{-\lambda_2 t})$$

$$+ A_2^0 e^{-\lambda_2 t} \qquad (8)$$

This equation is presented in its most general form and can be used for any parent-daughter relationship. In special cases, however, the mathematics can be simplified.

1. *Secular equilibrium*: $\lambda_2 \gg \lambda_1$

In secular equilibrium, the half-life of the parent is much longer than the half-life of the daughter. An example is the ^{113}Sn-^{113m}In generator. During the buildup period after separation (about 7 daughter half-lives), the general equation reduces to:

$$A_2 = A_1^0 (1 - e^{-\lambda_2 t}) \qquad (9)$$

At secular equilibrium, $A_2 = A_1$. Thereafter with decay of the parent nuclide:

$$A_2 = A_1^0 e^{-\lambda_1 t} \qquad (10)$$

2. *Transient equilibrium*: $\lambda_2 > \lambda_1$

In this case, the half-life of the parent is longer, but not greatly longer, than the daughter half-life. At equilibrium:

$$N_2 = \frac{k\lambda_1 N_1^0 e^{-\lambda_1 t}}{\lambda_2 - \lambda_1} \qquad (11)$$

From this time on, the daughter activity is greater than the parent activity. The ratio between daughter and parent remains constant, and the daughter activity appears to decline with the half-life of the parent. Combining equations (3) and (11):

$$\frac{N_2}{N_1} = \frac{k\lambda_1}{\lambda_2 - \lambda_1} \qquad (12)$$

for large values of t. Figure 9–1 shows the changing relationships in the ^{99}Mo-^{99m}Tc system. When the half-life of the daughter is short compared with that of the parent, approximately 50% of the equilibrium activity is reached within 1 daughter half-life, 75% at the end of 2 half-lives, and 99% after 6 half-lives.[11]

The curve shown in Figure 9–1 takes into account that only about 87% of Mo-99 disintegrations give rise to the metastable Tc-99m. Therefore, in calculating activity from equation (8), k = 0.87.

3. No equilibrium: $\lambda_1 > \lambda_2$

When the half-life of the parent is shorter than that of the daughter, no equilibrium exists. No commercial generator systems are currently used where $\lambda_1 > \lambda_2$. Brucer termed this case the "reverse cow" and described the production of I-131 ($T_{1/2} = 8.1$ day) from reactor-produced Te-131 ($T_{1/2} = 1.3$ day).[12] Spencer and Hosain have described potentially useful systems where $\lambda_2 \cong \lambda_1$.[13]

The usual means of separating the daughter from the parent takes advantage of the different valence states of the two nuclides. A common system uses a chromatographic column in which the parent is adsorbed onto some binder substance, such as ion exchange resin, alumina, or other inorganic exchanger. The daughter, having a different chemical form with a weaker affinity for the binder, is then washed off the column by a suitable eluting solution.

Figure 9–2 shows a simple "open" separation system consisting of a shielded glass column fitted with a porous fritted disc. Above this column, the chromatographic ion exchanger medium is placed and sealed with a retaining ring filter. Most commercial systems are "closed", that is, the top and bottom of the system are sealed to prevent bacteria from entering the column. This seal is usually effected by fitting a closed sterile source of eluting solution

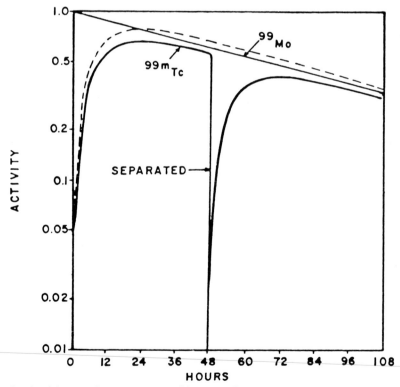

Fig. 9–1. The buildup and transient equilibrium of Tc-99m in a ^{99}Mo-^{99m}Tc generator. The dotted line indicates the theoretic Tc-99m activity if Mo-99 decayed 100% to Tc-99m, instead of only 87%.

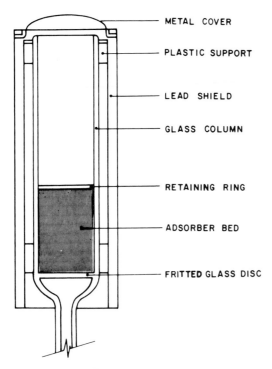

- METAL COVER
- PLASTIC SUPPORT
- LEAD SHIELD
- GLASS COLUMN
- RETAINING RING
- ADSORBER BED
- FRITTED GLASS DISC

Fig. 9–2. A chromatographic column used in open generator systems.

(bottle or plastic bag) and placing a Millipore filter in line with the outlet. Bacteriostatic agents such as 0.5% phenol may be used in this solution provided they do not interfere with either binding of the parent nuclide or the formation of radiopharmaceuticals for which the daughter is intended.

CLINICALLY USEFUL GENERATOR SYSTEMS

Table 9–1 lists several generator systems that either are currently used or have potential usefulness.

99Mo-99mTc Generator

The generator most frequently used is the 99Mo-99mTc generator, originally described by Powell. It was one of the earliest systems developed and in many respects remains one of the best. Molybdenum-99 may be obtained either as a carrier-free

product of U-235 fission in a reactor or by neutron irradiation of Mo-98 in a cyclotron: ^{98}Mo (n, γ) ^{99}Mo. The decay scheme of Mo-99 is shown in Figure 1–9. Because Tc-99 has a long half-life (2.15×10^5 yr), 10 mCi of Tc-99m completely retained in the body would yield only about 2.7×10^{-5} µCi (0.07 Bq) of Tc-99, a quantity too small to be considered significant in terms of radiation absorbed dose.

Most commercial Tc-99m generators are based on column chromatography, in which Mo-99 is adsorbed onto alumina and eluted with physiologic saline solution. The amount of alumina required depends upon the specific activity of the Mo-99 to be bound. This use of alumina is an important consideration because the efficiency of Tc-99m extraction is inversely proportional to the square root of the thickness of the alumina layer. For efficient elution systems, therefore, it is necessary to keep the alumina to a minimum.[15] This is easily accomplished with carrier-free fission Mo-99, although for several years this material was difficult to obtain without small but significant amounts of contaminants, including I-131, I-132, La-140, Ru-103, and Te-123.[16] Separation techniques now permit reasonably pure fractions of Mo-99.

With cyclotron-produced Mo-99, the quantity of contaminants is low, but the presence of residual Mo-98 reduces the specific activity.

Two other methods for separating Tc-99m from Mo-99 have been developed, although neither is used as often as the saline elution system. Perrier and Segré demonstrated that the difference in volatility of molybdenum and technetium oxides permits their separation.[17] A stream of oxygen passed over a bed of molybdenum trioxide heated to 800°C vaporizes the technetium oxide, which then condenses in a coil and can be dissolved in physiologic saline solution.[18] Separations as high as 99% can be achieved in an hour.[19] An efficient and completely auto-

TABLE 9–1. *Principal Characteristics of Currently and Potentially Useful Generators*

Daughter	Half-life (hr)	Mode of decay	Principal γ (keV)	Parent	Half-life	Column	Eluant
^{99m}Tc	6	Internal Transition (IT)	140	^{99}Mo	2.7 d	Alumina	Saline solution
^{113m}In	1.7	IT	393	^{113}Sn	118 d	Alumina, silica	0.05N HCl or HNO_3
^{87m}Sr	2.8	IT	388	^{87}Y	3.3 d	Dowex 1 × 8 resin	0.15M $NaHCO_3$
^{68}Ga	1.13	β^+	511	^{68}Ge	280 d	Alumina	0.005M EDTA
^{132}I	2.3	β^-	773	^{132}Te	78 h	Alumina	Saline solution
^{188}Re	17	β^-	155	^{188}W	69 d	Alumina	Saline solution
^{103}Rh	0.95	IT	20,10 (x-rays)	^{103}Pd	17 d	—	—
^{52m}Mn	0.30	β^+	511	^{52}Fe	8.2 h	Bio-Rad AG1 × 8	8N HCL
^{211}Pb	0.50	β^-	—	^{223}Ra	11.4 d	(^{219}Rn gas)	—
^{44}Sc	3.97	β^+, EC	511,1160	^{44}Ti	46 y	Dowex 1 × 8 resin	0.2M HCl

Adapted from Subramanian, G., and McAfee, J.G.[14]

mated system for the separation of Tc-99m by sublimation has been described by Colombetti.[20]

A fourth method, which has received somewhat greater attention, uses organic solvents to extract Tc-99m from Mo-99. Gerlit showed that Tc-99m (VII) could be efficiently extracted from Mo-99 (VI) with methylethylketone or pyridine.[21] After extraction, the solvent is evaporated off, and the remaining Tc-99m is dissolved in physiologic saline solution. Various investigators have tried to develop a completely automatic system.[15,22,23,24,25,26]

This system permits the elution of high concentrations of Tc-99m; however, the procedure is usually more complicated than the saline elution system. By fractionally eluting a column and using only the middle fractions, concentrations that are sufficiently high for most clinical studies can be obtained from most commercial generators. The chemistry of Tc-99m radiopharmaceuticals is discussed in detail in Chapter 10.

^{113}Sn-^{113m}In Generator

The decay scheme of Sn-113 is shown in Figure 9–3. The metastable In-113m decays with a half-life of 1.7 hr to stable In-113. The 393-keV gamma is somewhat high for scintillation cameras, but suitable for rectilinear scanners. The 118-day half-life of Sn-113 makes it a convenient generator system because it requires shipments only a few times per year instead of weekly, as for technetium.

The Sn-113 is bound either to hydrous zirconium oxide or to silica gel and is

eluted with 8 to 10 ml of HCl at pH 1.2 to 1.6. The first practical and sterile generator of In-113m, described by Colombetti, used a column of zirconium oxide, which produces a better eluate. Breakthrough of Sn-113 must be checked scrupulously at the beginning of each new generator and periodically during its life. This check can be made by letting the elution decay for 48 hr, after which all of the In-113m in the original elution will have decayed away. Any detectable In-113m may be assumed to be in equilibrium with eluted Sn-113.

Commonly used radiopharmaceuticals include In-113m transferrin as a blood pool agent. The eluted ionic indium is mixed with the patient's blood, in which it quickly binds to serum transferrin, and no chemical manipulations are required. Indium-113m forms stable complexes with DPTA and EDTA for brain and renal scanning.[26,31,32] In alkaline solutions, colloidal ^{113m}In(OH)$_2$ is formed.[33] Stabilized with gelatin, PVP, or mannitol, it is used to study the reticuloendothelial system.[34,35]

Albumin macroaggregates and microspheres have been labeled with In-113m for pulmonary perfusion studies.[36,37]

Phosphate compounds can be labeled for bone scanning.[38] Thus most of the radiopharmaceuticals that have been developed with Tc-99m can be adapted successfully for use with In-113m.

Other Generator Systems

Table 9–1 lists several other generator systems producing short-lived radionuclides suitable for radiopharmaceuticals. Besides Tc-99m and In-113m generators, only Ga-68 and Sr-87m systems have been used to any degree.

Gallium-68 is a useful source of positrons, and the generator system is attractive because of the long half-life (280 days) of the parent Ge-68 and the short half-life of Ga-68 (Fig. 9–4). Because of the limited use of positron emitters in nuclear medicine, this isotope has not been frequently

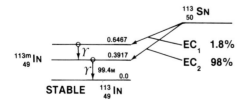

Fig. 9–3. Principal decay characteristics of Sn-113.

used; however, with the development of tomographic scanners, for which positron-emitting nuclides are ideal, interest in this radionuclide may be revived.

Organic as well as inorganic resins may be used as the chromatographic bed of the ^{68}Ge-^{68}Ga generator.[39,40,41] All of these new systems yield ionic Ga-68, a great advantage over the older systems yielding complexed gallium.

Strontium-87m has been used chiefly as a bone scanning agent and has some advantages (Fig. 9–5). Since the development of technetium phosphate radiopharmaceuticals, however, the ^{87}Y-^{87m}Sr generator has seldom been used.

Among other potentially useful generators, those of Pb-211, Mn-52m, and Ta-178 require special attention. Lead-211 is the granddaughter of Ra-223 and could be used for therapeutic purposes because it emits both alpha and beta particles.[42] Manganese-52m, the daughter of Fe-52, may have potential for use in positron tomography.[43,44]

A chemical separation that forms the basis of a generator of the short-lived Ta-178 ($T_{1/2}$ = 9.5 min) has been described by Neirinckx.[45] Tantalum-178 is a low-energy gamma emitter (93 KeV), but it has a strong tendency toward colloid formation, which may limit its applications. Compounds for lung and liver imaging have been tested in animals.[46]

ULTRASHORT-LIVED RADIONUCLIDE GENERATORS

A great diversity of readily available radiopharmaceuticals exists already, and new ones are continually being developed. Among these are radionuclides that have physical half-lives ranging from seconds to several minutes. Such ultrashort-lived radiotracers can be injected intravenously as a bolus, with the advantage that kinetic studies can be repeated numerous times with low radiation absorbed dose. Alternatively, ultrashort-lived radiotracers might be infused continuously into the circulatory system or inhaled. The direct production of these radionuclides is not usually practical because the activity would almost completely decay before it could be used. The preparation of generator systems has proved to be practical, however.

The first ultrashort-lived radionuclides were used to measure the velocity and relative volume of blood circulation through various organs. Bender and Blau used Ba-137m for this purpose.[47] Although Ba-137m has a physical half-life of only 2.6 min, the great disadvantage of this radio-

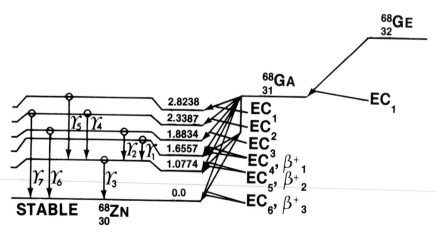

Fig. 9–4. Principal decay characteristics of Ge-68.

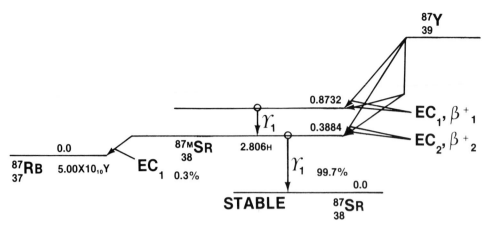

Fig. 9–5. Principal decay characteristics of Y-87.

nuclide is its high gamma-ray energy (660 keV), which makes it unsatisfactory for imaging purposes. Yano and Anger demonstrated the possibility of using ultrashort-lived radionuclides for dynamic function studies with Ag-109m and Ir-191m generators.[48]

A list of potentially useful generator-produced ultrashort-lived radionuclides is given in Table 9–2. Only radionuclide daughters with half-lives of less than 10 min are classified as ultrashort-lived. Not all radionuclides listed here can be used with the instrumentation available today, because many emit high-energy gammas, for example, Al-28 (1.78 MeV). Others are less practical because of short parent half-lives, such as Zn-62 (9.1 hr) and Rb-81 (4.7 hr). Both require a daily production of the parent and preparation of the generators. In spite of this problem, nuclear medicine has found useful applications for the [81]Rb-[81m]Kr generator and will probably do the same for the [62]Zn-[62]Cu generator.

Yano's first automated ultrashort-lived radionuclide generator system was designed to elute Ir-191 from its parent Os-191, but it was also used, with minor changes, for separation of other ultrashort-lived radionuclides.[49] The system was automated and furnished a continuous flow of sterile eluant solution. The resin column, inside a 5-cm thick lead shield, was connected to a 20-ml syringe, which was automatically filled from an eluant reservoir and emptied through the isotope generator by an electric motor drive and an automatic two-way valve. A second reservoir contained sterile water to dilute the highly saline concentration of the eluant before the radioactive solution reached the patient's vein. This generator system made it possible to deliver the radionuclide by direct intravenous infusion at the time intervals desired, before the radionuclide decayed appreciably. A Millipore bacterial filter at the end of the system guaranteed the sterility of the solution.

[82]Sr-[82]Rb Generator

Rubidium-82, the daughter of Sr-82, has a half-life of 1.2 min. The much longer half-life of the parent, 25 days, makes this system ideal for production of an ultrashort-lived radionuclide. Rubidium-82 decays by positron emission to stable Kr-82, as shown in Figure 9–6.

The chemistry of separation and binding of [82]SrCl$_2$ to a resin is quite simple. The generator system is shown in Figure 9–7. The column is eluted with 2% NaCl solution at a pH of 8. The flow of Rb-82 eluant can be controlled by the motor-driven Minarik system, and every 5 to 10 min, about 800 μCi of Rb-82 can be in-

TABLE 9–2. *Potentially Useful Ultrashort-Lived Radionuclide Generators*

	Daughter				Parent		
Isotope	$T_{1/2}$	Mode of decay	Photon MeV	Isotope	$T_{1/2}$	Mode of decay	Production
^{82}Rb	1.3 m	β^+ EC	0.511 0.777	^{82}Sr	25 d	EC	^{85}Rb(p,4n)
^{81m}Kr	13 s	IT	0.190	^{81}Rb	4.7 h	β^+ EC	^{79}Br(α,2n)
^{191m}Ir	4.9 s	IT	0.129	^{191}Os	15.0 d	β^-	^{190}Os(n,γ)
^{137m}Ba	2.55 m	IT	0.662	^{137}Cs	30.0 y	β^-	Fission
^{109m}Ag	39.2 s	IT	0.088	^{109}Cd	1.24 y	EC	^{108}Cd(n,γ) ^{109}Ag(d,2n)
^{28}Al	2.3 m	β^-	1.78	^{28}Mg	21.2 h	β^-	^{26}Mg(t,p) ^{26}Mg(α,2p)
^{62}Cu	9.8 m	β^+	0.511	^{62}Zn	9.1 h	β^+ EC	^{63}Cu(p,2n)
^{89m}Y	16.1 s	IT	0.91	^{89}Zr	3.3 d	β^+ EC	^{89}Y(p,n)
^{90m}Nb	24 s	IT	0.122	^{90}Mo	5.7 h	β^+ EC	^{93}Nb(p,4n)
^{178}Ta	9.5 m	EC	0.093	^{178}W	21.5 d	EC	^{181}Ta(p,4n)
^{195m}Au	30.6 s	EC	0.262	^{195m}Hg	41.6	EC	^{197}Au(p,3n)

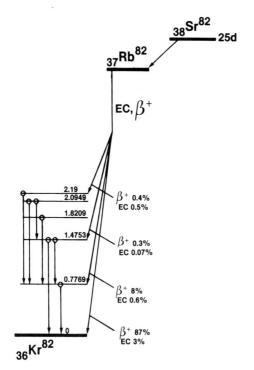

Fig. 9–6. Principal decay characteristics of [82]Sr-[82]Rb.

jected automatically with 7 to 8 ml of eluant.

This generator has been used in animal experiments, mostly to visualize the hearts of rabbits and dogs.[49,50,51,52] Images can be obtained about 1 min after the end of infusion, when the activity has cleared from the blood. Since Rb-82 accumulates to some extent in the liver, kidney, and spleen, these organs are also visualized.

[81]Rb-[81m]Kr Generator

Krypton-81m has a 13-sec half-life and decays by isomeric transition to Kr-81, emitting a 190-keV gamma ray (Fig. 9–8). Krypton-81 decays to Br-81, with a 2 × 10[5] yr half-life. A Kr-81m generator has two main problems. First, the parent radionuclide, Rb-81, has a half-life of only 4.7 hr. Second, krypton is a noble gas and therefore cannot be used to label any type of molecule. Rb-81 can be produced in a cyclotron reaction [79]Br (α, 2n) [81]Rb. The

development of Kr-81m generators was described by Jones and Clark and by Yano et al.[49,53,54,55] The generators, as described by these investigators, had some disadvantages, which were later corrected by Colombetti et al.[56] The main disadvantage was the presence of sodium ions in the target material. Sodium ions at greater than 1.5×10^{-4} molar concentration displace Rb-81 from the ion exchange resin. This problem was corrected by using Cu_2Br_2 as the target material. A yield of about 2 mCi of Rb-81/μA-hr can be produced, using alpha particles of 28 to 30 MeV. Total yields of 50 to 100 mCi (1.85 to 3.7 GBq) can be easily obtained in each bombardment. After purification of the target material, a generator can be prepared by binding the Rb-81 to a resin column. The system can be eluted with an isotonic glucose solution or with nonradioactive gases to produce a yield of approximately 80% of the available Kr-81m. The activity can be injected as a solution or inhaled as a gas.

This generator has been used clinically by Jones and Clark and by Yano et al. for lung ventilation studies,[49,53,54,55] and lately for organ perfusion studies by Kaplan et al. and by Jones et al.[57,58,59] Interestingly, when this generator is used for lung ventilation studies, environmental contamination is of little significance because of the short Kr-81m half-life.

[191]Os-[191m]Ir Generator

Iridium-191m has many characteristics of an ideal ultrashort-lived radionuclide. It has a half-life of only 4.9 sec and decays by isomeric transition to stable Ir-191, emitting two gamma rays of 40 and 129 keV (Fig. 9–9). About 70% of the 129-keV gamma rays are internally converted. The parent Os-191 has a half-life of 15.3 days, an excellent characteristic for a generator system because it has to be produced only about once a month. Osmium-191 can be produced by the [190]Os (n, γ) [191]Os reaction of 98% enriched Os-190. Naturally occur-

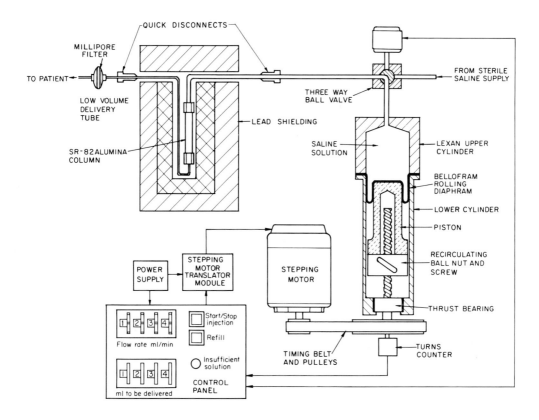

Fig. 9–7. Rubidium-82 closed generator system. (From Yano, Y., et al.[50])

ring osmium contains only 26.4% Os-190, while Os-192 is 41% abundant. Irradiation of a mixture of these two isotopes also produces large amounts of Os-193 by the reaction ^{92}Os (n, γ) ^{193}Os. This contamination is not important because Os-193 has a half-life of only 31 hr, but it will greatly reduce the yield of Os-191. Large yields of Os-191 in the 500 mCi range were obtained

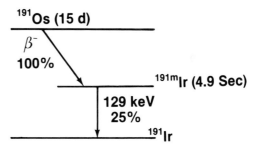

Fig. 9–9. Principal decay characteristics of ^{191}Os-^{191m}Ir.

using a neutron flux of 6.7×10^{13} n/cm²/sec by Hnatowich et al.[60]

The original development of an ^{191}Os-^{191m}Ir generator was reported by Yano and Anger.[48] These investigators used the method described by Campbell and Nelson to separate the decay product Ir-191m from its parent Os-191, which was ad-

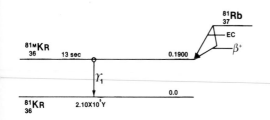

Fig. 9–8. Principal decay characteristics of ^{81}Rb-^{81m}Kr.

sorbed as $OsCl_6^{--}$ in anion exchange resin Ag 1 × 8, minus 400 mesh.[61] The mesh size of the resin is important since resin of 100 to 200 mesh size increases Os-191 contamination by a significant amount. The resin used by Yano allows a 0.1% osmium contamination, which is too large to be acceptable, and only a 10% elution of the available Ir-191m. Treves et al. recently modified the column system obtaining a generator with a slightly larger yield of Ir-191m (14%) while keeping the breakthrough of Os-191 below 0.001% over a long period of time and multiple elutions.[62]

The preparation of $OsCl_6^{--}$ can be achieved using the method of Gutbier and Mainsch.[63] Following its preparation, $OsCl_6^{--}$ can be bound in a strongly basic Bio-Rad AG1 resin column. Osmium breakthrough as well as iridium extraction

decreases with increasing cross-linking. Treves and associates reached a compromise using a system in which Bio-Rad AG1 × 4 and AG1 × 8 resins are used, as shown in Figure 9–10. The eluant from this generator has too high a saline concentration to be used in humans (about 4% NaCl), but has been used successfully in angiographic studies in monkeys, using a gamma camera and converging collimator. Approximately 15 mCi of Ir-191m in 1.5 ml of eluant were obtained from a 250- to 300-mCi generator. Since the elution time is less than 2 sec, most of the Ir-191 eluate can be infused.

If this generator can be modified to reduce the saline concentration of the eluate, human clinical studies will begin. Yano and Anger suggested that Ir-191m could be used to image veins, right heart, and lungs. The half-life may be too short to be used successfully in humans, but it may be acceptable for radionuclide angiography in newborns and small infants, because of the shorter circulation time.

^{109}Cd-^{109m}Ag Generator

Silver-109m has a 39-sec half-life, decaying by isomeric transition to Ag-109 with the emission of 87-keV gamma rays, 91% of which are converted internally to Auger electrons (Fig. 9–11).

Silver-109m has two parents: Pd-109, which has too short a half-life (13.5 hr) to be considered, and Cd-109, which has a half-life of 1.3 yr. The radiophysical characteristics of this parent-daughter system ^{109}Cd-^{109m}Ag are ideal for a generator.

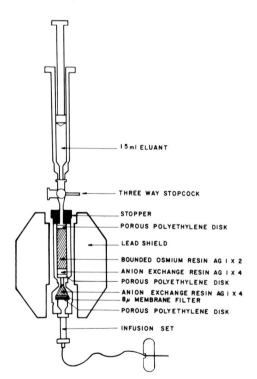

Fig. 9–10. Schematic diagram of the ^{191}Os-^{191m}Ir generator. (From Bodh, I., et al.: Circulation, 54:277, 1976. By permission of the American Heart Association, Inc.)

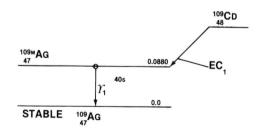

Fig. 9–11. Principal decay characteristics of ^{109}Cd-^{109m}Ag.

Three main problems exist, however: the energy of the Ag-109m gamma rays is low, 89 keV; photon yield is low owing to the high number of internal conversions; and finally, breakthrough of Cd-109 would be highly undesirable because of its long half-life. Chromatographic grade aluminum provides a satisfactory binding material for cadmium. Breakthrough of cadmium is usually small, but the separation of silver is less than satisfactory. Yields are approximately 34% when a 3% solution of NaI, which is not a physiologically suitable eluant, is used.

To produce counting rates equal to those obtained from a 10-mCi dose of Tc-99m, approximately 30 mCi of Ag-109m are required. This generator was prepared by Yano in the late sixties with some satisfactory results, but it was never tested for in vivo studies. An improvement of the silver elution system would make this a most suitable generator for clinical use.

^{137}Cs-^{137m}Ba Generator

Barium-137m decays by isomeric transition to stable Ba-137 with emission of energetic gamma rays (662 keV), as shown in Figure 9–12.

The half-life of Ba-137m is 2.6 min, longer than those of the radionuclides considered up to now, but still short enough to be useful for dynamic studies. As the daughter of Cs-137, which has a half-life of 30 yr, Ba-137m is an ideal generator system. Cesium-137 is a fission product of U-235 and can be produced in unlimited supply.

Barium-137m was used by Blau et al.

and by Vernejoul et al. in cardiac studies.[64,65,66] The first practical system for a sustained intravenous infusion was prepared by Castronovo et al. as a modification of the procedures of Van Smit et al. and Blau et al.[64,67,68] The column of the generator is made with Bio-Rad AMP-1 resin suspended in a washed asbestos powder. After a few mCi of carrier-free Cs-137m is added to the column, it is washed with the eluant solution containing 0.1N NH$_4$Cl in 0.1 N HCl. Because of possible breakthrough of Cs-137, a second column also containing Bio-Rad AMP-1 resin is connected at the bottom of the column of the generator; in this way, any Cs-137 freed from the generator is trapped, and eluate contamination is kept to a minimum. The yield of this generator per 10 ml of eluant is about 20% of the available Ba-137m, and breakthrough of Cs-137 approaches a constant value of approximately 3.5 μCi/10 ml of eluant, which is too high to be considered safe.

Castronovo connected the generator column to an ingenious system, as shown in Figure 9–13, to obtain a constant production of Ba-137m chelate and was therefore able to make constant infusions of this product. This system consists of a glass reservoir, which serves as a reaction vessel and sits on top of a magnetic stirrer. Reaction solutions, which are added continuously at a predetermined flow rate, are mixed in the vessel with the eluant by using a Teflon-covered magnetic bar. This closed system allows the eluants to be kept sterile and pyrogen free. Radiation exposure to the patients and technologists is minimal. This generator system has been used to study the cardiac blood pool in dogs, and it can also be used in humans.

^{195m}Hg-^{195m}Au Generator

Recently Panek et al. have described a reliable ^{195m}Hg-^{195m}Au-generator (Figs. 9–14 and 9–15).[69] The Hg-195m (T$_{1/2}$ = 41.6 hr) is prepared from a metallic gold target by a (p, 3n) reaction and loaded on

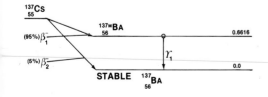

Fig. 9–12. Principal decay characteristics of Cs-137.

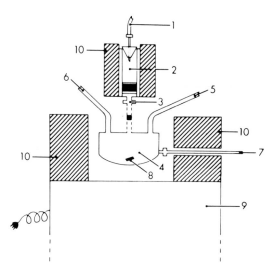

Fig. 9–13. Barium-137m chelate infusion system. *1*: eluting solution, *2*: generator, *3*: micropore filter, *4* : reaction vessel, *5* : buffer solution, *6*: chelating solution, *7*: outlet through a micropore filter to the biologic system, *8*: Teflon-covered stirring bar, *9*: magnetic stirrer, *10*: lead shielding. (From Castronovo, F.P., et al.[67])

a ZnS-coated silica gel column. Gold-195m ($T_{1/2}$ = 30.6 sec; γ = 262) is eluted with a 30 mg/ml thiosulfate solution. This generator is intended for cardiac and blood pool studies.[70] It can be eluted using either a bolus or a continuous infusion technique. Current production models contain approximately 200 mCi (7.4 GBq) of Hg-195m.

Current generator yields approach 30% of Au-195m flow rate of 12 ml/min. Mercury breakthrough remains a consideration and is the limiting factor for dosimetry considerations. At a 20% elution yield, the Hg-195m breakthrough is 2 × 10^{-3} to 3 × 10^{-3} % /ml. This results in an elution of about 1 µCi of Hg-195m per mCi of Au-195m. This breakthrough is nevertheless small enough to permit 10 to 12 successive first-pass cardiac studies while an acceptable radiation burden to the kidneys is maintained.

SPECIAL PROBLEMS ASSOCIATED WITH GENERATOR-PRODUCED ULTRASHORT-LIVED RADIONUCLIDES

The ultimate responsibility for quality control of these ultrashort-lived radionuclides must be assumed by the nuclear scientist in charge of the radiochemical laboratory in the nuclear medicine department, because the radionuclide daughter with an ultrashort half-life can be obtained only at the site of use. The short half-lives of such parent radionuclides as Rb-81 (4.7 hr), Zn-62 (9.1 hr), and Mo-90 (5.7 hr) make it almost mandatory that loading the parent in the generator's column be performed in the radiopharmacy. Special care should be taken in the preparation and use of these generators, because usual methods of testing sterility and pyrogenicity are time-consuming and consequently cannot be applied. These tests are carried out in trial runs during the development of the generator. Later, aliquots of all of the reagents used are tested. All solutions should be freshly made using distilled water for parenteral administration, and all chemicals must be pure and meet pharmacopeial standards. It is advisable to use only disposable syringes, needles, tubing, filtering surfaces, etc. to avoid possible contamination.

Most of the radionuclidic daughters mentioned here are not carrier-free, because they decay by isomeric transition to a ground state of the same species. Usually, a large proportion of the nuclide administered to the patient is the decay product of the daughter, but since the actual amount administered is in microgram or nanogram quantities, toxicity is not a hazard.

Radionuclidic impurities should be tested in advance, during the development of the column system. It is recommended that samples obtained from the generators be tested occasionally to detect possible breakthrough of the parent radionuclide.

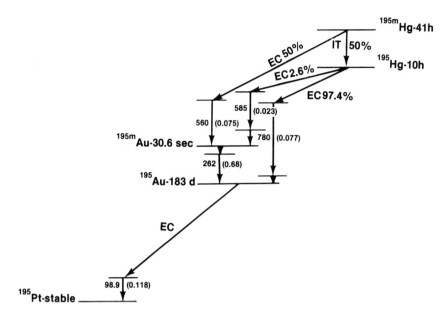

Fig. 9–14. Decay scheme for Hg-195m.

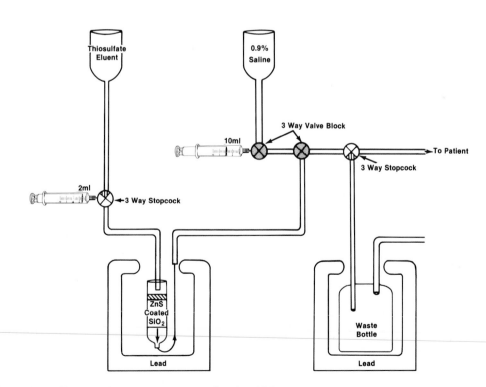

Fig. 9–15. Proposed generator system for Au-195m.

This test is performed after the daughter radionuclide has been used and serves only to control the behavior of the column involved. A column should not be used further if the test indicates larger than acceptable breakthrough of the parent radionuclide.

REFERENCES

1. Failla, G.: The development of filtered radium implants. Am. J. Roentgenol., *16*:507, 1926.
2. Richards, P.: Nuclide generators. *In* Radioactive Pharmaceuticals, Symposium No. 6, Conf 651111. Oak Ridge, U.S. Atomic Energy Commission, 1966, p. 155.
3. Stang, L.G., et al.: Production of iodine-132. Nucleonics, *12*:22, 1954.
4. Stang, L.G., et al.: Development of methods for the production of certain short-lived radioisotopes. *In* Radioisotopes in Scientific Research. London, Pergamon Press, 1958.
5. Tucker, W.D., et al.: Methods of preparation of some carrier-free radioisotopes involving adsorption of alumina. Trans. Am. Nucl. Soc., *1*:170, 1958.
6. Tucker, W.D., et al.: Practical methods of milking Y^{90}, Tc^{99m} and I^{132} from their respective parents. Trans. Am. Nucl. Soc., *3*:451, 1960.
7. Gleason, G.I.: A positron cow. Int. J. Appl. Radiat. Isot., *9*:90, 1960.
8. Greene, M.W., Doering, R.F., and Hillman, M.: Milking systems: Status of the art. Radiat. Technol., *1*:152, 1963–64.
9. Gillette, J.H.: Review of Radioisotope Progress. ORNL Report No. 3802. Oak Ridge, U.S. Atomic Energy Commission, 1965.
10. Gillette, J.H.: Review of Radioisotope Progress. ORNL Report No. 4013. Oak Ridge, U.S. Atomic Energy Commission, 1966.
11. Falconi, N.: Radioisotope generators. *In* Radioisotope Production and Quality Control. Technical Report Series, No. 128. Vienna, IAEA, 1971, p. 660.
12. Brucer, M.: One hundred and eighteen radioisotope cows. Isot. Radiat. Technol., *3*:1, 1965.
13. Spencer, R.P., and Hosain, F.: Radionuclide generators with equal decay constants for parent and daughter. Int. J. Appl. Radiat. Isot., *27*:57, 1976.
14. Subramanian, G., and McAfee, J.G.: Radioisotope generators. *In* Radiopharmacy. Edited by M. Tubis and W. Wolf. New York, Wiley Interscience, 1976.
15. Boyd, R.E.: Recent developments in generators of ^{99m}Tc. *In* Radiopharmaceuticals and Labelled Compounds. Vol. I. Vienna, IAEA, 1973, p. 3.
16. Smith, E.M.: Properties, uses, radiochemical purity and calibration of ^{99m}Tc. J. Nucl. Med., *5*:871, 1964.
17. Perrier, C., and Segré, E.: Chemical properties of element 43. J. Chem. Physiol., *5*:712, 1937.
18. Boyd, R.E., and Robson, J.: Report of study group on radioisotope production. Lucas Heights, IAEA, 1968, p.. 187.
19. Hallaba, E., and El-Asrag, H.A.: On the sublimation of ^{99m}Tc from irradiated molybdenum trioxide. Isotopenpraxis, *8*:290, 1975.
20. Colombetti, L.G.: Performance of ^{99m}Tc generating systems. *In* Quality Control in Nuclear Medicine. Edited by Buck A. Rhodes. St. Louis, C.V. Mosby, 1977.
21. Gerlit, J.B.: Some chemical properties of technetium. New York, Int. Conf. Peaceful Uses Atom. Energy (Proc. Conf., Geneva) *7*:145, 1956.
22. Lathrop, K.A.: Preparation and control of ^{99m}Tc radiopharmaceuticals. *In* Radiopharmaceuticals from Generator-Produced Radionuclides. Vienna, IAEA, 1971, p. 39.
23. Baker, R.J.: A system for the routine production of concentrated technetium-99m by solvent extraction of molybdenum. Int. J. Appl. Radiat. Isot., *22*:483, 1971.
24. Toren, D.M., and Powell, M.R.: Automatic production of technetium-99m for pharmaceutical use. J. Nucl. Med., *11*:368, 1970.
25. Charlier, R., Fallais, C., and Constant, R.: Apareil automatique pour l'extraction liquide du technetium-99m. I.R.E. 3. Belgium, Institut National des Radioéléments, 1973.
26. Mani, R.S., and Narasimham, D.V.S.: Development of kits for short-lived generator-produced radioisotopes. *In* Radiopharmaceuticals and Labelled Compounds. Vol. I. Vienna, IAEA, 1973, p. 135.
27. Stern, H., et al.: ^{133m}In, a short-lived isotope for lung scanning. Nucleonics, *24*:57, 1966.
28. Robles, A.M., Servian, J.L., and Touya, J.J.: Tests for the elution and eluates from ^{113m}In generators. *In* Radiopharmaceuticals from Generator-Produced Radionuclides. Vienna, IAEA, 1971, p. 91.
29. Colombetti, L.G., Goodwin, D.A., and Hinkley, R.L.: Preparation and testing of a sterile ^{113}Sn-^{113m}In generator. Am. J. Roentg. Rad. Ther. and Nucl. Med., CVI:745, 1969.
30. Colombetti, L.G., Barral, L.C., and Finston, R.A.: Experience with purity tests of ^{113}Sn-^{113m}In generators. Int. J. Appl. Radiat. Isot. *20*:714, 1969.
31. O'Mara, R.E., et al.: Comparison of ^{113m}In and other short-lived agents for cerebral scanning. J. Nucl. Med., *10*:18, 1969.
32. Hill, T., et al.: A simplified preparation of indium-DTPA brain scanning agents. J. Nucl. Med., *11*:28, 1970.
33. Colombetti, L.G., Barall, R.C., and Finston, R.A.: Distribution and dosimetry of ^{113m}In colloid used for bone marrow scanning. Int. J. Appl. Radiat. Isot., *21*:643, 1973.
34. Goodwin, D.A., Stern, H.S., and Wagner, H.N., Jr.: Colloidal indium-113m for liver, spleen and bone marrow scanning. J. Nucl. Med., *8*:304, 1967.
35. Sewaktar, A.B., et al.: A simple and safer ^{113m}In colloid preparation for scanning the liver. Int. J. Appl. Radiat. Isot., *21*:36, 1970.
36. Rodriguez, J., MacDonald, N.S., and Taplin, G.V.:

Preparation of [113mIn]-albumin aggregates for lung and liver scanning. J. Nucl. Med., *10*:368, 1969.

37. Raban, P., et al.: Two alternate techniques of labeling iron-free albumin microspheres with [99mTc] and [113mIn]. J. Nucl. Med., *14*:344, 1973.

38. Subramanian, G., et al.: Indium 113m labeled polyfunctional phosphonates as bone imaging agents. J. Nucl. Med., *16*:1080, 1975.

39. Neirinckx, R.D., and Davis, M.A.: Development of a generator for ionic Gallium-68. J. Nucl. Med., *20*:681, 1979.

40. Neirinckx, R.D., and Davis, M.A.: Potential column chromatography for ionic Ga68. II. Organic ion exchangers as chromatographic support. J. Nucl. Med., *21*:81, 1980.

41. Layne, W.W., and Davis, M.A.: Development of a Gallium-68 generator on alumina. J. Nucl. Med., *21*: P85, 1980.

42. Atcher, R.W., Friedman, A.M., et al.: Lead-211: A short-lived, generator produced alpha and beta emitting radionuclide suitable for therapeutic use. J. Nucl. Med., *21*:P85, 1980.

43. Ku, T.H., Richards, P., Stang, L.G., et al.: Generator production of manganese-52m for positron tomography. J. Nucl. Med., *20*:682, 1979.

44. Atcher, R.W., Friedman, A.M., et al.: Manganese-52m, a new short-lived generator produced radionuclide: A potential tracer for positron tomography. J. Nucl. Med., *21*:569, 1980.

45. Neirinckx, R.D., Jones, A.G., Davis, M.A., et al.: Tantalum-178, a short-lived nuclide for nuclear medicine: Development of a potential generator system. J. Nucl. Med., *19*:514, 1978.

46. Neirinckx, R.D., Holman, B.L., Davis, M.A., et al.: Tantalum-178 labeled agents for lung and liver imaging. J. Nucl. Med., *20*:1176, 1979.

47. Bender, M.A., and Blau, M.: The autofluoroscope. Nucleonics, *21*:52, 1963.

48. Yano, Y., and Anger, H.O.: Ultrashort-lived radioisotopes for visualizing blood vessels and organs. J. Nucl. Med., *9*:2, 1968.

49. Yano, Y., and Anger, H.O.: Visualization of heart and kidneys in animals with ultrashort-lived [82Rb] and the positron scintillation camera. J. Nucl. Med., *9*:412, 1968.

50. Yano, Y., Cahoon, J.L., and Budinger, T.F.: A precision flow-controlled Rb82 generator for bolus or constant infusion studies of the heart and brain. J. Nucl. Med., *22*:1006, 1981.

51. Yano, Y., et al.: Evaluation of rubidium-82 generators for imaging studies. J. Nucl. Med., *17*:536, 1976.

52. Yano, Y., Budinger, T.F., O'Brien, H.A., et al.: Evaluation and application of alumina column Rb-82 generators. J. Nucl. Med., *20*:684, 1979.

53. Jones, T., and Clark, J.C.: A cyclotron produced [81Rb]-[81mKr] generator and its uses in gamma camera studies. Br. J. Radiol., *42*:237, 1969.

54. Jones, T., et al.: [81mKr] generator and its uses in cardiopulmonary studies with the scintillation camera. J. Nucl. Med., *11*:118, 1970.

55. Yano, Y., McRae, J., and Anger, H.O.: Lung function studies using short-lived [81mKr] and the scintillation camera. J. Nucl. Med., *11*:674, 1970.

56. Colombetti, L.G., et al.: Continuous radionuclide generation. I. Production and evaluation of a krypton-81m mini-generator. J. Nucl. Med., *15*:868, 1974.

57. Kaplan, E., et al.: Continuous radionuclide generation. II. Scintigraphic definition of capillary exchange by rapid decay of krypton-81m and its applications. J. Nucl. Med., *15*:874, 1974.

58. Kaplan, E., et al.: Definition of myocardial perfusion by continuous infusion of krypton-81m. Am. J. Cardiol., *37*:878, 1976.

59. Jones, T., et al.: Use of [81Rb]-[81mKr] ratio for the measurement of spleen blood flow. J. Nucl. Med., *14*:414, 1973.

60. Hnatowich, D.J., Kulprathipanja, S., and Treves, S.: An improved [191Os]-[191mIr] generator for radionuclide angiography. Radiology, *123*:189, 1977.

61. Campbell, E.C., and Nelson, F.: Rapid ion-exchange techniques for radiochemical separations. J. Inorg. Nucl. Chem., *3*:232, 1956.

62. Treves, S., Kulprathipanja, S., and Hnatowich, D.J.: Angiocardiography with [191mIr]. Circulation, *54* :274, 1976.

63. Gutbier, A., and Mainsch, K.: Uber osmium. Ber Otsch Chem Ges., *42*:4239, 1909.

64. Blau, M., Zielinski, R., and Bender, M.: [137mBa] cow—a new short-lived isotope generator. Nucleonics, *24*:90, 1966.

65. Vernejoul, P., et al.: The importance of nuclear indicators of short half-life in the study of cardiac hemodynamics. Nucl. Med., *5*:3, 1966.

66. Vernejoul, P., Valeyre, J., and Kellershohn, C.: Dosimetry and technique for the use of [137mBa] in cardiac hemodynamics. C. R. Acad. Sci., *264*:10, 1967.

67. Castronovo, F.P., Reba, R.C., and Wagner, H.N.: System for sustained intravenous infusion of a sterile solution of [137mBa]-ethylenediaminetetraacetic acid (EDTA). J. Nucl. Med., *10*:242, 1969.

68. Van Smit, R., Robb, W., and Jacobs, J.: Cation exchange on ammonium-molybdo-phosphate-I. J. Inorgan. Nucl. Chem., *12*:1064, 1959.

69. Panek, K.J., Lindeyer, J., and van der Vlught, N.C.: A new generator system for production of short-living Au-195m radioisotope. J. Nucl. Med., *23*:P108, 1982.

70. Mena, I., Narahara, K.A., de Jong, R., and Maublaut, J.: Gold-195m, an ultra-short-lived generator-produced radionuclide: clinical application in sequential first-pass ventriculography. J. Nucl. Med., *24*:139, 1983.

Chapter 10

RADIOPHARMACEUTICAL CHEMISTRY

WILLIAM C. ECKELMAN

Radiopharmaceutical chemistry is the study of those aspects of chemistry, pharmacology, biochemistry, physiology, and associated disciplines that relate to the development of radiolabeled derivatives suitable for tracing biologic processes. Radiopharmaceuticals are generally labeled with gamma-emitting radionuclides and are used primarily as diagnostic agents. The ability to incorporate radionuclides with optimal decay characteristics into tracer molecules has been the foremost consideration in the development of most radiopharmaceuticals. In this respect, Tc-99m is the ideal choice.

The radioisotopes of iodine have played an established role in radiopharmaceutical chemistry since their early use in thyroid metabolism studies and radioimmunoassay. Because not one of the iodine isotopes has the ideal nuclear properties of Tc-99m, iodinated imaging agents have mostly been replaced by similar Tc-99m labeled radiopharmaceuticals. Nevertheless, radioiodine is constantly being rediscovered as constraints on the perturbations allowed in radiolabeled substrates become more stringent. Addition of a large chelating group to a steroid, peptide hormone, or drug might alter the size, the lipid solubility, the pK, or the surface topography to such an extent as to decrease the derivative's ability to act as a true tracer. In these cases, radioisotopes of iodine, especially I-123, are preferred. In this chapter, detailed discussion of the complex chemistry of technetium and iodine is presented, along with examples of clinically useful radiopharmaceuticals.

Other radionuclides with important applications, including short-lived cyclotron and other generator products, are reviewed with respect to their chemistry and quality assurance.

RADIOPHARMACEUTICAL CHEMISTRY OF TECHNETIUM

General Properties

Of the conveniently available radionuclides, technetium has by far the best nuclear properties for imaging with the Anger camera. The 6-hr half-life and absence of beta radiation result in a low-equilibrium dose constant ($\Delta = 0.303$ g-rad/μCi-hr).[1] The 140-keV gamma emission has satisfactory tissue penetration; 50% is absorbed in 4.6 cm of tissue, and yet the energy is low enough to be collimated easily. Technetium-99m is produced indirectly either by the neutron irradiation of Mo-98 or as a fission product of U-235:

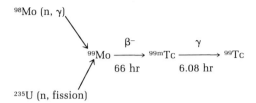

The generator system consists of Mo-99 adsorbed on an alumina column (see Chap. 9). Fission-produced Mo-99 is carrier free (sp. Act. $> 10^4$ Ci/g), which facilitates the adsorption of large amounts of radioactivity to small alumina columns. This lessens the chance of Mo-99 breakthrough and allows elution with a small volume of saline. Reactor-produced Mo-99 contains a high percentage of carrier Mo-98 (sp. act. ~10 Ci/g). More alumina is needed for the column, and consequently, more lead is required for shielding. With fractional elution of reactor-produced Mo-99, the same high specific concentration of Tc-99m can usually be achieved. For Tc-99m eluted from either fission- or cyclotron-produced Mo-99, the major radionuclidic impurity is Mo-99 itself. The acceptable limits of radionuclide purity are discussed in the section "Quality Assurance of Radiopharmaceuticals—General Considerations."

As use of Tc-99m radiopharmaceuticals has grown, larger generators have been manufactured. This has necessitated a return to high specific activity, fission-produced Mo-99, despite the increased difficulty of disposing of the fission waste material.[2] The higher specific activity is necessary because problems of size and shielding become more acute with multicurie generators.

With the larger generators, more attention must be given to details of the decay scheme. Molybdenum-99 decays partly to the Tc-99m (metastable) state and partly to the Tc-99g (ground) state directly (see Appendix B). This has three effects. First, the daughter activity of Tc-99m does not exceed that of the parent Mo-99 when the system reaches transient equilibrium.[3] In this discussion, transient equilibrium is defined as the time after elution when the ratio between daughter d and parent p activities becomes constant, that is:

$$\frac{A_d}{A_p} = \frac{\lambda_d}{\lambda_d - \lambda_p}$$

For the case of the ^{99}Mo-^{99m}Tc system, the branch to Tc-99m represents only 87.5% of the decay events. Therefore, the relationship at transient equilibrium is:

$$\frac{A(Tc\text{-}99m)}{A(Mo\text{-}99)} = \frac{.875\ \lambda(Tc\text{-}99m)}{\lambda(Tc\text{-}99m) - \lambda(Mo\text{-}99)}$$

Elimination of the time-dependent term $e^{-\lambda_2 t}$ in the transient equilibrium equation (see Chap. 9, equations 11 and 12) introduces a 1% error 42 hours after elution of the generator and a 0.17% error 63 hours after elution. Another definition of the transient equilibrium, a zero rate of change for technetium formation:

$$\frac{d(Tc\text{-}99m)}{dt} = 0$$

has been introduced but generally is not accepted in nuclear medicine.[4]

The second effect of the use of large generators is the formation of measurable amounts of Tc-99g in relatively short periods of time. The amount of Tc-99g produced (N_3) can be calculated from the expression:

$$N_3 = (N_1^0)\ [0.875(1 + \frac{\lambda_p}{\lambda_d - \lambda_p}\ e^{-\lambda_d t}$$

$$- \frac{\lambda_d}{\lambda_d - \lambda_p}\ e^{-\lambda_p t}) + 0.125\ (1 - e^{-\lambda_p t})]$$

where N_1^0 = atoms of Mo-99 at the time of the previous elution.

The contribution to N_3 (Tc-99g) from the 87% Tc-99m branch (^{99g}Tc from ^{99}Mo $\rightarrow$ ^{99m}Tc $\rightarrow$ ^{99g}Tc) and from the 13% Tc-99g branch (^{99g}Tc from Mo $\rightarrow$ ^{99g}Tc) can be calculated (Fig. 10–1). The relationships among the radioactive particles present

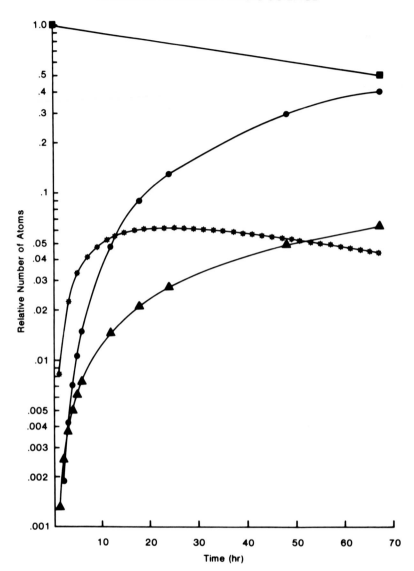

Fig. 10–1. The relative number of atoms of molybdenum and technetium as a function of time. Molybdenum atoms (■), Tc-99g from the 87% branch decay of Mo-99 via Tc-99m (●), Tc-99g from the 13% branch decay of Mo-99 directly (▲), and Tc-99m from the decay of Mo-99 (★).

are deceiving in that the Tc-99g appears to be insignificant. Because of the long half-life of Tc-99g, the radioactivity is low, but the mass is substantial. In a 1-Ci Mo-99 generator [2.1×10^{-8} mol of Mo-99], 4.7×10^{-10} mol of Tc-99g is produced 6 hr after the previous elution. If this Tc-99g is eluted in 10 ml, then the concentration of elemental Tc is 47 nM. At 67 hr after elution 0.09 μM of Tc is present. These are no longer "tracer" amounts of Tc; they can affect the chemistry of the radiopharmaceutical. Deutsch et al. have confirmed these theoretic results.[5]

The radiation field created by the larger amount of Mo-99, combined with the strong adsorption properties of alumina for Tc(VI) as TcO_4^{2-}, produces low yields under certain conditions. A "dry" column or the presence of oxidizing agents appears to prevent low elution yields.[6]

Reducing Agents for Tc(VII)

With the advent of the ^{99}Mo-^{99m}Tc generator system in the sixties,[7] "instant" technetium kits,[8] and innovations in chelation, use of Tc-99m labeled compounds has expanded. But the chemical form of Tc-99m eluted from the generator is pertechnetate—$^{99m}TcO_4^-$, or Tc(VII)—the most stable chemical state of technetium in aqueous solution.

Pertechnetate does not bind to chelating agents nor does it coprecipitate with particles necessary for bone, pulmonary, or renal imaging procedures. Consequently, a less stable, "positively-charged" reduced state of Tc-99m, capable of participating in chemical reactions, must be formed for these studies. The only exception to this is Tc-99m sulfur colloid, which is considered to have the Tc(VII) oxidation state, because the insolubility of the technetium sulfide stabilizes the Tc-99m in this oxidation state.[9]

Reduced states of technetium can be achieved by treatment with such reducing agents as stannous ion, the combination of ferric chloride and ascorbic acid, ferrous ion, sodium borohydride, concentrated hydrochloric acid, sodium dithionite, hypophosphorus acid, and hydrazine. The sulfhydryl group and the aldehyde group have been used as reducing agents, but both require heat and time to produce reasonable yields, which makes them somewhat less convenient. Pertechnetate can also be reduced electrolytically, i.e., electrons can be supplied by a voltage applied to inert electrodes. With zirconium and tin electrodes, metallic reducing species probably are responsible for the reduction. In the reduced state, the technetium binds readily to chelating agents, thereby forming such compounds as Tc-99m diethylenetriaminepentaacetic acid (DTPA), Tc-99m hydroxyethylidene diphosphon-

ate (HEDP), and Tc-99m glucoheptonate, which are commonly used in diagnostic imaging. Reduced technetium also coprecipitates with colloids to produce such compounds as Tc-99m stannous oxide or Tc-99m microaggregates and with particles to produce Tc-99m stannous macroaggregated albumin (MAA).

Many of the first Tc-99m chelates were formed using ferric chloride and ascorbic acid as the reducing agent.[10] Although these agents produced a suitable radiopharmaceutical, the need to use special equipment, such as a pH meter, and to prepare sterile buffers prevented their routine use in most nuclear medicine laboratories. The introduction of stannous ion as a reducing agent permitted pertechnetate to be added to the reaction vial with no pH adjustment or addition of other substances. Pertechnetate is reduced at pH 4 to 7 and then bound by the chelating agent. On a practical level, this use of stannous ion was a key development; most current radiopharmaceutical kits employ the stannous reduction technique. For blood cells, which are sensitive to changes in pH, stannous ion is also ideal.

The disadvantage of using a stannous or ferrous salt as the reducing agent is that at neutral pH it reacts readily with water to form colloids or large particles. These colloids and particles coprecipitate with reduced technetium, and in fact, this property has been used purposely to prepare imaging agents for liver and lung respectively. If the desired product is a Tc-99m chelate, however, these radiolabeled particles are unwanted radiochemical impurities. To avoid this side reaction, the metallic salt is kept soluble at neutral pH by binding it to a chelating agent, most often the same compound to be labeled with Tc-99m. For instance, in the preparation of Tc-99m DTPA, an excess of DTPA is added to the kit to bind all of the stannous ion present.

Equilibrium constants are known for the stannous chelates of pyrophosphate,[11,12]

DTPA,[13] and such organic ligands as acetate, oxalate, or citrate;[14] these constants determine the concentration of chelating agents needed to maintain the solubility of the metal at neutral pH.[15,16] Because metal oxides inhibit and competitively interfere with the desired binding of technetium,[17] the reducing agent must be in chelate form to prevent this side reaction from occurring.

Oxidation States of Tc-99m Radiopharmaceuticals

Although efforts to characterize Tc compounds have been considerable,[18] most have been carried out in nonaqueous solutions and therefore are not directly applicable to clinical Tc-99m radiopharmaceuticals. On the other hand, some recent work on Tc compounds in aqueous solution has involved thiol compounds that are not used routinely.[19] Efforts in both cases, however, have led to the discovery of important chemical information much needed in radiopharmaceutical chemistry.

Stannous Ion

Most Tc-99m radiopharmaceuticals in clinical use are treated with stannous ion, and therefore, studies with this reducing agent are relevant to the understanding of clinical Tc-99m radiopharmaceuticals. While it is desirable to know the exact oxidation state of technetium in clinically used radiopharmaceuticals, present methodology makes the determination of nanomolar concentrations difficult. Experiments with millimolar concentrations of Tc-99 have indicated that it is reduced by stannous ion to the V state, and then slowly to Tc(IV) at pH 7 in citrate buffer. In HCl also, Tc-99 is reduced by stannous ion to the IV state. With a DTPA buffer at pH 4, the ^{99}Tc(III) state prevails.[20] It is not known, however, whether these millimolar determinations can be extrapolated to the nanomolar concentrations used in diagnostic imaging procedures.

Investigators also have attempted to define the reduced oxidation state of Tc-99m in the DTPA chelate.[21] It is known that millimolar concentrations of ^{99}TcO$_4^-$, for which in vitro analysis can be made, form ^{99}Tc(IV) in the presence of the following reducing agents: (1) stannous ion, (2) ferric chloride and ascorbic acid, (3) ferrous ion, and (4) concentrated HCl-HI and ^{99}Tc(V) with concentrated HCl. In each case, and for concentrations ranging from millimolar Tc-99 to tracer Tc-99m, binding efficiency of the reduced technetium to DTPA is greater than 85% for those reducing agents producing Tc(IV). When the same measurements are performed with concentrated HCl alone as the reducing agent, only 10% of Tc-99, but 45% of Tc-99m, is bound to DTPA. Differences in the efficiency of compound formation almost certainly reflect a difference in oxidation state produced by concentrated HCl. When the same binding trend is evident for Tc-99m and Tc-99, the same oxidation state that occurs with Tc-99 also is found to occur with Tc-99m (10^{-9} M) utilized in nuclear medicine laboratories. Although in the absence of DTPA, Tc(IV) is produced with the first four reducing agents, any conclusions regarding the oxidation state of stannous-reduced technetium labeled to DTPA are unwarranted in view of the changes in the stannous-stannic electrochemical potential caused by the addition of DTPA.

A recent effort to extrapolate from millimolar to nanomolar chemistry by observing the biological behavior of the resulting radiopharmaceuticals has shown that Tc-99m HEDP and Tc-99m glucoheptonate (GHA) have the same biologic distributions as the Tc-99 compounds and therefore are probably in the same oxidation state, namely, Tc(IV).[22] On the other hand, Steigman has shown that a stable complex is formed with gluconate in the Tc(V) oxidation state at high pH.[23] He has also shown, using millimolar concentrations of Tc-99, that a mixture of Tc(III) and Tc(IV) pyrophosphate exists. Finally, Tc-

HIDA, a hepatobiliary agent, has been shown to be in the Tc(III) oxidation state when millimolar concentrations of Tc are used.[24]

Hydrochloric Acid

Hydrochloric acid has not been used in a clinically useful radiopharmaceutical because of the difficulty of handling concentrated acid. It interests researchers, however, because it provides one example of different oxidation states being produced at carrier-free levels of Tc-99m and at millimolar carrier levels of Tc-99. Hydrochloric acid was first reported to reduce Tc-99 by Gerlit, who showed that quantitative reduction could be achieved at 20° C in concentrated HCl in 1 hr or at 75° C in $9N$ HCl in 1/2 hr.[25] The exact oxidation state was not identified, but reduction was indicated by decreased extraction by diethyldithiocarbamate in $CHCl_3$. Busey identified the oxidation state as Tc(V) by titration with $SnCl_2$.[26] He showed that at room temperature, >80% yield of Tc(V) could be achieved immediately. The reduction to $TcCl_6^{2-}$ was slow.

Ossicini et al. developed a chromatographic method of separating the oxychlorocomplexes of Tc(IV), Tc(V), and Tc(VII) using HCl.[27]

Because oxidation states per se cannot be separated by chromatography there is the possibility of various complex oxychlorocompounds having the same R_f value of Tc(V) and Tc(IV). With development of this chromatographic system using $0.6N$ HCl on Whatman No. 3 MM paper, differences were noted between the rates of reduction for Tc-99m and Tc-99. Since 13% of Mo-99 decays to Tc-99 directly and Tc-99 is the decay product of Tc-99m, the actual concentration of Tc in any study using "Tc-99m" is usually unknown. With Tc-99, Ossicini et al. showed an immediate reduction to ^{99}Tc(V) in concentrated HCl.[27] At 100° C in concentrated HCl, ^{99}Tc(IV) is observed. At ½ hr, approximately 50% ^{99}Tc(V) remained. The

^{99}Tc(V) decreased to 30% after 1 hr. In HBr at room temperature, ^{99}Tc(VII), produced ^{99}Tc(V), but when heated at 100° C, it produced ^{99}Tc(IV).

Williams and Deegan varied the concentration of Tc-99 from 10 mg/ml to trace concentrations.[28] They found Tc(V) at higher concentrations but Tc(IV) at 0.05 mg/ml and at trace levels. Thus Tc is reduced to a lower oxidation state at trace levels, violating the generally accepted second-order kinetic rate dependence. The reducing agent Cl^- was held constant ($11N$) in these studies.

Cifka has shed some light on this system both by showing that trace impurities of ferric ion alter the chromatography on Whatman 3 MM paper and by adding ferric ion to accelerate the reduction of pertechnetate.[29]

Cifka has shown an HCl concentration dependence on the reduction of Tc-99m pertechnetate to Tc(IV). Above $5N$ HCl at 100° C, the reduction was quantitative. De Liverant and Wolf have confirmed this, using Tc-99m eluted from a commercial generator.[30] Cifka also observed Tc(IV) at 22° C in concentrated HCl, whereas de Liverant and Wolf found only ~20% Tc(V) under the same conditions. Earlier, Eckelman et al. observed that DTPA could bind up to 45% of the Tc-99m reduced by HCl but only 9% of the Tc-99 at 4×10^{-2}M in concentrated HCl, again implying that trace and millimolar concentrations of Tc are chemically different.[31] Based on Cifka's work with trace impurities and on the fact that the lower oxidation state is observed at lower concentrations, the parameters of the reduction of Tc with HCl need further study.

The reduction of millimolar concentrations of Tc(VII) to Tc(IV) can be achieved by using stronger reducing agents. Concentrated HCl in the presence of KI can reduce Tc(VII) to Tc(IV) quantitatively. Thomas et al. showed that at 25° C, concentrated HCl produces Tc(V) rapidly at carrier Tc levels but reduction to Tc(IV) is slow.[32] With concentrated HBr at 25° C, Tc(IV) is rapidly produced. At 0° C, HBr produces Tc(V). With HI, Tc(V) can be produced only at isopropanol-dry ice bath temperatures. The HCl system has been suggested as the reducing system of choice to produce $TcOCl_4^-$.

Electrolytic Reduction

The most popular electrolytic procedures for Tc-99m employ zirconium or tin electrodes.[33,34] For Tc-99, polarographic studies by Miller and co-workers,[35] and later by Terry and Zittel,[36] indicate that the pink Tc(IV) and the green or yellow Tc(III) can be attained electrolytically in the presence of phosphates. The reduction of Tc(IV) to Tc(III) seems slow, and the Tc(III) state is easily oxidized. Steigman has repeated these experiments and shown a similarity between pyrophosphates that are electrolytically produced and those that are stannous ion reduced.[23]

Other Reducing Agents

Sodium dithionate is an effective reducing agent for Tc at high pH, producing $TcO(SCH_2CH_2S)_2^{-1}$, a confirmed Tc(V) species.[37] This is also the structure for the secreted compound N,N'-*bis*(mercaptoacetamido)-ethylenediamine (Tc-DADS), a possible replacement for iodohippurate in kidney studies.[38]

The oxidation states produced by the other reducing agents mentioned have not been characterized. All experiments assuming a similarity of chemical behavior between Tc-99 and Tc-99m have considered the concentration of technetium as the only variable in the reaction. Unfortunately, variations exist in such other parameters as the quantities of reducing agent and chelating agent employed in chelate formation. The ratio of stannous and stannic ion to the amount of technetium has been considered responsible for reports of both $^{99}Tc(III)$ and $^{99}Tc(IV)$ in the chelate.[20] The quantity of reducing agent used in compound formation is therefore

crucial. Also, these findings strongly suggest that more than one oxidation state of technetium can bind to the same chelate, although the effect that this has on the in vivo distribution of the compound is unclear.

Another important consideration is the method used to determine the oxidation state of Tc-99 at millimolar concentrations. As an example of this, iodine titration could theoretically yield misleading information concerning the oxidation state of technetium if the iodine oxidizes not only the excess reducing agent, but also the reduced technetium itself.

Steigman et al. have shown that Tc-99 citrate and Tc-99 gluconate can be prepared as Tc(V) chelate quite readily,[20] but further reduction to Tc(IV) in the case of citrate requires time. If the work of Hambright et al. is compared with that of Steigman,[22,23] the final oxidation state of Tc-99 gluconate appears to depend on the chelating agent concentration. Both observations are difficult to apply to Tc-99m chemistry. Because of the chromatographic system available, a number of investigators have been able to show that concentrated HCl produces different oxidation states with Tc-99m and Tc-99. Whether this is due to trace iron impurities or to differences in rates of disproportionation has not been proven, but the need for caution is obvious. Many pitfalls are evident in comparing Tc-99 chemistry with Tc-99m chemistry.

Technetium Complexes

Determination of Equilibrium Constants

Just as information on the oxidation state prevalent in various chelates is limited, little is known about the aqueous chemistry of these reduced species of technetium. Electrophoretic and extraction studies with anionic chelating agents now provide indirect evidence for the existence of TcO^{2+}, $TcOOH^+$ and TcO_2, even though few equilibrium constants for chelates of Tc-99 have been reported.[39,40] Sundrehagen, however, has found it difficult to reproduce these findings and warns against polymer formation on the Tc-99 level.[41] The log equilibrium constants for Tc-EDTA (19.1), Tc-nitrilotriacetic acid (Tc-NTA) (K_1 = 13.8, K_2 = 25.7), and Tc-HEDTA (20.8) were determined by Gorski and Koch, using an electrophoretic technique and an ion exchange method.[42] Both determinations were carried out at low pH, and both analytic techniques are based on the fact that the rates of association and dissociation are rapid. Recently, Levin et al. have determined the equilibrium constant of Tc-DTPA to be log K_A = 26.[43]

Determination of Kinetic Parameters

Two recent studies have shown Tc(IV) to be kinetically slow with respect to ligand exchange at neutral pH. McRae and co-workers studied the kinetics of ligand exchange by mixing various chelating agents with Tc-99m radiopharmaceuticals and studying the distribution of Tc-99m in rats.[44] They reported that neither HEDP nor pyrophosphate can replace gluconate, although the concentrations of HEDP and pyrophosphate are low and these results could reflect an equilibrium situation. Technetium-99m HEDP and Tc-99m pyrophosphate were shown to be slow in exchanging with gluconate. That is, some exchange did occur with time, which indicates the inert nature, but the half-time for exchange was longer than the arbitrary time of 1 min chosen by Taube as the definition of inert.[45] This is attributed to the well-known inert character of d^3 states.

Loberg studied the exchange rate between Tc-HIDA and EDTA as a function of time and pH, using an electrophoretic separation.[46] The K_{eq} for Tc(HIDA)$_2$ is 10^{16}, using the log K of 19.1 for Tc(IV) EDTA, and the rate of dissociation occurs with a $T_{1/2}$ of 3.5 hr at pH 3.5 and of 9.0 hr at pH 6.0. Because Tc(III) is present in

Tc(HIDA)$_2$, the exchange experiment is complicated.

Deutsch et al. point out that some compounds that appear to follow first-order kinetics when labeled with Tc are independent of the Tc concentration.[5] Technetium diarsine complexes, e.g., Tc(diars)$_2$Br$_2$$^+$, seem to follow this kinetic order. In other cases, second order kinetics are evident, and the original concentration of the Tc then is important. An obvious example of the latter case is the reaction of two Tc species.

Types of Complexing Agents

Many colored compounds of reduced technetium have been prepared, to develop a spectrophotometric analysis of small quantities of technetium produced in fission.[47,48] In general, the analytic problem associated with counting the beta activity of Tc-99 led to the development of procedures that could detect microgram quantities of Tc-99. These compounds were not well defined since the purpose was to develop a sensitive analytic technique and not to isolate chelates of reduced technetium.

Crouthamel, using thiocyanate as a reducing and complexing agent, determined the existence of two species, which he confirmed by titration studies with titanium sulfate.[49] He observed that the "red complex," which he designated as Tc(V), is stabilized by acetone and reasonably inert, since in the study, it did not dissociate upon 50-fold dilution. The Tc(V) could not be oxidized by Br$_2$ or cerium (IV) sulfate.

Crouthamel also observed formation of Tc(VI), Tc(V), and Tc(IV) in the potentiometric titration of TcO$_4^-$ by Tc(III) in 12M H$_2$SO$_4$. In this medium, Tc(VI) disproportionates within 3 to 4 min to Tc(V) and Tc(VII), whereas Tc(V) disproportionates to Tc(VII) and Tc(IV) within 1 hr.

Howard and Weber later increased the speed of color development by adding ascorbic acid and ferric chloride to the Crouthamel preparation.[50] They still obtained the red Tc(V) in the presence of ferric chloride and ascorbic acid.

Although production of a colored species gives no indication of compound yield and at times can be misleading, it nevertheless suggests chelating groups that might be used.

The structure and properties of the cyanate and thiocyanate complexes were determined later by Schwochau.[51,52] The cyanate complex was prepared in basic media, and the thiocyanate in acidic media. In basic media, a tetracyano derivative, $Tl_3TcO(OH)_3(CN)_4$, was prepared and analyzed by elemental analysis, by molar conductivity, and by infrared, visible, and ultraviolet spectra. In acid solution, two compounds are prepared, $Tc^{IV}(NCS)_6^{2-}$ and $Tc^V(NCS)_6^-$, which form a reversible redox couple. All compounds contain Tc-N bonds, and none are stable at neutral pH. Trop et al. prepared $K_4Tc(CN)_7$, a Tc(III) complex that oxidized to $TcO(CN)_5^{2-}$ and $TcO_2(CN)_4^{3-}$, both Tc(V) complexes.[53] Their study provides evidence that Schwochau's complex, $Tl_3TcO(OH)_3(CN)_4$, should be reformulated as $TcO(CN)_5^{2-}$. Trop et al. also reinvestigated the thiocyanate complexes of Crouthamel and Schwochau and determined that the red complex, identified as a Tc(V) complex by Crouthamel and Schwochau, is actually at $Tc(NCS)_6^{2-}$, a Tc(IV) species.[54] Further reduction produces a yellow compound formulated as $Tc(NCS)_6^{3-}$.

Several other compounds have been prepared and studied as analogs to compounds already known for rhenium. Both Rulfs and Rajec have prepared the 8-hydroxyquinoline derivative of Tc(V).[55,56]

Extraction of Tc(V) prepared in concentrated HCl with a chloroform solution of 8-hydroxyquinoline produces a red organic layer. Technetium(IV) and Tc(VII) cannot be extracted. The Tc(V) chelate appears inert and cannot be stripped back into the aqueous phase in the range of 6N

HCl to 1N NaOH. The composition of the Tc(V) 8-hydroxyquinoline chelate was shown by titration, using $HClO_4$. From these data, a structural formula with a 1:1 complex was proposed, and the IR spectra indicated the formation of TcO_2 bands similar to those found for rhenium oxo-9-hydroxyquinoline. The stability constant appears to be between that of Co(II) and Mn(II), based on the relative shift of the visible absorption spectra. This would fix log K between 7.30 and 9.65.

Recently, Armstrong has prepared the trans-aquonitrosyl tetraamine technetium(I) compound.[57] Earlier, this compound was reported to contain a hydroxylamine moiety, but a crystal structure analysis of this compound indicated the presence of nitrosyl ligand. The one electron oxidation to Tc(II) is reversible, and the compound is stable in dilute acid. The stability of this compound is surprising for a metal with a formal charge of +1, and it may indicate the inert character of the d^6 state. A number of other interesting compounds in lower oxidation states have been described by Jones and Davison.[58] The major attraction of Tc(I), Tc(II), and Tc(III) chelates is the aqueous stability of many complexes.

In the last few years, several groups have concentrated on sulfhydryl ligands with Tc(V) cores. In general, the synthetic pathways have been carried out in nonaqueous chemistry, starting with the water-unstable $TcOCl_4^-$ core. If the chelating agent contains sulfhydryl groups, the TcO core is most likely present whereas if amines are present, the TcO_2 core is present.[37] Technetium cyclam is a recent example of the latter class.[59]

Ligand exchange also has been proposed as an efficient method of producing new radiotracers. For the preparation of Tc(V) compounds, Tc(V) gluconate appears to be a good starting material: for the preparation of Tc(IV) compounds, $TcCl_6^{2-}$ appears to be acceptable.[60]

Several Tc(V) compounds have been

isolated in the crystalline state.[37] They include:

TcOCl$_4$
TcO(SCH$_2$COS)$_2^-$
TcO(SCH$_2$CH$_2$S)$_2^-$
TcO(SCH$_2$CON(CH$_2$)$_2$NCOCH$_2$S)$^-$
TcO(Penicillamine)$_2$ complex
TcO(EDTA)$^-$
TcO$_2$(CN)$_4$ complex
TcO$_2$(cyclam)$^+$

Of the various oxidation states of Tc, the chemistry of Tc(V) has been emphasized to the greatest extent, even though from earlier work, Tc(IV) appeared to be the most stable. Of the clinically useful radiopharmaceuticals prepared on the Tc-99 level, the following oxidation states have been established:

Tc(III)
    Tc-Sn-DTPA
    Tc-Sn-bone agents
    Tc-HIDA
    Tc(diarsine)$_2$Cl$_2^+$ (potential myocardial agent)

Tc(IV)
    Tc-Sn-bone agents

Tc(V)
    Tc-gluconate
    Tc-DMSA

Whether the Tc-99m labeled compounds exist as these oxidation states, however, has not been determined absolutely.

Quality Assurance of Tc-99m Radiopharmaceuticals

Most radiopharmaceuticals cannot be studied by ultraviolet or infrared spectroscopy, nuclear magnetic resonance, or elemental analysis because they are carrier free. Accordingly, chromatography has become the major analytic tool for determining their radiochemical purity. The term *radiochemical purity,* however, is much abused. The strict definition is the percentage of the radionuclide in question in the desired chemical form. The common mistake is to use a chromatographic system that can separate only one radiochemical impurity, usually pertechnetate, and then to report the radiochemical purity on that basis. Certainly, pertechnetate is the most obvious impurity in Tc-99m radiopharmaceuticals, but as early as 1967, another impurity, commonly called *reduced unbound Tc-99m* or *reduced hydrolyzed Tc-99m,* had been identified. The exact nature of this species is not known; it may be a combination of impurities. Nevertheless, it is an impurity to be recognized.

Chromatographic Techniques

The most common method of separating radiochemical impurities in Tc-99m radiopharmaceuticals is *chromatography.* Paper chromatography and thin-layer chromatography (TLC) are simple methods of separation with closely related techniques for sample application, development, detection, etc. Column chromatography, which is a more complicated technique, offers a wider variety of solid supports (adsorption, gel filtration and permeation for molecular size, ion exchange, etc.) and is more adaptable to large-scale separations and to quantitation of the species present.[61,62] Recently, high-pressure liquid chromatography (HPLC) has been used for less polar Tc-99m chelates. This sensitive technique promises to make the definition of radiochemical purity more restrictive. With TLC and paper chromatography, only unchelated Tc-99m species have been identified as radiochemical impurities, but with HPLC, various chelated species are identified.

Paper and Thin-Layer Chromatography

These two chromatographic techniques, used primarily to determine the presence of pertechnetate in radiopharmaceuticals, can be completed within one hour, are simple to perform, and do not require expensive equipment. The procedure in each case consists of the application of microliter amounts of the radiochemical to a plate coated with a thin layer of absorbent, or to the paper chromatogram, at a point approximately 1 in. from the end that is to be immersed in the eluting solution. This point is called the *origin* and is marked at the lateral surface of the strip or plate for identification. The chromatogram then is immersed in the preferred solvent and the chromatographic tank is tightly covered (Fig. 10–2A and 10-2B). The solution level must be clearly below the point at which the radioactive sample is spotted. The solution ascends the strip by capillary action, carrying each radiochemical component according to its partition between the solid support material, e.g., the paper or silica gel, and the solution. When the solution has traveled the desired distance, the solvent front (S_f) is marked, and the plate or strip is removed from the container and allowed to dry.

The distance traveled by each radioactive component of the solution under analysis is the most important factor in these determinations. This distance, termed the R_f *value,* is defined as the ratio of the distance traveled by a given radiochemical component compared to the solvent front (S_f). It depends upon such conditions as temperature, quality of the support material, and pre-equilibration of the solution; because of these variables, R_f values are not always reproducible. For this reason, the suspected radiochemical impurity (e.g., pertechnetate) should be chromatographed simultaneously with the product being evaluated and in the same container as this product.

The radioactivity associated with the various components now can be determined by counting cut up portions of the chromatogram, or by counting on a radiochromatogram scanner, which gives the distribution of the radioactivity as a function of distance in a polygraph-like printout (Fig. 10–3A and 10-3B). Since glass-backed thin-layer strips must be scraped before counting the sectioned pieces,

which thus lengthens the procedure, fiber-backed or aluminum-backed thin layer plates are preferred when cutting is necessary.

One main source of error in the chromatographic analysis of Tc-99m radiochemical purity derives from the ease of oxidation of certain reduced states of technetium. For this reason, compounds should not be dried on the TLC plate or paper strip before elution in either chromatographic system. In the event that this is done inadvertently, oxidation may ensue with subsequent formation of pertechnetate not originally present in the radiopharmaceutical. In addition, nonspecific adsorption of the compound, as has been reported with ^{99m}Tc-Sn-HSA, may occur, owing to the small number of highly active sites on the chromatography strip or plate.[63] This phenomenon also has been observed in the preparation of high specific activity iodinated hormones used for radioimmunoassay.[64]

Column Chromatography

A more sophisticated chromatographic system is column chromatography (Fig. 10–2C). Larger samples of radiochemical (0.1 ml to 5% of the column volume) can be used, which is an advantage when analyzing for oxidation-sensitive compounds produced with Tc-99m. Each type of solid support, however, must be carefully prepared to obtain satisfactory performance, and the appropriate product manual must be consulted. Here, instead of measuring an R_f value, an *elution volume* is quantitated. Elution volume is defined as the volume of eluate required to elute the particular compound from the column (Fig. 10–3C). This volume also depends upon experimental conditions and must be calibrated using verified samples of the expected impurities.

Column chromatography requires more expensive equipment than do strip and TLC methods; fraction collectors and automatic gamma counters are needed. It is

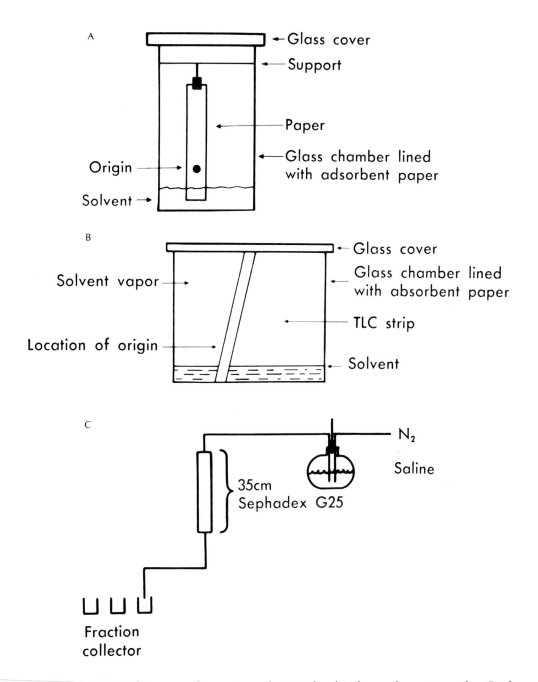

Fig. 10–2.   Apparatus for paper chromatography (A); for thin-layer chromatography (B); for column chromatography (C).

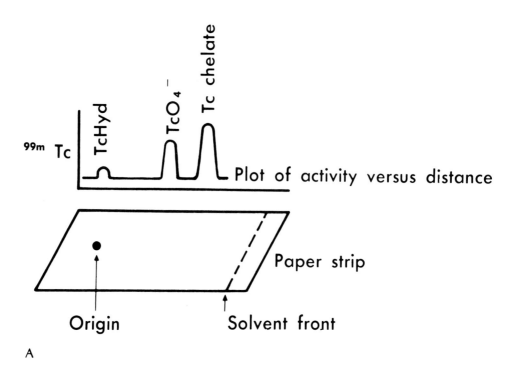

Fig. 10–3. Distribution of Tc-99m activity as a function of distance from the origin for a Tc-99m chelate chromatographed on Whatman No. 1 paper eluted with saline solution (*A*); for a Tc-99m chelate chromatographed on Silica Gel TLC eluted with acetone (*B*); for a Tc-99m chelate chromatographed on a Sephadex G25 column eluted with saline solution (*C*). The Tc-Hyd that adsorbs to the column is not represented here. This impurity must be determined from the percentage of total Tc-99m activity recovered in the eluted fractions.

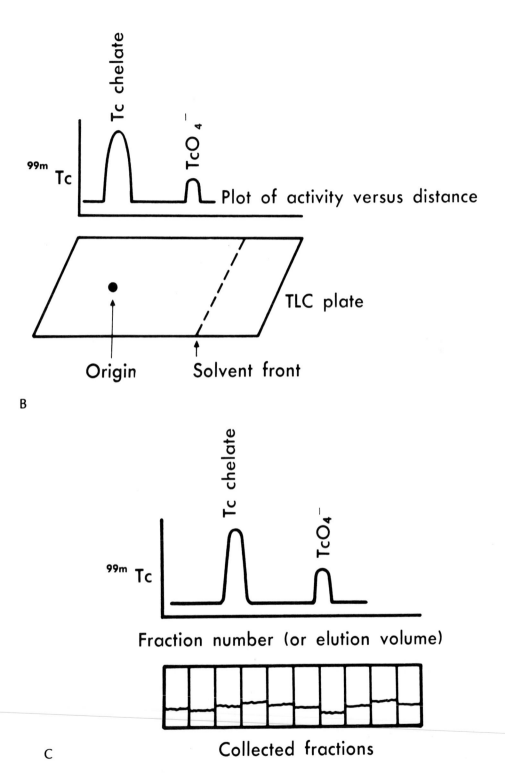

B

C

Fig. 10–3 *(continued).*

also more time consuming because of the large number of fractions that must be collected and counted. Finally, an attentive, competent technician is mandatory.

With these added complexities, however, determinations of radiochemical purity rather than pertechnetate contamination can be obtained. Short columns (10 cm) have been useful for relatively rapid determination of a certain impurity, whereas longer columns (greater than 30 cm) generally have been reserved for radiochemical purity determinations.

Another source of error may result from interaction between the solid phase of the chromatography system and the radiopharmaceutical. In this case, the solid support itself competes for the Tc-99m because of its own chelating ability. For example, the polysaccharide Sephadex can compete favorably for certain weak chelates, e.g., Tc-99m gluconate and Tc-99m mannitol.[20,65] Therefore, a Tc-99m radiopharmaceutical analyzed on such a chromatographic system might appear to contain a radiochemical impurity (a reduced form of technetium) that is not bound to the chelating agent. This shortcoming has been demonstrated for a number of weak chelates analyzed with Sephadex column chromatography. To avoid this artifact, the inert solid phase polyacrylamide, Bio Gel P-10, with which there is no competitive adsorption of Tc-99m to the base support, may be used.[66] Alternatively, the Sephadex column can be eluted with the same concentration of chelating agent that is used in the preparation of the radiopharmaceutical.[67,68] Both options provide reasonable assurance that the determination of radiochemical purity is accurate.

This same phenomenon also may occur with paper chromatographic systems. When radiochemically pure Tc-99m pyrophosphate (PYP) is eluted with saline, most of the reduced Tc-99m appears to be unbound; however, if the paper is eluted with a pyrophosphate solution, the chelate is found to be radiochemically pure.[69] With the dilutional effect of the saline solvent and the rapid dissociation constant of polyphosphate (TcPPi), the chelate can release the Tc-99m to another chelating compound. This property must be considered when evaluating radiochemical purity determinations with these systems.

Chelate stability on Sephadex and paper does not imply in vivo stability of the compound, but serves merely as an index of the competition (at the specific concentrations used) between the respective groups and the chelating agent.

HPLC

High-pressure liquid chromatography (HPLC) brings both improved column efficiency and high mobile-phase velocities to the separation procedures. Improved column efficiency is brought about by increased surface area per column length, which results from the use of decreased particle size (5 to 10 μm). The decreased particle size increases resistance to mobile-phase flow, however. This is overcome by using high pressure, usually on the order of 1000 psi. The most popular column packing consists of nonpolar chemically bonded phases. These columns are the "reverse" of the usual polar solid supports, such as silica gel and alumina. The reversed phase columns are better suited for separating the nonpolar molecules that characterize many biochemicals and drugs. The columns are eluted with such polar mobile phases as mixtures of water and methanol, tetrahydrofuran, or acetonitrile. As in classical liquid chromatography, the retention time t_R is measured relative to the retention time of a nonadsorbed component t_0 to determine the capacity factor $k' = t_R - t_0/t_0$. The relative retention of two components α is given by the equation:

$$\frac{t_{R2} - t_0}{t_{R1} - t_0} = \frac{k'_2}{k'_1}$$

Pertechnetate Generator Chromatography

The most important factor in the preparation of Tc-99m radiopharmaceuticals is the radiochemical purity of pertechnetate eluted from the generator.

Two primary paper chromatography systems (Table 10–1), based on the original work of Shukla, have been suggested to identify the various technetium species

TABLE 10–1. *Pertechnetate Generator Chromatography*

Solid support	Solvent	R_f (TcO_4^-)	R_f (Impurities)	Reference
Whatman No. 3 paper chromatography	0.3 M HCl	0.70	0.10 Tc(V) 0.90 Tc(IV)	Cifka, J., and Vesely, P.[71]
Whatman CC41 cellulose	90% CH_3OH	0.71	0.01–0.14 Tc(VI) 0.93 Tc(IV)	Müller, T., and Steinnes, E.[72]

present in the generator eluate.[70] These systems contrast with the majority of chromatographic systems, in which the sole purpose has been to identify pertechnetate in Tc-99m chelate and colloid preparations. Here, technetium species IV, V, and VII, which act as impurities with paper chromatography (in 0.3M HCl or 90% methanol solutions), can be identified.

Although these systems are capable of identifying the Tc(IV), Tc(V), and Tc(VII), only the Tc(V) state can be eluted with TcO_4^- directly from the alumina column in the generator.[71] This species does not bind to DTPA and can be implicated in certain instances of nonbonding by the effluent of the Mo-99 generator product.[21]

Pertechnetate Impurity Chromatography

Following the determinations for reduced Tc-99m species in generator pertechnetate, of major concern after the formation of Tc-99m compounds is reoxidation of the reduced state of TcO_4^-. This can be rapidly determined by several chromatographic systems, shown in Table 10–2. No information, however, is provided regarding the radiochemical purity of the reduced compound. Usually, nonradioactive kits for the various compounds are prepared properly; as a result, impurities that form most likely result from pertechnetate formed by oxidation of the reduced technetium in one's own laboratory. These systems are designed to adsorb all nonpertechnetate compounds at the origin in TLC or on the support in column chromatography. Only the presence or absence of TcO_4^- is evaluated.

Radiochemical Purity Chromatography

To assure that a Tc-99m radiopharmaceutical contains only the desired reduced species, at least two chromatographic systems in Table 10–3 must be used. Both systems used to assay for radiochemical purity should demonstrate a single band of radioactivity and possess a partition coefficient such that the compound is not freely eluted nor strongly adsorbed. Because of the complexity of these techniques, they are utilized primarily as research tools. Since pertechnetate is the most frequent impurity formed by Tc-99m chelate degradation, the previously described chromatographic systems usually suffice (Table 10–2).

Paper chromatography has been used for many years, whereas gel chromatography (Sephadex) was adopted in 1967. Richards and Atkins demonstrated the special advantage of the gel system, which strongly adsorbs reduced unchelated technetium.[88] Furthermore, Tc-99m HSA was shown not to be radiochemically pure, as was originally suggested by paper systems;[89] it only appeared so because of the limitations inherent in these earlier techniques. Since its introduction, gel chromatography has been widely used in combination with paper chromatographic systems to determine radiochemical purity.[31,90]

Other systems also are capable of separating radiochemical impurities, and by necessity, new systems will be developed with the ever-increasing number of chelating agents. These systems often can be adapted from methods used to purify nonradioactive chelates.[62] For example, a system is needed to separate DTPA from Tc-DTPA, compounds with obvious differences. Separations may be possible with compounds that show slow dissociation under high performance liquid chromatography.

The more polar Tc-99m chelates have been difficult to analyze on HPLC because of their poor retention. Russell and Majerik used a weak basic anion exchange column eluted with buffer-separated pertechnetate from

TABLE 10–2. Chromatographic Systems for the Determination of Pertechnetate

Compound*	Support	Solvent	Elution volume or R_f reduced	Elution volume or R_f of TcO$_4$	Reference
TcSc					
Tc-Sb$_2$S$_3$					
Tc-Sn(OH)$_2$	Silica Gel TLC	MEK or saline	0	1.0 or 0.85	Mitta, A., et al.[73]
TcHSA					
TcDTPA					
TcFe					
TcDTPA					
TcPPi	Silica Gel TLC	Acetone	0	1.0	Billinghurst, M.W.[74]
TcHEDP	Silica Gel TLC	Acetone	0	1.0	Billinghurst, M.W.[74]
Tc-Pen	Alumina TLC	Acetone	0	0.5	Billinghurst, M.W.[74]
Tc-mannitol	Alumina TLC	Acetone	0	0.5	Billinghurst, M.W.[74]
TcHSA	Alumina col. 3 cm × 0.5 cm	Acetone or MEK	Adsorbed	Eluted	Domek, N.S., and Loken, M.K.[75]
Tc-Tetracycline					Benjamin, P., et al.[33]
Tc-oxytetracycline					
TcHEDP	Acid washed alumina col. 10 cm × 0.6 cm	Saline	Adsorbed	Eluted	Colombetti, L.G., et al.[76]
TcMAA					
TcHAM					
TcDTPA					
TcPoly	Acid washed alumina col.	Saline	Adsorbed	Eluted	Colombetti, L.G., et al.[76]
Tc-phytate					
TcSC					

*See Appendix F for abbreviations.

such polar chelates as DTPA, EHDP, and glu-coheptonate, but since these chelates are not retained, they appeared to be radiochemically pure.[80] Wong et al. also studied a number of Tc-99m chelates on HPLC using a μ Bondagel column eluted with buffer and a μ Bondapak C-18 column eluted with buffer-acetonitrile.[78] There was good separation between Tc-HIDA or Tc-HSA and pertechnetate, but minimal separation between polar chelates (DTPA, MDP, and pyrophosphate) and pertechnetate.

Nonpolar chelates such as Tc-HIDA are more easily retained, especially on reversed phase columns, as first shown by Loberg and Fields.[81] They were able to separate Sn-HIDA, HIDA, and Tc-HIDA on HPLC, using a μ Bondapak C-18 column eluted with acetonitrile and buffer. In a subsequent study, Fields et al. were able to separate a number of chelate-containing Tc-99m HIDA radiochemical impurities when analogs were used with pKa values for the imino nitrogen of greater than 7.[91]

Fritzberg and Lewis also have discovered radiochemical impurities other than pertechnetate and reduced-hydrolyzed Tc in Tc-99m HIDA derivatives that have large substituents in the ortho position.[92] These impurities convert to the major component as a function of either time or increased pH. Pinkerton et al. were the first to develop a HPLC system to separate bone-imaging agents.[83] Using an anion exchange column eluted with buffer, they found as many as seven components in Tc-HEDP, in addition to pertechnetate and reduced hydrolyzed technetium. This result was observed using Tc-99 whereas with Tc-99m, only one major peak was found. Srivastava et al., however, found multiple peaks for Tc-99m MDP using reversed phase HPLC.[93]

Simple Compounds with Oxygen, Sulfur, and Halogens

The oxides, sulfides, and halides of technetium have received considerable attention. Of the oxides, oxo compounds are known to predominate in the higher oxidation states; the most common forms are TcO_2 and Tc_2O_7. The hydrated dioxide (TcO_2) is made by the addition of base to such Tc(IV) solutions as $TcCl_6^{2-}$ or $TcBr_6^{2-}$; alternatively, reduction of TcO_4^- in HCl with Zn may be used.

Technetium dioxide's relevance in ra-diopharmaceutical chemistry is that it represents a competitive pathway in the production of chelates. To prevent this adverse side reaction, an adequate amount of chelating agent, e.g., DTPA, must be present. The sequence and timing for the addition of pertechnetate, the chelating agent, and the reducing agent also are important.[21]

Simple halides of technetium have been reported, although they are unstable and hydrolyze in the presence of base. The complex fluoride of Tc(IV) resists hydrolysis and has been tried as a potential skeletal imaging agent,[94,95] but it demonstrates no bone localization. A hexachloro salt, $TcCl_6^{2-}$, also has been prepared by pertechnetate reduction with concentrated HCl. This salt hydrolyzes slowly in dilute acid.

Technetium forms sulfur compounds in the presence of H_2S or Tc_2S_7. Sodium thiosulfate can be obtained by saturation of a 2 to 6 N HCl solution of $^{99}TcO_4^-$ with H_2S, but precipitation of elemental sulfur as the colloid is often incomplete with this method. Consequently, sodium thiosulfate in acid, which is easier to prepare,[96,97] has become the sulfur colloid source for liver scintigraphy.

Direct Labeling of Chelating Agents

Radiopharmaceuticals

Technetium chelates are used to varying degrees in the study of three organ systems: the kidneys, liver, and bone. For the kidneys, Arnold documents 12 different chelating agents that have been combined with Tc-99m.[98] These include (1) EDTA,[99] (2) DTPA,[8,100] (3) mannitol,[101] (4) mannitol with gelatin,[102] (5) penicillamine-acetazolamide,[103,104] (6) caseidin,[105] (7) citrate,[106] (8) tetracycline,[107] (9) inulin,[101] (10) dimercaptosuccinic acid (DMSA),[108] (11) glucoheptonate, and (12) gluconate.[109] More recently, other compounds, mostly thiol derivatives, have been proposed: penicillamine,[110] cysteine,[111]

TABLE 10–3. Chromatographic Systems for Analysis of Radiochemical Purity

Compound	Support	Solvent	Compound*	Elution order or R_f value	Reference
TcBDD	Silica Gel TLC	Chloroform 50% Cyclohexene 40% Diethylamine 10%	TcO_4^- TcDD TcBDD (Tc-99m) TcBDD (Tc-99g)	0 0.13 0.89 0.91	Vigne, J.P.[77]
Tc Chelates	μ-Bondagel (HPLC) μ-Bondapak μ C-18 (HPLC)	Buffer Acetonitrile	Tc chelate TcO_4^-	Eluted 1st Eluted 2nd	Wong, S.H., et al.[78]
TcDTPA	Whatman No. 1	Saline	TcHyd TcO_4^- TcDTPA	0 0.75 0.9 to 1.0	Eckelman, W.C., et al.[31]
TcDTPA	Sephadex G25 0.9 × 30 cm	Saline	TcHyd TcO_4^- TcDTPA	Adsorbed Eluted 2nd Eluted 1st	Eckelman, W.C., et al.[31]
TcDTPA	Sephadex G25 20 × 1.5 cm	Saline	TcDTPA TcO_4^- TcHyd	Eluted 1st Eluted 2nd Adsorbed	Persson, R.B.R., and Strand, S.E.[79]
TcDTPA	Bio-Gel P-10	0.9% Saline	TcDTPA TcO_4^- TcHyd	Eluted 1st Eluted 2nd Adsorbed	Billinghurst, M.W., and Palser, R.F.[66]
TcDTPA (combination test)	(1) Silica Gel	Acetone	TcHyd TcDTPA TcO_4^-	0 0 1.0	Billinghurst, M.W.[74]
	(2) Silica Gel	Saline	TcHyd TcDTPA TcO_4^-	0 1.0 1.0	Billinghurst, M.W.[74]
TcDTPA	Anion exchange Column (HPLC)		Tc chelate TcO_4^-	Eluted 1st Eluted 2nd	Russell, C.D., and Majerik, J.[80]
TcHIDA	μ-Bondapak (HPLC)	Acetonitrile Buffer	TcO_4^- TcHIDA	Eluted 1st Eluted 2nd	Loberg, M.D., and Fields, A.T.[81]
TcFeAs	Sephadex G25 20 × 1.5 cm	Saline	TcFeAs TcO_4^- TcHyd	Eluted 1st Eluted 2nd Adsorbed	Persson, R.B.R., and Strand, S.E.[79]
TcGHA	Bio-Gel P-10	0.9% Saline	TcGHA TcO_4^- TcHyd	Eluted 1st Eluted 2nd Adsorbed	Billinghurst, M.W., and Palser, R.F.[66]

Compound	Support	Solvent	Species	Value	Reference
TcGHA	Anion exchange Column (HPLC)		TcGHA	Eluted 1st	Russell, C.D., and Majerik, J.[80]
			TcO$_4^-$	Eluted 2nd	
TcGluconate	Bio-Gel P-10	0.9% Saline	TcGluconate	Eluted 1st	Billinghurst, M.W., and Palser, R.F.[66]
			TcO$_4^-$	Eluted 2nd	
TcHEDP	Sephadex	0.9% Saline	TcHEDP	Eluted 1st	Castronovo, C.F., Jr., and Callahan, R.J.[82]
			TcO$_4^-$	Eluted 2nd	
			TcHyd	Adsorbed	
TcHEDP	Anion exchange Column (HPLC)	Acetate Buffer	TcHEDP	Eluted 1st	Pinkerton, T.C., et al.[83]
			TcO$_4^-$	Eluted 2nd	
			TcHyd	Adsorbed	
TcHSA	Whatman No. 1	Saline	Multiple Peaks	0	Eckelman, W.C., et al.[32]
			TcHyd	0.75	
			TcO$_4^-$	0.9 to 1.0	
TcHSA	G50 Sephadex 0.9 × 15 cm	Saline	TcHSA	Adsorbed	Billinghurst, M.W.[74]
			TcHyd	Eluted 2nd	
			TcO$_4^-$	Void volume	
TcMDP	μ-Bondapak C-18 (HPLC)	Dioxane Buffer	Multiple Peaks		Pinkerton, T.C., et al.[83]
TcPen	Whatman No. 1	n-butanol 4 Acetic acid 1 Water 1	TcO$_4^-$	0.25	Tubis, M., et al.[84]
			Pen	0.6	
			TcPen	0.7	
TcPen	Sephadex G25	0.9 Saline	TcPen	Eluted 1st	Domek, N.S., et al.[85]
			TcO$_4^-$	Eluted 2nd	
			TcHyd	Adsorbed	
TcHIDA	Paper	Acetonitrile 3 Water 1	TcHIDA	0.8	Loberg, M.D., et al.[86]
			TcO$_4^-$	0.9	
			TcHyd	0	
TcPPi	Bio-Gel P-10	0.9% Saline	TcPPi	Eluted 1st	Billinghurst, M.W., and Palser, R.F.[66]
			TcO$_4^-$	Eluted 2nd	
			TcHyd	Adsorbed	
TcPPi	Sephadex G50	0.9% Saline	TcPPi	Eluted 1st	Bowen, B.M., and Garnett, E.S.[87]
			TcO$_4^-$	Eluted 2nd	
			TcHyd	Adsorbed	
TcSC	Whatman No. 3	0.3 M HCl	TcSC	0	Cifka, J., and Vesely, P.[71]
			TcO$_4^-$	0.66	
			Tc(IV)	0.85	

*See Appendix F for abbreviations.

acetylcysteine,[112] glutathione,[113] and un-ithiol.[114] These are discussed in a recent review.[19]

Few of these compounds are used clinically to determine size, shape, and position of the kidneys because of the advent of computed tomography and ultrasound. The most common clinical agents for kidney studies are Tc-99m DTPA, Tc-99m glucoheptonate and Tc-99m DMSA. Three other important Tc-99m compounds also have been prepared: cyclam,[59] DADS [N,N' - *bis*(mercaptoacetamido) - ethylene-diamine],[115] and KTS [kethoxal-*bis*(thiosemicarbazone)].[116,117] Technetium-99m cyclam is important, not so much as a kidney agent per se, but as a positively charged chelate for bifunctional derivatives. Technetium-99m DADS is important because it is secreted by the renal tubules. Technetium-99m KTS is a neutral, lipophilic chelate useful for labeling structures that must cross cell membranes.

Hepatic and hepatobiliary Tc-99m chelates have been proposed as possible replacements for I-131 rose bengal, the advantage being the increased photon yield. They are as follows: (1) penicillamine,[84] (2) pyridoxylideneglutamate (PG), a Schiff base,[118] (3) dihydrothiotic acid,[119] (4) tetracycline,[107] (5) mercaptoisobutyric acid,[120] (6) 6-mercaptopurine,[121] and (7) HIDA, a lidocaine derivative containing iminodiacetic acid.[86,122] A convenient method has been developed to prepare various HIDA derivatives with substituents in the benzene ring.[123] Briefly, substituted anilines are reacted with the anhydride of nitrilotriacetic acid to produce chelating agents for Tc-99m. Several structure-distribution studies have been carried out.[124,125,126,127,128,129,130]

The final group of technetium chelates, those used for bone imaging, were developed in 1971. Prior to that, only the less desirable fluorine or strontium nuclides were available. Tripolyphosphate was the first of these.[101] Shortly thereafter, Tc-99m polyphosphate was introduced. The slow blood clearance and varying chain length, described by Subramanian et al.,[131] led to further investigation and subsequent synthesis of today's conventional skeletal imaging agents: pyrophosphate,[132] diphosphonate (HEDP),[133] methylene diphosphonate (MDP),[134] and hydroxymethylene diphosphonate (HMDP).[135,136] These compounds have been compared to other diphosphonate and imidodiphosphonate derivatives in terms of bone uptake and blood.[137,138,139]

In Vitro Radiochemical Purity

Of the chelating agents studied, ^{99m}Tc-Sn-DTPA is one that appears to be radiochemically pure.[31,80] By definition, this implies that only the chemical form stated is present in the compound. In contrast, most of the other chelating agents mentioned seem to have a low affinity (are weak chelates) for Tc; in these instances, the risk of radiochemical impurity (species other than those desired) is high.

The Tc-99m chelates suggested for renal scintigraphy are mostly weak chelates and may give confusing results if studied on certain chromatographic systems. One source of error, previously mentioned, can result from interaction with the solid phase of the system because chelating moieties in the solid support compete for the Tc-99m (see "Column Chromatography" in this chapter).

Among the agents suggested for hepatobiliary imaging, Tc-99m PG, Tc-99m penicillamine, and Tc-99m IDA compounds have been shown to be radiochemically pure. The absence of TcO_4^- or of Tc-99m pyridoxal can be demonstrated by electrophoresis, although because Tc-99m PG remains at the origin, radiochemical purity cannot be determined.[118] Nonetheless, similar behavior observed using other chromatography systems does seem to indicate radiochemical purity.[140] Use of the stannous reduction method appears to lead to a consistently purer product.[141]

Radiochemical purity tests were also performed on Tc penicillamine in a single system;[103] the R_f values of Tc-99m penicillamine, TcO_4^-, and unlabeled penicillamine were 0.7, 0.25, and 0.6 respectively. Technetium HIDA has been chromatographed in two systems and shown to be a single pure radiochemical.[86,122] There have been reports that various Tc-IDA compounds, e.g., N-(2,6-

diisopropylacetanilide) iminodiacetic acid and N-(p-isopropylacetanilide) iminodiacetic acid, showed two components on HPLC when prepared at low pH. Only a single peak was evident at neutral pH.[82]

Of the bone imaging agents, Tc-99m HEDP appears to be a strong chelate and has been chromatographed on Sephadex G25 eluted with saline.[92] Technetium pyrophosphate, on the other hand, dissociates on Sephadex G25 and on Whatman paper when saline is used. This artifact was described earlier and is remedied by eluting with a pyrophosphate solution; the change produces a single peak in both systems, which indicates a radiochemically pure product. Technetium polyphosphate also elutes from Sephadex G25 with saline, but presents an additional radiochemical purity analysis problem. Although one radioactive peak has been obtained in the chromatography of Tc-99m polyphosphate, the variations in phosphate chain length raise uncertainties concerning the identity of the localizing species.[142] It is hoped that the use of HPLC will clarify many of these and other questions concerning the radiochemical purity of chelates labeled with technetium.

In Vivo Radiochemical Purity

Renal Agents. Information about the chemical forms of Tc-99m renal imaging agents is sparse. Chromatography of plasma and urine samples after injection of Tc-Sn-DTPA indicates that at one hr after administration, the Tc-Sn-DTPA is 90% radiochemically pure in the plasma and 98% radiochemically pure in the urine. In contrast, only 38% of plasma and 18% of urine ^{99m}Tc-Fe-ascorbate remains as the original radiolabeled chelate.[143] These data emphasize the superior stability of the Tc-Sn-DTPA compound.

These chelates for kidney imaging fall into three categories: those that are filtered, those that are secreted, and those that exhibit a mixed behavior of filtration, secretion, and binding in the kidneys (Table 10–3). Technetium-99m DADS is largely secreted by the tubules. Although the mechanism is not certain, the secretion rate appears to be faster than DTPA and can be blocked by probenecid, which suggests that tubular secretion plays a dominant role in renal clearance of the chelate.[144] Although this tracer may not replace iodohippurate, it does offer hope that this last survivor of iodinated radiopharmaceuticals can be replaced by a technetium radiopharmaceutical.

Most of the chelates with mixed functions, such as Tc-ascorbate, Tc-glucoheptonate, and Tc-DMSA, have not been characterized chemically. Partly because the starting radiotracer is not a single component, researchers have been reluctant to investigate the chemical form in blood and urine. Renal extraction efficiencies were determined by McAfee et al. for a series of kidney agents.[145] Ortho-iodohippurate had the highest extraction efficiency. The Tc-99m complexes of DTPA and glucoheptonate have extraction efficiencies of 27 to 29%. Technetium-99m DMSA and Hg-197 chlormerodrin had lower extraction values of 8 and 14% respectively.

An interesting aspect of the mixed-function renal imaging agents is the effect of stannous ion on retention in the renal cortex. In the DMSA kit, the absolute amount of stannous ion is important in accelerating the formation of the kidney localizing component.[146] Both chromatographic and biologic differences were observed when Tc-99m DMSA was prepared with stannous ion, electrochemically or with sodium borohydride.[147] In the case of Tc-99m glutathione, increasing stannous ion concentration also increased retention in the kidneys.

A number of possible mechanisms were outlined but a causal relationship could not be extracted from the data.[148] Steigman et al. unified these concepts by showing that stannous ion increased the renal retention of Tc-99m for several chelating agents.[149] In general, for DTPA, pyrophosphate, and HEDP preparations, the kidney-to-background ratio was higher for the electrolytic kit than for the stannous ion kit. But with stannous-reduced Tc-99m gluconate, Tc-99m was retained longer in the kidney. The effect of stannous ion on renal physiology was demonstrated by injecting a stannous gluconate complex within 5 min of the electrolytic Tc-99m gluconate. The image showed the same high kidney retention observed with the Tc-99m(Sn)gluconate preparations. This can be explained by a change in membrane permeability.

Bone Agents. Some information concerning the in vivo fate of the skeletal imaging agents is also available. Krishnamurthy et al., in comparing Tc-99m pyrophosphate with diphosphonate, established the early binding properties of these compounds.[150,151,152] At 1 hr postadministration, approximately 80% of the serum Tc-99m activity was bound to serum proteins, most of which was associated with the globulin fraction. Red blood cell binding was also found. In another investigation, Bowen and Garnett determined that 1 hr following the intravenous administration of Tc-99m PYP, greater than 50% of the plasma activity was due to free Tc-99m polyphosphate;[87] this contrasts with the plasma clearance data obtained with Tc-99m PYP, which indicated that less than 33% of the total plasma activity was free Tc-99m pyrophosphate. Interestingly, the major urinary constituent after the administration of either Tc-99m PYP or Tc-99m PPi was Tc-99m PYP. This finding suggests that Tc-99m PYP was present in the Tc-99m PPi.

Recently, Schümichen et al. compared various methods of analyzing protein-bound Tc-99m labeled bone-imaging agents.[153] Using the ammonium sulfate precipitation method, the investigators found that bone-imaging agents had varying amounts of Tc-99m bound to plasma proteins. For example, Tc-99m HEDP had 8.6 and 24.5% of the Tc-99m bound to protein at 10 min and 5 hr respectively after a patient's injection. The comparable percentages were 13.3 to 48% for Tc-99m MDP; 18.2 to 79.3% for Tc-99m pyro-

phosphate; and 49.6 to 90.0% for Tc-99m tripolyphosphate. These are percentages of the radioactivity left in the blood at the time of sampling and are not related to the injected dose. When these human-plasma samples were injected in rats, the concentration of radioactivity in the bone at 1 hr was compared with the protein-bound concentration in the original sample. There was a good correlation between the nonprotein-bound Tc-99m in human plasma and the bone uptake in rats for all Tc-99m bone-imaging agents. Similar correlations were obtained when activity in the blood and urine of the rats was compared with the nonprotein-bound plasma fraction of Tc-99m from humans.

In 1971, Subramanian and McAfee published the first studies using a Tc-99m bone-imaging agent.[101] Since that time, criteria for Tc-99m uptake in bone have been determined almost entirely by organ distribution studies. In fact, the first phosphate, sodium tripolyphosphate, was not a pure ligand, and it prompted further studies on the effect of chain length on bone localization. For polyphosphates, bone uptake was found to be inversely proportional to the chain length, i.e., pyrophosphate gives the highest bone uptake.[138] The initial organ distribution studies focused on blood clearance, which did little to define the bone localizing species. In this respect, Tc-99m MDP appears to be one of the quickest bone-imaging agents in clearing the blood and is the most widely used, clinically. More recent organ distribution studies have focused less on blood clearance than on bone uptake. In two articles, Bevan et al. studied in vivo binding of technetium skeletal imaging agents.[135,136] Technetium-99m MDP and Tc-99m HMDP appear to clear the blood rapidly. On the other hand, Tc-99m HEDP has lower bone uptake but a higher ratio between areas of bone with different metabolic rates.

Buja et al. have shown that the uptake of Tc-99 HEDP is positively related to serum calcium levels.[154] Other proposed uptake mechanisms, such as high-affinity binding to organic matrix,[155,156] to tissue phosphatases,[157,158] or to various proteins of damaged tissue,[159] may play minor roles in Tc-99m localization in the bone.

Autoradiographic studies confirm that the growing face of the apatite crystal is the point of uptake of Tc-99m bone-imaging agents.[159,160] The chemical state of Tc-99m at the bone surface has not been determined. Christensen and Krogsgaard dissolved bone with EDTA and found that the Tc-99m labeled chemical form could not be distinguished from Tc-99m MDP.[161] Earlier theories had proposed that Tc-99m would be displaced on the bone surface by calcium to produce TcO_2.[138,162] Pinkerton et al. have shown that Tc-99m HEDP prepared with sodium borohydride contains many components before injection,[83] and Steigman et al. have suggested the possibility of polymeric species.[149] Therefore, in vivo radiochemical purity is uncertain until pure starting material is used.

The localization mechanism of Tc-99m phosphorus radiotracers in myocardial infarcts and in other soft-tissue abnormalities is probably due to microcalcification. Of the bone tracers, Tc-99m PYP is the most widely used in clinical evaluation of myocardial infarcts (see Vol. II, Chap. 18).[163] The reasons for the discrepancies between the relative uptakes of Tc-99m PYP and Tc-99m MDP in damaged myocardial tissue and the relative uptakes of these complexes in bone are not known.

Hepatobiliary Agents. The hepatocytes in the liver clear hepatobiliary agents from plasma by an active transport process. Most current Tc-99m hepatobiliary agents are cleared by the same general anionic mechanism operative for bilirubin. Therefore, in hyperbilirubinemia, there is competitive inhibition for transport of the Tc-99m agents. All hepatobiliary agents appear to have certain chemical characteristics that distinguish them from substances excreted by the kidney. The molecular weight of hepatobiliary agents is usually between 300 and 1000 daltons; the molecules contain at least two planar, lipophilic structures and a polar group. These hepatobiliary agents usually are protein bound, although neither Tc-99m PG nor Tc-99m HIDA are extensively protein bound in plasma.[164]

To optimize these chemical properties, many Tc-99m agents have been prepared and evaluated. As early as 1974, hepatobiliary Tc-99m chelates were proposed as possible replacements for I-131 rose bengal.[84] The early Tc-99m hepatobiliary agents were excreted by both kidney and liver. The first improvements focused on decreasing the kidney component; later, efforts to accelerate clearance were made. Loberg proposed a pharmacokinetic model that describes the competition between hepatobiliary clearance and renal clearance.[165]

Either an increase in hepatobiliary clearance or a decrease in renal clearance increases hepatobiliary specificity. When liver function is impaired, however, renal clearance becomes relatively more significant.[164] This effect is observed even when the Tc-99m HIDA derivative is one in which elimination by the hepatobiliary pathway is both efficient and rapid in normal patients and animals. Therefore, in addition to simply finding chelates that are rapidly cleared by the liver, chelates that more successfully compete with bilirubin are being sought so that these agents may be used in patients with high serum bilirubin.[166] For this reason, the most suitable chelates probably have a high affinity for anionic receptors or hepatocytes, compared to bilirubin, as well as normally rapid clearance rates.

The major tool for judging hepatobiliary specificity is chemical structure-distribution studies in vivo. Kato et al. have carried out extensive studies by varying the amino acid portion of the pyridoxylideneaminates (PA).[167,168] The authors overcame the earlier objection to PA by developing a stannous reduction technique to replace the tedious autoclaving method. They determined that Tc-99m(Sn) pyridoxylidene valine and Tc-99m(Sn) pyrodoxylidene isoleucine were relatively more hydrophobic. These compounds were cleared by the rat liver at a faster rate [$T_{1/2}$ = 15 sec for Tc-99m(Sn) pyrodoxylidene isoleucine] and excreted into the small intestine more rapidly [$T_{1/2}$ = 3.4 min for Tc-99m(Sn) pyrodoxylidene isoleucine]. Similar pharmacokinetics were observed in rabbits and human.

Several analogs of Tc-99m HIDA are sufficiently lipophilic and characterized by the other properties outlined by Firnau to be excreted by the hepatobiliary system.[169] Further refinements in the structure have been proposed to increase the blood and liver clearance.

Regarding the in vivo behavior of Tc-99m hepatobiliary chelates, Loberg et al. have shown that the Tc-99m activity in the bile has the same chromatographic behavior and distributes in rats in the same manner as the original compound.[86] The search continues for derivatives that are cleared from the blood and liver at a faster rate.

Direct Labeling of Colloids and Particles

Radiopharmaceuticals

Numerous radiolabeled colloids for use in hepatic scintigraphy have been reported. The one most commonly used is Tc-99m sulfur colloid prepared from the acid decomposition of sodium thiosulfate in the presence of a variety of stabilizing agents. Among these are gelatin (the most popular), albumin, PVP, and polyhydric alcohol.[170,171,172,173] Stabilizer-free preparations also have been proposed as well as compounds with carrier rhenium and antimony.[174,175,176] Other types of colloids include stannous oxide,[177] technetium oxide,[178] and microaggregated albumin.[179]

Several Tc-99m labeled particles can be used for lung scanning. Methods and types of preparations include macroaggregation

of Tc-99m labeled albumin,[180] the conversion of Tc sulfur colloids into HSA macroaggregates,[181] coprecipitation of Tc-99m with iron hydroxide,[182] macroaggregation of albumin in the presence of colloid,[183] and incorporation of Tc-99m sulfur colloid or reduced technetium into microspheres.[184] Macroaggregates are the most commonly used.

In Vitro Radiochemical Purity

The work of Cifka and Vesely is notable for having shown that premixing of pertechnetate with sodium thiosulfate could produce a nonpertechnetate radiochemical impurity.[185] In routine silica gel TLC systems, this impurity could not be identified because it remained at the origin and therefore was indistinguishable from Tc-99m sulfur colloid. On Whatman No. 3 paper with $0.3N$ HCl, however, this impurity did manifest itself. Differences in chromatographic behavior of technetium sulfur colloid preparations are known,[186] but they have not been related to biological behavior.

Determination of the particle size of colloids is important because the size may be related to the distribution. Methods of determining particle size differ, depending on whether the colloids are radioactive or nonradioactive. Traditionally, colloid chemists have used electron microscopy to determine particle size because it provides a direct measurement.[187] Steigman, however, has shown that Tc-labeled sulfur colloid has a different particle size distribution from that of cold sulfur colloid. Electron microscopy therefore may not be useful for measuring these particles.[60]

The major difference between Tc-99m colloid and sulfur colloid is in the size range < 100 nm, where a larger percentage of Tc-99m colloid particles fall.[60] Warbick et al., assuming no differences between labeled and nonlabeled colloid particle size distribution, compared several sizing methods (see Table 10–4).[188] Technetium-99m sulfur colloid prepared with perrhenate carrier showed at least three major size components: 22% particle < 100 nm; 39% between 200 and 400 nm; and 24% > 400 nm. Davis et al. also showed that such cellulose membrane filters as Millipore do not filter particles according to size because of the filter thickness and irregular path.[189] For the Tc sulfur colloid analyzed by Warbick et al., electron microscopy revealed the presence of aggregates as the cause of the bimodal distribution observed with Nucleopore filters.[188]

Warbick et al. chose electron microscopy because it allows direct observation of the particles and chemical components.[188] Technetium-99m antimony sulfur colloid was determined to have a smaller particle size (av = 10 nm) than thiosulfate-prepared sulfur colloid. The presence of aggregates makes data of antimony colloid difficult to interpret. Billinghurst and Jette used gel filtration to measure particle size because of the general unavailability of electron microscopes and the evaporation of sulfur that occurs with that technique.[190] They proposed gel filtration for colloidal particles below 100-nm diameter because larger particles are above the maximum operating range. In addition, based on the relationship between percentage radioactivity and number of particles, they proposed that the surface area, not the volume, is the relevant variable. Only certain particle size ranges can be analyzed on these columns, and the elution time is long.

Pedersen and Kristensen have compared several techniques, including filtration, photon correlation spectroscopy, and light microscopy.[191] They confirmed by these methods that several Tc-99m colloid preparations change with time, especially the Tc-99m colloids. They reemphasize that the Nucleopore filtration technique measures the distribution of radioactivity in particles of different sizes, whereas photon correlation spectroscopy (Nanosizer) measures particle size. For example, for rhenium-sulfur gelatin, the mean particle size by Nanosizer measurement was 420 ± 40 nm, whereas only 30% of the Tc-99m radioactivity was retained on a 400-nm filter, 33% on a 200-nm filter, and 36% on a 100-nm filter. The lower level of size detection for the spectroscopic method can also create inconsistencies.

In some preparations of Tc-99m sulfur colloid, the colloid adheres to the walls of the glass vial in which it has been prepared. If the total vial is assayed, an aliquot removed may not represent the true fraction removed. It is therefore necessary to assay the dose in the syringe. Unless the syringe containing colloid is flushed with the patient's blood, a substantial fraction of the dose remains in the syringe.

Microspheres are particles formed by extrusion of albumin into hot oil, as opposed to macroaggregates, which are formed by heating albumin in water.[192] After sieving, they are uniformly sized and can be readily labeled. Microspheres have also been prepared from gelatin and amylose by modification of the albumin methods.[193] Other microspheres of various compositions are available for diagnostic and therapeutic purposes.[194]

It is important that labeled particles be of nearly uniform size and that a small proportion of unbound radionuclide exist. Microspheres are supplied presieved and have a narrow size range. Unbound radionuclides may be determined by washing or incubating with the fluid to be used, filtering the mixture of spheres and fluid through a 0.45-μm filter to retain the spheres, and determining the activity of the filtrate. The U.S. Pharmacopeia (USP) specifies that no less than 90% of Tc-99m macroaggregated albumin (MAA) have diameters between 10 μm and 90 μm, and none may have a diameter greater than 150 μm.[195] On some occasions, the spheres may break under rough handling. For a general reference to albumin microspheres, the reader is referred to Rhodes and Bolles.[196]

In Vivo Radiochemical Purity

The chemical form of Tc-99m following the intravenous administration of either radiolabeled particles or colloids is not known. Radiochemical impurities are easily demonstrated by chromatography,[185] but their relationship to the biologic behavior of the compound is not well understood.

In further support of Steigman's contention that the particle size of the Tc-99m particles differs from the sulfur colloid itself, two groups have studied the distribution of sulfur colloid doubly labeled with Tc-99m and S-35 and found 86% of the Tc-99m in the liver at 4 min but only 11% of S-35 at the same length of time. With longer heating time, only 29% of the Tc-99m concentrated in the liver, while a much greater percentage concentrated in the lung. Clearance rates were also different. Technetium-99m remained in the liver (87% at 36 hr), but the S-35 cleared more rapidly (4% at 36 hr). Frier et al. observed similar pharmacokinetics.[197] When they used Tc-99 in equimolar amounts, they observed high liver uptake with both Tc-99m and S-35. They suggest that sulfur colloid is broken down by serum whereas Tc colloid is not. Although this may occur in sera, accelerated breakdown also occurs in the liver, as shown in the first case. Both groups removed soluble sulfur by dialysis. The S-35 can be incorporated in either of the nonequivalent sulfur atoms in thiosulfate.[198]

Many experiments have been carried out to determine the effect of size, number of particles, surface charge, and stabilizer on the distribution. Most of these have been designed to increase the concentration of colloid in the bone marrow. Atkins et al. studied the distribution of sulfur colloid produced by H_2S and by thiosulfate.[143] Increasing either the number of colloid particles or the gelatin concentration increased the marrow uptake. Pretreatment of animals with either gelatin or nonradioactive colloid also decreased liver uptake and increased bone marrow uptake. At large doses, relatively more H_2S-produced colloid than thiosulfate-produced colloid goes to the marrow.

Quantitative studies of the effect of particle size and number by Cohen et al. and by Caro and Ciscato revealed that the clearance $T_{1/2}$ could be described by the Michaelis-Menten equation for enzyme reactions.[199,200]

$$T_{1/2} = \frac{.693}{V_m}(N_{op}) + \frac{.693}{V_m}K_s$$

where:

(N_{op}) = number of particles per kilogram body weight,

V_m = maximum rate of phagocytosis,

K_s = overall rate constant.

The colloid disappears from the blood by an exponential function, is adsorbed on the surface of Kupffer's cells, and then is bound irreversibly. Caro and Ciscato used gold colloid stabilized by PVP or gelatin.[200] The hepatic clearance time was not affected by the mean size of the particles that were at least in the range of 2.5 to 30 nm. The overall rate constant is greater for PVP-protected colloids than for gelatin-protected colloids. The gelatin-protected particles have a greater affinity for the cell sites, but their entry into the cell is slower. Smaller particles seem to be cleared from the blood faster,[201,202] but a kinetic analysis using the methods of Caro and Ciscato has not been applied; therefore, the surface charge and the rate of binding and internalization still may be determining factors.

McAfee et al. have recently compared several colloids to determine relative bone marrow uptake.[145] No significant increase in uptake was observed among different colloids such as antimony sulfur colloid, stannous oxide colloid, microaggregated albumin, and small albumin microspheres. McAfee et al. showed that minimicroaggregated albumin had the highest marrow concentration in dogs, and this was confirmed by comparative imaging.[203] The mean particle sizes of several colloids are listed in Table 10–4.

Several factors must be kept in mind during discussion of colloid distribution as a function of physicochemical properties. The measurement of size can be misleading because the radioactive particles may not have the same size distribution as the nonradioactive particles, and the extrapolation from one physical measurement to another is beset with difficulties. Emphasis on particle size may be incorrect, based on the work of Caro and Ciscato and Myers.[200,204] Also, the difference in relative distribution between the liver and bone marrow might best be explained by a difference in mechanism of sequestration. Martindale et al. conclude that small colloids, such as Tc-99m antimony sulfur colloid, concentrate in the subendothelial dendritic phagocytes of the bone marrow.[205] The actual route to these cells may be by micropinocytosis across the endothelial lining of the sinusoid, through the junctions between adjoining endothelial cells. Only occasionally was the radiocolloid found in the endothelial cells lining the bone-marrow sinusoids. Thus small colloids are better suited to localization in the bone marrow.

TABLE 10–4. *Particle Size of Common Radiocolloids*

Material	Diameter (nm)
^{99m}Tc-phytate	In vivo formation
^{99m}Tc-antimony sulfide	4–14
^{113m}In-colloid	10–20
^{198}Au colloid	10
^{99m}Tc-Sn-phosphate	In vivo
^{99m}Tc-liposomes (neutral)	33
^{99m}Tc-minimicroaggregates (HSA)	90
^{99m}Tc-sulfur colloid (thiosulfate)	200–500

From Spencer, R.P.: Reticuloendothelial compounds. *In* Radiopharmaceuticals: Structure-Activity Relationships. Edited by R.P. Spencer. New York, Grune & Stratton, 1981. Reprinted by permission of the publisher.

Direct Labeling of Cells and Blood Elements

Radiopharmaceuticals

The two blood components erythrocytes and albumin (HSA) have received the most attention in radiolabeling with Tc-99m.[206] Although in vitro labeling of RBC appears to be superior to in vivo labeling (injecting tin intravenously, followed 20 min later by injecting Tc-99m pertechnetate), many laboratories still use the latter because of technical ease. In vitro methods, especially those using the pretinning kit developed by Brookhaven National Laboratory,[207] appear to produce quantitative retention of radioactivity.[208] The problem with the in vivo labeling technique, as described by Pavel and Zimmer,[209] is the low labeling yield in some patients..[210] Gottchalk et al. have suggested that the two techniques can be combined as follows: Stannous pyrophosphate is injected as in the in vivo technique, but instead of injecting pertechnetate 15 min later, blood is withdrawn and labeled in vitro.[211] This permits determination of the labeling yield before reinjection.

Attempts have also been made to label leukocytes,[212] lymphocytes,[213] and platelets,[145,214] although little success has been achieved with these blood cells. Many tumor cells have been labeled with technetium, including murine fibrosarcoma, human carcinoma of the breast, lung, colon, and malignant melanoma.[215] Thymocyte labeling with Tc-99m also has been reported.[216]

Because of the frequency of thromboembolic disorders, great interest has surrounded labeled fibrinogen and urokinase for thrombus localization.[217,218,219] Streptokinase, although not found in humans, has been studied for the same reasons,[220] as has plasmin.[221] For these and all other blood products and cells mentioned, the labeling procedure is based on the stannous chloride method developed for RBCs and HSA.

In Vitro Radiochemical Purity

The best method of determining labeling yield of cells is by centrifugation, which readily separates unbound radioactivity from the labeled cells. It does not separate Tc-99m labeled colloids or particles, because they sediment also.

For blood protein components, the most widely employed means of separation is by gel filtration with Sephadex G25 using saline solution.[222] Radiochemical impurities do exist. Early investigators erroneously assumed that pertechnetate is the only possible impurity. This led to much confusion when the in vivo stability of Tc-HSA was determined. In the production of Tc-99m HSA by the iron ascorbate reduction method, impurities include not only pertechnetate, but also Tc-ascorbate, which is excreted rapidly and therefore overestimates plasma volume.

With development of the highly efficient tin reduction method for preparing Tc-99m HSA, not only is the production of ascorbate avoided, but the probability of a pertechnetate impurity is remote.[222] Those labeling procedures that use stannous chelate and HSA at neutral pH, however, may result in formation of small colloids with slow blood clearance.[202] The clearance of Tc-HSA and small colloid is similar, so that the clinical observation is not affected.

The binding of Tc-99m to blood clot agents is variable. Persson et al. demonstrated that even under optimal reaction conditions, Tc-99m streptokinase was only 70 to 80% radiochemically pure.[223] With fibrinogen, 85% labeling occurred following electrolysis using zirconium electrodes.[34] Duffy and Duffy obtained the same yield using stannous chloride and streptokinase at pH 1 to 2.[224] But upon increasing the pH to 7, approximately 15 to 20% of the Tc-99m was released. Streptokinase also can be labeled by using stannous pyrophosphate as the reducing agent, yielding between 50 and 60% for a 2-hr labeling time at neutral pH. The radiochemical purity of radiolabeled streptokinase was determined on TLC, Sephadex column chromatography, and polyacrylamide gel electrophoresis. The commercially available streptokinase contains gelatin, which is also labeled. To obtain radiochemically pure streptokinase, pure streptokinase must be used. The product is labeled at neutral pH and must be purified on a Sephadex column eluted with saline.

In Vivo Radiochemical Purity

Demonstrating radiochemical purity of labeled blood products is a minor task compared with the problem of proving that the radiolabeled product truly represents its natural blood counterpart.

For RBCs, red cell volume determinations have indirectly confirmed 95% radiochemical purity as much as 1 hr after injection.[225] Similar studies with Tc-99m HSA remain in doubt because they are not accompanied by in vitro radiochemical purity data.

Two problems complicate labeling of cells other than RBCs. First, conclusively determining the chemical form of technetium in vivo is difficult. The second problem pertains to cell fragility. Labeling such cells as leukocytes, platelets, and thymocytes necessitates an evaluation of cell viability following the labeling procedure. Although such viability tests as trypan blue staining or determinations of cellular ability to incorporate thymidine and amino acids can indicate that the function tested is intact, the in vivo distribution does not represent that of native cells. A possible explanation is that the cell membrane is compromised during the labeling process, which changes the cell characteristics and behavior.

Nevertheless, even large quantities of radiochemical impurities may not frustrate the clinical objective. Acceptable thrombus visualization has been achieved with as little as 18% of Tc-99m fibrinogen migrating electrophoretically with the clotting fractions.[34]

New Directions in Tc-99m Radiopharmaceuticals

Future progress in nuclear medicine appears to rest upon more specific approaches to compound localization, mechanisms that depend upon the use of radiolabeled biologically active compounds or synthetic drugs. In spite of the potential suggested by this type of application, major difficulties are encountered in directly radiolabeling the functional groups of such compounds as hormones, enzymes, and drugs. First, the native functional group(s) may be essential to interaction with the active biological site responsible for compound localization; second, the affinity binding the radionuclide to the molecule may be insufficient to produce a stable chelate.

The importance of both of these factors is exemplified by radiolabeled bleomycin. Bleomycin is a mixture of closely related antibiotics that have been used successfully to treat a variety of malignancies. Chemically, this antibiotic acts as a chelating agent and binds a number of divalent and trivalent cations with varying affinities.[226] Although chelates of indium, gallium, and copper have not demonstrated the necessary in vivo and in vitro stability, cobalt-labeled bleomycin is more stable.[227] A technetium-labeled bleomycin would be more useful. While inspection of the bleomycin structure indicates that the disaccharide moiety is the most likely chelating group, it is unfortunately a low affinity site for Tc-99m.[9] The sugar moiety has a high affinity for Tc-99m at pH 10 to 12, but a weak affinity at neutral pH. Therefore, the use of the native functional groups of bleomycin to bind technetium results in a weak chelate with poor stability.

The biologic activity of a drug may also change with the addition of a radiolabel. For example, the chelation of copper to bleomycin destroys its ability to cleave strands of DNA.[228] When labeled with cobalt, the antibacterial activity of bleomycin is deleteriously affected and becomes negligible when tested against the usually responsive Bacillus Subtilis ATC 6633.[229] In this instance, cobalt appears to alter the biologic effectiveness of the bleomycin because of its bond to the functional groups responsible for maintaining the antibiotic integrity of this drug.

Another approach for labeling biochemicals (for which there have been many precedents) is derivatization. Drug derivatives have been prepared to increase absorption, eliminate bitterness and odor, diminish gastric upset, increase or decrease metabolism, and improve stability of the parent compound both in vivo and in vitro. Derivatives might also be developed that will accept a radiolabel without altering biologic activity.

Increasingly, specific *site-directed* synthetic derivatives are being developed. These are molecules that concentrate within the body by virtue of their physiologic action. Examples are (1) steroid hormones, (2) peptide hormones, (3) adrenergic substances, (4) vitamins, and (5) certain synthetic drugs. The ideal properties for any site-directed derivative were outlined by Paul Ehrlich approximately seventy years ago and more recently have been enumerated by Sinkula and Yalkowsky as follows:[230]

1. Exclusive and complete transport to the diseased tissue or target organ, including high binding affinity and interaction with these cell systems and tissues.
2. Absence of binding by the derivative to protein or tissue not specifically diseased and absence of degradation or metabolism of the derivative prior to contact with the diseased bioenvironment.
3. Lack of toxicity for normal tissue in the body.
4. Complete elimination from the body of the nonlocalized pharmaceutical.

Because these criteria are so stringent, the "ideal" site-directed drug derivative has yet to be synthesized. Even with radioiodide, perhaps the best example of a physiologic site-directed radiopharmaceutical, the normal 24-hr thyroid uptake is only 15 to 25% of the administered dose. Localization also occurs in the stomach and salivary glands, with most of the dose excreted in the urine.

Regarding the use of radiopharmaceut-icals, certain other factors must be considered. One factor is the time frame during which a radiopharmaceutical must maintain its integrity. During evaluation of pharmacokinetics, no absolute criteria exist, but rather a medical tracer needs to remain stable in vivo only for the duration of the study. For example, if a blood pool label reflects the vascular pool size accurately for only 30 min after injection, then it fulfills the criteria for a stable in vivo derivative, and its use is valid during that period of time.

Chelate-Containing Derivatives

In the reduced oxidation states, technetium usually requires an octahedral coordination structure, i.e., up to six coordination sites in a target molecule are bound directly to the radionuclide. This structure can prevent the biologic molecule's expected interaction with the active site responsible for localization. Technetium-99m probably is not bound directly to many molecules with affinities able to withstand in vivo dilution or ligand substitution. As a result, the radiolabeled tracer in many cases may not reflect the biologic behavior of the parent molecule. In addition, the ready oxidation of certain reduced weak chelates interferes with studies of radiochemical purity and in vivo metabolism. To avoid the problems encountered with direct labeling of a biologically active molecule, derivatives are formed by covalent bonding of a chelating agent to a molecule known to act on a specific organ or to follow a specific pathway.

Labeling derivatives of biologically active compounds for use as tracers is a recent procedure. For reasons already elucidated, technetium appears to be the most logical of the radioactive metals for development of agents with widespread applicability. To bind such "positively charged" metal ions as Tc-99m requires a relatively large chelating agent. The che-late, however, adds a large polar group to the molecule, altering its biologic activity.

An example of this chelate derivative approach is the synthesizing of an EDTA derivative that contains a diazonium group [1-(p-benzenediazonium)-ethylene-diamine-N,N,N',N', tetraacetic acid].[231,232] This chelating agent can be reacted with a molecule that contains an activated benzene ring, i.e., phenol or aniline, and in fact was used to chelate derivatives of fibrinogen, albumin, and bleomycin. Although these compounds were subsequently labeled with In-111 only, their potential applicability to technetium is evident.

Other chelate derivatives include structural analogs of tolbutamide;[233] of fatty acids chelated with DTPA, EDTA, and diethylenetriamine (DTA);[234,235] and analogs of the antiarrhythmic drug lidocaine.[86,122] Recently, fatty acids have been labeled with other Tc-99m chelates, but to no avail.[24,236] Synthetic pathways are available to produce DTPA-like chelating agents that can be easily reacted with biologic molecules.[237] In addition, the Mannich reaction has been proposed as a single method of incorporating chelating agents without destroying functional groups.[238]

At present, the optimal type of chelating agent is undefined. Interaction of the chelating group with the active site responsible for the biologic effect cannot be predicted for DTPA, IDA, or DTA from the preliminary data available. The most successful derivatives, however, probably will bind the chelating agent distant from the site-interacting functional groups of the biologic molecule. Another more subtle consideration is the chelating agent's effect on the resultant charge of the molecule. If a particular chelating agent is found to stabilize a certain oxidation state of technetium, one chelate derivative may be more suited to reduce the charge of the chelate. This derivative then would allow minimal polar disruption to the lipophilic character of the biologically active molecule. To this end, a number of investigators have proposed neutral chelates that would cross cellular membranes with a higher efficiency than would the charged chelates. Technetium-99m KTS was first proposed in 1976 but has not yet been attached to a biochemical or drug. Kramer et al. have produced a Tc(V) neutral chelate, but it, too, has yet to be incorporated into a bifunctional chelate.[239]

Pitfalls

Factors that can affect the integrity of technetium radiopharmaceuticals adversely and deteriorate the quality of the scan image are due primarily to (1) improper preparation of nonradioactive components, (2) improper technique in the introduction of pertechnetate, and (3) differences in patient biophysiology.

In the first case, oxidation of stannous chloride (Sn^{2+}) to Sn^{4+}, inadequate binding of the stannous ion to the chelating agent, or binding of stannous ion to a degradation product of the chelating agent fails either to reduce technetium or to introduce a competitive binder involving the degradation product. Should any of these problems occur during the manufacturing of stannous pyrophosphate or macroaggregated albumin particles, for example, the desired product will not be obtained.

Improper technique in the addition of pertechnetate to stannous-labeled chelating agents also degrades image quality. Careless contamination with O_2 during the addition of pertechnetate can prevent technetium reduction and ruin the Tc-99m bone scanning agent.

Metabolic variations among patients receiving technetium-labeled compounds affect tracer distribution. For example, both prospective and retrospective evaluations of Tc-99m diphosphonate following bone scans with excess soft tissue activity have demonstrated no chromatographic irregularities in the administered

compound or in analyzed samples of the patient's urine and blood. Local variations in tissue metabolism probably are responsible for distributional variations. Several of these so-called iatrogenic effects on radionuclide distribution have been reviewed.[240,241]

Any of these factors can produce ineffective agents, and all have been responsible for suboptimal scintigraphs. Although the incidence of these problems is low, nuclear medicine laboratories should be capable of differentiating between these sources of error, particularly now that university and community hospitals are preparing, at least in part, their own technetium radiopharmaceuticals.

The most significant factor in successful Tc-99m chromatography is a complete understanding of each system's function and limitations. Of those methods presented in Table 10–2 for the determination of pertechnetate, there are no distinct advantages to either the column or the TLC systems. Each system has certain attributes that become apparent after extensive use. As new radiopharmaceuticals are developed, the chromatographic system must be validated with pure radiopharmaceutical. A case in point is the use of the silica gel:acetone system for analyzing Tc-99m HIDA compounds. Because of the increased lipophilicity, Tc-99m HIDA is not retained at the origin as is Tc-99m DTPA; rather, it spreads over the entire strip in a broad peak. With 75% $CHCl_3$ and 25% acetone as the solvent, the Tc-99m HIDA is retained at the origin in a sharp peak and TcO_4^- migrates with the solvent front. As in most areas of quality control, baseline reference determinations of the radiopharmaceutical are imperative. When the question of radiochemical purity arises, the chromatographic methods in Table 10–3 can be utilized.

With these concepts, a rational approach to Tc-99m compound chromatography can be adopted. If the presence of pertechnetate is suspected from a bone scan, e.g., gastrointestinal visualization, then the systems in Table 10–2 should be used exclusively for the detection of pertechnetate; those in Table 10–3 should be used to determine the presence of reduced but unchelated technetium.

Unsatisfactory Images and Their Causes

Unexpected distribution of a radiopharmaceutical may be attributed to the radiopharmaceutical or to an altered physiologic or pathologic process in the patient. As mentioned in the last section, unsatisfactory Tc-99m radiopharmaceuticals can easily result from adding oxygen (air bubbles) along with pertechnetate to the kit. The oxidation produces pertechnetate, which results in thyroid and stomach localization. More subtle changes in distribution are observed when the nonradioactive kit is prepared in such a fashion that stannous oxide colloid is produced in a chelate kit. When some colloid is formed, soft tissue background or liver uptake occurs. This same effect is observed when too little chelating agent is used or when the kit is diluted excessively.

Many reports have been published in which an abnormal physiologic state of the patient was believed to cause the poor image. The following list includes examples of some abnormalities to be considered in the differential diagnosis of a poor image.

1. Brain Imaging Agents
   Physiologic Causes
   a. Slow blood clearance of pertechnetate, due to previous bone scan. Stannous ion in the bone kit remains with the red blood cells, reducing the pertechnetate and thereby labeling the cells.
   b. Abnormal areas of pertechnetate concentration due to incomplete suppression of the choroid plexus, uptake by perchlorate or by previous angiographic contrast injection.

   c. Abnormal areas of concentration or radioactivity due to contamination with saliva, sweat, or urine.

2. Kidney Imaging Agents
   Physiologic Causes
   a. Radioactivity above the left kidney on the flow study due to splenic blood pool.
   Radiopharmaceutical Causes
   a. Radioactivity above the left kidney due to gastrointestinal activity resulting from oxidation to pertechnetate.
   b. Radioactivity above the right kidney due to hepatic activity resulting from colloid formation.

3. Liver Imaging Agents
   Physiologic Causes
   a. Radioactivity in the lung due to liver disorders and pulmonary reticuloendothelial activation.
   b. Radioactivity in the bone marrow due to compromised hepatic function.
   Radiopharmaceutical Causes
   a. Radioactivity in the kidneys due to preparation of soluble forms of reduced Tc-99m.
   b. Radioactivity in the lungs due to increased particle size.
   c. Radioactivity in the bone marrow due to decreased particle size.

4. Lung Agents
   Physiologic Causes
   Radioactivity in the kidney due to right-to-left intracardiac or pulmonic shunt.
   Radiopharmaceutical Causes
   a. Radioactivity in the kidney due to formation of a soluble chelate.
   b. Unequal perfusion or apparent perfusion defects due to nonrandom distribution of too few injected particles.
   c. Symmetric foci of increased activity due to clumping of the particle during preparation or injec-

tion, especially injection into polyethylene tubing.

5. Bone Imaging Agents
   Physiologic Causes
   a. Soft-tissue accumulation due to
      numerous causes (see Table 8–2
      Vol. II, Chap. 8).
   b. Localization of radioactivity in
      the calyceal collecting systems of
      a kidney overlying bone.
   Radiopharmaceutical Causes
   a. Radioactivity in the liver due to
      formation of colloids.
   b. Radioactivity in the stomach and
      gastrointestinal tract due to for-
      mation of pertechnetate.
   c. Radioactivity in the blood due to
      formation of small colloids or
      protein-binding species.

Conclusion

The nuclear properties of Tc-99m have
led to many successes not attained by nuclides with less ideal properties. For example, mercury chlormerodrin has better
biologic characteristics (according to the
ideal qualities outlined earlier for site-directed derivatives) than do the Tc-99m
agents suggested for kidney imaging.[98] Because of the poor nuclear properties of the
mercury nuclides, however, Tc-99m chelates are usually chosen for kidney imaging. Until recently, the extraordinary
succcess of Tc-99m radiopharmaceuticals
had led to the neglect of the chemical
properties of Tc-99m. The first compounds developed were based on removal
of foreign substances from the blood, and
many such factors as binding affinities,
equilibrium constants, and oxidation state
were not crucial to the efficacious application of these imaging agents.

The binding of technetium to biologically active compounds or drugs, however, necessitates a clear understanding of
both the nuclide's effect on the biologic
behavior of the radiopharmaceutical and
the affinity with which this radionuclide
is bound. As exemplified by bleomycin,
direct binding of technetium may be quite
limited and really only applicable to labeling proteins and cells of large molecular weight. By analogy with research
efforts in pharmaceuticals, chemothera-
peutics, and radiolabeled antigens for radioimmunoassay and radioreceptor assay,
synthesis of a chelate-containing derivative of a biologically active molecule has
been suggested as the most promising approach; however, further research is necessary. The chemistry of Tc-99m is being
investigated,[242] but insufficient data regarding present radiopharmaceuticals
have been collected.

Indirect labeling of chelate-containing
derivatives of biologically active molecules seems promising in that it guarantees stable chelates of Tc-99m and the Tc-
99m does not interfere with those functional groups interacting with the active
site. Also, the problem of air oxidation of
reduced technetium can be overcome to
some extent by the formation of stable chelates. The primary obstacle to success is
synthesis of a derivative sufficiently similar to the parent molecule for it to retain
the desired biologic action. This problem
cannot be overemphasized, based on the
precedent available from other efforts to
prepare derivatives that retain the biologic
activity of the parent.

RADIOPHARMACEUTICAL CHEMISTRY OF IODINE

Radionuclides of Iodine

The radionuclides of iodine having the
best nuclear properties for gamma-ray detecting systems are I-123, I-125, and I-131.
Both I-125 and I-131 are reactor produced
and therefore less expensive and more
readily available than the cyclotron product, I-123. The radiation absorbed dose to
the patient from both I-131 and I-125 is
high, however. Iodine-123 is a superior
radionuclide for imaging systems, with a
159-keV gamma ray and low radiation ab-

sorbed dose. This gamma ray has a half-thickness in water of 4.7 cm and therefore affords satisfactory tissue penetration, yet its energy is low enough to be collimated easily. This radionuclide, though, can be produced only in a cyclotron and currently cannot easily be made free of I-124 and/or I-125. High-energy protons or helium particles produce the purest I-123, but they are not readily available.[243] The most frequently used reaction to produce I-123 of high purity is the $^{127}I(p,5n)^{123}I$ reaction (see Chapter 8).

Iodine-124 is an undesirable radionuclide impurity because of its long half-life (4.2 days) and its positron and high-energy protons (511 keV, 603 keV, and 723 keV). A 1% concentration of I-124 at time of production usually results in ~5% contamination at an imaging time 24 hr later. The I-124 degrades resolution because a significant fraction of the high-energy gamma rays are detected as scattered radiation in the 159-keV energy window. With a low-energy collimator, the scatter contribution is about 28%. With a high-resolution, medium-energy collimator, the contribution is 10%. With a high-energy collimator, only 3% is scattered radiation, but the sensitivity is greatly reduced. The need for high radionuclidic purity is obvious.[244]

Chemistry of Iodine

Of the halogens, iodine is most likely to support a positive charge and thus is the least reactive toward electrophilic addition or substitution. The chemical properties of iodine stem from the decreasing ionization potential, larger atomic radii, larger van der Waals forces, and increased polarizability that are found as the atomic number in the group VII congeners increases. Also, iodine forms the weakest bonds to carbon and the other first-row elements. Despite its anticipated stability, the I^+ ion does not exist alone but usually forms a complex with a nucleophilic species, such as water or pyridine.

Target Molecules for Electrophilic Substitution by Iodine

In electrophilic substitution, the most reactive aromatic compound is phenol, followed by aniline, methoxybenzene, and imidazole. The anion seems to be the reactive species, so close attention must be paid to the pKa and pH values of the reaction. Imidazole and pyrazole are iodinated in the 4-position, and therefore, such fused ring compounds as benzimidazole are not easily iodinated. Iso-oxazole, oxazole, and thiozole are less reactive than imidazole. In other heterocyclic compounds, the order of iodination at a specific reaction site is 2-thiophen≈3-furan <3-benzofuran≈2-benzothiophen <3-benzothiophen≈2-benzofuran <<2-thiophen<<2-furan. For benzothiophen and indole the 3-position is preferred, although in the heterocyclic alone (thiophen and pyrole), the 2-position is more reactive. The 2-position is most reactive in furan and benzofuran.[245]

Pyridine is not easily iodinated at a carbon atom, but rather, it forms charge transfer complexes with the halogen at nitrogen. Aliphatic unsaturated compounds can be iodinated, but the carbon-iodine bond is much less stable than the bond in aromatic compounds, although the mode of deiodination differs in each case.

The most popular iodinating agents used to produce electrophilic addition or substitution in activated aromatic rings are (1) iodine,[246] (2) iodine monochloride,[247] (3) chloramine-T,[248] (4) lactoperoxidase,[249] (5) electrolysis,[250] and (6) prelabeled ligands.[251]

Iodination Using Iodine

The reaction mechanism for the electrophilic aromatic substitution has been studied extensively. Reactions with phenols and imidazole generally show an isotope effect, indicating that the rate-determining step involves removal of hydrogen from the intermediate. In this case, the rate of catalysis seems to be determined by the type of base used. Where no isotope effect is observed, as in the iodination of dimethylaminobenzenesulfonic acid, the rate of reaction appears to be related to the basicity of the catalyst. This observation suggests that the formation of a complex iodinating agent may be involved in a rate-determining step.

Papers by Grovenstein et al. showed a definite effect of iodide on the rate of iodination.[252] This effect is consistent with I_2 as the reactive species:

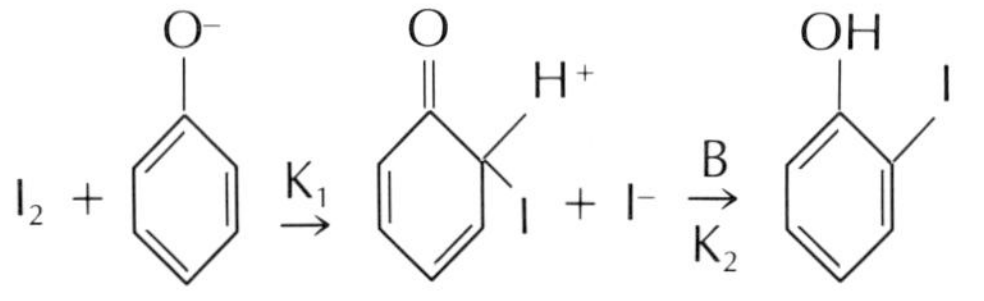

These same authors observed that as the iodide concentration decreased, the kinetic isotope effect also decreased, and the first step involving the attack of the iodine became rate-determining. At high concentrations of iodide, the removal of hydrogen became the rate-determining step.

In radioiodination, half of the radioisotope is converted to the iodide chemical form after the reaction of the positive iodinating species. This process limits the theoretic yield.

Iodination Using Iodine Monochloride

McFarland showed that compared to I_2 solutions, ICl increases the iodination efficiency because all iodine atoms can be incorporated.[247] Radioiodide is mixed with ICl and then added to the target molecule. Since carrier ICl is added, the specific activity of the product is lower than that obtained with chloramine-T. Lambrecht et al. have proposed a recoil method for preparing carrier free *ICl,[253] but because of the complicated techniques involved, it is not in common use.

The mechanism of ICl iodination has been studied by Berliner.[254] He suggested that either H_2OI^+ or ICl might be the electrophile in the rate-determining step. Batts and Gold, by studying the reverse reaction, i.e., deiodination, showed that the chloride concentration affected the rate of reaction, and that ICl must therefore be the electrophile.[255] The deiodination was also acid catalyzed and the iodine released could be trapped by either chloride or dimedone. A substantial catalysis by chloride was observed, but the deiodination rate approached zero as the pH approached 7.

Iodination Using Chloramine-T

Chloramine-T, the sodium salt of N-chloro-p-toluenesulfonamide, has been used as an oxidant since its discovery by F.D. Chattaway in 1905. It is not widely used at present because it has few advantages over a standard iodine solution. Chloramine-T is unstable when exposed to light, but a 0.05 M solution in water decreases in oxidizing power by only 0.02% per month when stored in the dark. The major equilibria of chloramine-T as given by Jennings are:[256]

$$RNClNa = RNCl^- + Na^+$$
$$RNCl^- + H^+ = RNClH$$
$$2\ RNClH = RNCl_2 + RNH_2$$
$$RNCl_2 + H_2O = RNHCl + HOCl$$
$$RNHCl + H_2O = RNH_2 + HOCl$$
$$HOCl = H^+ + OCl^-$$

with the following constants, respectively:

$$K_A = 2.38 \times 10^{-3}$$
$$K_1 = 6.1 \times 10^{-2}$$
$$K_H = 8 \times 10^{-7}$$
$$K_H = 4.9 \times 10^{-8}$$
$$K_A = 3.3 \times 10^{-8}$$

The free acid and $RNCl_2$ exist at pH 1; at pH 2.6, the concentrations of $RNCl^-$ and RNClH are equal, and at pH 4, only $RNCl^-$ exists. The rate of reaction for the hydrolysis at pH 3.7 and 25° C is 10.10 l/mol/sec, and the reverse reaction is 2.5 l/mol/sec.

In addition to being a powerful oxidizing agent, chloramine-T can act also as a chlorinating agent in electrophilic substitution of aromatic molecules. Huguchi and Hussain describe the active species as the N,N-dichloro p-toluenesulfonamide (dichloramine-T).[257] The rate of disproportionation to produce dichloramine-T at pH 6.4 is 1.3 l/mol/sec and at pH 6.9 is 0.40 l/mol/sec. When the amide is added to the reaction, the rate of disproportionation drops to one half of the expected value. This drop indicates that dichloramine-T is probably the active chlorinating agent, not HOCl as previously proposed.

When phenol is used as the target molecule and the chloramine-T to phenol ratio is 10, chlorophenol is found in the reaction mixture after 3 min in a yield of 10 to 19%, in the pH range of 9.6 to 6.5. In the presence of radioiodide, the average yield of iodophenol based on radioiodide is 50% whereas the average yield of chlorophenol based on phenol is approximately 10%. In attempts to produce iodinated molecules with maximum specific activity, equimolar amounts of chloramine-T, iodide, and target molecule can produce mixed chloroiodo-compounds which are difficult to separate and identify from the desired radioiodine compounds.

The use of chloramine-T has been discouraged because of these possible side reactions. Nevertheless, use of appropriate molar ratios can produce satisfactory products even with the most sensitive target molecules. Freychet et al. have reported that equimolar amounts of either chloramine-T or chloramine-T added in small aliquots produces radiolabeled insulin that retains its biological activity.[258] Eckelman et al. found that bleomycin can be radiolabeled by the chloramine-T method and that this sensitive molecule retained its antibacterial activity after iodination.[229]

To use chloramine-T, the target molecule must contain a tyrosine or imidazole moiety. The major advantages of iodination using chloramine-T are the simplicity and high reactivity that allow rapid preparation of products with high specific activity.

Iodination Using Lactoperoxidase

Iodide can be enzymatically oxidized to active iodine.[249] Immunoglobulin and bovine serum albumin were iodinated at low specific activity. Later, Thorell and Johansson improved the method to prepare high specific activity iodinated polypeptides and proteins.[259] This method is claimed to be less destructive to the target molecule but involves the usual problems encountered when dealing with enzymes, such as purification, determination of enzymatic activity, and separation from the reaction mixture. It is advantageous, however, in that carrier-free iodide, which yields products with high specific activity, can be used.

Iodination Using Electrolysis

Although the reaction conditions needed for the electrolytic oxidation of iodide are generally mild, carrier iodine is needed, and the reaction volumes are usually larger than needed for other methods.[250] Miller and Watkins proposed a method of electrolytic iodination in acetonitrile that is effective for molecules as unreactive to electrophilic substitution as ethyl benzoate.[260] This reaction apparently proceeds through a nitrogen iodine intermediate.

Iodination Using Prelabeled Ligands

Bolton and Hunter proposed iodinated 3-(4-hydroxyphenyl)propionic acid N-hydroxysuccinimide ester as an indirect iodinating reagent that avoids many of the problems of direct iodination.[251] In this indirect method of iodination, the active ester is iodinated and purified from oxidizing and reducing agents before being mixed with the target molecule. In this way, the impurities inherent in other iodination methods, e.g., chloramine-T and metabisulfate, do not come into contact with the target molecule. The reaction results in the formation of an amide bond with lysine groups of the target molecule. This method permits iodination of molecules that do not contain tyrosine or whose biologic activity might be lowered by alteration at the tyrosine rather than at the lysine moiety. The specific activity obtained is usually lower than that obtained with chloramine-T. The Bolton-Hunter reagent is the most popular, although two other prelabeled ligands—iodoaniline, which is converted to a reactive diazonium ion, and methyl-3,5-diiodo-p-hydroxybenzimilate—have been offered as equally effective reagents.[261,262] This indirect iodination method has been practiced for some time in preparing iodinated tracers for use in radioimmunoassay. Iodinated histamine-, tyramine-, and tyrosine-methyl ester can be reacted with carboxymethyl groups to produce iodinated derivatives.[263]

Other Iodination Agents

Several methods of electrophilic halogenation of aromatic compounds that are less activated by substitution than are phenol and aniline have been proposed.[245] These methods are not usually necessary for labeling peptides and proteins but are important for labeling smaller drugs and biochemicals. Nucleophilic substitution has been used in a few cases to introduce iodine, e.g., by the diazonium ion reaction or the triazene reaction, but in general, use of this method has been limited. Iodination of drugs and biochemicals is discussed in the section "Radiopharmaceuticals."

Purification

In the past, high specific activities were attained by using one or more iodine molecules per target molecule. Heavily iodinated species are present even at low molar ratios,[264] and chlorocompounds might be present with chloramine-T. Discouraged with these findings, most investigators iodinate low molecular weight compounds at high target-to-iodide ratios and then separate the iodinated target molecule by high pressure liquid chromatography (HPLC) to attain maximum specific activity. When carrier-free radioiodine is used and one iodine atom per molecule is assumed, the maximum specific activity is 2200 Ci/mmol for I-125, 16,000 Ci/mmol for I-131, and 23,600 Ci/mmol for I-123. This specific activity is not reached for I-131 prepared from natural tellurium, because I-127 and I-129 are also produced.[265] Depending on the irradiation time and the time after irradiation, various specific activities can be obtained.[266] Iodine-131 with higher specific activity is obtained by uranium fission. Using enriched tellurium, maximum specific activity is produced by the $^{130}Te(n,\gamma)^{131}I$ reaction, and this is now the method of choice.

Radiopharmaceuticals

A recent review enumerates the iodinated radiopharmaceuticals that have been tested.[267] Labeled dyes, macromolecules, steroids, heterocyclics, and other labeled compounds have been studied as tracers of the parent molecule. Few have been used routinely.

Iodoalbumin is used extensively for plasma volume determinations. Iodohippuric acid is still the only radiopharmaceutical used to measure tubular secretion, and iodinated rose bengal is used occasionally to study the patency of the hepatobiliary tract, although Tc-99m radiopharmaceuticals are now preferred. Iodo-oleic acid has been used for fat absorption studies and myocardial imaging, although the aliphatic carbon iodine bond is quite unstable in this compound.[268] These are usually labeled with I-131, although I-123 has been suggested for iodohippuric acid.

An interesting iodinated radiopharmaceutical is 6-iodomethyl-19-norcholest-5(10)-en-3-ol,[269] which is used for imaging the adrenal cortex (see Vol. II, Chap. 3). The original method of preparing 19-iodocholesterol produced apparently as much as 30% of 6-iodomethyl-19-norcholesterol, and this "impurity" is now thought to be the adrenal concentrating species. The latter compound has higher adrenal uptake and less in vivo deiodination and is now the agent of choice. Iodine-131 must be used because the gamma camera images are taken several days after injection to allow clearance of nonadrenal activity.

Iodinated fibrinogen has been studied extensively by Welch and Krohn,[270] and numerous parameters that affect in vitro and in vivo characteristics have been identified.[271]

Iodinated fibrinogen was developed to detect deep vein thrombosis.[272] Labeled fibrinogen accumulates quickly in thrombi but is slow to clear the blood. Of the labeling methods, iodine monochloride is preferred, because it causes the fewest side reactions and therefore produces a radiopharmaceutical that behaves most like native fibrinogen.[270] Tracer fibrinogen usually contains 0.5 iodine atoms per molecule. Fibrinogen can be heavily iodinated (25 to 100 iodine atoms per molecule) so that it clears more rapidly from the blood and allows earlier diagnosis.[273] Commercially available fibrinogen is labeled with I-125, which cannot be imaged on the gamma camera but can be used for uptake studies. To image the fibrinogen distribution, I-123 should be used;[34,274] however, if the material is to be injected before surgery to detect thrombosis after surgery, I-125 is the label of choice.

Iodine-125 is used most often as a label for in vitro radioimmunoassays and radioreceptor assays. Its long half-life, high specific activity, and low energy make it ideal for this application.

Quality Assurance of Iodinated Radiopharmaceuticals

In 1969, the International Atomic Energy Agency organized a symposium on analytical controls for radiopharmaceuticals. This contained chromatographic systems for many of the iodinated radiopharmaceuticals, including hippuran, rose bengal, thyroxine, and triolein. For hippuran, the major contaminations are o-iodobenzoic acid, sodium 2,4,6-triiodohippurate, and iodide. In the preparation of rose bengal, a number of iodinated products are possible, owing to the many activated sites in rose bengal. Labeled proteins also have been analyzed. In general, the protein is destroyed by the chromatographic solvent, and iodide is determined. Quality control for all radiopharmaceuticals except those containing Tc-99m has become less important because use of these compounds has decreased, and they possess relative stability.

MECHANISMS OF RADIOTRACER LOCALIZATION

The greatest strength of nuclear medicine lies in its capacity to detect and quantify physiologic function rather than to record fixed anatomic properties, which are often better detected by other imaging techniques. The nuclear medicine image depicts dynamic physiologic processes inherent in the living system. This approach is advantageous because pathologic processes are often more accurately characterized by functional rather than structural differences. Furthermore, functional abnormalities usually precede gross structural changes within organs.

Many early radiopharmaceuticals were developed because of a particular radionuclide's availability and certain chemical characteristics of the element. With the discovery of the Tc-99m pertechnetate generator system, more stringent requirements were placed on radiopharmaceuticals. On the other hand, technetium does not readily allow study of biochemical pathways because of poor chemical properties and the necessity of combining a Tc-99m chelate with the parent structure.

Radiopharmaceuticals can be divided into two general classes; those with *substrate specific* and those with *substrate nonspecific* mechanisms of localization.

Substrate Nonspecific Radiopharmaceuticals

These radiopharmaceuticals do not require a specific chemical reaction to effect distribution, i.e., no discrete chemical structure is responsible for their localization. Clinical utility of these compounds is not lessened by their nonspecificity; in fact, most radiopharmaceuticals used routinely in nuclear medicine belong to this class of compounds.

Regional blood flow can be measured by the particle distribution method, but the agent is not a specific substrate. Several different radiolabeled particles of the appropriate size are trapped in capillary beds regardless of their chemical composition. Colloids are trapped by reticuloendothelial cells, but the liver phagocytes do not discriminate among such colloids as sulfur colloid, gold colloid, and antimony sulfur colloid. Liposomes, produced by sonicating aqueous solutions of lipids to form microvesicles that contain radionuclide tracers, are newer examples of nonspecific tracer transport and localization.[275]

Substrate Specific Radiopharmaceuticals

Substrate specific radiopharmaceuticals involve a specific chemical reaction, or a chemical interaction at a specific, high-affinity site. The interaction demands a discrete chemical structure for localization. Incorporation of P-32 into cell nucleotides and I-131 into thyroid hormones are examples of substrate specific biochemical pathways. Several similar tracers have been developed through the years, e.g., Se-75 selenomethionine, but only recently has this approach been reemphasized.

Isotopically Substituted Substrates

Radionuclide labels have been incorporated into such natural biochemical substances as glucose, ammonia, fatty acids, catecholamines, and neurotransmitter agents and antagonists. When these substances are used in combination with tomographic imaging, quantitative differences in regional metabolism following various stimuli, i.e., drug or surgical manipulation, can be determined.

In tracing the entire biochemical pathway, such positron-emitting radiopharmaceuticals as C-11 labeled tracers have a special advantage. Carbon-11 palmitic and I-123 hexadecanoic acid have been prepared for the study of fatty acid metabolism in the heart. Carbon-11 carboxyl label is released slowly as CO_2. Iodine-123 iodide is released from the myocardium into the bloodstream. As with many nonisotopically substituted analogs, measurement of fatty acid metabolism has not been calibrated using I-123 hexadecanoic acid.[276]

Carbon-11 labeled amino acids have been used to measure discrete structural and functional components of the pancreas as well as to identify and measure metabolic rates of malignant cells.[277] Radiolabeled gases, such as CO, CO_2, O_2 and NH_3 have been used to study distribution of the gas as a function of blood flow and biochemical changes.

Nonisotopically Substituted Substrates

Nonisotopic substitution using positron-emitting radionuclides is also possible. Fluorine-18 fluoro-DOPA (3,4-dihydroxy-5-fluorophenylalanine) has many of the biochemical properties of DOPA.[278] An important area of investigation is metabolic trapping. Fluorine-18 2-deoxy-2-fluoro-D-glucose (FDG) is a suitable substrate for hexokinase, but the resulting hexose phosphate is a poor substrate for subsequent metabolic steps. Neurons in the brain have been demonstrated to concentrate glucose in proportion to their metabolic activity. FDG has been validated as a marker for glucose and has been used to measure regional glucose metabolism.[279] Fluorine-18 FDG also has been used to measure regional rates of myocardial glucose metabolism. Iodine-131 6-iodomethyl-19 norcholesterol (IMC) also is metabolically trapped. IMC behaves similarly to cholesterol in that it is taken up by the adrenal glands and incorporated into lipoproteins. IMC, however, is trapped in the adrenals as the ester, whereas native cholesterol is not. This metabolic trapping of IMC leads to sufficient adrenal-to-nonadrenal ratios for external imaging.[280]

M-iodobenzylguanidine, another interesting compound, appears to follow catecholamines in many aspects of uptake and storage, but not in metabolism.[281] This compound is taken up by both the heart and the adrenal medulla.

Several biochemicals and drugs cause a highly specific reaction in the body when administered in relatively low doses. Evidence from several sources suggests that the primary event in the action of many peptides and steroid hormones and drugs is the binding to a specific site, a receptor, on the plasma membrane or in the cytosol. The receptor determines the biochemical action, and the response is controlled by the amount of unchanged biochemical or drug acting as a substitute in the biophase surrounding the receptor. Because receptors are involved in the action of the drug or biochemical, concentration of the receptor would be expected to change as a function of the disease state.[282] Examples of receptor-binding radiotracers are estrogens,[283] muscarinic acetylcholine ligands,[242] and neuroleptics.[284]

Several antibodies and antineoplastic agents have been labeled on the basis that the therapeutic effect indicates a concentration difference between the abnormal tissue, surrounding tissue, and blood. Concentration gradients do not seem to exist in most cases, and therefore, therapeutic drugs do not generally make good diagnostic agents with high target-to-blood ratios. Radiolabeled antibodies, however, have been used with some success. Radiolabeled carcinoembryonic antigen (CEA) antibody has been used with varying success to image tumors.[285,286,287]

All radiotracers in the substrate specific class offer hope that specificity will be added to the already sensitive and noninvasive character of radiopharmaceuticals.

QUALITY ASSURANCE OF RADIOPHARMACEUTICALS—GENERAL CONSIDERATIONS

Quality assurance of radiopharmaceuticals is the system of controls that guarantees their constant composition, repro-

ducible biologic behavior, and safety for human use. The diversity of radiopharmaceuticals and ancillary materials, including kits for radiopharmaceutical preparations, radioimmunoassays, and the many short-lived radionuclides, has greatly expanded the role of quality control. Short-lived radionuclides require rapid chemical, physical, and biologic control methods. Among the quality assurance procedures unique to radiopharmaceuticals is the control of such radioisotopic contaminants as I-124 and I-125 in I-123 labeled compounds. The responsibility for quality assurance falls not only upon the manufacturer, but also upon the radiopharmaceutical chemist, the technicians dispensing labeled compounds, and the nuclear physician.

Purity

Radionuclidic Purity

The definition of radionuclidic purity is that proportion of total radioactivity in the form of the designated radionuclide. For example, Tc-99m sodium pertechnetate, according to the USP XX,[195] must not contain more than 0.15 μCi of Mo-99 per mCi of Tc-99m and not more than 2.5 μCi of Mo-99 per administered dose of the solution at the time of administration. Other gamma-emitting radionuclide impurities must not exceed 0.5 μCi per mCi Tc-99m or 2.5 μCi per administered dose at the time of administration.

A dramatic example of the importance of radionuclidic purity is cited by Hoppes, who has observed that when the activity of an I-125 sample is measured in a steel-walled ionization chamber, a 0.5% I-126 impurity can cause an error of 50%.[288] While this is an extreme case, it is not unique. For example, the greatest contribution of the radiation dose to the thyroid may come from its I-124 and I-126 impurities if the I-123 has decayed more than a few half-lives after production. Some common impurities are listed in Table 10–5.

TABLE 10–5. *Some Common Radionuclidic Impurities*

Radionuclide	Common impurities
F-18	H-3
Na-24	K-42
P-32	P-33
K-42	Na-24
Co-58	Co-60, Co-57
Fe-59	Fe-55
Tc-99m	Mo-99
In-113m	Sn-113
I-123	I-124, I-125, I-126
I-125	I-126
Hg-197	Hg-203
Au-198	Au-199

Radionuclidic purity may be determined by radiospectrometric analysis, half-life determinations, and absorbers to eliminate low-energy interference. Gamma scintillation spectrometry is best performed with a multichannel analyzer and a germanium detector that has been carefully calibrated with known radionuclidic standards.

Radionuclides with high-energy beta rays produce bremsstrahlung in the container; however, the energy spectrum is much too broad to identify the beta emitter. It is important to check all beta emitters with a gamma spectrometer for contamination by gamma emitters.

Radiochemical Purity

Radiochemical purity is that proportion of the total radioactivity in the specified chemical form. Radiochemical purity is usually expressed as a percentage and is determined by chemical and physical separation techniques and by counting the fractions associated with known standards of the compound. Customary methods of separation include solvent extraction; resin separation; column, paper, and gel chromatography; electrophoresis; and co-precipitation.

Radiochemical contaminants may arise from self-radiolysis, heat and light degradation, and the presence of interacting chemical species. Chemical reactions may occur in the solvents used because of irradiation of the solvent molecules. For example, one product of the irradiation of water is hydrogen peroxide, which readily oxidizes radioiodide to radioiodate, or selenomethionine to methionine selenone and methionine selenoxide. Oxidation is also enhanced by dissolved oxygen. In the case of kits for the preparation of Tc-99m compounds that depend upon the reduction of pertechnetate by stannous chloride, it is essential to purge oxygen from the solutions using nitrogen gas and to overlay the contents with nitrogen.

Chemical Purity

Chemical purity is that proportion of material in the specified chemical form regardless of any isotopic substitution. For example, in Tc-99m pertechnetate solutions prepared from reactor-produced Mo-99, the aluminum content should not exceed 20 µg per ml or 0.5 mg per 10 mCi Tc-99m.

For fission-produced Mo-99, the aluminum content should not be greater than 10 µg per ml.[196] Although the aluminum content poses no problem of toxicity, Tc-99m generator eluates containing as little as 5 µg/ml may cause agglutination when labeling erythrocytes.[289] Excess aluminum causes flocculation of some radiopharmaceuticals at alkaline pH and may cause variations in the particle size of preparations of Tc-99m sulfur colloid. Solvents, additives, preservatives, and buffers in a radiopharmaceutical are not considered impurities.

Chemical impurities may be produced during labeling. For example, rose bengal, which should contain at least 90% tetrachlorotetraiodofluorescein, may contain excessive amounts of trichloro- and dichloro-analogs, which upon radioiodination produce fractions having different clearance rates by the liver. Metallic impurities, upon neutron irradiation, may produce undesirable and unwanted radionuclides, e.g., Pt-198 that will produce

Au-199. Impurities may also affect the labeling process. In the production of radioiodinated albumin, for example, globulin impurities acquire a disproportionate amount of the radioiodine.

Purity Criteria

Tc-99m Sodium Pertechnetate

The limits and significance of aluminum and molybdenum breakthrough have already been described. Technetium-99m pertechnetate eluted from parent Mo-99 produced by uranium fission may contain other radionuclides. The limits permitted by the USP are:

I-131

    Not more than 0.05 μCi per mCi Tc-99m at time of administration

Ru-103

    Not more than 0.05 μCi per mCi

Sr-89

    0.0006 μCi per mCi

Sr-90

    0.00006 μCi per mCi

All other beta and gamma emitters

    0.1 μCi total per mCi

All alpha emitters

    0.001 nCi total per mCi

Molybdenum breakthrough can be detected by a color test using filter paper impregnated with zinc or cadmium xanthate. A red coloration or ring appears when the acid test solution is applied. The lower limit of identification is 0.01 μg molybdenum.[290]

Aluminum is detectable by a rapid technique based on a reaction on test paper impregnated with quinalizarin.[290] The test is sensitive to as little as 0.005 μg aluminum.

In-113m Generator Eluate and Compounds

Indium-113m generators contain a matrix of hydrous zirconium oxide or silica gel on which is adsorbed Sn-113 in the stannic form. The generated In-113m is eluted with 0.05 NHCl. For at least 10 days after its preparation, the generator is tested for leakage by washing at 24-hr intervals and checking the eluate spectrometrically for Sn-113 and other radioactive species, such as Sn-117m, Sb-125, and its daughter Te-125m. In addition, the quality control includes testing for zirconium, silica, and stable tin, all of which can be determined by analytic techniques.

Inasmuch as Sn-113 is not easily detected by gamma spectrometry, the eluate is allowed to decay for at least 48 hr, and then the sample is counted for the In-113m that will be in transient equilibrium with its parent Sn-113. Because of the short half-life of the In-113m (100 min), all of the In-113m eluted decays during the 48 hr, and whatever is then present must have come from Sn-113 leaked during elution. The Sn-113 should not exceed 0.2 μCi/mCi of In-113m. This procedure should be repeated for each new generator prior to clinical use. Most commercial generators yield less than 0.02% Sn-113, over a 6-mo period which is the maximum permissible concentration.

A control test for the breakthrough of tin is desirable because it detects breakdown and leakage of the parent carrier. The test is performed by adding 2 drops of a 0.1% solution of hematoxylin in slightly acidic alcohol to 2 drops of eluate in a spot plate. A pink-red to purplish color indicates approximately 0.1 ppm of tin. The test is considered sensitive to 30 μg tin/ml eluate.

Tin can be separated from In-113m by ascending chromatography on Whatman No. 3 MM paper using a solvent of ammonia: ethanol: water (0.1:50:125). The R_f of In-113m is zero and the R_f of Sn-113 is 0.6.

The zirconium breakthrough test is based on the development of a red coloration by the zirconium and alizarin sulfide (sodium alizarinesulfonate). This chemical is used in a spot test: 1 drop of eluate plus 1 drop of 0.05% alizarin S aqueous solution produces a yellow-purple color if the quantity of zirconium is greater than 0.7 μg. This reaction can be made quantitative by determining the color spectrophotometrically at 520 nm.

Indium-113m labeled radiopharmaceuticals include labeled colloidal iron hydroxide, DTPA, EDTA, gelatin, human transferrin complexes, iron hydroxide macroaggregates, and microspheres.[291] The radiochemical purity of these materials is based on the isolation, identification, and estimation of the unbound ionic In-113m. For example In-113m DTPA is tested by Sephadex gel filtration using 0.15 N NaCl followed by paper chromatography using ammonia: ethanol:

water (0.1:50:125). After ascending migration for 3 hr, the R_f of the complex is 0.88 and for ionic In-113m, zero.[292]

Sterility

The method of sterilizing a radiopharmaceutical depends on the character of the product itself, the solvent, any additives or buffers, the effect of heat on these constituents, and the container and stopper. Biologic indicators such as bacteria and fungi may be added to containers of control samples to test and monitor the efficacy of sterilization processes except when the method used is membrane filtration. The organisms and manner of use are described in further detail in the USP.[195] The sterilization process requires constant supervision of the equipment, application of procedures for obtaining and maintaining sterility, and adequate proof of the effectiveness of these procedures. Heat-labile radiopharmaceuticals require sterile filtration, while microaggregates and macroaggregates that cannot be heated or sterile-filtered, must be prepared and dispensed using rigid aseptic techniques.

Heat Sterilization

This method uses steam under pressure at 121°C for 15 min for thin-walled vessels whereas thick-walled vessels and large volumes require more time. Lower-temperature sterilization may be feasible for some compounds, e.g., sodium iodohippurate, which can be sterilized at 100°C for 60 min. Some radiopharmaceuticals that do not have growth supporting compositions can be sterilized at 100°C for 15 min.

Among the heat-labile preparations are (1) colloids, microaggregates and macroaggregates that may change particle size and composition; (2) such heat-sensitive molecules as rose bengal; and (3) such organic compounds and biochemicals as carbohydrates and proteins.

Membrane Filtration

Membrane filters are available in a variety of compositions and porosities. A pore size of 0.22 μm is recommended for removal of smaller organisms.

Occasionally, membrane filters may be defective because of a rupture or poor fit in their holders. The user of these filters must develop a sense of "feeling" for the pressure required to force through a solution of the viscosity of normal saline solution. Whenever too little pressure is required, the filter is suspect, and the solution should be refiltered. A more elaborate test procedure using known pressures has been reported.[293]

Sterility Testing

Procedures for sterility testing are described in the USP and other pharmacopeias. The number of containers of radiopharmaceuticals prepared in a small institution is usually limited, especially if prepared from kits. If a single preparation of one compound is made daily, aliquots can be composited aseptically, and an adequate single sample of the composite for the week (5 to 6 days) can be tested. Sufficient individual daily samples should be retained for a possible retest. It is convenient to collect samples for sterility testing in sterile multidose vials or in sterile rubber-capped evacuated tubes, dividing the samples later for testing with thioglycollate and soybean-casein digest media.

For bulk solution preparations, such as are used in making "kits," the prescribed numbers of individual containers should be tested.[195] Adequate samples also should be reserved for pyrogen testing of bulk solutions.

The usual sterility test can only be "after use" in the case of short-lived radiopharmaceuticals. In the case of long-lived or experimental radiopharmaceuticals, samples should be incubated for at least 10 days under the conditions specified by the USP. Some radiopharmaceuticals may be dispensed or distributed prior to completion of the sterility test, the latter being started the day of final preparation. The USP should be consulted in each particular case. The volume requirements to be tested are also waived. Complete records of sterility tests are necessary to assure compliance.

Automated methods have been developed for detecting bacterial contamination based on the production of $^{14}CO_2$ from C-14 labeled glucose.[294] This system is described in detail in Chapter 15.

Pyrogenicity

Pyrogens are the products of growth and metabolism of microorganisms, which when injected into man and animals, are believed to act on the temperature control center of the hypothalamus to cause a rise in body temperature. They are lipids or phospholipids, are attached to a polysaccharide or amino acid moiety, and are particulate, being less than 1 μm in size. Although many organisms produce pyrogens, those produced by gram-negative bacilli are the most potent.[295] Pyrogens are produced in solutions and on moist surfaces by the growth of organisms or are introduced by way of salts, or such growth-supporting chemicals as organic acids, buffers, and distilled water that is not freshly prepared. Containers, glassware, plastic tubing, and syringes not dried immediately after autoclaving can support development of pyrogens.

Pyrogenic contamination can be prevented by using the cleanest chemicals and keeping them dry and sterile-filtered as soon as possible after solution. Stable chemicals like sodium chloride can be made pyrogen-free by dry heat sterilization at 175°C for 3 hr. All water must be freshly distilled or come from freshly opened containers. The remaining portion should not be used for parenteral preparations. Glassware, glass syringes, and needles are rendered pyrogen-free by hot air sterilization at 175°C for 3 to 4 hr or at 250°C for not less than 30 min.

Manifestations of Pyrogenic Reactions in Humans. A latent period of 45 to 90 min occurs after intravenous injection. The initial reaction may be chills, a cool skin, dilated pupils, hypertension, and sometimes leukopenia. The most common symptoms are a slight fever and pain in the back and in the legs. The fever may reach a peak at 2 to 3 hr, and with this fever may come flushing and sweating, constricted pupils, hypotension, and leukocytosis. Symptoms resemble a mild protein shock. A pyrogenic material producing a febrile response in rabbits usually produces a response of chills and fever in man. Pyrogenic reactions in man are rarely fatal, but their presence in a radiopharmaceutical or parenteral is contraindicated physiologically and is indicative of poor manufacturing conditions, contamination, and inadequate quality control.

Pyrogen Testing. Current testing measures the febrile response in rabbits following injection of a suitable test dose of the pharmaceutical, after 1, 2, and 3 hr. The details are presented in the USP.[195] The USP procedure stipulates a dose related to the volume injected into a patient but not greater than 10 ml per body weight of the rabbit; however, this dose level refers to the usual parenterals and is not feasible for radiopharmaceuticals, which are administered in much smaller doses, usually 1 ml or less. A more rational dose would be the equivalent of the human dose based on relative body weights or on some multiple of the relative dose. In some instances, aliquots of several successive generator eluates may be combined and diluted if necessary. Because three rabbits are injected initially and the possibility of a repeat test exists, dilution of the original liquid may be necessary to provide sufficient volume of the parenteral. Rabbits used to test products containing gelatin or other proteins should not be used again for pyrogen testing because previous injections may cause an anaphylactic reaction with pyrexia, leading to a false-positive result. The rabbit test is important because it is an effective screening test and because it indicates a failure of adequate sterilization and compliance with aseptic technique.

It has, however, several important undesirable features: the time required, especially if a retest is necessary; the volume of test material needed; the exposure of the personnel to radiation; the tendency of rabbits to become febrile from fright or struggling; and the need for expensive animal housing. These factors indicate the need for a reliable, rapid test that can be used "in house" by adequately trained personnel. Such a test, the Limulus test, is now widely used.

Limulus Amebocyte Lysate (LAL) Test for Endotoxins and Pyrogens. The principle of this test is the formation of a firm gel in a solution of the lysate of amebocytes from the blood of Limulus polyphemus, the horseshoe crab, by reaction with very small quantities of bacterial or fungal endotoxins and pyrogenic substances.[296] The rate of gel formation depends on the concentration of pyrogenic substances under proper conditions of pH and temperature. The exact mechanism of the reaction is not understood. The major limitation is that the test will not respond to such nonendotoxin pyrogens as particulate contamination or to certain chemicals.

The LAL reagent must produce a positive reaction with 0.1 ng of the reference endotoxin and give a negative reaction with 0.0125 ng of the reference endotoxin.

The time required for the test is short; gel formation occurs within 25 min after mixing and incubating 0.1 to 0.2 ml of the sample being tested. The Limulus test is at least five times more sensitive to purified endotoxin than is the rabbit pyrogen test. If the product is injected into man at 0.1 ml/kg and into the rabbit at 1 ml/kg, the safety factor of the LAL compared with rabbit testing is 50 because man and rabbit

are equally sensitive to threshold levels of pyrogen on a dose-per-weight basis. This increased safety becomes more important when screening intrathecal drugs for pyrogen because endotoxin is at least 1000 times more potent in producing toxic reactions by this route of administration.[297]

REFERENCES

1. Dillman, L.T.: Radionuclide decay schemes and nuclear parameters for use in radiation dose estimation. J. Nucl. Med., Suppl. 2, *10*:1, 1969.
2. Boyd, R.E.: Technetium-99m generators: The available options. *In* Technetium-99 Generators, Chemistry, and Preparation of Radiopharmaceuticals. Edited by W.C. Eckelman and B.M. Coursey. Int. J. Appl. Radiat. Isot., *33*:801, 1982.
3. Lamson, M., Hotte, C.F., and Ice, R.D.: Practical generator kinetics. J. Nucl. Med. Tech., *4*:21, 1975.
4. Prince, J.R.: Comments on equilibrium, transient equilibrium, and secular equilibrium in serial radioactive decay. J. Nucl. Med., *20*:162, 1979.
5. Deutsch, E., Heineman, W.R., Zodda, J.P., et al.: Preparation of "no-carrier-added" technetium-99m complexes: Determination of the total technetium content of generator eluents. *In* Technetium-99m Generators, Chemistry, and Preparation of Radiopharmaceuticals. Edited by W.C. Eckelman and B.M. Coursey. Int. J. Appl. Radiat. Isot., *33*:843, 1982.
6. Steigman, J.: Chemistry of the alumina column. *In* Technetium-99m Generators, Chemistry, and Preparation of Radiopharmaceuticals. Edited by W.C. Eckelman and B.M. Coursey. Int. J. Appl. Radiat. Isot., *33*:829, 1982.
7. Richards, P., Tucker, W.D., and Srivastava, S.C.: An historical perspective. *In* Technetium-99m Generators, Chemistry, and Preparation of Radiopharmaceuticals. Edited by W.C. Eckelman and B.M. Coursey. Int. J. Appl. Radiat. Isot., *33*:793, 1982.
8. Eckelman, W.C., and Richards, P.: Instant 99mTc-DTPA. J. Nucl. Med., *11*:761, 1970.
9. Richards, P., and Steigman, J.: Chemistry of technetium as applied to radiopharmaceuticals. *In* Radiopharmaceuticals. Edited by G. Subramanian, B.A. Rhodes, J.F. Cooper, and V.J. Sodd. New York, Society of Nuclear Medicine, 1975, p. 23.
10. Harper, P.V., Lathrop, K., and Gottschalk, A.: Pharmacodynamics of some technetium-99m preparations. *In* Radioactive Pharmaceuticals. U.S. Atomic Energy Commission, 1964, p. 335.
11. Davis, J.A.: A study of the behavior of the tin (II) ion in pyrophosphate solution. Thesis, Indiana University, 1955.
12. Mesmer, R.E., and Irani, R.R.: Metal complexing by phosphorus compounds VIII complexing of tin (II) by polyphosphates. J. Inorg. Nucl. Chem., *28*:493, 1966.

13. Smith, D.: The chelates formed by tin (II) with certain amino polycarboxylic acids. J. Chem. Soc., 2:2554, 1961.

14. Elbourne, R.G.P., and Buchanan, G.S.: A potentiometric study of complexes of tin (II) with some carboxylic acids. J. Inorg. Nucl. Chem., 32:3559, 1970.

15. Martell, A.E.: *In* Stability Constants. Special Publication No. 17. The Chemical Society, Burlington House, London WIV OBN, 1964.

16. Martell, A.E.: *In* Stability Constants. Special Publication No. 25, Suppl. No. 1 to Special Publiction No. 17. The Chemical Society, Burlington House, London WIV OBN, 1971.

17. Lin, M.S. and Winchell, H.S.: A "kit" method for the preparation of a technetium-tin(II) colloid and a study of its properties. J. Nucl. Med., 13:58, 1972.

18. Cotton, F.A., and Wilkinson, G.: Advanced Inorganic Chemistry. 3rd ed. New York, Interscience, 1976.

19. Johannson, B., and Spies, H.: Chemie und radiopharmakologie von technetium komplexen. Akademie der Wissenschaften der DDR. Dresden, DDR, 1981.

20. Steigman, J., Meinken, G., and Richards, P.: The reduction of pertechnetate-99 by stannous chloride. I. The stoichiometry of the reaction in HCl, in a citrate buffer and in a DTPA buffer. Int. J. Appl. Radiat. Isot., 26:601, 1975.

21. Eckelman, W.C., Meinken, G., and Richards, P.: The chemical state of ^{99m}Tc in biomedical products. II. The chelation of reduced technetium with DTPA. J. Nucl. Med., 13:577, 1972.

22. Hambright, P., McRae, J., Valk, P.E., et al.: Chemistry of technetium radiopharmaceuticals. I. Exploration of the tissue distribution and oxidation state consequences of technetium (IV) in Tc-Sn-gluconate and Tc-Sn-HEDP using carrier ^{99}Tc. J. Nucl. Med., 16:478, 1975.

23. Steigman, J.: Scintiphotos in rabbits made with Tc-99m preparations reduced by electrolysis and by $SnCl_2$: concise communication. J. Nucl. Med., 20:766, 1979.

24. Loberg, M.D.: Abstracts of the Eighth Northeast Regional Meeting of the American Chemical Society. Boston, MA. June 25, 1978.

25. Gerlit, J.B.: Some chemical properties of technetium. *In* Proc. Intern. Conf. Peaceful Uses of Atomic Energy. Geneva, 1965. 1:145, 1965.

26. Busey, R.M.: Chemistry of technetium in hydrochloric acid solution. U.S. Atomic Energy Commission, Document ORNL-2782:13, 1959.

27. Ossicini, L., Saracino, F., and Lederer, M.: The solution, chemistry and chromatographic behavior of technetium in aqueous HCl and HBr. J. Chromatogr., 16:524, 1964.

28. Williams, M.J., and Deegan, T.: The process involved in the binding of technetium-99m to human serum albumin. Int. J. Appl. Radiat. Isot., 22:767, 1971.

29. Cifka, J.: Lower-oxidation-state technetium-99m in the generator product: Its determination and occurence. *In* Technetium-99m Generators, Chemistry, and Preparation of Radiopharma-

ceuticals. Edited by W.C. Eckelman and B.M. Coursey. Int. J. Appl. Radiat. Isot., 33:849, 1982.

30. De Liverant, J., and Wolf, W.: Studies on the reduction of ^{99m} Tc-TcO$_4^-$ by hydrochloric acid. *In* Technetium-99m Generators, Chemistry, and Preparation of Radiopharmaceuticals. Edited by W.C. Eckelman and B.M. Coursey. Int. J. Appl. Radiat. Isot., 33:857, 1982.

31. Eckelman, W.C., Meinken, G., Richards, P., et al.: Methods for ^{99m}Tc localization in bone. Brookhaven National Laboratory Report, 1972.

32. Thomas, R.W., Davison, A., Trap, H.S., and Deutsch, E.: Technetium radiopharmaceuticals development. II. Preparation, characterization and synthetic utility of the oxotetrahalotechnetate (V) species. Inorg. Chem., 19:2840, 1980.

33. Benjamin, P., Rejali, A., and Friedell, H.: Electrolytic complexation of ^{99m}Tc at constant current: its application in nuclear medicine. J. Nucl. Med., 11:147, 1970.

34. Harwig, S.S.L., Harwig, J.F., Coleman, R.E., et al.: In vivo behavior of ^{99m}Tc-fibrinogen and its potential as a thrombus-imaging agent. J. Nucl. Med., 17:40, 1976.

35. Miller, H.H., Kelley, M.T., and Thomason, P.E.: Polarographic studies of the reduction of pertechnetate ion in aqueous solutions. Adv. Polarog., 1:716, 1960.

36. Terry, A.A., and Zittel, H.E.: Determination of technetium by controlled-potential coulometric titration in buffered sodium tripolyphosphate medium. Anal. Chem., 35:614, 1963.

37. Davison, A., and Jones, A.G.: Chemistry of technetium-V. *In* Technetium-99m Generators, Chemistry, and Preparation of Radiopharmaceuticals. Edited by W.C. Eckelman and B.M. Coursey. Int. J. Appl. Radiat. Isot., 33:875, 1982.

38. Klingensmith, W.C., Gerhold, J.P., Fritzberg, A.R., et al.: Clinical comparison of Tc-99m N,N'-Bis(mercaptoacetamido)ethylenediamine and ^{131}I ortho-iodohippurate for evalution of renal tubular function: Concise communication. J. Nucl. Med., 23:377, 1982.

39. Gorski, B., and Koch, H.: Zur chemie des technetium in wasseriger Iosung-I. J. Inorg. Nucl. Chem., 31:3465, 1969.

40. Guennec, J.Y., and Guilloumont, R.: Behavior of technetium (IV) in a noncomplexing medium at tracer concentrations. Radiochem. Radioanal. Letters, 13:33, 1973.

41. Sundrehagen, E.: Polymer formation and hydrolysation of Tc(IV). Int. J. Appl. Radiat. Isot., 30:739, 1979.

42. Gorski, B., and Koch, H.: Technetium complex formation with chelate forming ligands. II. J. Inorg. Nucl. Chem., 32:3831, 1970.

43. Levin, V.I., Gracheva, M.A., and Ilyushchenko, O.N.: The stability constant of ^{99}Tc-DTPA complexes. Int. J. Appl. Radiat. Isot., 31:382, 1980.

44. McRae, J., Hambright, P., Valk, P., and Bearden, A.J.: Chemistry of Tc tracers. II. In vitro conversion of tagged HEDP and pyrophosphate (bone-seekers) into gluconate (renal agent). Effects of Ca and Fe(II) on in vivo substitution. J. Nucl. Med., 17:208, 1976.

45. Taube, H.: Rates and mechanisms of substitution in inorganic complexes. Chem. Rev., *50*:69, 1952.

46. Loberg, M.D., and Fields, A.T.: Stability of ^{99m}Tc labeled N-substituted iminodiacetic acids: ligand exchange reaction between ^{99m}Tc-HIDA and EDTA. J. Label. Comp. Radiopharm., *13*:163, 1977.

47. Al-Kayssi, M., Magee, R., and Wilson, C.L.: Spectrophotometric studies on technetium and rhenium. Talanta, *9*:125, 1962.

48. Salaria, G.B.S., Rulfs, C.L., and Elving, P.J.: Spectrophotometric studies of lower oxidation states of technetium. Talanta, *10*:1159, 1963.

49. Crouthamel, C.E.: Thiocyanate spectrophotometric determination of technetium. Anal. Chem., *29*:1756, 1957.

50. Howard, O.H., and Weber, C.W.: Rapid spectrophotometric determination of technetium in uranium materials. Anal. Chem., *34*:530, 1962.

51. Schwochau, K., and Herr, W.: Darstellung und eigenschaften von cyanotechnetat (IV). A. Anorg. Allg. Chem., *318*:198, 1962.

52. Schwochau, K.: Thiocyanato-komplex des 4- und 5 wertigen technetiums. Inorg. Nucl. Chem. Letters, *4*:711, 1968.

53. Trop, H.S., Davison, A., Jones, A.G., et al.: Synthesis and physical properties of hexakis (isothiocyanoto) technetate (III) and (IV) complexes: Structure of the Tc(NCS) ion. Inorg. Chem., *19*:1105, 1980.

54. Trop, H.S., Jones, A.G., and Davison, A.: Technetium cyanide chemistry: Synthesis and characterization of technetium (III) and (V) cyanide complexes. Inorg. Chem., *19*:1993, 1980.

55. Rulfs, C.L.: Recent developments in the analytical chemistry of rhenium and technetium. CRC Crit. Rev. Anal. Chem., *1*:335, 1970.

56. Rajec, P., and Mikulaj, V.: Preparation of dioxo-(8-hydroxyquinolate) technetium (V). Chelate by extraction method. Radiochem. Radioanal. Letters, *17*:375, 1974.

57. Armstrong, R.A., and Taube, H.: Chemistry of trans-aquonitrosyl-tetraamine technetium (I) and related studies. Inorg. Chem., *15*:1904, 1976.

58. Jones, A.G., and Davison, A.: Chemistry of technetium I, II, III, and IV. *In* Technetium-99m Generators, Chemistry, and Preparation of Radiopharmaceuticals. Edited by W.C. Eckelman and B.M. Coursey. Int. J. Appl. Rad. Isot., *33*:867, 1982.

59. Troutner, D.E., Simon, J. Ketring, A.R., et al.: Complexing of Tc-99m with cyclam: concise communication. J. Nucl. Med., *21*:443, 1980.

60. Steigman, J., and Eckelman, W.C.: Tc Chemistry as Applied to Medicine. National Research Council, Technical Information Center, U.S. Dept. of Energy, Washington, D.C., in press.

61. Karger, B.L., Snyder, L.R., and Horvath, C.: An Introduction to Separation Science. New York, John Wiley & Sons, 1973.

62. Zweig, G., and Sherma, J. (Eds.): Handbook of Chromatography. Vols. 1 and 2. Cleveland, CRC Press, 1972.

63. Lin, M.S., Kruse, S.L., Goodwin, D.A., et al.: Albumin loading effect: a pitfall in saline paper analysis of ^{99m}Tc-albumin. J. Nucl. Med., *15*:1018, 1974.

64. Yalow, R.S., and Berson, S.A.: Immunoassay of plasma insulin. *In* Methods of Biochemical Analysis. Vol. 12. Edited by D. Glick. New York, Interscience, 1964.

65. Valk, P.E., Dilts, C.A., and McRae, J.: A possible artifact in gel chromatography of some ^{99m}Tc-chelates. J. Nucl. Med., *14*:235, 1973.

66. Billinghurst, M.W., and Palser, R.E.: Gel chromatography as an analytical tool for ^{99m}Tc radiopharmaceuticals. J. Nucl. Med., *15*:722, 1974.

67. Schneider, P.B.: A simple "electrolytic" preparation of a ^{99m}Tc (Sn) citrate renal scanning agent. J. Nucl. Med., *14*:843, 1973.

68. Steigman, J., and Williams, H.P.: Letter: Gel chromatography in the analysis of ^{99m}Tc-radiopharmaceuticals. J. Nucl. Med., *15*:318, 1974.

69. Eckelman, W.C., Reba, R.C., Kubota, H., and Stevenson, J.S.: ^{99m}Tc-pyrophosphate for bone imaging. J. Nucl. Med., *15*:279, 1974.

70. Shukla, S.K.: Ion exchange paper chromatography of Tc (IV), Tc (V), and Tc (VII) in hydrochloric acid. J. Chromatogr., *21*:92, 1966.

71. Cifka, J., and Vesely, P.: Some factors influencing the elution of technetium-99m generators. Radiochimica Acta, *16*:30, 1971.

72. Müller, T., and Steinnes, E.: On the purity of eluates from Tc generators. Scand. J. Clin. Lab. Invest., *28*:213, 1971.

73. Mitta, A.E.A., Alvarez, J., and Rabin, P.: Determination of free ^{99m}Tc in labeled compounds by means of thin layer chromatography. Int. J. Appl. Radiat. Isot., *22*:223, 1971.

74. Billinghurst, M.W.: Chromatographic quality control of ^{99m}Tc labeled compounds. J. Nucl. Med., *14*:793, 1973.

75. Domek, N.S., and Loken, M.K.: Rapid quality control test for ^{99m}Tc-DTPA. Radiology, *113*:393, 1974.

76. Colombetti, L.G., Pinsky, S., and Moerlien, S.: A rapid column-chromatographic determination of unreacted pertechnetate ^{99m}Tc in labeled radiopharmaceuticals. Radiochem. Radioanalyt. Letters, *20*:77, 1975.

77. Vigne, J.P.: Synthése de composés marques au technetium-99^m utilisables comme traceurs en gammagraphie. *In* Radiopharmaceuticals and Labeled Compounds. Vol. 1, Vienna, IAEA, 1973, p. 73.

78. Wong, S.H., Hosain, P., Zeichner, S.J., et al.: Qualiity control studies of ^{99m}Tc-labeled radiopharmaceuticals by high performance liquid chromatography. Int. J. Appl. Radiat. Isot., *32*:185, 1981.

79. Persson, R.B.R., and Strand, S.E.: Labeling processes and short term biodynamic behavior of different types of ^{99m}Tc labeled compounds. *In* Radiopharmaceuticals and Labelled Compounds. Vol. 1. Vienna, IAEA, 1973, p. 169.

80. Russell, C.D., and Majerik, J.: Determination of

pertechnetate in radiopharmaceuticals by high-pressure liquid, thin layer and paper chromatography. Int. J. Appl. Radiat. Isot., 29:109, 1978.

81. Loberg, M.D., and Fields, A.T.: Chemical structures of technetium-99m labeled N-(2,6-dimethylphenylcarbamoylmethyl)-iminodiacetic acid (Tc-HIDA). Int. J. Appl. Radiat. Isot., 29:167, 1978.

82. Castronovo, C.F., Jr., and Callahan, R.J.: A new bone scanning agent: Tc labeled 1-hydroxyethylidene-1, 1-disodium phosphonate. J. Nucl. Med., 13:823, 1972.

83. Pinkerton, T.C., Heineman, W.R., and Deutsch, E.: Separation of technetium diphosphonate complexes by anion exchange high performance liquid chromatography. Anal. Chem., 52:1106, 1980.

84. Tubis, M., Krishnamurthy, G.T., Endow, J.S., and Blahd, W.H.: Tc-penicillamine, a new cholescintigraphic agent. J. Nucl. Med., 13:652, 1972.

85. Domek, N.S., Custer, J.R., and Loken, M.K.: 99mTc-penicillamine: preparation using electrolytic methods and rapid analysis of products. Private communication.

86. Loberg, M.D., Cooper, M., Harvey, E., et al.: Development of new radiopharmaceuticals based on N-substitution of iminodiacetic acid. J. Nucl. Med., 17:633, 1976.

87. Bowen, B.M., and Garnett, E.S.: Analysis of the relationship between Tc-Sn-Polyphosphate and 99mTc-Sn-Pyrophosphate. J. Nucl. Med., 15:652, 1974.

88. Richards, P., and Atkins, H.L.: 99mTc technetium labeled compounds. In Proc. 7th Annual Meeting of the Japanese Society of Nuclear Medicine. Tokyo Radioisotope Association, 1968, p. 165.

89. Stern, H.S., McAfee, J.G., and Zolle, I.: Technetium-99m-albumin. In Radioactive Pharmaceuticals. Edited by G.A. Andrews, R.M. Kniseley, and H.N. Wagner, Jr. U.S. Atomic Energy Commission Conf. 651111, 1966.

90. Persson, R.B.R., and Liden, K.: 99mTc-labeled human serum albumin: a study of the labeling procedure. Int. J. Appl. Radiat. Isot., 20:241, 1969.

91. Fields, A.T., Porter, D.W., Callery, P.S., et al.: Synthesis and radiolabeling of technetium radiopharmaceuticals based on N-substituted iminodiacetic acid. J. Label. Compd. Radiopharm., 15:387, 1978.

92. Fritzberg, A.R., and Lewis, D.: HPLC analysis of Tc-99m iminodiacetate hepatobiliary agents and a question of multiple peaks: Concise communication. J. Nucl. Med., 21:1180, 1980.

93. Srivastava, S.C., Bandyopadhyay, D., Meinken, G., and Richards, P.: Characterization of Tc-99m bone agents (MDP, EHDP) by reverse phase and ion exchange high performance liquid chromatography. J. Nucl. Med., 22:P69, 1981.

94. Eckelman, W.C., and Richards, P.: Analytical pitfalls with 99mTc-labeled compounds. J. Nucl. Med., 13:202, 1972.

95. Chervu, L.R., Novich, I., and Blaufox, M.D.: Fluorotec: a new bone seeker. Radiology, 107:435, 1973.

96. La Mer, V.K., and Dinegar, R.H.: Theory, production and mechanism of formation of monodispersed hydrosols. J. Am. Chem., Soc., 72:4848, 1950.

97. Zaiser, E.M., and La Mer, V.K.: The kinetics of the formation and growth of monodispersed sulfur hydrosols. J. Am. Chem. Soc., 1948, p. 571.

98. Arnold, R.W., et al.: Comparison of 99mTc complexes for renal imaging. J. Nucl. Med., 16:357, 1975.

99. Fleay, R.F.: 99mTc-labeled EDTA for renal scanning. Aust. Radiol., 12:265, 1968.

100. Hauser, W., Atkins, H.L., Nelson, K.G., et al.: Technetium-99m DTPA: a new radiopharmaceutical for brain and kidney scanning. Radiology, 94:679, 1970.

101. Subramanian, G., and McAfee, J.G.: A new complex of 99mTc for skeletal imaging. Radiology, 99:192, 1971.

102. Lebowitz, E., Atkins, H.L., Hauser, W., et al.: 99mTc-gelatin: a "compound" with high renal specificity. Int. J. Appl. Radiat. Isot., 27:786, 1971.

103. Halpern, S.E., Tubis, M., Endow, S.J., et al.: TcPAC, a new renal scanning agent. J. Nucl. Med., 13:45, 1972.

104. Halpern, S.E., Tubis, M., Golden, M., et al.: 99mTcPAC, a new renal scanning agent. II. Evaluation in humans. J. Nucl. Med., 13:723, 1972.

105. Winchell, H.S., Lin, M., Shipley, B., et al.: Localization of polypeptide caseidin in the renal cortex: a new radioisotope carrier for renal studies. J. Nucl. Med., 12:678, 1971.

106. Kountz, S.L., Yeh, S.H., Wood, J., et al.: Technetium-99m(V)-citrate complex for estimation of glomerular filtration rate. Nature, 215:1397, 1967.

107. Fliegel, C.P., Dewanjee, M.K., and Holman, L.B.: 99mTc tetracycline as a kidney and gallbladder imaging agent. Radiology, 110:407, 1974.

108. Lin, T.H., Khentigan, A., and Winchell, H.S.: A 99mTc-chelate substitute for organoradiomercurial renal agents. J. Nucl. Med., 15:34, 1974.

109. Charamza, O., and Budikova, M.: Herstellungsmethode eines 99mTc-zinn-komplexes für die nierenszintigraphie. Nucl. Med., 8:301, 1969.

110. Lichte, H., and Hor, G.: Nierenszintigraphie mit Tc-99m penicillamine. Fortschr. Geb. Rontgenstr. Nuklearmed., 122:119, 1975.

111. Ikeda, I., Inoue, O., Uchida, J., et al.: New renal scanning agents of Tc-99m compounds. World Congress Nucl. Med. Tokyo, 1974.

112. Subramanian, G., Singh, M.V., Chander, J., and Singh, B.: Tc-99m-Sn-acetylcysteine: a new renal scanning agent. Eur. J. Nucl. Med., 1:243, 1976.

113. Johannson, B., Syhre, P., and Spies, H.: Analytische untersuchungen zer markierung von cystein und glutathion mit technetium-99m.

Jahresbericht des Zentralinstitutes fur Kernforschung Rossendorf, Zfk-*312*:53, 1976.

114. Oginski, M., and Rembelska, M.: Tc-99m-unithiol complex, a new pharmaceutical for kidney scintigraphy. Nucl. Med., *15*:282, 1976.

115. Davison, A., Sohn, M., Orvig, C., et al.: A tetradentate ligand designed specifically to coordinate technetium. J. Nucl. Med., *20*:641, 1979.

116. Yokoyama, A., Saji, H., Tanaka, H. et al.: Preparation of chemically characterized ^{99m}Tc-penicillamine complex. J. Nucl. Med., *17*:810, 1976.

117. Yokoyama, A., Terauchi, Y., Horiuchi, K., et al.: Technetium - 99m - kethoxalbis(thiosemicarbazone), an uncharged complex with a tetravalent ^{99m}Tc state and its excretion into the bile. J. Nucl. Med., *17*:816, 1976.

118. Baker, R.J., Bellen, J.C., and Ronai, P.M.: Technetium 99m-pyridoxylideneglutamate: a new hepatobiliary radiopharmaceutical. J. Nucl. Med., *16*:720, 1975.

119. Dugal, P., Eikman, E.A., Natarajan, T.K., and Wagner, H.W., Jr.: A quantitative test for gallbladder function. J. Nucl. Med., *13*:428, 1972.

120. Lin, T.H., Khentigan, A., and Winchell, H.S.: A ^{99m}Tc-labelled replacement for ^{131}I-rose bengal in liver and biliary tract studies. J. Nucl. Med., *15*:613, 1974.

121. Hunt, F.C., Maddalena, D.J., and Yeates, M.G.: Technetium-99m-6 mercaptopurine, a new radiopharmaceutical for cholescintigraphy. *In* Recent Advances in Nuclear Medicine. Tokyo, First World Congress of Nuclear Medicine, 1974.

122. Callery, P.S., Faith, B., Loberg, M.D., et al.: Tissue distribution of technetium-99m and carbon-14 labeled N-(2,6-dimethylphenylcarbamylmethyl) imino-diacetic acid. J. Med. Chem., *19*:962, 1976.

123. Burns, H.D., Sowa, D.T., and Marzilli, L.G.: Improved synthesis of N(2,6-dimethylphenylcarbamoylmethyl)iminodiacetic acid and analogs. J. Pharm. Sci., *67*:1434, 1978.

124. Wistow, B.W., Subramanian, G., Van Heertum, R.L., et al.: An evaluation of ^{99m}Tc-labeled hepatobiliary agents. J. Nucl. Med., *18*:455, 1977.

125. Burns, H.D., Worley, P., Wagner, H.N., Jr., et al.: Design of technetium radiopharmaceuticals. *In* Chemistry of Radiopharmaceuticals. Edited by N. Heindel. New York, Masson, 1978.

126. Van Wyke, A.J., Fourie, P.J., Van Zyl, W.H., et al.: Synthesis of five new ^{99m}Tc-HIDA isomers and comparison with ^{99m}Tc-HIDA. Eur. J. Nucl. Med., *4*:445, 1979.

127. Molter, M., and Kloss, G.: Studies of the pharmacokinetics of various Tc-99m-IDA derivatives. Third Int. Sym. Radiopharm., Abstract *19*:9, 1980.

128. Hunt, F.C., Wilson, J.G., and Maddalena, D.J.: Structure-Activity Relationships for Technetium-99m-Benzimidazolyl Methylimino-Diacetic Acid Hepatobiliary Radiopharmaceutical. Third Int. Symp. Radiopharm., Abstract *19*:7, 1980.

129. Nunn, A.D.: Preliminary structure-distribution relationships of ^{99m}Tc hepatobiliary agents. I. Protein binding of HIDA's. Third Int. Symp. Radiopharm., Abstract *18*:12, 1980.

130. Nunn, A.D., and Loberg, M.D.: Hepatobiliary agents. *In* Radiopharmaceuticals: Structure-Activity Relationships. Edited by R.P. Spencer. New York, Grune & Stratton, 1981, p. 539.

131. Subramanian, G., McAfee, J.G., Bell, E.G., et al.: ^{99m}Tc-labeled polyphosphate as a skeletal imaging agent. Radiology, *102*:701, 1972.

132. Perez, R., Kohen, Y., Henry, R., et al.: A new radiopharmaceutical for ^{99m}Tc bone scanning. J. Nucl. Med., *13*:788, 1972.

133. Yano, Y., McRae, J., Van Dyke, D.C., et al.: Technetium-99m-labeled stannous ethane-1-hydroxy-1-diphosphonate: a new bone scanning agent. J. Nucl. Med., *14*:73, 1973.

134. Subramanian, G., McAfee, J.G., Blair, R.J., et al.: Technetium-99m methylene diphosphonate— a superior agent for skeletal imaging: Comparison with other technetium complexes. J. Nucl. Med., *16*:744, 1975.

135. Bevan, J.A., Tofe, A.J., and Benedict, J.J.: Tc-99m HMDP (Hydroxymethylene diphosphonate): A radiopharmaceutical for skeletal and acute myocardial infarct imaging. II. Comparison of Tc-99m hydroxymethylene diphosphonate (HMDP) with other technetium-labeled bone-imaging agents in a canine model. J. Nucl. Med., *21*:967, 1980.

136. Bevan, J.A., Tofe, A.J., and Benedict, J.J.: Tc-99m HMDP (Hydroxymethylene diphosphonate): A radiopharmaceutical for skeletal and acute myocardial infarct imaging. I. Synthesis and distribution in animals. J. Nucl. Med., *21*:961, 1980.

137. Subramanian, G., McAfee, J.G., Blair, R.J., et al.: Technetium-99m-labeled stannous imidodiphosphate, a new radiodiagnostic agent for bone scanning: comparison with other ^{99m}Tc complexes. J. Nucl. Med., *16*:1137, 1975.

138. Jones, A.G., Francis, M.D., and Davis, M.A.: Bone scanning: radionuclide reaction mechanisms. Semin. Nucl. Med., *6*:3, 1976.

139. Davis, M.A., and Jones, A.L.: Comparison of ^{99m}Tc labeled phosphate and phosphonate agents for skeletal imaging. Semin. Nucl. Med., *6*:19, 1976.

140. Kubota, H., Eckelman, W.C., Poulose, K.P., and Reba, R.C.: Technetium-99m-pyridoxylideneglutamate: a new agent for gallbladder imaging. Comparison with ^{131}I-rose bengal. J. Nucl. Med., *17*:36, 1976.

141. Kato, M., and Hazue, M.: Tc-99m(Sn)pyridoxylideneaminates: preparation and biologic evaluation. J. Nucl. Med., *19*:397, 1978.

142. King, A.G., Christy, B., Hupf, H.B., et al.: Polyphosphates: a chemical analysis of average chain length and the relationship to bone deposition in rats. J. Nucl. Med., *14*:695, 1973.

143. Atkins, H.L., Cardinale, K.G., Eckelman, W.L., et al.: Evaluation of ^{99m}Tc-DTPA prepared by three different methods. Radiology, *98*:674, 1971.

144. Fritzberg, A.R., Klingensmith, W.C., Whitney,

W.P., et al.: Chemical and biological studies of Tc-99m N,N'-Bis(mercaptoacetamido)-ethylenediamine: A potential replacement for I-131 iodohippurate. J. Nucl. Med., 22:258, 1981.

145. McAfee, J.G., Subramanian, G., Aburano, T., et al.: A new formulation of Tc-99m minimicroaggregated albumin for marrow imaging: Comparison with other colloids, In-111 and Fe-59. J. Nucl. Med., 23:21, 1982.

146. Ikeda, I., Inoue, O., and Kurata, K.: Chemical and biological studies on ^{99m}Tc-DMS-II: Effect of Sn(II) on the formation of various Tc-DMS complexes. Int. J. Appl. Radiat. Isot., 27:681, 1976.

147. Ikeda, I., Inoue, O., and Kurata, K.: Preparation of various Tc-99m dimercaptosuccinate complexes and their evaluation as radiotracers. J. Nucl. Med., 18:1222, 1977.

148. Fritzberg, A.R., Lyster, D.M., and Dolphin, D.H.: Tc-glutathione: role of reducing agent on renal retention. Int. J. Nucl. Med. Biol., 5:87, 1978.

149. Steigman, J., Meinken, G., and Richards, P.: The reduction of pertechnetate-99 by stannous chloride. II. The stoichiometry of the reaction in aqueous solutions of several phosphorus (V) compounds. Int. J. Appl. Radiat. Isot., 29:653, 1978.

150. Krishnamurthy, G.T., Tubis, M., Endow, J.S., et al.: Clinical comparison of the kinetics of ^{99m}Tc-labeled polyphosphate and diphosphonate. J. Nucl. Med., 15:848, 1974.

151. Krishnamurthy, G.T., et al.: Comparison of ^{99m}Tc-polyphosphate and 18-F. I. Kinetics. J. Nucl. Med., 15:832, 1974.

152. Krishnamurthy, G.T., Hoebotter, R.L., and Walsh, C.E.: Kinetics of Tc-labeled pyrophosphate and polyphosphate in man. J. Nucl. Med., 16:109, 1975.

153. Schümichen, C., Koch, K., Kraus, A., et al.: Binding of technetium-99m to plasma proteins: Influence on the distribution of Tc-99m phosphate agents. J. Nucl. Med., 21:1080, 1980.

154. Buja, L.M., Tofe, A.J., Kulkarni, P.V., et al.: Sites and mechanisms of localization of technetium-99m phosphorus radiopharmaceuticals in acute myocardial infarcts and other tissues. J. Clin. Invest., 60:724, 1977.

155. Rosenthall, L., and Kaye, M.: Technetium-99m-pyrophosphate kinetics and imaging in metabolic bone disease. J. Nucl. Med., 16:33, 1975.

156. Kaye, M., Silverton, S., and Rosenthall, L.: Technetium-99m-pyrophosphates. Studies in vivo and in vitro. J. Nucl. Med., 16:40, 1975.

157. Schmitt, G.H., Holmes, R.A., and Isitman, A.T.: A proposed mechanism for ^{99m}Tc-labeled polyphosphate and diphosphonate uptake by human breast tissue. Radiology, 112:733, 1974.

158. Zimmer, A.M., Isitman, A.T., and Holmes, R.A.: Enzymatic inhibition of diphosphonate: A proposed mechanism of tissue uptake. J. Nucl. Med., 16:352, 1975.

159. Dewanjee, M.K., and Kahn, P.C.: Mechanism of localization of ^{99m}Tc-labeled pyrophosphate and tetracycline in infarcted myocardium. J. Nucl. Med., 17:639, 1976.

160. Francis, M.D., Ferguson, D.L., Tofe, A.J., et al.: Comparative evaluation of three diphosphonates: in vitro absorption (C-14 labeled) and in vivo osteogenic uptake (Tc-99m complexed). J. Nucl. Med., 21:1185, 1980.

161. Christensen, S.B., and Krogsgaard, O.W.: Localization of Tc-99m MDP in epiphyseal growth plates of rats. J. Nucl. Med., 22:237, 1981.

162. Van Langevelde, A., Driessen, O.M.J. Pauwels, E.K.J., et al.: Aspects of ^{99m}technetium binding from an ethane-1-hydroxy-1,1-diphosphonate-^{99m}Tc complex to bone. Eur. J. Nucl. Med., 2:47, 1977.

163. Lyons, K.P., Olson, H.G., and Aronow, W.S.: Pyrophosphate myocardial imaging. Semin. Nucl. Med., 10:168, 1980.

164. Loberg, M.D., and Porter, D.W.: Review and current status of hepatobiliary imaging agents. In Radiopharmaceuticals II. New York, Society of Nuclear Medicine, 1979, p. 519.

165. Loberg, M.D.: Radiotracer distribution by active transport. In Principles of Radiopharmacology. Edited by L. Colombetti. Vol. 3. Boca Raton, FL, CRC Press, 1979, p. 43.

166. Loberg, M.D., Ryan, J.W., and Porter, D.W.: Hepatic clearance mechanisms of Tc-99m-N-(Acetanilido)-Iminodiacetic acid derivatives (letter to the editor). J. Nucl. Med., 21:1111, 1980.

167. Kato, M., and Hazue, M.: Tc-99m(Sn) pyridoxylideneaminates: preparation and biological evaluation. J. Nucl. Med., 19:397, 1979.

168. Kato-Azuma, M., and Hazue, M.: Tc-99m(Sn) pyridoxylidenephenylalanine and its lipophilic derivatives: An approach to structure/bio-distribution relationship of technetium complexes. J. Nucl. Med., 21:P14, 1980.

169. Firnau, G.: Why do Tc-99m chelates work for cholescintigraphy? Eur. J. Nucl. Med., 1:137, 1976.

170. Harper, P.V., Lathrop, K.A., and Richards, P.: ^{99m}Tc as a radiocolloid. J. Nucl. Med., 5:382, 1964.

171. Larson, J.M., and Bennett, L.R.: Human serum albumin as a stabilizer for ^{99m}Tc-sulfur suspension. J. Nucl. Med., 10:294, 1969.

172. Ege, G.N., and Richards, L.P.: Introducing PVP as a stabilizer in the preparation of technetium sulphur colloid. Br. J. Radiol., 42:552, 1969.

173. Hunter, W.W., Jr.: Stabilization of particulate suspensions with nonantigenic polyhydric alcohols: application to ^{99m}Tc-sulfur colloid. J. Nucl. Med., 10:607, 1969.

174. Webber, M.M., Victery, W., and Cragin, M.D.: Stabilizer reaction-free ^{99m}Tc-sulfur suspension for liver, spleen, and bone-marrow scanning. Radiology, 92:170, 1969.

175. Larson, S.M., and Nelp, W.R.: Radiopharmacology of a simplified technetium-99m-colloid preparation for photo scanning. J. Nucl. Med., 7:817, 1966.

176. Garzon, O.L., Palcos, M.C., and Radicella, R.: A technetium-99m labeled colloid. Int. J. Appl. Radiat. Isot., 16:613, 1965.

177. Maas, R., Alvarez, J., and Arriaga, C.: On a new

tracer for liver scanning. Int. J. Appl. Radiat. Isot., *18*:653, 1967.

178. Johnson, A.E., and Gollan, F.: ^{99m}Tc-technetium dioxide for liver scanning. J. Nucl. Med., *11*:564, 1970.

179. Yamada, H., Johnson, D.E., and Griswold, M.L.: Radioalbumin macroaggregates for reticuloendothelial organ scanning and function assessment. J. Nucl. Med., *10*:453, 1969.

180. Gwyther, M.M., and Field, E.O.: Aggregated Tc 99m-labeled albumin for lung scintiscanning. Int. J. Appl. Radiat. Isot., *17*:485, 1966.

181. Cragin, M.D., Webber, M.M., and Victery, W.K.: Technique for the rapid preparation of lung scan particles using Tc-sulfur and human serum albumin. J. Nucl. Med., *10*:621, 1969.

182. Yano, Y., McRae, J., Honbo, D.S., et al.: ^{99m}Tc-ferric hydroxide macroaggregates for pulmonary scintiphotography. J. Nucl. Med., *10*:683, 1969.

183. Lin, M.S., and Winchell, H.S.: Macroaggregation of an albumin-stabilized technetium-tin (II) colloid. J. Nucl. Med., *13*: 928, 1972.

184. Rhodes, B.A., Stern, H.S., Buchanan, J.A., et al.: Lung scanning with ^{99m}Tc-microspheres. Radiology, *99*:613, 1971.

185. Cifka, J., and Vesely, P.: Non-pertechnetate radiochemical impurity in sulfur colloid labeled with ^{99m} technetium. *In* Radiopharmaceutical and Labelled Compounds. Vol. 1. Vienna, IAEA, 1973, p. 53.

186. Kristensen, K., and Pedersen, B.: Letter: Lung retention of ^{99m}Tc-sulfur colloid. J. Nucl. Med., *16*:439, 1975.

187. Enüstün, B.V., and Turkevich, J.: Coagulation of colloidal gold. J. Am. Chem. Soc., *85*:3317, 1963.

188. Warbick, A., Ege, G.N., Henkelman, R.M., et al.: An evaluation of radiocolloid sizing technique. J. Nucl. Med., *18*:827, 1977.

189. Davis, M.A., Jones, A.G., and Trindale, H.: A rapid and accurate method for sizing radiocolloids. J. Nucl. Med., *15*:923, 1974.

190. Billinghurst, M.W., and Jette, D.: Colloidal particle size determination by gel filtration. J. Nucl. Med., *20*:133, 1979.

191. Pedersen, B., and Kristensen, K.: Evaluation of methods for sizing of colloidal radiopharmaceuticals. Eur. J. Nucl. Med., *6*:521, 1981.

192. Rhodes, B.A., et al.: Radioactive albumin microspheres for studies of the pulmonary circulation. Radiology, *92*:1453, 1969.

193. Subramanian, L.G., Bell, E.G., and McAfee, J.G.: Preparation and labeling of gelatin, amylose and human serum albumin microspheres for in vivo use in nuclear medicine. J. Nucl. Med., *10*:373, 1969.

194. Tubis, M.: Hospital preparation and dispensing of radiopharmaceuticals. *In* Radiopharmacy. Edited by M. Tubis and W. Wolf. New York, Wiley Interscience, 1976.

195. The United States Pharmacopeia: 20th rev. U.S. Pharmacopeial Convention, Rockville, MD, 1975.

196. Rhodes, B.A., and Bolles, T.E.: Albumin mi-crospheres: current methods of preparation and use. *In* Radiopharmaceuticals. Edited by G. Subramanian, B.A. Rhodes, J.F. Cooper, and V.J. Sodd, New York, Society of Nuclear Medicine, 1974.

197. Frier, M., Griffiths, P., and Ramsey, A.: The biological fate of sulfur colloid. Eur. J. Nucl. Med., *6*:371, 1981.

198. Szymendera, J., Zoltowski, T., Radwan, M., and Kaminska, J.: Chemical and electron microscope observations of a safe PVP-stabilized colloid for liver and spleen scanning. J. Nucl. Med., *12*:212, 1971.

199. Cohen, Y., Ingrand, J., and Caro, R.: Kinetics of the disappearance of gelatin protected radiogold colloids from the bloodstream. Int. J. Appl. Radiat. Isot., *19*:703, 1968.

200. Caro, R.A., and Ciscato, V.A.: Kinetics of the phagocytosis of radiogold colloids by the reticuloendothelial system in the rat. Int. J. Appl. Radiat. Isot., *21*:405, 1970.

201. Dobson, E.L., Goffman, J.W., Jones, H.B., et al: Studies with colloids containing radioisotopes of yttrium, zirconium, columbium, and lanthanum in bone marrow, liver, and spleen. J. Lab. Clin. Med., *34*:306, 1949.

202. Kyker, G.C., and Rafter, J.J.: Colloid properties of the lanthanides. *In* Radioactive Pharmaceuticals. U.S. Atomic Energy Commission, 1966.

203. Heyman, S., Davis, M.A., Shulkin, P.M., et al.: Biologic evaluation of radiocolloids for bone marrow scintigraphy. *In* Radiopharmaceuticals II: Proc. 2nd Intl. Symp. on Radiopharmaceuticals, New York, Society of Nuclear Medicine, 1981, p. 593.

204. Myers, W.G.: Radioisotopes of iodine. *In* Radioactive Pharmaceuticals. Edited by G.A. Andrews. U.S. Atomic Energy Commission, 1966, p. 217.

205. Martindale, A.A., Papadimitrion, J.M., and Turner, J.H.: Technetium 99m antimony colloid for bone-marrow imaging. J. Nucl. Med., *21*:1035, 1980.

206. Eckelman, W.C.: Technical considerations in labeling of blood elements. Semin. Nucl. Med., *5*:3, 1975.

207. Smith, T., and Richards, P.: A simple kit for the rapid preparation of ^{99m}Tc red blood cells. J. Nucl. Med., *15*:534, 1974.

208. Hegge, F.N., Hamilton, G.W., Larson, S.M., et al.: Cardiac chamber imaging: a comparison of red blood cells labeled with Tc-99m in vitro and in vivo. J. Nucl. Med., *19*:129, 1978.

209. Pavel, D.G., and Zimmer, A.M.: In vivo labeling of red cells with Tc pertechnetate. J. Nucl. Med., *19*:972, 1978.

210. Leitl, G.P., Drew, H.M., Kelly, M.E., and Alderson, P.O.: Interference with Tc-99m labeling of red blood cells (RBCs). J. Nucl. Med., *21*:P44, 1980.

211. Gottchalk, A., Armas, R., and Thakur, M.: Reply to spleen scanning with Tc-99m-labeled red blood cells (RBC). J. Nucl. Med., *21*:1000, 1980.

212. Dugan, M.A., Kozar, J.J. Ganse, G., and Quap,

C.: New radiopharmaceuticals for thrombosis localization. J. Nucl. Med., *13*:782, 1972.

213. Barth, R.F., Singla, O., and Gillespie, G.Y.: Use of ^{99m}Tc as a radioisotopic label to study the migratory patterns of normal and neoplastic cells. J. Nucl. Med., *15*:656, 1974.

214. Uchida, T., Yasunaga, K., Kariyone, S., et al.: Survival and sequestration of ^{51}Cr- and ^{99m}TcO$_4^-$-labeled platelets. J. Nucl. Med., *15*:801, 1974.

215. Gillespie, G.Y., Barth, R.E., and Goburty, A.: Labeling of mammalian nucleated cells with ^{99m}Tc. J. Nucl. Med., *14*:706, 1973.

216. Barth, R.F., and Singla, O.J.: Organ distribution of ^{99m}Tc and ^{51}Cr labeled thymocytes. J. Nucl. Med., *16*:633, 1975.

217. Wong, D.W., and Mishkin, F.S.: Technetium-99m-human fibrinogen. J. Nucl. Med., *16*:343, 1975.

218. Jonckheer, M.H., Abramovici, J., Jeghers, O., et al.: The interpretation of phlebograms using fibrinogen labeled with ^{99m}Tc. Eur. J. Nucl. Med., *3*:233, 1978.

219. Millar, W.T., and Smith, J.F.: Localization of deep-venous thrombosis using technetium-99m-labelled urokinase. Lancet, *2*:695, 1974.

220. Dugan, M.A., Kozar, J.J., Ganse, G., and Charkes, N.D.: Localization of deep vein thrombosis using radioactive streptokinase. J. Nucl. Med., *14*:233, 1973.

221. Deacon, J.M., En, P.J., Anderson, P., and Khan, O.: Technetium 99m-plasmin: a new test for the detection of deep vein thrombosis. Br. J. Radiol., *53*:673, 1980.

222. Eckelman, W.C., Meinken, G., and Richards, P.: ^{99m}Tc human serum albumin. J. Nucl. Med., *12*:707, 1971.

223. Persson, R.B.R., and Kempi, V.: Labeling and testing of ^{99m}Tc-streptokinase for the diagnosis of deep vein thrombosis. J. Nucl. Med., *16*:474, 1975.

224. Duffy, M.F., and Duffy, G.J.: Studies on the labeling of streptokinase with ^{99m}Tc for use as a radiopharmaceutical in the detection of deep vein thrombosis: concise communication. J. Nucl. Med., *18*:483, 1977.

225. Korubin, V., Maisey, M., and McIntyre, P.: Evaluation of technetium-labeled red cells for determination of red cell volume in man. J. Nucl. Med., *13*:760, 1972.

226. Renault, H., Henry, R., Rapin, J., and Hegesippe, M.: Chelation de cations radioactifs par un polypeptide: la bleomycine. *In* Radiopharmaceuticals and Labeled Compounds. Vol 2. Vienna, IAEA, 1973, p. 195.

227. Reba, R.C., Eckelman, W.C., Poulose, K.P., et al.: Tumor-specific radiopharmaceuticals: radiolabeled bleomycin. *In* Radiopharmaceuticals. Edited by M. Subramanian, B.A. Rhodes, J.F. Cooper, and V.J. Sodd. New York, Society of Nuclear Medicine, 1974.

228. Asakura, H., Hori, M., and Umezawa, H.: Characterization of bleomycin action on DNA. J. Antibiot., *28*:537, 1975.

229. Eckelman, W.C., Kubota, H., Siegel, B.A., et al.:

Iodinated bleomycin: an unsatisfactory radiopharmaceutical for tumor localization. J. Nucl. Med., *17*:385 1976.

230. Sinkula, A.A., and Yalkowski, S.H.: Rationale for design of biologically reversible drug derivatives: prodrugs. J. Pharm. Sci., *64*:181, 1975.

231. Sundberg, M.W., Mears, C.F., Goodwin, D.A., et al.: Selective binding of metal ions to macromolecules using bifunctional analog of EDTA. J. Med. Chem., *17*:1304, 1974.

232. Goodwin, D.A., Sundberg, M.W., Diamanti, C.I., et al.: In labeled radiopharmaceuticals and their clinical use. *In* Radiopharmaceuticals. Edited by G. Subramanian. New York, Society of Nuclear Medicine, 1975, p. 80.

233. Heindel, N.D., Risch, V.R., Burns, H.D., et al.: Synthesis and tissue distribution of ^{99m}Tc sulfonylureas. J. Pharm. Sci., *64*:687, 1975.

234. Eckelman, W.C., Karesh, S.M., and Reba, R.C.: New compounds: fatty acid and long chain hydrocarbon derivatives containing a strong chelating agent. J. Pharm. Sci., *64*:704, 1975.

235. Karesh, S.M., Eckelman, W.C., and Reba, R.C.: Biological distribution of chemical analogs of fatty acids and long chain hydrocarbons containing a strong chelating agent. J. Pharm. Sci., *66*:225, 1977.

236. Livni, E., Davis, M.A., and Warner, V.D.: Synthesis and biologic distribution of mercapto derivatives of palmitic acid. J. Med. Chem., *22*:580, 1979.

237. Rzeszotarski, W.J., Eckelman, W.C., and Reba, R.C.: Application of Mannich reaction to introduction of chelating groups into a biologically active carrier. J. Label. Compd. Radiopharm., *13*:175, 1977.

238. Rzeszotarski, W.J., Paik, C., Eckelman, W.C., and Reba, R.C.: The synthesis of chelating agents for the preparation of drug derivatives. J. Label. Compd. Radiopharm., *13*:172, 1977.

239. Kramer, A.V., Epps, L.A., Ranganathan, N., et al.: Synthesis and characterization of neutral aminoethanol complexes of technetium. Fourth Int. Symp. Radiopharm. Chem., 1982, p. 323.

240. Lentle, B.C., Schmidt, R., and Nonjaim, A.A.: Iatrogenic alterations in the biodistribution of radiotracers. J. Nucl. Med., *19*:743, 1978.

241. Hladik, W.B., Nigg, K.K., and Rhodes, B.A.: Drug-induced changes in the biologic distribution of radiopharmaceuticals. Semin. Nucl. Med., *12*:184, 1982.

242. Eckelman, W.C.: Radiolabeled adrenergic and muscarinic blockers for in vivo studies. *In* Receptor Binding Radiotracers. Vol. 1. Edited by W.C. Eckelman. Boca Raton, FL, CRC Press, 1982, p. 69.

243. Lambrecht, R.M., and Wolf, A.P.: Cyclotron and short-lived halogen isotopes for radiopharmaceutical applications. *In* Radiopharmaceuticals and Labeled Compounds. Vol 1. Vienna, IAEA, 1973, p. 275.

244. Wellman, H.N., Anger, R.T., Jr., Sodd, V., and Paras, P.: Properties, production and clinical uses of radioisotopes of iodine. CRC Crit. Rev. in Clin. Radiol. and Nucl. Med., *6*:81, 1975.

245. De La Mare, P.B.D.: Electrophilic Halogenation. New York, Cambridge University Press, 1976.

246. Clayton, J.C., and Hems, B.A.: The synthesis of thyroxine and related substances. Part VI. The preparation of some derivatives of DL-thyroxine. J. Chem. Soc., 1950, p. 840.

247. MacFarland, A.S.: Efficient trace-labeling of proteins with iodine. Nature, *182*:53, 1958.

248. Hunter, W.M., and Greenwood, F.C.: Preparation of iodine-131 labeled human growth hormones of high specific activity. Nature, *194*:495, 1962.

249. Marchalonis, J.J.: An enzymic method for the trace iodination of immunoglobulins and other proteins. Biochemistry, *113*:299, 1969.

250. Katz, J., and Bonorris, G.: Electrolytic iodination of proteins with ^{125}I and ^{131}I. J. Lab. Clin. Med., *72*:966, 1968.

251. Bolton, A.E., and Hunter, W.M.: The labeling of proteins to high specific radioactivities by conjugation to a ^{125}I-containing acylating agent. Biochem. J., *133*:529, 1973.

252. Grovenstein, E., Jr., Aprahamian, N.S., Bryan, C.S., et al.: Aromatic halogenation. IV. Kinetics and mechanism of iodination of phenol and 2,6 dibromophenol. J. Am. Chem. Soc., *75*:4261, 1973.

253. Lambrecht, R.M., Montescu, C., Redvanly, C., and Wolf, A.P.: Preparation of high purity carrier free ^{123}I-iodine monochloride as iodination reagent for synthesis of radiopharmaceuticals. IV. J. Nucl. Med., *13*:266, 1972.

254. Berliner, E.: Kinetics of aromatic halogenation. V. The iodination of 2,4 dichlorophenol and anisole with iodine monochloride. J. Am. Chem. Soc., *80*:856, 1958.

255. Batts, B.D., and Gold, V.: The kinetics of aromatic protio- and deuterio-deiodination. J. Chem. Soc., 1964, p. 5753.

256. Jennings, V.J.: Analytical applications of chloramine-T. CRC Crit. Rev. Anal. Chem., *3*:407, 1974.

257. Huguchi, T., and Hussain, A.: Mechanism of chlorination of cresol by chloramine-T. Mediation by dichloramine-T. J. Chem. Soc., 1967, p. 549.

258. Freychet, P., Roth, J., and Neville, D.M., Jr.: Monoiodoinsulin: demonstration of its biological activity and binding to fat cells and liver membranes. Biochem. Biophys. Res. Commun., *43*:400, 1971.

259. Thorell, J.I., and Johansson, B.G.: Enzymatic iodination of polypeptides with ^{125}I to high specific activity. Biochim. Biophys. Acta, *251*:363, 1971.

260. Miller, L., and Watkins, B.F.: Scope and mechanism of aromatic iodination with electrochemically generated iodine (I). J. Am. Chem. Soc., *98*:1515, 1976.

261. Hayes, C.E., and Goldstein, I.S.: Radioiodination of sulfhydryl-sensitive proteins. Anal. Biochem., *67*:580, 1975.

262. Wood, F.T., Wu., M.M., and Gerhart, J.C.: The radioactive labeling of proteins with an iodinated amidination reagent. Anal. Biochem., *69*:339, 1975.

263. Hunter, W.M.: Preparation and assessment of radioactive tracers. Br. Med. Bull., *30*:18, 1974.

264. Rosa, U., Pennisi, G.E., and Scarsellati, G.A.: Factors affecting protein iodination. *In* Labeled Proteins in Tracer Studies. Edited by L. Donato, G. Milhard, and J. Sirchis. Brussels, Euratom, 1966.

265. Bale, W.F., Helmkamp, R.W., Davis, T.P., et al.: High specific activity labeling of proteins with ^{131}I by the iodide monochloride method. Proc. Soc. Exp. Biol. Med., *122*:407, 1966.

266. Bale, W.F., Contreras, M.A., and Grady, E.D.: Factors influencing localization of labeled antibodies in tumor. Cancer Res., *40*:2965, 1980.

267. Wolf, A.P., et al.: Synthesis of radiopharmaceuticals and labeled compounds using short-lived isotopes. *In* Radiopharmaceuticals and Labeled Compounds. Vol 1. Vienna, IAEA, 1973, p. 345.

268. Poe, N., Robinson, G.D., and Graham, L.S.: Experimental basis for myocardial imaging with ^{123}I-labeled hexadecanoic acid. J. Nucl. Med., *17*:1077, 1976.

269. Kojima, M., and Maeda, M.: Homoallylic rearrangement of 19-iodocholesterol. J. Chem. Soc. Commun., 1975, p. 47.

270. Welch, M.J., and Krohn, K.A.: Critical review of radiolabeled fibrinogen: its preparation and use. *In* Radiopharmaceuticals. Edited by G. Subramanian, B.A. Rhodes, J.F. Cooper, et al. New York, Society of Nuclear Medicine, 1975.

271. Krohn, K.A., and Knight, L.C.: Radiopharmaceuticals for thrombosis detection, selection, preparation and critical evaluation. Semin. Nucl. Med., *7*:219, 1971.

272. Charkes, N.D., Dugan, M.A., Maier, W.P., et al.: Scintigraphic detection of deep vein thrombosis with ^{131}I fibrinogen. J. Nucl. Med., *15*:1163, 1974.

273. Harwig, J.F., Colman, R.E., Harwig, S.S.L., et al.: Highly iodinated fibrinogen: a new thrombus localizing agent. J. Nucl. Med., *16*:756, 1975.

274. Harwig, J.F., Welch, M.J., and Coleman, R.E.: Preparation and use of ^{123}I labeled highly iodinated fibrinogen for imaging deep-vein thrombi. J. Nucl. Med., *17*:397, 1976.

275. Hnatowich, D.J., and Clancy, B.: Investigations of a new, highly negative liposome with improved biodistribution for imaging. J. Nucl. Med., *21*:662, 1980.

276. Kloster, G., and Stocklin, G.: Determination of the rate-determining step in halofatty acid-turnover in the heart. *In* Radioaktive Isotope in Klinik und Forschung 15. Band. Verlag H. Egermann, 1982, p. 235.

277. Spencer, R.P.: Reticuloendothelial compounds. *In* Radiopharmaceuticals: Structure-Activity Relationships. Edited by R.P. Spencer, New York, Grune & Stratton, 1981, p. 549.

278. Garnett, E.S., Firnau, G., Chang, P.K.H., et al.: (^{18}F) Fluoro-dopa, an analogue of dopa, and its use in direct external measurement of storage,

degradation and turnover. Proc. Natl. Acad. Sci., USA, *75*:464, 1978.

279. Gallagher, B.M., Fowler, J.S., Gutterson, N.I., et al.: Metabolic trapping as a principle of radiopharmaceutical design. Some factors responsible for the biodistribution of ^{18}F 2-deoxy-2-fluoro-D-glucose. J. Nucl. Med., *19*:1154, 1978.

280. Counsell, R.E., and Korn, N.: Radioiodinated cholesterol as a radiotracer in biochemical studies. *In* Receptor Binding Radiotracers. Vol. 1. Edited by W.C. Eckelman. Boca Raton, FL, CRC Press, 1982, p. 147.

281. Wieland, D.M., Brown, L.E., Rogers, W.L., et al., Myocardial imaging with a radioiodinated norepinephrine storage analog. J. Nucl. Med., *22*:22, 1981.

282. Gibson, R.E.: Quantitative changes in receptor concentration as a function of disease. *In* Receptor Binding Radiotracers. Vol. 2. Edited by W.C. Eckelman. Boca Raton, FL, CRC Press, 1982, p. 185.

283. Katzenellenbogen, J.R., Heiman, D.E., Carlson, K.E., and Lloyd, J.E.: In vivo and in vitro steroid receptor assays in the design of estrogen radiopharmaceuticals. Vol 1. *In* Receptor Binding Radiotracers. Edited by W.C. Eckelman. Boca Raton, FL, CRC Press, 1982, p. 93.

284. Kulmula, H.K., Huang, C.C., Dinerstein, R.J., and Friedman, A.M.: Specific in vivo binding of ^{77}Br-p-bromospiroperidol in rat brain. A potential tool for gamma ray imaging. Life Sciences, *28*:1911, 1981.

285. Goldenberg, D.M., Kim, E.E., DeLand, F., et al.: Clinical studies on the radioimmunodetection of tumor containing alpha-feto protein. Cancer, *45*:2500, 1980.

286. Goldenberg, D.M., Kim, E.E., DeLand, F.H., et al.: Clinical radioimmunodetection of cancer with radioactive antibodies to human chorionic gonadotropin. Science, *208*:1284, 1980.

287. Mach, J.P., Buchegger, F., Forni, M., et al.: Use of radiolabeled monoclonal anti-CEA antibodies for the detection of human carcinomas by external photoscanning and tomoscintigraphy. Immunology Today, 1981, p. 239.

288. Hoppes, D.D.: Radionuclide purity. *In* Quality Control in Nuclear Medicine. Edited by B.A. Rhodes. St. Louis, C.V. Mosby, 1977, p. 164.

289. Weinstein, M.B., and Smoak, W.M.: Technical difficulties in ^{99m}Tc-labeling of erythrocytes. J. Nucl. Med., *11*:41, 1970.

290. Oniciu, L., and Cook, G.B.: Preliminary study of quality control of ^{99m}Tc from ^{99}Mo generators. Radioanal. Chem., *13*:247, 1973.

291. Cohen, Y., and Besnard, M.: Analytical methods of radiopharmaceutical quality control. *In* Radiopharmaceuticals. Edited by G. Subramanian et al. New York, Society of Nuclear Medicine, 1975, p. 207.

292. Besnard, M., Gaucher, C., and Merlin, L.: Pureté radiochimique du complexe ^{113m}In acide diethylene-triaminopentaacétique. J. Radioanal. Chem., *9*:73, 1971.

293. Leach, K.G.: A simple method of checking filters used for sterilization. J. Nucl. Med., *13*:285, 1972.

294. DeLand, F.J., and Wagner, H.N., Jr.: Early detection of bacterial growth with carbon-14-labeled glucose. Radiol.,*92*:154, 1969.

295. Avis, K.E., Miller, W.A., and Phillips, G.B.: Parenteral medications. *In* Dispensing of Medication. 8th ed. Edited by J.E. Hoover. Easton, PA, Mack, 1976.

296. Cooper, J.F., Levin, J., and Wagner, H.N., Jr.: Quantitative comparison of in vitro and in vivo methods for the detection of endotoxin. J. Lab. Clin. Med., *78*:138, 1971.

297. Cooper, J.F., and Avis, K.E.: Control of microbial contamination. *In* Radiopharmaceuticals. Edited by G. Subramanian, B.A. Rhodes, J.F. Cooper and V.J. Sodd. New York, Society of Nuclear Medicine, 1975, p. 256.

Chapter 11

RADIOPHARMACEUTICAL DOSE CALCULATION

ROGER J. CLOUTIER,
EVELYN E. WATSON, AND
JACK L. COFFEY

The technique for calculating radiation dose recommended by the Medical Internal Radiation Dose (MIRD) Committee of the Society of Nuclear Medicine has now become widely accepted. This chapter describes the MIRD technique and the various data that are available to assist the user of MIRD reports in calculating radiation doses. Additional information concerning the MIRD technique can be found in several textbooks and reports.[1,2,3]

The basic principles of calculating radiation dose can be understood by first examining the relationship between dose rate and activity. Imagine a container of almost infinite dimensions filled with soft tissue, throughout which a radioactive material is uniformly distributed. In this situation, the dose rate to the tissue varies directly with the activity per unit mass and the amount of energy released per nuclear transformation.*

Mathematically this relationship may be expressed:

$$\dot{D} = k \cdot \frac{A}{m} \cdot E$$

where:

$\dot{D}$ = the absorbed dose per unit time

k = a constant whose value depends on the units used for the other factors in the equation

A = the amount of activity

m = the tissue mass so that A/m is the activity per unit mass

E = the average energy released per transformation.

If $\dot{D}$ is expressed in rads per hour, A in microcuries, m in grams, and E in million electron volts per nuclear transformation, the constant k is 2.13, and the dose rate equation becomes:

$$\dot{D} = 2.13 \frac{A}{m} E$$

Because the MIRD Committee has not yet published any tables that use the In-

---

*A transformation is almost synonymous with disintegration but is more general since it includes other modes of decay, e.g., isomeric transition and K-capture.

ternational System of Units (SI units), the more familiar units of rad, hour, microcurie, gram, and MeV will be used for calculating radiation dose. Dose values can be converted from these units to SI units by the following relationship: one gray (Gy) equals 100 rad. Similarly, activity can be converted to SI units by the following relationship: one microcurie equals 3.7×10^4 becquerel (Bq). Table 11–1 lists the principal quantities used in the MIRD schema with both traditional and SI units.

The two constants k and E can be combined into one constant, Δ, because the average energy E released per transformation is a constant for each radionuclide.

$$\Delta = 2.13 \, E$$

Hence,

$$\dot{D} = \frac{A}{m} \Delta$$

In reality, a Δ value exists for each type of radiation: beta particle, positron, gamma photon, etc. These values have been published for most radionuclides of general interest in MIRD Pamphlet 10.[5] Figure 11–1 shows the data for Tc-99m. In our example of activity in a large container, the dose rate to tissue from all types of radiation can be expressed as:

$$\dot{D} = \frac{A}{m} (\Delta_1 + \Delta_2 + \ldots + \Delta_n)$$

TABLE 11–1. *Principal Quantities Used in MIRD Schema with Symbols and Units*

Symbol	Quantity	Traditional units	SI units
Functions of Radiation Type Only			
E	Mean energy per particle or photon	MeV	kg · Gy (≡J)
n	Mean number of particles or photons per nuclear transformation	1	1
Δ	Mean energy emitted per unit cumulated activity*	$\dfrac{\text{g} \cdot \text{rad}}{\mu\text{Ci} \cdot \text{h}}$	$\dfrac{\text{kg} \cdot \text{Gy (≡J)}}{\text{Bq} \cdot \text{s}}$
λ	Decay constant	h^{-1}	s^{-1}
T	Half-life or half-time	h	s
Functions of Radiation Type and Absorbing Material			
$\Phi(x)$	Point isotropic specific absorbed fraction	g^{-1}	kg^{-1}
Ben(μx)	Point isotropic energy-absorption buildup factor	1	1
μ_{en}	Linear energy-absorption coefficient	cm^{-1}	m^{-1}
μ	Linear attenuation coefficient	cm^{-1}	m^{-1}
Functions of Radiation Type, Absorbing Material, and Source and Target			
$\dot{D}$, D ≡ R	Absorbed dose	rad	Gy
	Absorbed dose rate†	rad/h	Gy/s
ϕ	Absorbed fraction	1	1
Φ	Specific absorbed fraction	g^{-1}	kg^{-1}
S	Mean absorbed dose per unit cumulated activity	rad/μCi·h	Gy/Bq · s (≡Gy)
Quantities Characterizing Source and Target			
A	Activity	μCi	Bq
$\tilde{A}$	Cumulated activity	μCi · h	Bq · s (≡1)
α	Fractional distribution function	1	1
τ	Residence time	h	s
λ_j	Biologic disappearance constant	h^{-1}	s^{-1}
m	Mass	g	kg
r	Region, i.e., point, line, surface, or volume	—	—

*This quantity was given the name "equilibrium dose constant" in MIRD Pamphlet 1.[4]
†The symbol R was used in MIRD Pamphlet 1 for absorbed dose rate.[4]

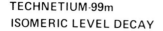

TECHNETIUM-99m
ISOMERIC LEVEL DECAY

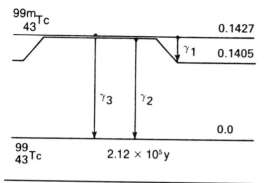

	OUTPUT DATA		
RADIATION	MEAN NUMBER/ DISINTE- GRATION	MEAN ENERGY/ PAR- TICLE	EQUI- LIBRIUM DOSE CONSTANT
	n_i	$\bar{E}_i$ (MeV)	Δ_i (g-rad/ μCi-h)
GAMMA 1	0.0000	0.0021	0.0000
P INT CON ELECT	0.9860	0.0016	0.0035
GAMMA 2	0.8787	0.1405	0.2630
K INT CON ELECT	0.0913	0.1194	0.0232
L INT CON ELECT	0.0118	0.1377	0.0034
M INT CON ELECT	0.0039	0.1400	0.0011
GAMMA 3	0.0003	0.1426	0.0001
K INT CON ELECT	0.0088	0.1215	0.0022
L INT CON ELECT	0.0035	0.1398	0.0010
M INT CON ELECT	0.0011	0.1422	0.0003
K ALPHA-1 X-RAY	0.0441	0.0183	0.0017
K ALPHA-2 X-RAY	0.0221	0.0182	0.0008
K BETA-1 X-RAY	0.0105	0.0206	0.0004
KLL AUGER ELECT	0.0152	0.0154	0.0005
KLX AUGER ELECT	0.0055	0.0178	0.0002
LMM AUGER ELECT	0.1093	0.0019	0.0004
MXY AUGER ELECT	1.2359	0.0004	0.0011

Fig. 11–1. Radiations emitted by Tc-99m and Δ values.

or:

$$\dot{D} = \frac{A}{m} \Sigma \Delta$$

Each particle or photon released during a nuclear transformation has unique characteristics that determine its range in tissue. Their principal dosimetric characteristics are given in Table 11–2.

Because of their short range, charged particles emitted during the transformation of an atom lose their energy close to their origin. X-rays and gamma rays, which are not electrically charged, may deposit their energy at considerable distances from their origin. When radiation absorbed doses are calculated, the model used must be capable of reflecting the distribution of this energy deposition in man. Snyder et al. have designed such a phantom for dosimetry calculations and, by means of mathematical equations, have also incorporated most body organs, as shown in Figure 11–2.[6] This heterogeneous phantom has organs with atomic composition and density that approximate those of Reference Man.[7] Table 11–3 gives masses for the phantom and those for Reference Man.

ABSORBED FRACTIONS

Because of the phantom's finite dimensions, some photons originating within the phantom are not absorbed within the phantom. Thus the dose rate to the phantom will be less than the dose rate calculated on the assumption that all energy is absorbed. To calculate the proper dose rate, the fraction of the available energy absorbed by the phantom must be known. This term is called the *absorbed fraction*, ϕ, and depends upon the energy and other characteristics of the radiation emitted and upon the size and shape of the phantom. If the radionuclide is in a specific organ rather than in the entire phantom, the absorbed fraction depends on the size and shape of both the organ containing the radioactive material (*source organ*) and the organ absorbing the radiation (*target organ*).

Radiation may be classified as *nonpenetrating* or *penetrating*. Nonpenetrating radiation includes all forms that are readily attenuated; hence, they deposit their energy in the immediate vicinity of their origin. This means that except for extremely small organs, energy emitted by electrons, positrons, internal conversion electrons, and Auger electrons is depos-

TABLE 11–2. *Principal Dosimetric Characteristics of Radiation Emitted During a Nuclear Transformation*

Radiation	Relative mass	Electric charge	Usual energy	Range in soft tissue
α	7400	+2	4 to 8 MeV	Micrometers
β−	1	−1	<2 MeV	Millimeters
β+	1	+1	<2 MeV	Millimeters
Internal Conversion Electrons (ICE)	1	−1	<2 MeV	Millimeters
Auger Electrons (AE)	1	−1	<50 keV	Millimeters
X-rays	0	0	<80 keV	Millimeters to centimeters
γ-rays	0	0	<2 MeV	Centimeters to meters

ited within the organ containing the radionuclide. Because the energy absorbed in the source organ equals the amount of energy released, the absorbed fraction for the source organ equals one. The absorbed fraction for all other organs is assumed to be zero.

Photons (x-rays and gamma rays) are termed *penetrating radiation* because they can travel long distances before interacting and depositing their energy. The absorbed fraction for penetrating radiation depends upon the energy of the photon and the size and shape of the source organ. For example, Brownell in MIRD Pamphlet 3 has shown that for a sphere of 2000 g (the approximate mass of the liver), the absorbed fraction varies from close to 1.0 for photons below 20 keV to less than 0.15 for photons greater than 1.5 MeV (Fig. 11–3).[8] In practice, such low-energy photons as characteristic x-rays usually are included with nonpenetrating radiations.

CALCULATION OF ABSORBED FRACTIONS FOR PHOTONS

Several methods are used to calculate absorbed fractions for photons. Perhaps the most useful is the Monte Carlo computer technique, which requires a geometric model of the source organ and target organ. Information about their density

and atomic composition as well as knowledge about the probability of photon interactions is also needed. To initiate a Monte Carlo calculation, a photon is created at a random position within the source organ, and the photon's initial direction is randomly determined. The distance that the photon travels before interacting is based on a random selection from a distribution that is weighted according to the probability of a photon interacting within the phantom. The type of interaction—photoelectric, Compton, or pair production—and the initial energy of the photon determine the amount of energy absorbed. The computer notes the location of the interaction and the amount of energy absorbed. Whenever an interaction requires the creation of a secondary photon, as in Compton scattering, a new photon is created at the point of interaction according to the rules of the interaction. The initial photon and any subsequent photons are followed until they are totally absorbed or escape from the phantom.

Knowing the life history of a *single* photon is not very useful since the energy it carries is quite small and the location of its energy deposition is statistically quite variable. If the paths of many photons are followed, however, the distribution of energy absorption within the body can be determined accurately. The absorbed frac-

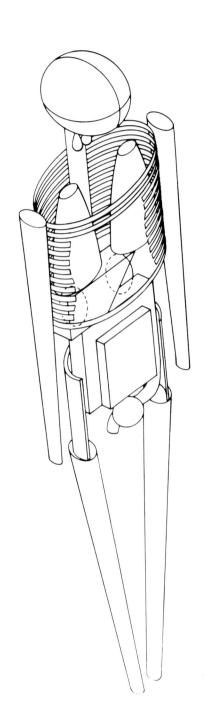

Fig. 11–2. Reference Man phantom showing some internal organs. (From Snyder, W.S., et al.[6])

tion for a target organ is thus the amount of energy absorbed within that organ divided by the total amount of energy liberated within a source organ.

The Monte Carlo technique is especially useful for calculating the amount of energy absorbed by an organ at some distance from the radioactivity, e.g., the spleen being irradiated by activity in the liver. Because the distance between the liver (source organ) and spleen (target organ) is greater than the range of the nonpenetrating radiation, the absorbed fraction for nonpenetrating radiation would be zero. The absorbed fractions for photons are generally greater than zero because they have sufficient penetrability to reach the target. The exact value depends on the energy of the photons, the distance between source and target, and the composition of the material that must be penetrated. Figure 11–4 shows the absorbed fractions for the liver as a source organ and the spleen as a target organ as a function of photon energy.

MIRD Pamphlet 5 provides more than 4000 absorbed fractions for 16 source organs, 25 target organs, and 12 photon energies.[6] Table 11–4 abstracted from MIRD Pamphlet 5, gives some of the absorbed fractions when the radioactivity is distributed uniformly throughout the liver. The full table includes absorbed fraction values for photon energies of 0.01, 0.015, 0.02, 0.03, 0.05, 0.10, 0.20, 0.50, 1.0, 1.5, 2.0, and 4.0 MeV.

Because the absorbed fraction tables for photons are for discrete energies, interpolation and extrapolation are necessary to obtain ϕ values for specific radionuclides. Linear interpolation is usually adequate for obtaining absorbed fractions for energies between published values. Absorbed fractions below 10 keV are obtained by extrapolation. When the source and target are the same, the value of ϕ at zero energy is assumed to be one. If the source and target are not the same, the value of ϕ at zero energy is assumed to be

TABLE 11–3. *Masses of Body Organs of Reference Man and of Anthropomorphic Phantom*

Body organs	Mass (g)	
	Reference Man	Phantom
Adrenals	14	15.5
Bladder		
Wall	45	45.1
Contents	200	200
Gastrointestinal tract		
Stomach		
Wall	150	150
Contents	250	247
Small intestine		
Wall	640	640*
Contents	400	400*
Upper large intestine		
Wall	210	209
Contents	220	200
Lower large intestine		
Wall	160	160
Contents	135	137
Kidneys (both)	310	284
Liver	1,800	1,810
Lungs (both, including blood)	1,000	999
Other tissue	48,000	48,500 (2,800 g suggested for muscle; 12,500 g for separable adipose tissue)
Ovaries (both)	11	8.27
Pancreas	100	60.3
Salivary glands	85	Not represented
Skeleton	10,000	10,500
Cortical bone	4,000	4,000
Trabecular bone	1,000	1,000
Red marrow	1,500	1,500
Yellow marrow	1,500	1,500
Cartilage	1,100	1,100
Other constituents	900	1,400
Spleen	180	174
Testes	35	37.1
Thyroid	20	19.6
Uterus	80	65.4
Total body	70,000	69,900

*Small intestine wall and contents not separated in phantom.

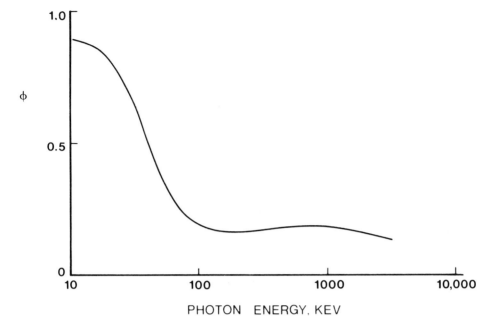

Fig. 11–3.   Absorbed fractions in a 2000-g sphere as a function of photon energy.

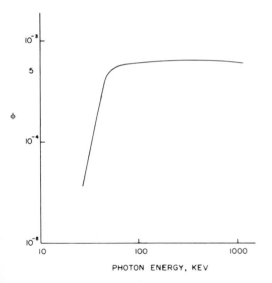

Fig. 11–4.   Absorbed fractions for the liver as a source organ and the spleen as a target organ as a function of photon energy.

zero since at low energies little or none of the energy is absorbed by the target. For the special situation in which the source is uniformly distributed in the total body, values of φ for energies below 10 keV can be obtained by assuming the value of φ at

zero energy to be equal to m_T/m_{TB}, where m_T is the mass of the target and m_{TB} the mass of the total body.

Because each target-source organ pair has a different absorbed fraction for each type of radiation, the dose-rate equation becomes:

$$\dot{D}(T \leftarrow S) = \frac{A_S}{m_T} \Sigma \, \Delta \, \phi \, (T \leftarrow S)$$

where (T←S) refers to a target organ irradiated by a source organ.* Note that the activity present in the source is divided by the mass of the target.

Also included in Table 11–4 is the coefficient of variation, $100 \, \sigma_\phi/\phi$. This value is a measure of the statistical reliability of the absorbed fractions. For large target organs, a coefficient of variation of less than 50% is usually obtained with 30,000 or fewer photons. Absorbed fractions with

---

*In MIRD Pamphlet 1, Revised, r_k and r_h are used to represent the target and source regions;[4] however, in this introduction, (T←S) can be used because the full generalization included in the MIRD notation is not yet required.

TABLE 11–4. *Absorbed Fractions and Coefficients of Variation with Uniform Source in Liver*

	Photon energy, E (MeV)							
	0.200		0.500		1.000		1.500	
Target organ	ϕ	$\frac{100\,\sigma_\phi}{\phi}$	ϕ	$\frac{100\,\sigma_\phi}{\phi}$	ϕ	$\frac{100\,\sigma_\phi}{\phi}$	ϕ	$\frac{100\,\sigma_\phi}{\phi}$
Adrenals	0.237E–03	16.	0.198E–03	25.	0.221E–03	23.	0.235E–03	29.
Bladder	0.389E–03	15.	0.358E–03	17.	0.521E–03	16.	0.515E–03	17.
GI (Stom)	0.271E–02	5.6	0.280E–02	6.9	0.240E–02	8.4	0.254E–02	8.9
GI (SI)	0.100E–01	3.2	0.971E–02	3.7	0.925E–02	4.4	0.904E–02	4.6
GI (ULI)	0.387E–02	4.9	0.364E–02	5.9	0.320E–02	7.2	0.287E–02	7.8
GI (LLI)	0.211E–03	17.	0.391E–03	19.	0.268E–03	22.	0.286E–03	24.
Heart	0.570E–02	4.1	0.573E–02	4.9	0.501E–02	5.9	0.498E–02	6.3
Kidneys	0.390E–02	4.7	0.386E–02	5.8	0.335E–02	7.2	0.294E–02	8.0
Liver	0.158	0.79	0.157	0.93	0.144	1.1	0.132	1.2
Lungs	0.923E–02	3.0	0.838E–02	3.8	0.825E–02	4.5	0.696E–02	5.2
Marrow	0.133E–01	1.7	0.107E–01	2.2	0.935E–02	2.7	0.924E–02	2.8
Pancreas	0.102E–02	8.2	0.822E–03	12.	0.864E–03	14.	0.587E–03	18.
Sk. (Rib)	0.111E–01	2.7	0.867E–02	3.8	0.760E–02	4.7	0.748E–02	5.
Sk. (Pelvis)	0.216E–02	6.0	0.182E–02	7.7	0.171E–02	9.1	0.181E–02	9.7
Sk. (Spine)	0.108E–01	3.1	0.857E–02	3.9	0.694E–02	4.8	0.670E–02	5.3
Sk. (Skull)	0.140E–03	25.	0.187E–03	27.	0.262E–03	23.	0.360E–03	23.
Skeleton (Total)	0.324E–01	1.7	0.260E–01	2.2	0.231E–01	2.6	0.229E–01	2.8
Skin	0.507E–02	3.8	0.561E–02	4.6	0.581E–02	5.2	0.567E–02	5.7
Spleen	0.645E–03	10.	0.619E–03	13.	0.633E–03	15.	0.396E–03	21.
Thyroid								
Uterus	0.136E–03	22.	0.130E–03	33.	0.127E–03	30.	0.729E–04	44.
Trunk	0.413	0.47	0.404	0.51	0.377	0.58	0.351	0.64
Legs	0.716E–03	14.	0.141E–02	10.	0.208E–02	9.6	0.248E–02	9.0
Head	0.867E–03	11.	0.106E–02	11.	0.179E–02	10.	0.225E–02	9.5
Total body	0.415	0.47	0.407	0.51	0.381	0.58	0.355	0.64

The digits following the symbol E indicate the powers of ten by which each number is to be multiplied.
A blank in the table indicates that the coefficient of variation was greater than 50%.
Total body = head + trunk + legs.
Abstracted from Snyder, W.S., et al.[6]

coefficients of variation greater than 50% were not included in the tables because of their large statistical uncertainty. The coefficient of variation is large when the number of interactions and the amount of energy absorbed in the target organ are so small that even one additional photon interaction could drastically change the absorbed fraction estimate. This situation occurs when the target is small and distant from the source organ. An example would be liver to thyroid (Table 11–4). To obtain a statistically reliable absorbed fraction, 120,000 or more photons might need to be followed, a costly and time-consuming effort. Fortunately, several different tech-

niques that are reasonably accurate can be used to calculate absorbed fractions under these circumstances.

One technique makes use of the reciprocity principle described in MIRD Pamphlet 1, Revised.[4] According to this principle, the fraction of energy absorbed per unit mass is independent of which organ is designated the source and which the target as long as both organs are contained within a large homogeneous medium.

$$\frac{\phi(1{\leftarrow}2)}{m_1} = \frac{\phi(2{\leftarrow}1)}{m_2}$$

Since three of the factors are generally known, the fourth can easily be calculated.

Thus, whenever the Monte Carlo technique fails to provide a statistically significant absorbed fraction for a source-target pair, the reciprocity principle may be used.

The ratio of ϕ/m is called the *specific absorbed fraction*, Φ, i.e., the fraction of energy absorbed per gram of target tissue.

$$\Phi(1 \leftarrow 2) = \frac{\phi(1 \leftarrow 2)}{m_1}$$

$$\text{or } \Phi(T \leftarrow S) = \frac{\phi(T \leftarrow S)}{m_T}$$

and

$$\Phi(1 \leftarrow 2) = \Phi(2 \leftarrow 1)$$

$$\text{or } \Phi(T \leftarrow S) = \Phi(S \leftarrow T)$$

Hence, the dose-rate equation can be given as:

$$\dot{D} = A_S \Sigma \Delta \Phi(T \leftarrow S)$$

By reciprocity, the equation may be written as:

$$\dot{D} = A_S \Sigma \Delta \Phi(S \leftarrow T)$$

In spite of the nonhomogeneity of the phantom, application of the reciprocity principle to Reference Man is usually valid to within a factor of two.[9] For example, when the coefficient of variation is less than 50%, the ratio of the two values of Φ obtained for a specific energy and organ pair is less than 1.8 for more than 90% of the soft-tissue organ-pair combinations tested (ratios ordered to give a value greater than 1.0).

If neither the Monte Carlo nor the Monte Carlo reciprocity principle technique provides a reliable estimate of the absorbed fraction, an estimate can be obtained by using standard attenuation equations with dose buildup factors, published by Berger for an infinite homogeneous medium (MIRD Pamphlet 2):[10]

$$\Phi = \left[\frac{\mu_{en}}{\rho} \cdot \frac{1}{4\pi x^2} \cdot e^{-\mu x} \right] \cdot B_{en}(\mu x)$$

Although Berger's buildup factors were calculated for a homogeneous medium, this technique provides values that lie between 0.5 and 2 times the absorbed fractions calculated by the Monte Carlo technique using the heterogeneous phantom.[11] Hence, within these limits, the technique is valid for calculating absorbed fractions that cannot be calculated by the Monte Carlo method (Fig. 11–5).

DOSE

The total dose, D, is the sum of the instantaneous dose rates $\dot{D}$ for the time period of interest:

$$D = \int \dot{D} \, dt$$

or

$$D = \int A \Sigma \Delta \Phi \, dt$$

where D is expressed in rads. For simplicity, the $(T \leftarrow S)$ notation and the integration limits have been omitted.

Since in this equation only A generally varies with time,*

$$D = \Sigma \Delta \Phi \int A \, dt$$

The time integral of activity, $\tilde{A}$, is called the *cumulated activity:*

$$\tilde{A} = \int A \, dt$$

Cumulated activity is directly proportional to the number of nuclear transformations and is expressed in terms of microcurie-hours. The dose equation becomes $D = \tilde{A} \Sigma \Delta \Phi$.

The value of $\tilde{A}$ depends not only on the physical half-life of the radionuclide but also on the biologic uptake and excretion of the material. Sometimes the value of $\tilde{A}$ can be calculated relatively easily, such as

---

*If the phantom size changes during the period of interest, Φ may also vary and a more general equation would be required.

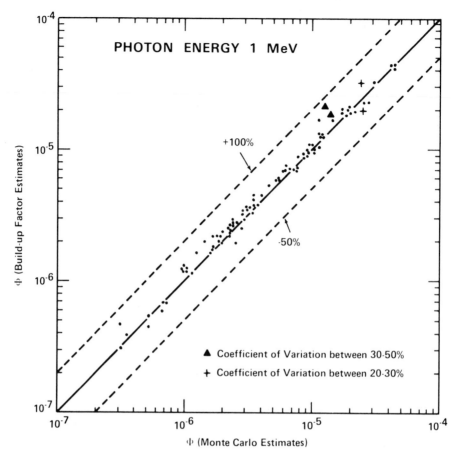

Fig. 11–5. Comparison of specific absorbed fractions calculated by the buildup technique with those calculated by the Monte Carlo technique.

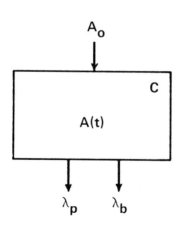

Fig. 11–6. Diagram of single-compartment model.

when the activity enters a single compartment "instantaneously" and the amount leaving the compartment is proportional to the amount of activity within the compartment. In the simple model diagrammed in Figure 11–6, activity leaves compartment C by two routes: physical transformation and biologic excretion. It is convenient to discuss these processes in terms of the effective elimination constant, $(\lambda_j)_{\text{eff}}$, and the effective half-time, $(T_j)_{\text{eff}}$.

$$(\lambda_j)_{\text{eff}} = \lambda + \lambda_j \text{ and } (T_j)_{\text{eff}} = \frac{T \cdot T_j}{T + T_j}$$

where λ is the physical decay constant and is equal to $0.693/T$ (T is the physical half-life). The biologic disappearance constant,

λ_j, represents that fraction of the jth component of the remaining activity excreted per unit time, and $\lambda_j = 0.693/T_j$.[4] The biologic half-time of the material is T_j.

The equation describing the amount of activity in compartment C is:

$$A_h(t) = A_o e^{-(\lambda + \lambda_j)t} = A_o e^{-(\lambda_j)_{eff} t}$$

$$= A_o e^{-\frac{0.693}{(T_j)_{eff}} \cdot t}$$

Figure 11–7 shows the change in activity with respect to time. For this simple model, Ã could be calculated by the following equation:

$$\tilde{A} = \int_o^t A_o e^{-\frac{0.693}{(T_j)_{eff}} \cdot t} \, dt$$

$$= 1.44(T_j)_{eff} \, A_o \left(1 - e^{-\frac{0.693}{(T_j)_{eff}} \cdot t} \right)$$

If t is infinity (∞) or at least 10 times the effective half-time, $\tilde{A} = 1.44 \, A_o (T_j)_{eff}$. Note that Ã is proportional to the area under the curve in Figure 11–7.

Unfortunately, the change in activity with time in most biologic systems is not as simple as in the preceding example; hence, more complex models and mathematical equations are required.[12] The equations must take into account the distribution and retention of the radionuclide in each region of the body. A typical equation describing the amount of activity $A_h(t)$ in source region r_h is:

$$A_h(t) = A_o \sum_j \alpha_{hj} \, e^{-(\lambda_j)_{eff} \cdot t}$$

where A_o is the initial activity present in the body and α_{hj} is the fraction of A_o in region h associated with the jth biologic compartment.

MIRD Pamphlet 12, "Kinetic Models for Absorbed Dose Calculations," describes how kinetic models can be handled to provide Ã for complex biologic models and how residence time τ is used in dose calculations.[12] Residence time, i.e., the average time that administered activity remains in a specific region, depends on the kinetic model and on the physical decay constant of the radionuclide, and for tracers, is independent of the administered activity (Fig. 11–8). Using τ allows the cumulated activity to be expressed as a function of the administered activity A_o. Thus:

$$\tilde{A}_{(o,\infty)} = A_o \tau_h$$

and

$$\tau_h = \frac{\tilde{A}}{A_o}$$

For a simple model, as in Figure 11–6:

$$\tau_h = \frac{A_o(1.44) \, (T_j)_{eff}}{A_o}$$

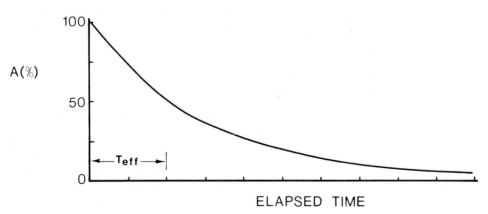

Fig. 11–7.   Amount of activity in compartment C with respect to time.

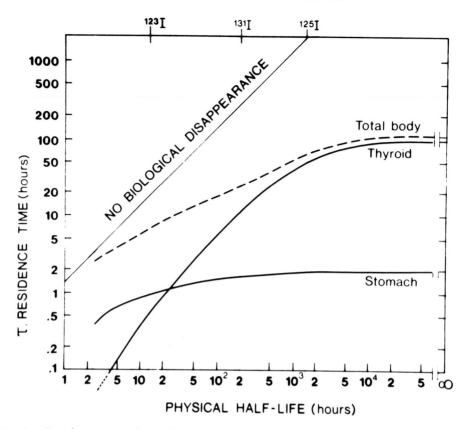

Fig. 11–8. Residence time for iodide in total body, thyroid, and stomach as a function of the physical half-life.

Thus:

$$\tau_h = 1.44(T_j)_{eff} = \frac{1}{(\lambda_j)_{eff}}$$

Even when values of $\bar{A}$ are available, dose calculation can be a tedious task because of the necessity of finding each value of Δ and Φ and then summing their products for each target-source combination. Because $\Sigma \Delta \Phi$ is uniquely specified for a given radionuclide and target-source pair, MIRD has developed a term called the *absorbed dose per unit cumulated activity*, S, expressed in the following equation:

$$S = \Sigma \Delta \Phi$$

The general dose equation becomes:

$$D = \bar{A} \cdot S$$

Values of S for over 100 radionuclides have been published in MIRD Pamphlet 11.[13] Each table provides S values for 20 source organs and 20 target organs. Table 11–5 shows part of the S table for Tc-99m.

Published values of τ are not yet available from MIRD. When these become available, the dose equation can be expressed as follows:

$$D(r_k \leftarrow r_h) = A_o \cdot \tau_h \cdot S(r_k \leftarrow r_h)$$

EXAMPLES OF DOSE CALCULATIONS

Most of the facts and data needed to calculate the radiation dose to a Reference Man phantom have been presented. This dose serves as an estimate of the dose that a patient might receive from administration of a radionuclide. Consider a simple

TABLE 11–5.   S, Absorbed Dose per Unit Cumulated Activity (rad/μCi·h) for Tc-99m

Target organs	Source organs					
	Adrenals	Kidneys	Liver	Lungs	Spleen	Total body
Adrenals	3.1E–03	1.1E–05	4.5E–06	2.7E–06	6.3E–06	2.3E–06
Bladder wall	1.3E–07	2.8E–07	1.6E–07	3.6E–08	1.2E–07	2.3E–06
Bone (total)	2.0E–06	1.4E–06	1.1E–06	1.5E–06	1.1E–06	2.5E–06
GI (Stom wall)	2.9E–06	3.6E–06	1.9E–06	1.8E–06	1.0E–05	2.2E–06
GI (SI)	8.3E–07	2.9E–06	1.6E–06	1.9E–07	1.4E–06	2.5E–06
GI (ULI wall)	9.3E–07	2.9E–06	2.5E–06	2.2E–07	1.4E–06	2.4E–06
GI (LLI wall)	2.2E–07	7.2E–07	2.3E–07	7.1E–08	6.1E–07	2.3E–06
Kidneys	1.1E–05	1.9E–04	3.9E–06	8.4E–07	9.1E–06	2.2E–06
Liver	4.9E–06	3.9E–06	4.6E–05	2.5E–06	9.8E–07	2.2E–06
Lungs	2.4E–06	8.5E–07	2.5E–06	5.2E–05	2.3E–06	2.0E–06
Marrow (red)	3.6E–06	3.8E–06	1.6E–06	1.9E–06	1.7E–06	2.9E–06
Muscle	1.4E–06	1.3E–06	1.1E–06	1.3E–06	1.4E–06	1.9E–06
Ovaries	6.1E–07	1.1E–06	4.5E–07	9.4E–08	4.0E–07	2.4E–06
Pancreas	9.0E–06	6.6E–06	4.2E–06	2.6E–06	1.9E–05	2.4E–06
Skin	5.1E–07	5.3E–07	4.9E–07	5.3E–07	4.7E–07	1.3E–06
Spleen	6.3E–06	8.6E–06	9.2E–07	2.3E–06	3.3E–04	2.2E–06
Testes	3.2E–08	8.8E–08	6.2E–08	7.9E–09	4.8E–08	1.7E–06
Thyroid	1.3E–07	4.8E–08	1.5E–07	9.2E–07	8.7E–08	1.5E–06
Uterus (nongravid)	1.1E–06	9.4E–07	3.9E–07	8.2E–08	4.0E–07	2.6E–06
Total body	2.2E–06	2.2E–06	2.2E–06	2.0E–06	2.2E–06	2.0E–06

Based on MIRD Pamphlet 11.[13]

example in which 1 mCi of Tc-99m in a "unique" chemical form is administered, resulting in a uniform distribution throughout the body without any biologic excretion. In this case, $(T_j)_{eff} = T$. The dose to the total body, TB, is:

$$A_o = 1000 \ \mu Ci$$
$$\tilde{A}_{TB(\infty)} = 1.44 \ (T_j)_{eff} A_o = (1.44)(6)(1000) = 8.64 \times 10^3 \ \mu Ci\text{-hr}$$
$$S(TB \leftarrow TB) = 2.0 \times 10^{-6} \ rad/\mu Ci\text{-hr (Table 11–5)}$$
$$D_{TB(\infty)} = \tilde{A}_{TB(\infty)} S(TB \leftarrow TB) = (8.64 \times 10^3)(2.0 \times 10^{-6}) = 1.7 \times 10^{-2} \ rad$$

The dose to other body organs as a result of the activity uniformly distributed throughout the body can also be estimated. For example, the dose to the liver is calculated as follows:

A_o and $\tilde{A}_\infty$ are the same as in the previous example because the total body remains the source organ. Thus:

$$S(LI \leftarrow TB) = 2.2 \times 10^{-6} \ rad/\mu Ci\text{-hr}$$
$$D_{LI(\infty)} = \tilde{A}_{TB(\infty)} S(LI \leftarrow TB) = (8.64 \times 10^3)(2.2 \times 10^{-6}) = 1.9 \times 10^{-2} \ rad$$

The value of S for the total body irradiating the liver includes a nonpenetrating radiation component for only those transformations that occur within the liver. In the calculation of S, this part is done automatically by setting the cumulated activity in the liver at $(m_{LI}/m_{TB})\tilde{A}_{TB}$ when the

activity is uniformly distributed in the total body as in the example. The penetrating radiation contribution to S(LI←TB) includes transformations occurring both in the liver and in the remainder of the body.

A more complex dose problem is encountered when the administered activity is unevenly divided among several organs. For simplicity, assume that immediately after administration of 1 mCi of Tc-99m, 30% of the activity is located in the liver, 40% is located in the spleen, and 30% is uniformly distributed in the remainder of the body. If no further distribution of the Tc-99m takes place and no excretion occurs, the dose to the liver would be calculated as follows:

$$D_{LI} = D(LI \leftarrow LI) + D(LI \leftarrow SP)$$
$$+ D(LI \leftarrow RB)$$

where SP is the spleen and RB is the remainder of the body.

$$D_{LI} = \tilde{A}_{LI}S(LI \leftarrow LI) + \tilde{A}_{SP}S(LI \leftarrow SP)$$
$$+ \tilde{A}_{RB}S(LI \leftarrow RB)$$

Until the final term, the solution of this equation is straightforward:

$$D_{LI} = (1.44)(6)(.3)(1000)(4.6 \times 10^{-5})$$
$$+ (1.44)(6)(.4)(1000)(9.8 \times 10^{-7})$$
$$+ (1.44)(6)(.3)(1000) [S(LI \leftarrow RB)]$$

$$D_{LI} = 1.2 \times 10^{-1} + 3.4 \times 10^{-3}$$
$$+ 2600[S(LI \leftarrow RB)]$$

The value of $S(LI \leftarrow RB)$ is not available in MIRD Pamphlet 11.[13] In fact, the S tables probably will never contain values for the "remainder of the body" because the remainder of the body represents the entire body minus those source organs in-

cluded in the calculations. In this example, the remainder of the body represents the entire body minus liver and spleen.

Since the S value for $(LI \leftarrow RB)$ is not available in the tables, the temptation to use $S(LI \leftarrow TB)$ might arise. This value would be a good first approximation, but because $S(LI \leftarrow TB)$ was calculated from the assumption that the activity was distributed throughout the entire body, it is not exact for $S(LI \leftarrow RB)$.

Cloutier et al. solved the problem of calculating the dose to an organ from the remainder of the body by correcting values of ϕ.[15] Snyder et al. and Roedler and Kaul have shown that a similar technique can be used to obtain S values for specific organs being irradiated by the remainder of the body.[16,17] The general equation for the S value of a target r_k from the remainder of the body ($RB = TB - \sum_h r_h$) is:

$$S(r_k \leftarrow RB) = S(r_k \leftarrow TB) \frac{m_{TB}}{m_{RB}}$$
$$- \sum_h S(r_k \leftarrow r_h) \frac{m_{r_h}}{m_{RB}}$$

or

$$S(r_k \leftarrow RB)$$
$$= \frac{S(r_k \leftarrow TB) m_{TB} - \sum_h S(r_k \leftarrow r_h)m_{r_h}}{m_{RB}}$$

where r_h is a source region. In this example, $S(LI \leftarrow RB)$ would be:

$$S(LI \leftarrow RB) = \frac{S(LI \leftarrow TB)m_{TB} - [S(LI \leftarrow SP) \, m_{SP} + S(LI \leftarrow LI) \, m_{LI}]}{m_{TB} - (m_{SP} + m_{LI})}$$

$$S(LI \leftarrow RB) = \frac{(2.2 \times 10^{-6})(70,000) - [(9.8 \times 10^{-7}((174) + 4.6 \times 10^{-5})(1800)]}{70,000 - (174 + 1800)}$$

$$= 1.0 \times 10^{-6} \text{ rad/}\mu\text{Ci-hr}$$
$$\text{and } D_{LI} = 1.2 \times 10^{-1} + 3.4 \times 10^{-3} + (2600)(1.0 \times 10^{-6})$$
$$= 1.2 \times 10^{-1} + 3.4 \times 10^{-3} + 2.6 \times 10^{-3} = 0.13 \text{ rad}$$

As would be expected, the energy absorbed from transformations occurring in the liver contributed most of the radiation dose to the liver. Although $S(LI \leftarrow TB)$ is

approximately a factor of two higher than $S(LI \leftarrow RB)$, transformations occurring in the remainder of the body do not greatly influence the total dose to the liver.

Although MIRD has provided considerable data for dose calculations, more are still required. Values of S, Φ, or ϕ are needed for different-sized phantoms. Without these data, radiation dose estimates are almost impossible to calculate for patients that do not resemble Reference Man. Phantoms that will be used to generate S values for the newborn, 1-, 5-, 10-, and 15-year-olds have been described by Poston.[18] Cloutier et al. have designed a model for pregnant women that has been used to provide values of ϕ for the developing fetus.[19]

In an attempt to solve part of the problem of changing values of Φ with time, Snyder and Ford and Smith and Warner have reported on the effect that changing bladder size and voiding schedule have on Φ.[20,21]

Several groups have examined changes in Φ for nonpenetrating radiation when the source is located in small organs.[22,23,24] The more difficult problem of handling dose calculations when activity within an organ is distributed nonuniformly remains to be solved. Blau has discussed this problem for bone-seeking radionuclides.[25]

Regardless of now much physical data are provided, the greatest need for dose estimation is still good biologic data on the distribution and retention of a radionuclide in normal and diseased patients. To help correct this deficiency, MIRD has established several task groups. Each group has the goal of collecting all available information on a specific radiopharmaceutical and preparing a dose estimate report. Several task groups have completed dose estimate reports.[26,27,28,29,30,31,32,33]

The proceedings of three symposia on radiopharmaceutical dosimetry held in Oak Ridge also contain considerable biologic data useful in dose estimation.[34,35,36] With the help of nuclear medicine departments, good biologic data can be obtained on new radiopharmaceuticals. Use of these data ensures the proper risk assessment and the continued safe use of radionuclides in medicine.

REFERENCES

1. Loevinger, R.: Distributed radionuclide sources. *In* Radiation Dosimetry. Vol. 3. 2nd ed. Edited by F.H. Attix and E. Tochlin. New York, Academic Press, 1969.
2. Loevinger, R.: Some remarks on the MIRD schema for absorbed-dose calculations for biologically distributed radionuclides. *In* Medical Radionuclides: Radiation Dose and Effect. Edited by R.J. Cloutier et al. USAEC Symposium Series 20, CONF-691212. Springfield, VA, National Technical Information Service, 1970.
3. Rohrer, R.H.: Physics of internal dosimetry. *In* Radiopharmaceutical Dosimetry Symposium, HEW Publication (FDA) 76-8044, 1976.
4. Loevinger, R., and Berman, M.: A revised schema for calculating the absorbed dose from biologically distributed radionuclides. NM/MIRD Pamphlet 1, Revised. New York, Society of Nuclear Medicine, 1976.
5. Dillman, L.T., and Von der Lage, F.C.: Radionuclide decay schemes and nuclear parameters for use in radiation dose estimation. NM/MIRD Pamphlet 10. New York, Society of Nuclear Medicine, 1975.
6. Snyder, W.S., et al.: Estimates of absorbed fractions for monoenergetic photon sources uniformly distributed in various organs of a heterogeneous phantom. J. Nucl. Med./Suppl. 3, MIRD Pamphlet 5, August 1969.
7. ICRP No. 23, Report of the Task Group on Reference Man, adopted by the International Commission on Radiological Protection, October 1974. New York, Pergamon Press, 1975.
8. Brownell, G.L., Ellett, W.H., and Reddy, A.R.: Absorbed fractions for photon dosimetry. J. Nucl. Med./Suppl. 1, MIRD Pamphlet 3, p. 27, February 1968.
9. Snyder, W.S.: Estimation of absorbed fraction of energy from photon sources in body organs. *In* Medical Radionuclides: Radiation Dose and Effect. Edited by R.J. Cloutier et al. USAEC Symposium Series 20, CONF-691212. Springfield, VA, National Technical Information Service, 1970.
10. Berger, M.J.: Energy deposition in water by photons from point isotropic sources. J. Nucl. Med./Suppl. 1, MIRD Pamphlet 2, p. 15, February 1968.
11. Snyder, W.S., Ford, M.R., and Warner, G.G.: Estimates of absorbed fractions for photon emitters within the body. Part III. Internal dosimetry. *In* Oak Ridge National Laboratory Health Physics Division Annual Progress Report, period ending July 31, 1972, ORNL-4811. Springfield, VA, National Technical Information Service, September 1972.
12. Berman, M.: Kinetic models for absorbed dose calculations. NM/MIRD Pamphlet 12. New York, Society of Nuclear Medicine, 1976.

13. Snyder, W.S., et al.: "S" absorbed dose per unit cumulated activity for selected radionuclides and organs. NM/MIRD Pamphlet 11. New York, Society of Nuclear Medicine, 1975.

14. Reference deleted.

15. Cloutier, R.J., et al.: Calculating the radiation dose to an organ. J. Nucl. Med., 14:53, 1973.

16. Snyder, W.S., et al.: A tabulation of dose equivalent per microcurie-day for source and target organs of an adult for various radionuclides. ORNL-5000. Springfield, VA, National Technical Information Service, November 1974.

17. Roedler, H.D., and Kaul, A.: Dose to target organs from remaining body activity: results of the formally exact and approximate solution. In Radiopharmaceutical Dosimetry Symposium, HEW Publication (FDA) 76–8044, 1976.

18. Poston, J.W.: The effects of body and organ size on absorbed dose: There is no standard patient. In Radiopharmaceutical Dosimetry Symposium, HEW Publication (FDA) 76-8044, 1976.

19. Cloutier, R.J., Watson, E.E., and Snyder, W.S.: Dose to the fetus during the first three months from gamma sources in maternal organs. In Radiopharmaceutical Dosimetry Symposium, HEW Publication (FDA) 76-8044, 1976.

20. Snyder, W.S., and Ford, M.R.: Estimation of dose to the urinary bladder and to the gonads. In Radiopharmaceutical Dosimetry Symposium, HEW Publication (FDA) 76-8044, 1976.

21. Smith, E.M., and Warner, G.G.: Practical methods of dose reduction to the bladder wall. In Radiopharmaceutical Dosimetry Symposium, HEW Publication (FDA) 76-8044, 1976.

22. Cloutier, R.J., and Watson, E.E: Radiation dose from radioisotopes in the blood. In Medical Radionuclides: Radiation Dose and Effects. Edited by R.J. Cloutier et al. USAEC Symposium Series 20, CONF-691212, Springfield, VA, National Technical Information Service, 1970.

23. McEwan, A.C.: Dosimetry of radionuclides in blood. Br. J. Radiol., 47:652, 1974.

24. Ford, M.R., Snyder, W.S., and Warner, G.G.: Variation of the absorbed fraction with shape and size of the thyroid. Part V. Medical physics and internal dosimetry. In Oak Ridge National Laboratory Health Physics Division Annual Progress Report, period ending June 30, 1975, ORNL-5046. Springfield, VA, National Technical Information Service, September 1975.

25. Blau, M.: Problems of dose calculations for technetium-99m bone scanning agents. In Radiopharmaceutical Dosimetry Symposium, HEW Publication (FDA) 76-8044, 1976.

26. Lathrop, K.A., et al.: MIRD/Dose Estimate Report 1. Summary of current radiation dose estimates to humans from ^{75}Se-L-selenomethionine. J. Nucl. Med., 14:49, 1973.

27. Lathrop, K.A., et al.: MIRD/Dose Estimate Report 8. Summary of current radiation dose estimates to humans from ^{99m}Tc as sodium pertechnetate. J. Nucl. Med., 17:74, 1976.

28. Cloutier, R.J., et al.: MIRD/Dose Estimate Report

29. 2. Summary of current radiation dose estimates to humans from [66]Ga-, [67]Ga-, [68]Ga-, [72]Ga-citrate. J. Nucl. Med., 14:755, 1973.

29. Cloutier, R.J., et al.: MIRD/Dose Estimate Report 4. Summary of current radiation dose estimates to humans from [198]Au-colloidal gold. J. Nucl. Med., 16:173, 1975.

30. Atkins, H.L., et al.: MIRD/Dose Estimate Report 3. Summary of current radiation dose estimates to humans from ^{99m}Tc-sulfur colloid. J. Nucl. Med., 16:108, 1975.

31. Berman, M., et al.: MIRD/Dose Estimate Report 5. Summary of current radiation dose estimates to humans from ^{123}I, [124]I, ^{125}I, [126]I, [130]I, ^{131}I, and [132]I as sodium iodide. J. Nucl. Med., 16:857, 1975.

32. Blau, M., et al.: MIRD/Dose Estimate Report 6. Summary of current radiation dose estimates to humans from [197]Hg- and [203]Hg-labeled chlormerodrin. J. Nucl. Med., 16:1095, 1975.

33. Freeman, L.M., et al.: MIRD/Dose Estimate Report 7. Summary of current radiation dose estimates to humans from ^{123}I, [124]I, [126]I, and ^{131}I as sodium rose bengal. J. Nucl. Med., 16:1214, 1975.

34. Cloutier, R.J., Edwards, C.L., and Snyder, W.S. (Eds.): Medical Radionuclides: Radiation Dose and Effects. USAEC Symposium Series 20, CONF-691212, Springfield, VA, National Technical Information Service, 1970.

35. Cloutier, R.J., Coffey, J.L., Snyder, W.S., and Watson, E.E. (Eds.): Radiopharmaceutical Dosimetry Symposium, HEW Publication (FDA) 76-8044, 1976.

36. Watson, E.E., Schlafke-Stelson, A.T., Coffey, J.L., and Cloutier, R.J.: Third International Radiopharmaceutical Dosimetry Symposium, HEW Publication FDA 81-8166, 1981.

ADDITIONAL MIRD REPORTS

Dillman, L.T.: Radionuclide decay schemes and nuclear parameters for use in radiation-dose estimation. J. Nucl. Med./Suppl. 2, MIRD Pamphlet 4, March 1969.

Berger, M.J.: Distribution of absorbed dose around point sources of electrons and beta particles in water and other media. J. Nucl. Med./Suppl. 5, MIRD Pamphlet 7, March 1971.

Ellett, W.H., and Humes, R.M.: Absorbed fractions for small volumes containing photon-emitting radioactivity. J. Nucl. Med./Suppl. 5, MIRD Pamphlet 8, March 1971.

Snyder, W.S., Ford, M.R., and Warner, G.G.: Estimates of specific absorbed fractions for photon sources uniformly distributed in various organs of a heterogeneous phantom. NM/MIRD Pamphlet 5, Revised. New York, Society of Nuclear Medicine, 1977.

Coffey, J.L., Cristy, M., and Warner, G.G.: Specific absorbed fractions for photon sources uniformly distributed in the heart chambers and heart wall of a heterogeneous phantom. NM/MIRD Pamphlet 13. J. Nucl. Med., 22:65, 1981.

Chapter 12

RADIATION EFFECTS IN NUCLEAR MEDICINE

KENNETH L. MOSSMAN

This chapter addresses the biologic effects of radiation as they pertain to nuclear medicine. An understanding of these effects is important for the nuclear medicine physician, who has an obligation to his patients to balance what he can accomplish with a given procedure against a wide spectrum of possible biologic effects, many of which remain poorly defined.

Biologic effects of radiation from radioactive substances were noted soon after the discovery of radioactivity in 1896. Becquerel observed reddening of the skin under his pocket where he had been carrying a vial of radium; Pierre Curie exposed his arm to radium and observed the burn's healing process. The biologic effects of ionizing radiation were poorly understood in those early days, and consequently, many radiation workers (medical and industrial) died or were seriously injured from overexposure to radiation.

Early animal experiments showed that radiation produced a variety of effects besides the skin lesions seen by Curie and others, and a relation between quantity of radiation and degree of damage was demonstrated for many biologic systems. Realization of the dangers of radiation exposure resulted in the formulation of guidelines for safe handling of radioactive preparations. By 1946, when reactor-produced radioisotopes became available for medical purposes, knowledge of the biologic effects of radiation had expanded, and levels of permissible exposure were set.

The spectacular growth of nuclear medicine and the impressive safety record of the discipline reflect an understanding of the hazards of radiation exposure and the efforts to enforce strict guidelines for safe handling and use of radionuclides. In this chapter, the basic concepts of radiobiology are reviewed, with emphasis on those concepts of importance in nuclear medicine.

INITIAL PHYSICAL AND CHEMICAL EVENTS

Development of tissue injury from radiation exposure is a complex series of physical, chemical, and biologic events, the first of which is absorption of radiation by the tissues. The radiations are listed in Table 12–1. Collectively, these are called *ionizing radiations* because the principal means of energy dissipation is ejection of electrons from the atoms with which they interact.

TABLE 12–1. *Ionizing Radiations of Biologic Importance*

Type	Description	Production	Mode of interaction*	Range in soft tissue*
X-rays	High-energy electromagnetic waves (uncharged)	X-ray tubes	Energy transfer resulting in ejection of high-speed electrons	Centimeters
Gamma rays	High-energy electromagnetic waves (uncharged)	Radioactive decay	Energy transfer resulting in ejection of high-speed electrons	Centimeters
Beta particles (electrons, positrons)	Particulate; charged; light	Radioactive decay; accelerators	Direct interaction with orbital electrons	Millimeters
Alpha particles	Particulate; charged; heavy	Radioactive decay; accelerators	Direct interaction with orbital electrons	Micrometers
Protons, deuterons, heavy nuclei	Particulate; charged; heavy	Accelerators	Direct interaction with orbital electrons	Micrometers
Neutrons	Particulate; uncharged; heavy	Nuclear Fission Accelerators	Interaction with light atomic nuclei	Centimeters
Negative pi mesons (pions)	Particulate; charged; heavier than beta but lighter than proton	Accelerators	Direct interaction with orbital electrons	Centimeters

*Other modes of interaction may be important, and range in tissue may vary depending on the energy of the radiation.

Of particular interest in nuclear medicine are gamma rays and beta particles. Although these radiations, as well as the others listed in Table 12–1, differ radically in many characteristics, including their initial reactions with matter, the majority of their effects are similar.

In the ionization process, an orbital electron is completely stripped from the atom. Because chemical bonds that hold molecules together are made up of electrons shared between atoms, the removal of binding electrons causes dissociation of atoms within the molecules. Thus, when an atom is ionized, the molecule of which it is a part undergoes chemical changes.

A second method of energy dissipation by radiation in tissue is excitation. In this process, the electrons are not completely removed from the atom but are raised to a higher energy level, so that the atom or molecule is in an excited state. In dissipating this excess energy, excited molecules undergo reorganization of the electrons that hold the constituent atoms together, and often, these chemical bonds rupture with destruction of the molecule and release of stable and unstable molecular fragments.[1] Thus, the ultimate effect of ionization and excitation is the disruption of stable molecules with release of chemically reactive species. The actual physical process of radiation absorption lasts approximately 10^{-16} seconds. Ionization and excitation follow rapidly, occurring in about 10^{-12} seconds.

Chemical change can occur by two mechanisms—direct and indirect action. In direct action, the molecule undergoing change absorbs energy directly from the radiation. In indirect action, energy is absorbed from another molecule, which acts as an intermediary in energy transfer. The intermediary in the cell is usually H_2O. Highly reactive ions and free radicals (e.g., H^+, $OH^\cdot$, OH^- are produced when H_2O is ionized, and their products (e.g., H_2O_2) can be powerful oxidizing agents that react with biologically important molecules to alter their function.

The net result of chemical alteration is twofold: essential chemical constituents in the cells, such as DNA, RNA, and enzymes, may be changed and their functions altered, and new toxic compounds (e.g., powerful oxidizing agents from the radiolysis of water) may be produced in the cell. These initial chemical reactions occur quickly, usually within milliseconds.

Because of the random nature of the absorption of ionizing radiation, any type of molecule within the cell can be altered. Molecular damage may or may not be of consequence to the cell depending upon the abundance of the particular molecule affected. For example, water molecules are abundant in the cell; the alteration of a small percentage of them by radiation is unlikely to affect the cell. When damage is incurred by certain rare and essential cellular molecules, however, it becomes important to cell survival. Some of these critical molecules are complex structural lipids of cell membranes, enzymes, and nucleic acids. Damage to just a few of these molecules may seriously hamper normal cell function or cause cell death. Table 12–2 lists some essential cellular macromolecules and the effects of their alteration.

Development of molecular lesions within the cell and subsequent effects at higher levels of biologic organization may take seconds to years to develop, depending upon the dose of radiation and the nature of the damage. Some key effects of radiation at different levels of biologic complexity are presented in Table 12–3. At low doses of radiation (less than 10 centigray; 1 cGy = 1 rad), which are usually encountered in radiodiagnostic procedures, principal effects include cancer induction, genetic damage, and damage to the developing embryo and fetus. Some of these effects may first become apparent years after the radiation exposure. At high

TABLE 12–2. *Radiation Effects on Some Key Cellular Molecules*

Molecule	Radiation effect	Possible cellular effect
DNA	Disruption of linear arrangement of bases by base substitution, deletion, or addition; cross linking; single-strand break; double-strand break	Temporary or permanent inhibition of DNA synthesis; synthesis of incorrect DNA; inhibition or prevention of mitosis; synthesis of incorrect protein
Enzymes	Alteration in tertiary structure of molecule because of disruption of chemical bonds	Inhibition of enzymatic activity with resultant changes in cellular metabolism
Structural lipids composing cell membranes	Disruption of molecular bonds	Increased permeability to K^+, Na^+, etc. with resultant alteration in normal intracellular/extracellular environment

TABLE 12–3. *Biologic Effects of Radiation*

Level of organization	Type of damage	Important effects
Cell	Chromosomal aberrations; mutations	Cell death; inhibition of cell division; transformation to malignant state
Tissue	Hypoplasia; transformation of cells to malignant state	Disruption in tissue function; death, induction of cancer
Whole body	Disruption of hemopoietic, gastrointestinal, central nervous systems	Death
	Transformation of tissue to malignant state	Cancer

doses of radiation (typically 1000 to 10,000 cGy for radiotherapy), principal effects include cell death and tissue dysfunction. These effects may be apparent within a few days following radiation exposure.

LOW DOSES OF RADIATION: BIOLOGIC EFFECTS OF DIAGNOSTIC NUCLEAR MEDICINE PROCEDURES

Radiodiagnostic procedures usually involve patient doses of a few cGy or less. Exposures to such low doses are thought to be associated with genetic effects, cancer induction, and damage to the developing embryo or fetus. Direct evidence of radiation effects at low dose levels in man, however, has not been found; thus quantification of radiation effects cannot be precise. Estimates of the probability of effects (risks) at low doses must be extrapolated from the better known effects at high doses. Most of the estimates are derived from studies involving external radiation, e.g., studies of the Japanese survivors of the atomic bombings, or of radiotherapy patients.[2,3] The prevailing view among radiation scientists has been that risk is directly proportional to radiation dose even at low doses, and that any dose, no matter how small, is potentially damaging (linear, no-threshold model). Some scientists postulate a threshold dose below which the risk is zero, while others contend that risk is disproportionally lower or higher than expected from the linear, no-threshold model. Distinguishing among these models is difficult because the effects predicted by each theory are small, and because insufficient data at low doses have been collected, which makes it almost impossible to verify the correct model.

Table 12–4 lists risk estimates for the major low-dose radiation effects. Risk estimates have been predicted using linear, no-threshold; quadratic; and linear-quadratic models.

Carcinogenesis

The major effect in somatic tissues following low doses of radiation is the induction of cancer. Production of tumors by radiation has been observed from the earliest uses of radiation. Undoubtedly, ionizing radiation can induce cancer in man; the type depends on the tissue irradiated, the sex and age of the individual, and other factors. Evidence for radiation carcinogenesis in humans is shown in Table 12–5.

The appearance of leukemia following radiation exposure is documented in reports of the Japanese A-bomb survivors and the British ankylosing spondylitis patients. From over 100,000 individuals studied at Hiroshima and Nagasaki, there is clear evidence that the risk of leukemia is increased in exposed individuals even at doses as low as 25 to 50 cGy. Acute lymphocytic and acute and chronic myeloid leukemias were most prevalent. In Hiroshima survivors and in the spondylitis patients, no cases of chronic lymphocytic leukemia due to radiation were observed.[6]

Thyroid cancer has an increased incidence in Japanese A-bomb survivors, in individuals given radiation during childhood for treatment of lymphoid hyperplasia in the head and neck, and in Marshall Islanders exposed to fallout radiation from the 1954 nuclear tests. Within these three groups, excess thyroid cancer occurred more frequently in women than in men. Apparently, however, there is no age dependence with respect to susceptibility to thyroid cancer induction.[3]

In humans, the female breast is probably the tissue most susceptible to cancer induction by radiation. Excess breast cancer has been observed in Japanese A-bomb survivors, in women given multiple fluoroscopic examinations during artificial pneumothorax for pulmonary tuberculosis, and in women treated by x-ray for postpartum mastitis. In these studies, women exposed before the age of 30 appeared to have higher risk, and fractionation of the radiation dose did not significantly affect the risk.[7]

One characteristic of radiation-induced cancer is a long latent period, that is, the

TABLE 12–4. *Risk Estimates for Low-Dose Radiation Effects*

Effect	Risk	Reference
Carcinogenesis	10^{-4} per cGy*	UNSCEAR[2] BEIR[3]
Mutagenesis	10^{-4} per cGy†	UNSCEAR[2] BEIR[3]
In utero effects	$<10^{-3}$ per cGy‡	UNSCEAR[2] Mole, R.[4]

*Risk of death due to cancer.
†Risk of severe dominant, X-linked, and other genetic conditions.
‡Risk primarily for postnatal neoplasia.

TABLE 12–5.   *Cancers Associated with Radiation Exposure*

Exposed population	Strong associations*	Weak associations†
Japanese A-bomb survivors	leukemia, thyroid, breast, lung	stomach, esophagus, bladder, lymphoma, salivary gland, etc.
Marshall Islanders		thyroid
Radium-dial painters	bone	colon
Pioneer radiologists	leukemia, skin	lymphoma, brain
Ankylosing spondylitis patients	leukemia, lung, bone	breast, stomach, esophagus, lymphoma
Multiple chest fluoroscopy patients	breast	
Enlarged thymus patients (infants)	thyroid	leukemia, skin, salivary gland
Thorotrast patients	leukemia, liver	lung, lymphoma, kidney
In utero x-ray patients	leukemia	
Thyroid cancer patients (I-131)		leukemia

*Strong associations between radiation exposure and induction of cancer.
†Weak associations, or suggestive but unconfirmed associations, between radiation exposure and induction of cancer.
From Interagency Task Force on the Health Effects of Ionizing Radiation: Report of Work Group on Science, Dept. HEW.[5]

time between exposure and the appearance of cancer, which for some cancers may be 30 years or longer. This long latency, plus the fact that radiation-induced cancers are no different clinically from cancers resulting from other causes, makes it extremely difficult to study the effects of radiation, especially at low doses, on cancer incidence. Leukemias appear to have the shortest latent period, sometimes as short as 2 to 3 years; thyroid and breast cancer may have latencies of 25 years or more.

The risks of cancer induced by low doses of radiation are not known, because most available data in humans has resulted from exposures at high doses. As discussed earlier, several mathematical dose-response models have been used to predict the risks at low doses. Different cancers may have different dose responses, however. Table 12–6 lists the lifetime risks for various cancers, based on a linear, no-threshold model. For all cancers combined, the lifetime risk is about one excess cancer death in 10,000 persons each given 1 cGy of whole-body x-ray or gamma radiation.[2,3] In an unexposed population of 10,000 people, approximately 1600 are expected to die of cancer.

The mechanisms by which radiation carcinogenesis occur are not known. Cancer may result from radiation-induced somatic mutations. In another theory, radiation may activate a latent carcinogenic virus in cells. Another possible mechanism is that radiation acts indirectly by creating body conditions that favor growth of tumors.

Cancers following high levels of radionuclide exposure have been reported in several studies. Sources of exposure include radionuclide therapy, industrial exposures, and military activities. Some examples follow:

1. Evidence suggests that patients

TABLE 12–6. *Radiation Risks for Various Cancers*

Cancer	Risk estimate* (cases/million persons/cGy)
Leukemia	10–60
Thyroid cancer (external radiation)	20–150
Breast cancer	30–200
Lung cancer	20–100
Bone cancer	3
Other	10–15
Deaths due to all cancers	approximately 100

*Risk estimates are for x-rays or gamma rays. Estimates obtained from UNSCEAR and BEIR reports.[2,3]

treated with P-32 orthophosphate for polycythemia have a higher incidence of leukemia than patients treated with chemotherapeutic agents.[8]

2. Study of radium-dial painters has conclusively shown that alpha-emitting radionuclides can cause osteosarcomas when deposited in bone.

3. Inhalation of radioactive dust can undoubtedly induce lung cancer; the most notable evidence is given by the study of uranium miners.[6]

4. Cholangiomas and hemangioendotheliomas of the liver have been associated with the use of colloidal thorium dioxide (Thorotrast) in diagnostic radiology.[9]

Genetic Effects

In 1927, H.J. Muller discovered that x-rays could induce permanent changes, called *mutations,* in hereditary material. For this work, he was awarded the Nobel Prize in 1946. Mutations, like cancer, can occur spontaneously or as a result of actions by chemicals, viruses, or radiation. Mutations can arise in somatic or germ cells. Somatic cell mutations are harmful only to the individual carrying them, whereas mutations in germ cells may be harmful to succeeding generations. Mutations can occur as a result of either gross structural changes in chromosomes or changes in chromosome number, or they can occur as point mutations that result from small changes in the DNA base composition or sequence.

Breakage of chromosomes *(aberrations)* can be induced by radiation with doses of 10 cGy or lower.[9,10] Aberrations are of two general types: those that occur in the chromosome after mitosis but before DNA synthesis *(chromosome breaks)* and those that occur after DNA synthesis (i.e., when the DNA content of the cell has doubled) but before mitosis *(chromatid breaks).* Breaks can behave in several ways:

1. The break may restitute, i.e., repair the damage.
2. The break may fail to rejoin, giving rise to an aberration.
3. Fragments may realign and rejoin, giving rise to aberrations.

Aberrations have been classified according to the portion of the chromosome or chromatid involved and to the number of breaks. Some possibilities are:

1. Chromosome terminal deletions
2. Chromosome interstitial deletions
3. Chromosome exchanges
4. Chromatid deletions
5. Isochromatid deletions
6. Intrachanges
7. Interchanges

Chromosomal aberrations can be significant to the cell. Extensive chromosomal changes probably result in cell death. If the alterations do not cause cell death, they may nevertheless change heritable characteristics of cells, a process that results in mutation.

A comprehensive radiation genetics study with mice was performed by W.L. Russell's group at the Oak Ridge National Laboratory.[10] Russell's experiments form the foundation for most of what is now believed about genetic effects in man, because little data on man himself are available. In these experiments, a specific locus method was used to study mutation rates produced in mice by a variety of dose rates, fractionation patterns, and germ cell stages. Seven specific loci were studied, including coat color and ear shape.

From early work on genetic effects of radiation in the fruit fly, it had been assumed that the frequency of point mutations increases linearly with increasing radiation dose and that there is no dose-rate effect. Russell's studies have shown that both of these assumptions are wrong. In male mice, the dose-response curve for point mutations appears linear down to doses of about 25 cGy. In female mice, however, the frequency of point mutation is much lower at 50 cGy than would be predicted by extrapolating the dose-response curve from high doses. No evidence was found for a threshold dose, i.e., any dose of radiation may cause a mutation. Furthermore, mutation rate decreased as dose rate is decreased. This dose-rate effect was more pronounced in female mice. According to a model proposed by Russell, the repair process of premutational damage becomes inactivated at high dose rates. Thus a given dose delivered at a low dose rate interferes with the repair process to a lesser degree than the same dose delivered at a high dose rate. At lower dose rates, greater repair of premutational damage and fewer mutations occur.[11]

In addition, Russell's studies showed that mutation rate varied with the stage of germ cell development. In fully developed sperm, the frequency of mutation was essentially independent of dose rate. Irradiation of immature oocytes and spermatogonia, however, resulted in fewer mutations, and mutation rate was dose-rate dependent. These findings were attributed to the fact that mature germ cells are incapable of repairing premutational damage.

It is difficult to extrapolate human mutation rates from the mouse data of Russell's study. Recently, Schull et al. reported a 34-year follow-up study of children born to survivors of the Japanese atomic bombing.[12] They found no statistically significant effects of parental exposures on characteristics of the offspring studied. The various indicators of possible genetic damage used, however, including indicators of major congenital defects and sex chromosome aneuploidy, were all in the direction expected if an effect had been produced. These results suggest that the genetic data collected in experimental studies of the mouse may not accurately reflect human sensitivities. Nevertheless, the following aspects of Russell's studies of the mouse may be important for man:

1. No evidence exists of a threshold dose for genetic damage. Any dose of radiation may be capable of causing mutation.
2. All genetic damage may not be cumulative with radiation dose. Some premutational damage may be reparable at low dose rates.
3. In general, mutations are permanent.

If a lethal mutation occurs in a germ cell, the zygote that inherits it will probably be nonviable or at least will not survive embryonic life. Other mutations, such as that giving rise to hemophilia, are severely detrimental but are not lethal immediately. Individuals carrying such mutations can survive into adulthood if considerable care is taken. Other mutations, such as albinism, may be less detrimental. Like gene mutations, chromosomal aberrations in germ cells result in genetic imbalances that may be lethal or result in severe disabilities.

When a large population is exposed to ionizing radiation, some cell mutation occurs in some of the individuals exposed. The hazard associated with medical radiation exposure is that too many mutations introduced into the population at the same time can be detrimental to the population as a whole.

The deleterious genes found within a population make up the *genetic load.* The size of the genetic load depends on the rate of production of deleterious genes through mutations and the rate at which the deleterious genes are removed from the population via natural selection processes. When these two rates are equal, *genetic equilibrium* is reached. At genetic equilibrium, the number of deleterious genes in the population is stable. Increased medical radiation levels increase the genetic load of the population and raise the level of genetic equilibrium.

Genetic effects from low levels of radiation are considered a population hazard because it is difficult to express genetic risk in terms of the individual or his offspring.

One measure of possible genetic damage to the population is the *genetically significant dose,* or GSD.[13] The GSD is an index of presumed genetic impact of radiation on the whole population from radiation received by individuals and is determined by the gonadal dose to the exposed populations, population size, and the number of children to be expected from this population. For 1964, the GSD for radiodiagnostic procedures was calculated to be .016 cSv. (One centisievert equals 1 rem.) In 1970, the GSD was .020 cSv, despite increases in the number of radiodiagnostic procedures performed. Natural background radiation contributes approximately .090 cSv to the GSD.[13]

Another measure of genetic effects is the *doubling dose,* or the dose of radiation to a population that results in a 100% increase over the spontaneous mutation rate. In man, the doubling dose for acute x-ray or gamma radiation is approximately 160 cSv; this is approximately four times higher than the doubling dose calculated for the mouse (40 cSv).[12] Risk estimates for genetic damage following radiation (x or gamma) are not well known, but esti-mates have been made.[2,3] The total genetic risk over the next several generations is approximately 10^{-4} per cGy, which is about the same as the cancer death rate because of radiation-induced cancer in one generation.[14] The genetic effects that define risk include chromosomal and recessive diseases and congenital anomalies.[2,3]

Genetic changes have been observed following nuclear medicine procedures:

1. Cantolino et al. reported that standard doses of I-131 used in treating hyperthyroidism produced chromosomal abnormalities. The doses averaged 5 mCi (185 MBq) of I-131 and resulted in a whole body dose of about 5 cGy.[15]

2. Boyd et al. found that chromosomal abnormalities were significantly increased in former radium-dial painters, who retained small quantities of radium in their bones for many years. The frequency of aberrations was directly related to the body burden of the radium.[16]

3. Lisco and Conard studied the effects of radioactive fallout on the Marshallese. Aberrations in peripheral blood cells and bone marrow were observed. Clones of cytogenetically abnormal cells in the bone marrow were also demonstrated. Strontium and radioiodine were the major sources of radiation exposure in these people.[17]

4. Fischer et al. found that 95% of patients who had received Thorotrast 19 to 27 years earlier had peripheral blood cell aberrations in direct proportion to body burden.[18]

These examples demonstrate that chromosomal damage in humans can occur after exposure to radionuclides. Of additional interest is the repeated epidemiologic finding of an association between radioactivity in a specific tissue and an increase in neoplasms in that tissue (e.g., bone tumors and radium, liver tumors and thorium). This association raises the possibility that chromosomal aberrations within the cells of a given tissue are related in some way to the malignant process.[19]

Effects in Utero

Pregnancy is a major contraindication for radiodiagnostic procedures. The developing embryo and fetus are extremely sensitive to ionizing radiations.[20] Irradiation of the uterine contents can occur from nuclear medicine procedures in which radiopharmaceuticals are concentrated in maternal organs or in the embryo or fetus itself, the latter occurring when the radiopharmaceutical can cross the placenta.[21,22,23,24] The major effects following substantial radiation exposure of the developing embryo or fetus include gross congenital malformations, growth retardation, postnatal neoplasia, and death. Several recent articles provide detailed reviews of the subject.[4,20,22,23,24,25]

A critical determinant of the nature of the bioeffects following radiation exposure is the time following conception, in which the irradiation occurred. In the preimplantation period (first week postconception), the embryo is sensitive to the lethal effects of radiation but has a low probability of sustaining teratogenic or growth-retarding effects if implantation and continued development occur. During the period of major organogenesis (2 to 8 weeks postconception), the embryo is sensitive to the teratogenic, growth-retarding, lethal, and postnatal neoplastic effects of radiation. During the fetal period (8 to 40 weeks postconception), radiosensitivity for multiple organ teratogenesis decreases, but growth retardation, functional abnormalities (especially of the central nervous system), and postnatal neoplastic effects can occur.[20,21,22,23,24] The period of radiation exposure in an unsuspected pregnancy is often during major organogen-

esis, one of the most sensitive periods of development.

The type of radiodiagnostic examination and the exposure factors are important in estimating embryonic or fetal dose. For nuclear medicine procedures, the type of radiopharmaceutical, total activity administered, effective half-life, metabolic pathway of the labeled compound in the mother, rate of placental transfer, and fetal uptake must be evaluated in determining fetal dose.[23] Methods for estimating fetal dose following nuclear medicine procedures have been described by Cloutier et al. and by Husak and Wiedermann.[26,27] Typical values of embryonic doses for various radiopharmaceuticals are shown in Table 12–7.

Most nuclear medicine procedures result in embryonic or fetal doses of less than 1 cGy.[27] A dose of 10 cGy or less to the embryo probably results in little, if any, increase in the incidence of congenital malformations, growth retardation, or fetal death, but carcinogenic or mutagenic effects are possible.[22,24,28] The probability of these effects occurring is estimated to be less than 1/1000 per cGy.[2,4]

Obviously, radiation exposure is not the only risk confronting the developing embryo and fetus. Factors contributing to risk include smoking, alcohol consumption, drugs, maternal age and size, parity, socioeconomic status, placental abnormali-

TABLE 12–7.   Doses to Embryo from Various Radiopharmaceuticals

Radiopharmaceutical	Administered activity mCi (MBq)*	Dose to embryo (cGy)
Tc-99m pertechnetate	10 (370)	0.27
Tc-99m polyphosphate	10 (370)	0.25
Tc-99m DTPA	10 (370)	0.35
Tc-99m sulfur colloid	2 (74)	0.014
Ga-67 citrate	2 (74)	0.50
Se-75 methionine	0.25 (9)	0.95

*1 mCi = 37 MBq.
From Husak, V. and Wiedermann, M.[27]

ties, toxemia, diabetes, and malnutrition.[29] Though difficult to quantitate, these risks should be considered together with the risks of radiation exposure. Depending on radiation dose, the radiation risk may be small compared to other possible risks of pregnancy.[30]

Some nuclear medicine procedures are potentially dangerous to the embryo and fetus. A critical factor is the degree of placental permeability for a given radiation carrier. The placenta can be completely permeable to small molecules of sugars, amino acids, etc. and impermeable to large protein molecules, colloidal suspensions, or small molecules that attach themselves to protein carriers during metabolism. Radiopharmaceuticals hazardous to the developing embryo or fetus include Se-75 selenomethionine, radioactive noble gases, ionic Ca-47, Sr-85, and Tl-201, all of which readily cross the placental barrier.[23]

Probably the most dangerous procedure is thyroid imaging and function studies carried out with radioiodine. Iodine freely crosses the placental barrier; in addition, the fetal thyroid concentrates iodine six to seven times more avidly than the maternal thyroid.[23] There have been reports of complete destruction of the fetal thyroid with severe exophthalmos and microcephaly associated with therapeutic doses (millicuries) of radioiodine in unknown pregnancies.

In many cases, the placenta is impermeable to the radiopharmaceutical and consequently less dangerous. Examples include liver scanning with radiocolloids, kidney and brain scanning with chelates and lung scanning with macroaggregates.

Organ imaging with radiopharmaceuticals appears to bear relatively little danger to the fetus with the exception of thyroid scanning with I-131. For radiopharmaceuticals that are confined to the maternal compartment, fetal irradiation by gamma rays is approximately equal to or less than the amount received in most x-ray diagnostic procedures.[23]

Therapeutic applications of radiopharmaceuticals, especially radiophosphorus and radioiodine, can result in serious problems during pregnancy. Radiocontamination with megabecquerel (millicurie) doses of P-32 may produce severe damage to the developing central nervous system.

Exposure of the embryo or fetus represents a serious problem not only from medical considerations but also because of parents' concern and anxiety. When it is learned that irradiation occurred early in pregnancy, serious questions arise regarding the consequences to the baby and the necessity of abortion.

The referring physician is the key individual in preventing irradiation of the pregnant or potentially pregnant patient. He initiates the diagnostic process and is likely to know of the patient's pregnancy status. Nuclear medicine request forms should have clearly marked sections dealing with pregnancy status, to heighten the awareness of the referring physician and to alert the nuclear medicine physician and technicians to inquire further about the possibility of pregnancy. Bureau of Radiologic Health posters are available to inform patients about the importance of pregnancy status.[30]

When a pregnant or potentially pregnant patient is a candidate for radiodiagnostic examination, the referring physician, in consultation with the nuclear physician, has several possible courses of action open to him, depending upon the examination required and patient's needs. (1) The pregnancy status may be disregarded and the full examination performed. (2) The procedure may be modified to include only selected studies; however, in this instance, modification should not compromise diagnostic value. (3) The examination may be deferred until after delivery, or in the case of a suspected, but unconfirmed pregnancy, until pregnancy is ruled out. (4) The examination may be canceled altogether. Detailed considerations of procedures to minimize radiation exposure of the fetus and management of the pregnant or potentially pregnant patient have been published by the Bureau of Radiologic Health.[31]

Despite efforts to eliminate accidental exposures of the embryo, there are situations, e.g., during a clinical emergency, in which the fetus will be exposed to radiation. In such cases, after-the-fact dose estimation is essential. As discussed earlier, making dose estimates may be difficult. Furthermore, it is impossible to attribute a given effect in a baby to a small dose of radiation received by the mother during pregnancy. Many other maternal and environmental factors influence the health of the child.[30] All that can be said about radiation exposure is that it increases the probability of damage and that the probability increases with dose.

Frequently, physicians have relied on the "Danish Rule" as a guideline in reaching a clinical decision on the necessity of therapeutic abortion.[32] This rule suggests that therapeutic abortions are advised when the fetal dose exceeds 10 cGy but gives no consideration to other biomedical or personal factors. Since a fetal dose of 10 cGy is rarely encountered in nuclear medicine procedures, and since other pregnancy risk factors are important considerations, the "Danish Rule" is not useful in the evaluation of most cases. Each case must be considered individually, and all pregnancy risks and personal factors weighed appropriately.[30]

HIGH DOSES OF RADIATION: BIOLOGIC EFFECTS OF RADIOTHERAPEUTIC NUCLEAR MEDICINE PROCEDURES

Radiotherapeutic procedures are usually associated with organ doses in excess of 1000 cGy. High radiation doses to specific body areas, as in the treatment of neoplastic diseases, result in destruction of tissues in the irradiated volume. Whole body radiation exposure, which is biologically more effective than partial body exposure, can be lethal with doses as low as 200 cGy, as a consequence of dysfunction of such critical normal tissues as bone marrow and the gastrointestinal tract. These effects at high doses are usually attributed to cell killing.

Effects on Cells

A variety of effects has been observed in the division process of cells. Mitosis may be delayed or completely inhibited with doses of radiation as low as 50 cGy.[33] The specific response depends on the type of cell, its mitotic rate, and irradiation factors. The results of many experiments indicate the following:

1. Most cells in division at the time of irradiation complete the division.
2. Those cells irradiated just prior to division may be delayed in entering division.
3. Synthesis of DNA may be partially or completely inhibited.
4. Cells may be inhibited from entering DNA synthesis.
5. Cells in early prophase (first stage of mitosis) may be delayed or caused to revert to the premitotic configuration.

Cells can also be killed by radiation. For the purposes of this discussion, differentiated cells, such as nerve cells and muscle cells, may be considered killed if a particular function has been lost. For cells that divide, such as hemopoietic stem cells and crypt cells of the small intestine, death means the loss of proliferative capacity, sometimes referred to as *reproductive death*.

Though other definitions may be proposed for cell death, reproductive death for proliferating cells is the most relevant for several reasons: (1) proliferative capacity is an easy endpoint to measure, (2) the radiation responses of whole animals and their tissues may be explained by the loss of proliferative capacity of cells in certain critical cell populations, and (3) in the radiation therapy of tumors, the primary objective is to sterilize tumorigenic cells, that is, to prevent tumorigenic cells from dividing indefinitely and causing further growth and spread of disease.

In general, doses greater than 1000 cGy are needed to destroy cell function in nonproliferating systems, such as the central nervous system, whereas doses of 50 cGy can result in loss of proliferative capacity in dividing cells.[34] Cells that have lost their reproductive integrity, however, may still retain the capacity to metabolize.

Figure 12–1 shows the relation between radiation dose and surviving fraction of a population of cells when survival is measured by proliferative capacity. The survival curve has a characteristic shape—an initial shoulder region followed by a straighter and steeper portion on a semilogarithmic plot. The shoulder region implies that damage must be accumulated before the lethal effect is evident. Several targets or key sites in the cell must be damaged for the cell to lose its proliferative capacity.

Low doses of radiation inactivate some, but not all, of the target sites. As the dose increases, more target sites are inactivated. Finally, in the exponential part of the curve, all but one of the critical sites have been hit. Further increase in dose results in *exponential cell killing* (the same proportion of cells is killed with each dose increment), which may be interpreted to mean that an inactivating event in the last remaining target site kills the cell. The slope of the survival curve reflects the sensitivity of the cells: the steeper the slope, the greater the sensitivity. Slope is expressed in terms of the dose required to reduce the number of surviving cells by a factor of 0.37, usually designated D_0. For most mammalian cells (normal and neoplastic), D_0 lies between 100 and 200 cGy, indicating little, if any, difference in radiosensitivity among proliferating mam-

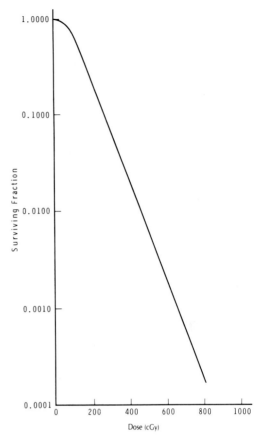

Fig. 12–1. A typical survival curve for mammalian cells exposed to radiation, such as x-rays or gamma rays. The fraction of cells surviving (measured by colony formation) is plotted on a logarithmic scale against dose on a linear scale.

malian cells in which reproductive capacity is the end point.

The mechanism by which cells lose their reproductive capacity is not entirely clear. The sensitive sites in the cell responsible for this effect have not been identified, but much evidence indicates that they reside in the nucleus rather than in the cytoplasm. Furthermore, there is evidence for regarding the chromosome as the primary target for radiation, and chromosomal damage is widely believed to be the major cause of reproductive death.[13]

Chromosomes contain DNA, the cell's

primary information system, which directs cell activity. The sequence of bases within DNA molecules constitutes the code for this information system. If the linear base sequence is altered, the DNA may transfer incorrect information, resulting in synthesis of a wrong protein that may be toxic to the cell. Alternatively, a damaged DNA molecule may be unable to transfer information for synthesis of a critical protein. The shortage of such a protein could delay mitosis, alter some metabolic pathway important in cell function, or cause cell death.

If a portion of a chromosome is broken, inverted, or exchanged, the cell may survive for a long time because it has a full complement of DNA. If the cell divides, however, some of the genetic information may not be transmitted to the daughter cells. The lost genetic information may lead to dysfunction (such as transformation to a cancerous state) or death of one or both of the daughter cells. Extensive chromosomal aberrations are usually lethal to the cell as soon as it attempts to enter mitosis.

Not all mammalian cells respond to radiation in the same way. In general, cells that divide regularly, such as hemopoietic stem cells, are relatively sensitive to radiation damage. Differentiated cells, such as muscle and nerve, do not divide and are radiation-resistant. As early as 1906, the French radiobiologists Bergonié and Tribondeau, recognized this difference. They studied the effect of radiation on rat testes and observed that dividing germinal cells were markedly affected by radiation while nondividing interstitial cells appeared undamaged. On the basis of these observations, Bergonié and Tribondeau formulated a law that broadly states that radiosensitivity varies *directly* with the mitotic activity and with the number of future divisions the cells will undergo and *inversely* with the degree of morphologic and functional differentiation.

Although many exceptions to this law are now known (e.g., the small lymphocyte and oocyte), it may still be used as a general guide for predicting the relative sensitivity of cells. In Table 12–8 cells are listed in order of decreasing relative sensitivity. A close look at the table reveals that radiosensitivities predicted by the law are consistent with the observed relative radiosensitivities.

Effects on Tissues

Tissues differ in their response to radiation. The hemopoietic tissues are extremely sensitive in showing effects (e.g., leukopenia) after whole-body doses as low as 25 cGy.[35] Other tissues, such as muscle or nerve, can withstand massive doses (1000 cGy) without apparent injury. Part of this variation in tissue sensitivity may be attributed to different cell sensitivities that make up the tissues. Other factors, such as cell turnover time, various cell interactions, and capacity to repopulate, also influence tissue response to radiation. In Table 12–9, sensitivity of various tissues in order of decreasing sensitivity is presented.

For many tissues, the principal radiation effect is hypoplasia resulting in altered tissue function. Depending on the particular tissue and dose of radiation, functional alteration can occur within hours or days of exposure. Of particular interest in nuclear medicine is the effect upon thyroid tissue following I-131 administration for thyrotoxicosis or thyroid carcinoma. Thyroid tissue is relatively radioresistant to direct cytocidal actions of radiation (Table 12–9). Massive doses of radiation are usually needed to produce thyroid ablation.[35] The histologic and functional effects of I-131 administration on the thyroid has been studied extensively in both man and laboratory animals.[36] In human thyroids studied within 2 months of administration of a therapeutic dose of I-131, the changes observed included nuclear pyknosis, cellular necrosis, breakdown of follicles, development

TABLE 12–8. *Relative Radiosensitivities of Mammalian Cells*

Relative radiosensitivity	Cell type	Characteristics
High	Hemopoietic stem cells, spermatogonia, intestinal crypt cells	Short-lived; undifferentiated; divide regularly
Fairly high	Precursor cells of hemopoietic series	Divide limited number of times; differentiate to some degree
Medium	Endothelial cells, fibroblasts	Divide irregularly; life span highly variable
Fairly low	Epithelial cells of liver, kidney, salivary gland, etc.	Long-lived; do not divide often; variable degree of differentiation
Low	Neurons, erythrocytes, muscle cells, etc.	Do not divide; highly differentiated

Based on Rubin, P., and Casarett, G.[35]

TABLE 12–9. *Relative Tissue Radiosensitivity*

Relative sensitivity	Tissues
High	Lymphoid, hemopoietic, spermatogenic epithelium, intestinal epithelium
Fairly high	Oropharyngeal stratified epithelium, epidermal epithelium
Medium	Interstitial connective tissue, fine vascular, growing cartilage and bone
Fairly low	Mature cartilage and bone; hepatic, renal, pancreatic, thyroid, and adrenal epithelium
Low	Muscle, neuronal tissue

Based on Rubin, P. and Casarett, G.[35]

of bizarre cell forms, capillary thrombosis, and stromal edema. Chronic radiation effects include development of abnormal cell forms, derangement of the follicles, reduction of colloid, and small-vessel telangiectasia.[36] Shrinkage of gland size results from the failure of thyroid cells to reproduce. Rubin and Casarett, and Wilson have written excellent reviews of thyroid radiopathology.[35,36]

Effects on the Whole Body

When an individual is exposed to a sufficient amount of radiation, changes occur in many tissues and organs of the body, depending on the radiation dose, extent of exposure, age, and state of health. Most of the information regarding effects in man come from the Japanese survivors at Hiroshima and Nagasaki, from radiation accidents, and from radiation therapy patients.

In Table 12–10, the most common sources of radiation exposure in man are listed. Background radiation exposure and medical radiodiagnosis involve low doses of radiation. As previously discussed, the biologic effects of low doses are mutagenesis, carcinogenesis, and in utero effects; the extent to which these effects occur is not well known. Radiotherapy exposures involve approximately 500,000 patients per year. As discussed earlier, cell death and tissue (neoplastic and normal) destruction result.

In whole-body radiation exposures at high doses, which may occur in industrial accidents or nuclear explosions, the total

TABLE 12–10. *Radiation Exposure in Man*

Source	Population exposed	Duration of exposure	Exposure conditions	Radiation effects
Medical radiodiagnosis (incl. nuclear medicine)	150,000,000 per yr	intermittent throughout life	low dose to part of body (~1 cGy)	mutations? cancer? in utero effects?
Natural background radiation	entire population	throughout life	low dose to whole body (0.1 cGy/yr)	mutations? cancer? in utero effects?
Radiotherapy	500,000 per yr	2 mo	high dose to part of body (>1,000 cGy)	tumor control; normal tissue effects
Industrial accidents; military activities	tens of thousands may be exposed	seconds to days	high dose to whole body (doses vary widely)	normal tissue dysfunction; death

body is as sensitive as the most sensitive of vital tissues, i.e., the hemopoietic tissues. The whole body dose-response curve for acute radiation lethality is sigmoid in shape (Fig. 12–2).

As the dose of radiation increases, the probability of survival decreases. Doses below about 200 cGy are nonlethal to any individual; intermediate doses in the range of about 200 to 600 cGy are lethal in a fraction of the exposed population, and lethality is directly proportional to dose; doses in excess of 600 cGy are lethal in 100% of the population. The lack of a sharp transition from 0 to 100% lethality indicates that many factors, some unknown, determine the response of the individual to a specific radiation dose.

It is customary when considering acute radiation lethality to refer to the LD_{50} value, or *median lethal dose*. This dose of radiation kills 50% of exposed individuals. For man, the LD_{50} is not known exactly but is believed to be in the range of 250 to 450 cGy (x-ray or gamma radiation). Comparison of LD_{50} doses between man and other mammals indicates that man is relatively sensitive to whole-body radiation.

Following radiation exposure, a variety of tissue and organ changes may be grossly visible or visible only at the microscopic level. In Table 12–11 the various syndromes as they occur in man are described. The syndrome latency period is a

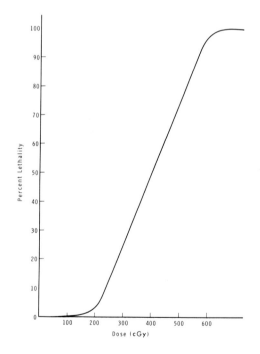

Fig. 12–2. The sigmoid dose-response curve describes the relation between radiation dose and percent lethality in the exposed population. Low doses result in no lethality; intermediate doses result in lethality in a fraction of the population directly proportional to dose; and high doses result in 100% lethality in the exposed population.

time after exposure when no signs or symptoms are manifest. This does not mean that nothing is happening; on the contrary, radiation damage is developing.

It should not be inferred from Table 12–11 that a dose of radiation produces effects in only one organ system. An individual receiving an exposure of 5000 cGy or more will die from damage to the central nervous system. Damage has also been done to the bone marrow and gastrointestinal tract, however. Because this exposure results in death from central nervous system damage in 1 or 2 days, bone marrow and gastrointestinal effects hardly have time to develop fully, let alone contribute to the death of the individual. With lower doses of radiation, such that the individual may survive for at least a week or two, the effects on several systems contribute to the overall radiation damage. The major systems involved are the gastrointestinal, hemopoietic, vascular, and endocrine.[34]

At the tissue level, perturbations in cell population kinetics have been implicated as the major pathophysiologic disturbance resulting in the bone marrow and gastrointestinal syndromes.[37] The critical cells involved are the *progenitor cells*, or *stem cells*, from which all functional cells of the

tissue are derived. If cell production stops in stem cell populations, normal losses of the mature functioning elements are not replaced. Temporary inhibition or complete cessation of mitosis in stem cells, which give rise to the formed elements of the blood, or in the cells lining the villi in the gastrointestinal mucosa results in rapid deterioration of function in these systems.

Unlike gastrointestinal and hemopoietic tissues, the central nervous system is a nonproliferating tissue. The exact and immediate cause of the central nervous system syndrome is not fully understood, but vasculitis, encephalitis, meningitis, and edema have been suggested as the major underlying pathologic processes of the syndrome.[35]

FACTORS INFLUENCING BIOLOGIC EFFECTS

Several factors influence the biologic effects of radiation discussed so far. The most important physical factor is radiation dose. To reduce the risk of adverse biologic effects in nuclear medicine procedures as well as in diagnostic radiology, the absorbed dose should be the minimum

TABLE 12–11.   *Acute Radiation Syndromes after Whole-Body Irradiation*

Aspects	Central nervous system syndrome	Gastrointestinal syndrome	Hemopoietic syndrome
Chief determining organ	Brain	Small intestine	Bone marrow
Syndrome threshold	2000 R	500 R	100 R
Syndrome latency	¼ hr–3 hr	3–5 days	2–3 weeks
Death threshold	5000 R	1000 R	200 R
Death time	Within 2 days	3–14 days	3–8 weeks
Characteristic signs and symptoms	Lethargy, tremors, convulsions, ataxia	Malaise, anorexia, nausea, vomiting, diarrhea, GI malfunction, fever, dehydration, electrolyte loss, circulatory collapse	Malaise, fever, dyspnea on exertion, fatigue, leukopenia, thrombopenia purpura

Based on Rubin, P. and Casarett, G.[35]

amount consistent with the acquisition of adequate diagnostic information.

A radiation dose may be defined as minimal when the radionuclide has an effective average time in the body equal to the time of the nuclear medicine procedure, that is, from administration of the radionuclide to completion of scanning, sampling, or counting.[38] During the last several years, the greatest advances in minimizing radiation dose have resulted from the introduction of (1) metastable radionuclides, such as Tc-99m, that emit mainly gamma rays, (2) radionuclides with short physical half-lives, and (3) radiopharmaceuticals with rapid biologic elimination.

The radiation dose rate also contributes to the severity of the biologic effect. In general, for a given radiation dose, the biologic effect is greater at high dose rates than at low dose rates, and single or acute exposures produce greater effects than do fractionated exposures. Another factor is the volume of tissue irradiated: the greater the volume, the greater the biologic effect. For instance, whole body doses greater than 200 to 300 cGy may be lethal, whereas doses greater than 1000 cGy directed to only a small part of the body may be readily tolerated.

The type of radiation delivered greatly affects biologic response. The spatial distribution of ionizing events is determined by the average rate of energy loss per unit path length (the linear energy transfer, or LET). Radiations with high LET are densely ionizing and biologically more effective than low LET radiations, which are sparsely ionizing. Table 12–12 lists some types of radiations and their LET values. Gamma rays and beta particles, the two radiations of principal interest in nuclear medicine, have relatively low LET and are generally less biologically effective than neutrons or alpha particles.

In this chapter, risks of radiation exposure have been described. At low doses, the major risks are carcinogenesis, genetic

TABLE 12–12. *LET Values for Several Types of Radiations*

Radiation	LET (keV/μ)	Biologic effectiveness
Co-60 gamma	0.3	Low
0.6-keV beta	5.5	↓
Fission neutrons	45.0	
Alpha	110.0	High

Based on Casarett, A.[33]

effects, and in utero effects. At high doses, cell killing, tissue effects, and lethality may occur. The risks and benefits associated with high doses of radiation, e.g., as used in cancer therapy, are often obvious. Risks of radiodiagnostic procedures (low doses of radiation) are not as obvious. The extent of radiation damage at low doses (in the diagnostic range) has yet to be determined. Estimates of risk by extrapolation from effects at high radiation doses indicate that for carcinogenesis, the hazard is small when compared with such risks as cigarette smoking and automobile travel.[39] The radiation risk, however small, should always be weighed against potential benefits to the patient.

How can nuclear medicine physicians reduce the potential radiation risk to the patient? The following are a few measures that can be taken:

1. The amount of radionuclide should be kept as small as possible, consistent with obtaining statistically valid diagnostic information.

2. Tc-99m and other metastable radionuclides reduce the radiation dose because they emit mainly gamma rays and lack beta particles.

3. The effective half-time of the radionuclide should be about equal to the total time of the procedure. Radioactivity remaining in the patient after the conclusion of the nuclear medicine procedure needlessly contributes to dose.

4. Needless radiation occurs when radiopharmaceuticals are concen-

trated in nontarget tissues (i.e., regions of the body not involved in the study). Such concentrations can be reduced by diluting the radioisotope with large quantities of nonradioactive isotope, and by decreasing uptake of the radiopharmaceuticals by administering nonradioactive agents chemically identical or similar to the particular radiopharmaceutical. An example is the use of Lugol's solution to block uptake of free I-131 when administering I-131 labeled radiopharmaceuticals.

REFERENCES

1. Lea, D.: Actions of Radiation on Living Cells. London, Cambridge University Press, 1956.
2. United Nations Scientific Committee on the Effects of Atomic Radiation (UNSCEAR): Sources and Effects of Ionizing Radiation. New York, United Nations, 1977.
3. Biological Effects of Ionizing Radiations, Committee (BEIR): The Effects on Populations of Exposure to Low Levels of Ionizing Radiation: 1980. National Research Council, Washington, D.C., National Academy Press, 1980.
4. Mole, R.: Radiation effects on prenatal development and their radiological significance. Br. J. Radiol., *52*:89, 1979.
5. Interagency Task Force on the Health Effects of Ionizing Radiation: Report of the Work Group on Science. Washington, D.C., U.S. Dept. of Health, Education, and Welfare, June 1979.
6. Miller, R.: Radiation induced cancer. J. Nat. Cancer Inst., *49*:1221, 1972.
7. Boice, J., et al.: Risk of breast cancer following low-dose exposure. Radiology, *131*:589, 1979.
8. Krauss, S., and Wasserman, I.: Leukemia in patients with polycythemia vera treated with radioisotopes. *In* Medical Radionuclides: Radiation Dose and Effects (AEC Symposium 20), U.S. Atomic Energy Commission, Division of Technical Information, 1970, p 441.
9. Swarm, R.: Late effects following the medical uses of colloidal thorium dioxide. *In* Medical Radionuclides: Radiation Dose and Effects (AEC Symposium 20), U.S. Atomic Energy Commission, Division of Technical Information, 1970, p. 387.
10. Gaulden, M.: Genetic effects of radiation. *In* Medical Radiation Biology. Philadelphia, W.B. Saunders, 1973.
11. Yuhas, J., and Storer, J.: Radiation hazards. *In* Primer of Radiobiology. New York, GAF Corporation, 1971.
12. Schull, W., et al.: Genetic effects of the atomic bombs: A reappraisal. Science, *213*:1220, 1981.
13. Hall, E.: Radiobiology for the Radiologist. 2nd ed. Hagerstown, MD, Harper & Row, 1978.
14. Crow, J.: Can we assess genetic risk? *In* Radiation Research: Proceedings of the Sixth International Congress of Radiation Research, Tokyo, Japanese Association for Radiation Research, 1979, p. 70.
15. Cantolino, S., et al.: Persistent chromosomal aberrations following radioiodine therapy for thyrotoxicosis. N. Engl. J. Med., *275*:739, 1966.
16. Boyd, J., et al.: Chromosome studies on women formerly employed as luminous-dial painters. Br. Med. J., *1*:377, 1966.
17. Lisco, H., and Conard, R.: Chromosome studies on Marshall Islanders exposed to fallout radiation. Science, *157*:445, 1967.
18. Fischer, P., et al.: Chromosomal aberrations in thorium dioxide patients. Ann. N.Y. Acad. Sci., *145*:759, 1967.
19. Bloom, A.: Cytogenetic effects of low-dose internal and external radiations. *In* Medical Radionuclides: Radiation Dose and Effects (AEC Symposium 20), U.S. Atomic Energy Commission, Division of Technical Information, 1970, p. 245.
20. Hoffman, D., et al.: Effects of Ionizing Radiation on the Developing Embryo and Fetus: A Review. U.S. Dept. of Health and Human Services, Public Health Service, Food and Drug Administration, Bureau of Radiological Health, Rockville, Maryland. HHS Publication FDA 81-8170, 1981.
21. Dekaban, A.: Abnormalities in children exposed to x-radiation during various stages of gestation: Tentative timetable of radiation injury to the human fetus. Part I. J. Nucl. Med., *9*:471, 1968.
22. Brent, R., and Gorson, O.: Radiation exposure in pregnancy. Current Problems in Radiology, *2*:1, 1972.
23. Sternberg, J.: Radiation risk and pregnancy. Clin. Obstet. Gynecol., *16*:235, 1973.
24. Brent, R.: Radiation teratogenesis. Teratology, *21*:281, 1980.
25. Gaulden, M.: Possible effects of diagnostic x-rays on the human embryo and fetus. J. Arkansas Med. Soc., *70*:424, 1974.
26. Cloutier, R., et al.: Radiation dosimetry. *In* Textbook of Nuclear Medicine: Basic Science. Philadelphia, Lea & Febiger, 1978.
27. Husak, V., and Wiedermann, M.: Radiation absorbed dose estimates to the embryo from some nuclear medicine procedures. Eur. J. Nucl. Med., *5*:205, 1980.
28. National Council on Radiation Protection and Measurements: Medical Radiation Exposure of Pregnant and Potentially Pregnant Women. Report 54. Washington, D.C., NCRP, 1977.
29. Brown, A., and Freehafer, J.: Prenatal risks—a pediatrician's point of view. *In* Risks in the Practice of Modern Obstetrics. 2nd ed. St. Louis, C.V. Mosby, 1975.
30. Mossman, K., and Hill, L.: Radiation risks in pregnancy. Obstet. Gynecol., *60*:237, 1982.
31. Bureau of Radiological Health: Radiation Recommendation Series. Procedures to Minimize Diagnostic X-ray Exposure of the Human Embryo and Fetus. U.S. Dept. of Health and Human Serv-

ices, Food and Drug Administration, Rockville, MD, HHS Publication FDA 81-8178, 1981.

32. Hammer-Jacobsen, E.: Therapeutic abortion on account of x-ray. Dan. Med. Bull., *6*:113, 1959.

33. Casarett, A.: Radiation Biology. Englewood Cliffs, NJ, Prentice-Hall, 1968.

34. Cox, R., and Masson, W.: X-ray survival curves of cultured human diploid fibroblasts. *In* Proceedings of the Sixth L.H. Gray Conference. Cell Survival After Low Doses of Radiation. London, John Wiley & Sons, 1975.

35. Rubin, P., and Casarett, G.: Clinical Radiation Pathology. Philadelphia, W.B. Saunders, 1968.

36. Wilson, G.: The treatment of thyrotoxicosis by radioiodine. *In* The Thyroid. Physiology and Treatment of Disease. New York, Pergamon Press, 1979.

37. Bond, V., Fliedner, T., and Archambeau, J.: Mammalian Radiation Lethality: A Disturbance in Cellular Kinetics. New York, Academic Press, 1965.

38. Mitchell, T.: Practical factors in radiation dose reduction. *In* Pediatric Nuclear Medicine. Philadelphia, W.B. Saunders, 1974.

39. Mossman, K.: Analysis of risk in computerized tomography and other diagnostic radiology procedures. Computerized Radiology, *6*:251, 1982.

Chapter 13

RADIATION SAFETY

ROGER L. AAMODT AND
JOHN HARBERT

Radiation safety, health physics, radio-logic health, and radiation protection are all terms that denote the discipline devoted to the protection of individuals from the hazards of ionizing radiation. The health physicist must protect workers from the possible adverse effects of ionizing radiation while, at the same time, ensuring the beneficial application of radiation sources. In practice, this rule means that the cost of protection should never be allowed to exceed the benefits in terms of increased protection to the worker, and that the risk to the worker should never be allowed to exceed the benefits of the application.

A large body of experimental and observational data has been gathered relating to the biologic effects of radiation (see Chapter 12). Much of this information is derived from animal studies. The remainder comes from the relatively few cases of accidental human exposure and from medical applications of atomic energy. While these studies provide much knowledge of the dangers of exposure to high doses of ionizing radiation, the effects of low doses are still incompletely understood. The balancing of benefits versus risks is difficult when the ranges of doses

concerned are those for which biologic effects have not yet been observed.

Radionuclides and other radiation sources have made possible many important advances in biology and medicine, but they have also created a unique set of problems associated with their increasing use. Soon after the discovery of x-rays by Roentgen in 1895 and Becquerel's nearly simultaneous discovery of natural emissions from certain minerals, it became apparent that these radiations could produce serious harmful biologic effects. This recognition and the resulting attempts to define the magnitude of the dangers and to restrict radiation exposure marked the real beginning of health physics.

During the first 50 years of radiation development, exposure limits were somewhat arbitrary, generally voluntary, and related to easily observed acute effects. Initial attempts to develop guidelines for exposure to external radiation sources were based on the production of erythema, or reddening of the skin. Since 1925, when Mutscheller suggested a limit of 1/100 of an erythema dose in 30 days (0.2 R/day), various erythema-based limits have been suggested by several individuals and committees. As more penetrating x-rays came into use and better measurement systems were developed, the tolerance dose was further reduced to 100 mR/day by 1936.

The modern era of health physics really began with the Manhattan Project. Just prior to the construction of the first nuclear reactor at the University of Chicago in 1942, a group primarily composed of physicists was assembled to deal with the safety problems posed by the production of large amounts of fission products and then later by the chemical processing plants associated with the development of nuclear weapons. The early health physicists were given the task of creating a discipline with all of the associated technology required to maintain safe working conditions. It is a tribute to the skills and intelligence of these pioneers that the nuclear industry has maintained one of the best safety records of any industry (Table 13–1). The National Council on Radiation Protection and Measurements (NCRP) reduced the maximum permissible occupational exposure limits in 1945. Exposure to blood-forming organs was limited to 300 mrem/week, skin exposure was limited to 600 mrem/week, and exposure to hands and feet was limited to 1.5 rem/week. Individuals over 45 years of age were allowed exposures of twice these

limits. These limits were adopted by the International Commission on Radiation Protection (ICRP) in the following year. A further reduction in maximum permissible dose levels to 100 mrem/week to the total body was recommended by the ICRP in 1956 and by the NCRP in 1957. Although each reduction in the radiation dose to occupationally exposed workers was probably based on the availability of new data, and specifically on an awareness of the increased genetic risk to the population as more and more workers entered the nuclear industry, the NCRP has stressed that the reductions were not the result of positive evidence of damage due to the use of earlier recommendations. Recommendations of the ICRP and NCRP since 1958 have related primarily to exposures to the general population, pregnant women, and persons under 18 years of age. A summary of current NCRP recommendations is shown in Table 13–2.

The current philosophy of radiation protection is based upon two major premises: (1) All exposure to radiation may be harmful; thus all doses must be minimized. (2) Exposure of large numbers of people to small amounts of radiation can produce the same genetic effects in a population as the exposure of a small number of people to large doses of radiation.

These two tenets have led to the "as low as reasonably achievable" (ALARA) philosophy, which now governs the approaches of the U.S. Nuclear Regulatory Commission (NRC) and many other national regulatory agencies. Under this approach, each exposure situation should be evaluated, not in terms of how to avoid exceeding maximum permissible exposure values, but rather in terms of how to achieve the lowest exposure commensurate with reasonable cost and effort.

A recent review of the various federal agencies that regulate radioactive materials in medicine is given by Sodd.[4]

RADIATION UNITS

The development of well-defined units of radioactivity and of energy deposition

TABLE 13–1. *Work Related Injury Rates for Selected Industries*

Industry	Frequency* rate	Severity† rate
All	8.1	668
Atomic workers‡	0.9	200
Aerospace	2.2	166
Steel	3.5	709
Machinery	4.7	317
Electric utilities	5.9	1072
Petroleum	7.2	736
Printing and publishing	10.0	434
Food	13.2	719
Air transport	22.1	508
Undergound mining (except coal)	28.1	4320

*Frequency rate—injuries per million man-hours.
†Severity rate—days lost per million man-hours.
‡Data from Morgan, K.Z., and Turner, J.E.[1]

TABLE 13–2. *Current NCRP Dose Limits*

	Maximum Permissible Dose Equivalent for Occupational Exposure
Combined whole body occupational exposure	
Prospective annual limit	5 rems (50 mSv) in any one year
Retrospective annual limit	10–15 rems (100–150 mSv) in any one year
Long-term accumulation	(N − 18) × 5 rems, where N is age in years
Skin	15 rems (150 mSv) in any one year
Hands	75 rems (750 mSv) in any one year (25/qtr)
Forearms	30 rems (300 mSv) in any one year (10/qtr)
Other organs, tissues and organ systems	15 rems (150 mSv) in any one year (5/qtr)
Fertile women (with respect to fetus)	0.5 rem (5 mSv) in gestation period
	Dose Limits for the Public, or for Occasionally Exposed Individuals
Individual or Occasional	0.5 rem (5 mSv) in any one year
Students	0.1 rem (1 mSv) in any one year

From NCRP Reports No 39, 1971, and No 43, 1975.[2,3]

by ionizing radiation in matter was essential for the establishment of clear standards for the use of radionuclides. The International Commission on Radiological Units and Measurements (ICRU) originally defined four special radiation units: the roentgen (R) to be used only as a measure of exposure, the *rad* (D) to be used as a measure of radiation absorbed dose, the rem (H) to be used as a measure of dose equivalent, and the curie (Ci) to be used as a measure of activity. These units have now been replaced with radiation units in the International System of Units (SI), which are given in Appendix A. New SI units include the gray (Gy = 1 J kg^{-1} = 100 rad), the sievert (Sv = 1 J kg^{-1} = 100 rem), and the becquerel (Bq = 1 d sec^{-1} = 2.703 × 10^{-11} Ci). The unit to replace the roentgen has not yet been named. The ICRU intends for these new special radiation units to be adopted completely by 1985.

The roentgen was first defined in 1928 as a measure of the energy deposition of x-rays in air. The restriction to x-rays has since been dropped, and the definition of R expanded to include all photons with energy below 3 MeV. *Exposure* is defined as the total electrical charge of all ions of one sign produced in a unit mass of air. The roentgen is defined as 2.58 × 10^{-4} coulombs/kg in dry air at standard temperature and pressure. This amount is equivalent to 87 ergs/g of air at standard temperature and pressure.

The rad was designed to fill the need for a unit of energy deposition that was not restricted to air and would be applicable to radiations other than photons. It is a measure of *radiation absorbed dose,* which is defined as the energy imparted to a unit mass of matter. The rad is specifically defined as the deposition of 100 ergs/g to the volume of interest. This is equal to 62.4 × 10^6 MeV per gram and 0.01 gray. As a general rule of thumb, 1 rad is approximately equal to the dose to soft tissue resulting from exposure to 1 R of intermediate-energy x-rays or gamma rays.

The rem was developed in response to a considerable body of evidence that indicated that the biologic effects of exposure to different types or distribution patterns of radiation were often different for the same radiation absorbed dose. The *dose equivalent* is defined as the absorbed dose times two other factors: the *quality factor*, Q, a defined unit related to linear energy transfer used to express differences in biologic effectiveness of various ionizing radiations; and the *distribution factor,* N, which is used to correct for differences in the distribution of internally deposited radionuclides on the observed biologic effects. The distribution factor and all other factors used in weighting the absorbed dose are currently assigned the value of 1. Thus the dose equivalent, H, is the product of D and Q, or:

$$H = DQ$$

The unit of dose equivalent is assigned the special name *sievert* (Sv) where 1 Sv = 100 rem (see Appendix A).

The curie is a measure of activity that was originally based on the disintegration rate of 1 g of radium but is now defined as the amount of any radionuclide that has an activity equal to 3.7×10^{10} dps. When multiple events occur following the emission of a particle, the whole process is considered to be one disintegration.

Recently, the ICRU has designated the becquerel (Bq) the special unit of radioactivity.[5] Throughout this book, activity is given in both curies and becquerels for convenience.

PRINCIPLES OF RADIATION PROTECTION

The responsibilities of the health physicist can be divided into three categories: (1) personnel protection, (2) area control activities, and (3) waste disposal. All of these activities have as their primary goal the prevention of unnecessary exposure or dose commitment from the use of atomic energy.

Control of External Exposure

In general, the health physicist cannot control all uses or sources of external exposure. What he can and must do is insist that all workers be aware of applicable regulations and means of controlling radiation exposure, that adequate procedures be available for measurement of personnel radiation exposures, and that work areas be designed for optimum control. The degree of control required in any specific situation depends on the probability of exposure and the balancing of benefits and risks by the health physicist. Control of exposure to sources of ionizing radiation includes the establishment of areas of restricted occupancy, limitations on the time an employee may spend in the radiation area, and shielding to minimize exposure to the source. Work areas should be designed with exposure factors in mind and may include areas designed to prevent either unauthorized access or access when the source is in an unsafe condition.

Three methods of reducing the hazard from radiation sources are time, distance, and shielding. *Time* refers to reducing the time of exposure to the source, *distance* refers to maintaining as much distance as possible between the source and anyone working in the area, and *shielding* refers to surrounding the source with enough material to reduce the potential for exposure. Essentially, all systems for protection from external radiation sources use one or more of these three methods.

The simplest and cheapest method is to increase distance. The intensity of gamma ray or x-ray exposure decreases roughly as the inverse of the distance squared. Although this inverse square law holds rigorously only for the case of a point source and a point target, it is, in practice, a good approximation whenever the distance is much larger than the dimensions of the radiation source. Thus, moving from a position 1 m from a source to one 10 m away reduces the exposure by a factor of 100.

Whenever possible, areas that contain radiation sources should be controlled. The degree of control required depends on the hazard and can range from conspicuously posted radiation area signs to complicated interlock systems that bar all unauthorized access. In a typical nuclear medicine laboratory, control can be provided by limiting access to dosing and radionuclide storage areas and arranging patient waiting areas so that they are remote from all sources of external radiation. On the other hand, protection from a multicurie therapy source requires extremely stringent restrictions to access. In handling radionuclides in the laboratory, the distance principle can be applied by requiring the use of forceps whenever possible.

Reducing the time of exposure is another effective way to decrease radiation exposures. In general, this reduced exposure time can be accomplished by careful planning of all activities involving radiation sources. Whenever possible, planning should include not only detailed instructions for the operation, but also dry runs using nonradioactive materials until all aspects of the planned operation are familiar.

The use of shielding to reduce exposure has become a common practice. In general, the optimal shielding material has a high density and a large atomic number. Enclosing the source in a small container is the most efficient use of shielding. Examples of this approach include small lead containers for transport and storage of radionuclides and radiopharmaceuticals, and syringe shields to reduce exposure to patients and personnel during injection.[6] Other approaches include lead and leaded glass barriers to reduce exposure during radiochemical and radiopharmaceutical processing, shielding of walls surrounding x-ray equipment, and heavy shielding surrounding radiation therapy and other high-radiation facilities. Shielding for alpha and beta radiation is much simpler because of their lower penetra-

tion. Most alpha particles can be completely absorbed by a sheet of paper, while a few millimeters of nearly any material are sufficient to absorb all but the highest-energy beta radiation. High-energy beta rays can be hazardous because of the production of bremsstrahlung radiation from interaction with high Z materials. Shielding in these cases (e.g., P-32, Sr-90) is best accomplished by absorbers with a low atomic number, such as lucite, to absorb beta particles with little bremsstrahlung production.

Surveys and Measurements

To ensure that exposures meet the ALARA criteria, it is necessary to measure radiation levels and to carry out routine surveys to map the distribution of radiation levels within the facility. Such surveys are required in 10 CFR 20.201.[7] Appendix I of the NRC Regulatory Guide 10.8 lists the following area survey procedures:[8]

1. All elution, preparation, and injection areas are to be surveyed daily with a low-range, thin-window G-M survey meter.
2. Laboratory areas in which only small quantities of radioactive material are used (less than 200 μCi) are surveyed monthly.
3. All other laboratory areas are surveyed weekly.
4. Weekly and monthly surveys must consist of:
   a. Measurement of radiation levels with a survey meter sufficiently sensitive to detect 0.1 mrem/hr (1 mSv/hr).
   b. Wipe tests sufficiently sensitive to detect 200 dpm/100 cm^2 for the contaminant involved.
5. A permanent record is to be kept of all survey results, including negative results, noting:
   a. Location, date, and type of equipment used.

b. Name of person conducting survey.

c. Area surveyed, identifying such relevant features as active storage areas, active waste areas, etc.

d. Measured exposure rates and contamination levels.

e. Corrective action taken in the case of contamination or excessive exposure rates and reduced contamination levels, or exposure rates after corrective action.

Work areas must be cleaned if the contamination level exceeds 200 dpm/100 cm^2.

Selection of specific instruments or devices depends on the type and energy of the radiation to be detected and the range of exposure likely to be encountered.

Whenever radiation exposure levels exceed a preselected value (0.75 mR/hr), that area should be designated a controlled area and appropriate precautions taken.[10] All personnel entering controlled radiation areas should wear a personnel dosimeter to record their radiation exposure. Careful records of area surveys and personnel exposure are required by law.

Ionization chamber instruments have been used in a wide variety of applications. When care is given to the size, shape, and composition of the chamber, the instruments can be calibrated for accurate measurement of absorbed dose. Pocket dosimeters (see "Gas-Filled Detectors," Chap. 2) designed to measure exposure make use of the ionization chamber concept and can be obtained with ranges from 0.1 to 50 R. Several portable ionization chamber survey meters are available. They have the advantage of being relatively independent of the energy of incident radiation and are not paralyzed at high counting rates. Disadvantages include slow response times, which may interfere with measurement of short bursts of radiation, and low sensitivity.

For most survey applications, the Geiger-Müller detector is used. When the covering around a G-M tube is made very thin, beta radiation can be measured. Usually, a sliding shield over the thin area is used to remove the beta contribution, and the composition of the radiation is determined by $\beta^- = (\beta^- + \gamma) - \gamma$. Two potential disadvantages of G-M tube instruments are their strong energy dependence and their tendency to give erroneously low readings at high exposure rates. The primary advantages of G-M instruments are their good sensitivity, stability to variations in high voltage, simplicity, and low cost.

Scintillation detectors can be used for the measurement of a wide variety of radiations, including alpha, gamma, beta, and neutron. Sodium iodide detectors are usually used for detection of gamma radiation. The resulting signal can be processed to produce a display related to the exposure or dose rate of all incident radiation or to discriminate between photons of different energy by pulse-height analysis. Scintillation detectors for beta measurement usually are made using anthracene as the phosphor. Zinc sulfide is used for alpha detection. Fast neutrons can be detected by organic phosphors with a high hydrogen content, or by $^{10}B(n,\alpha)$ ^7Li or ^6Li $(n,\alpha)^3H$ reactions followed by measurement of the resulting alpha particles by a detector containing neutron-sensitive atoms with the scintillator material. Since the development of semiconductor detectors, a thin coating of boron or lithium over the semiconductor material has been used to detect fast neutrons.

In most large facilities, removable contamination wipe tests are performed by the radiation protection office of that institution. If such tests are to be conducted completely by the nuclear medicine laboratory, special radiation measuring equipment may be required, such as gamma-radiation well counters. Selection of such equipment depends on the types of radionuclides used in the laboratory and the requirements for detection sensitivities cited in Appendix I of the NRC Regulatory Guide 10.8.[8] Records of all surveys must be kept and maintained for inspection by the NRC.

Personnel Monitoring

To ensure that radiation exposures to personnel remain as low as possible and to fulfill legal and administrative requirements, some system must be available for measuring individual radiation exposures. Personnel monitoring devices use a variety of detectors, including film badges, thermoluminescent dosimeters (TLDs), photoluminescent dosimeters and various types of ionization chamber dosimeters. In a complex working environment, there are few cases in which personnel monitoring devices accurately reflect total body exposure. Dosimeters can measure only exposure to the area of the body in which they are worn. Personnel monitoring devices do, however, reflect the exposure history of the worker, and when these results are considered in conjunction with area monitoring data, they can provide a basis for radiation control actions.

Guidelines as to who should wear personnel dosimeters are given in 10 CFR 20.202.[7] In general, these guidelines include all workers likely to receive more than 320 mrem whole body, 4690 mrem extremity, or 1880 mrem skin exposures in any 3-month period. Additional special personnel monitors, such as finger or wrist dosimeters, may be necessary for adequate measurement of exposure higher than that near the dosimeter.

Film badges are the most widely used detectors for personnel monitoring. They consist of a sealed packet of photographic film contained in a holder that includes a series of filters to aid in the separation of dose components from different types or energies of radiation. The degree of darkening in various areas of the shielded film can be related to radiation exposure from x-ray and gamma radiation, beta particles, and slow neutrons. Also, special films are available for measuring exposure to fast neutrons.

The TLD uses a radiation-sensing element that when heated emits light in proportion to the radiation exposure it has received.[9] This instrument has an advantage over photographic film in that it is reusable, but a disadvantage in that it does not provide a permanent record, because once it has been read, no further readout of the dose can be made.

While film badges and TLDs provide accurate, sensitive measurements of personnel exposure, their results are not available to either the worker or radiation safety personnel until they can be developed or read. Ionization chamber devices, such as pocket electroscope dosimeters and integrating radiation meters (often equipped with audible alarms to signal a preset dose level), can be used to indicate radiation exposure while it is occurring. In general, these devices are used in addition to film badges or TLDs to provide rapid information about exposure levels or warnings of exposure hazards. They are, in general, more subject to damage and accidental loss of data than are film or TLD monitors and thus are unsuitable for long-term monitoring of personnel exposure levels.

Selection and Calibration of Detectors

Various instruments are available for measuring exposure or absorbed dose. Each of these instruments has its own distinctive advantages and disadvantages, so selecting the correct instrument for a particular application is important. An ideal instrument for radiation monitoring is small, light, rugged, stable over a wide range of environmental conditions, capable of measuring all types of radiation that might be encountered, capable of operating for long periods without depleting its batteries, and insensitive to intensity, pulse rate, and beam shape of the incident radiation. At present, no single instrument meets all of these requirements. Careful selection of meters for measuring low-energy x-rays is especially important, since both time- and energy-integrating response characteristics can be critically important.

Once the instrument has been selected, proper calibration is necessary to ensure meaningful results. Because of energy dependence and variations in response to different types of radiation, calibration should always be done with standardized sources, under conditions that are as much as possible like those encountered in actual use. Separate calibration may be necessary for each type of radiation that might be encountered. Routine calibration of instruments also ensures that instruments are operating properly and are accurate and reliable over all instrument ranges.

A calibration facility should be designed so that a variety of instruments and dosimeters can be reliably positioned in a field of known dose rate under relatively scatter-free conditions. When this situation cannot be arranged, then either an absolute standard should be used, or a secondary standard instrument should be compared to the instrument being calibrated. A number of factors can complicate calibration measurements, and the reader would be well advised to consult standard works on the subject before establishing a calibration program.[9]

Control of Internal Radiation Exposure

Radionuclides may be incidentally taken into the body by inhalation of aerosols or gases, by ingestion, through wounds or breaks in the skin, and in some cases, directly through the skin. Internal contamination with radionuclides results in radiation exposures that may continue for long times after the contaminating event. The nuclide may concentrate preferentially in specific organs or tissues, thus complicating evaluation of the hazard.

Once a radionuclide is deposited within the body, it may be difficult to remove. The radiation dose from internally deposited isotopes contributes to the lifetime dose and so must be taken into consideration when determining whether an individual has exceeded the recommended dose limits. The ICRP has developed methods for determining maximum permissible levels for internally deposited radionuclides. The development of these standards is explained in ICRP Publications Nos. 2 and 6 and current recommendations can be found in ICRP Publication No. 30.[11,12,13]

The ICRP Publication No. 2 calculates the amount of a radioactive isotope that can be present in the body throughout a working lifetime without exceeding the maximum permissible dose to specific organs or tissues.[11] This amount is the maximum permissible body burden (MPBB). A related concept is the maximum permissible concentration (MPC) of radionuclide. These MPC values are the concentrations of a radionuclide in air or water that would result in acquisition of an MPBB over the course of a working lifetime.

The revised recommendations of ICRP Publication No. 30 are based on new information and changes in the Commission's methods for determining risk.[13] The concepts of MPC and MPBB have been replaced by that of Annual Limit of Intake (ALI), a value equivalent to 0.05 Sv (5 rem) per year from all tissues irradiated. Complete details of methodology are available in ICRP Publication No. 26[14], and with limits for 187 radionuclides of 21 elements in part 1 of ICRP Publication No. 30.[13] Limits for the remaining radionuclides can be found in parts 2 and 3 of ICRP Publication No. 30. These limits have been adopted by many state and national regulatory agencies to form the basis for control of internal and environmental radionuclide contamination.

Prevention of Internal Exposure

Because of the difficulty of reducing radiation exposure from internally deposited radionuclides, most effort should be concentrated on preventing their entry into the body. The development and enforcement of rules for safe handling of radionuclides can, in most cases, nearly eliminate the potential for hazard from either internal deposition or external contamination. Some commonsense rules for working safely with unsealed radionuclide sources include the following:

1. Always work in areas designed for handling radionuclides.
2. Never open sealed bottles or vials in open areas, especially if they contain such a volatile material as radioiodine. Use a well-designed hood or glove box. Volatilization of radioiodine is greatly reduced by buffering solutions at pH 7.5 to 9.0 and by such antioxidants as sodium bisulfite and disodium edetate.[15]
3. Work areas should be covered with a plastic, glass, or stainless steel tray, preferably with absorbent paper covering the tray, to catch any spills and to prevent the spread of contamination.
4. Plan all procedures in advance to increase awareness of problem areas. A test run using nonradioactive materials prevents delays and pinpoints problems.
5. Do not eat or drink in areas where unsealed radionuclides are being used or stored.
6. Do not smoke in areas where radionuclides are being used or stored.
7. Clearly label all containers of radionuclides with isotope, date, and activity.
8. Work in a well-ventilated area, and use a hood or glove box designed for radiation control for all procedures that might release activity into the air.
9. Do not pipette by mouth.
10. Be aware of hazards and use good judgment.
11. Wear protective clothing and surgical gloves while working, and dispose of gloves before leaving the area.
12. Do not wear protective clothing outside the work area.
13. Keep all radionuclides in sealed containers when they are not in use.
14. Maintain high standards of cleanliness in the laboratory. Promptly clean up spills and dispose of wastes properly.
15. Survey the work area regularly for both contamination and exposure hazards. Conduct special surveys after operations that might result in contamination.
16. Wash hands thoroughly before eating, drinking, or smoking.

Additional precautions to be considered by the individual responsible for radiation safety include area air sampling where airborne contamination is possible, especially during radionuclide procedures; a routine program of personnel monitoring, including bioassay and whole body counting as appropriate; and routine education programs for all employees before they are allowed to use radionuclides. It is especially important for employee training programs to include detailed information about isotope handling techniques, radiation safety support, and specific steps to be taken in the event of spills or other emergencies.

Assessment of Internal Radionuclide Contamination

A radiation safety program for detecting the presence of internal contamination should have two components: a routine detection program for all employees who work near sources of contamination and a special program for cases in which contamination is suspected.

Three methods are available for the detection and evaluation of internal contamination. The least accurate method is the calculation of body burden from such environmental measurements as air sampling, surface contamination levels, and ratemeter measurements of skin contamination. All of these sources of data require a number of assumptions with resulting uncertainty in the final estimate. Air sampling, especially in the breathing zone of workers throughout each procedure, probably yields the most accurate measurements in this indirect method.

The second method, bioassay, involves measurments of radioactivity concentration in accessible body fluids or tissues. These measurements generally include urine, stool, hair, and blood. The translation of these values into internal body burdens requires knowledge of the metabolism of the radionuclide. Since metabolism is a dynamic process, uncertainties arise from such factors as lack of detailed knowledge of pool or organ sizes and the difficulty of determining when the contaminating event occurred. A number of commercial sources are available for analysis of bioassay samples. ICRP Publications Nos. 10 and 10A provide much information relating to methods of assessing internal contamination for occupational exposure.[16,17]

The NRC requires that bioassays be performed on individuals handling volatile— or large quantities of bound, nonvolatile— I-125 or I-131.[18] This includes physicians preparing and administering therapy doses of 10 mCi (370 MBq) or more of I-131. Urine analyses may be required by the NRC as a condition of obtaining license to use large quantities of H-3, C-14 and P-32.

Whole body counting, the third method, involves direct measurement of the emission from internally deposited gamma or x-ray emitters and highly energetic beta emitters (by means of bremsstrahlung x-rays produced in the body). Whole body counters, in general, do not provide good data about the distribution pattern of the nuclide, but they do provide rapid and ac-

curate measurement of total body burden. Other advantages include relatively high sensitivity and comfort for the subject. Whole body counters are available in nearly every region of the United States and in 30 other countries. Since most of the counters are primarily research installations, access for routine radiation monitoring measurements may be difficult to obtain.

The frequency of routine employee measurements must be related to several factors, including the effective half-times of nuclides in use, the amounts used, the degree to which controls on usage are being applied, and the history of the employee with respect to contamination. Adequate controls on the use of radionuclides can essentially eliminate the need for expensive routine bioassay programs in some installations.

Treatment for the Removal of Internally Deposited Radionuclides

Whenever the possibility of serious internal uptake of radionuclides is suspected, rapid determination of the extent of the problem and of the need for treatment is essential. The first priorities are to identify both the radionuclide involved and the probable route of entry and to determine the amount of radionuclide that entered the body. Identification of the radionuclide and route of entry can be provided by the employee or from survey of the laboratory. The amount of radionuclide can be determined by whole body counting or bioassay, or if these methods are not immediately available, by calculation based on air sample results or on knowledge of how much activity was involved in the procedure and how much of that remains.

The effectiveness of procedures for the removal of radionuclides from the body often depends directly on how soon treatment is initated. Treatment to remove activity from the stomach or to minimize absorption must be made before the material has left the stomach or been absorbed. The use of chelating agents or other means to increase the rate of removal of the substance from the body is often far more effective if initiated soon after entry. In all cases, competent medical consultation is required to determine whether the benefits of such treatment outweigh the risks.

When a radionuclide has been ingested, several steps may be taken to remove the material or to decrease its absorption. Removal from the stomach can be accomplished by either inducing vomiting or using a stomach pump. Methods for decreasing absorption include administration of precipitating agents or antacids to favor the formation of insoluble compounds. Use of chelating agents during the absorptive phase may lead to increased absorption and should be avoided. Elimination from the gastrointestinal tract may be enhanced through the use of bowel cleansing procedures in order to reduce the radiation dose to these organs.

When intake occurs by inhalation, removal may be accomplished by rinsing the mouth and nose with saline solution and administering expectorants to increase removal via the ciliary escalator system. Soluble substances are rapidly absorbed and must be dealt with by systemic treatments.

Once a material is absorbed into the body, treatment becomes much more difficult, and the possibility of a toxic reaction to the treatment agent exists. Chelating agents may be used to increase the excretion of some substances. Recent evidence suggests that the use of Zn-DTPA (diethylenetriamine pentaacetic acid) instead of Ca-DTPA provides equivalent effectiveness with considerably less toxicity. Administration of stable forms of the material or other stable compounds that compete metabolically with the substance may reduce deposition in critical organs and result in more rapid elimination of the radionuclide. Stable iodine, if administered early enough, may interfere with thyroid uptake of radioiodine. Diuretics, beer,

or increased water intake may hasten the elimination of tritium.

Treatment of contaminated wounds requires removal of radioactive materials by washing, abrasion, or surgical removal of embedded material. If radioactive material is left on a wound site, it can become solubilized or cause local radiation damage to the affected area.

When radionuclides are spilled or escape into the air, they may be deposited on skin surfaces. Unless it is quickly removed, external contamination of the skin can result in large radiation doses to the affected area. Beta-emitting radionuclides are especially hazardous in this respect. The initial step in removal of skin contamination is gentle washing with a mild detergent. It is important not to abrade the skin while removing the contamination since this abrasion may facilitate entry of the material into the body. A soft brush may be helpful for removing activity from hands and wrists, especially around the fingernails. Particular attention should be given to thorough washing of hair using a mild shampoo. In all cases, rinsing with ample amounts of clean water should ensure that all loose activity is removed. During rinsing, it is important that material removed from one part of the body not be deposited on another.

Xenon Gases. The use of xenon gases imposes additional radiation control requirements. Xenon-133 is commonly used in nuclear medical laboratories for pulmonary ventilation studies. The use of Xe-127 is not common, but it is increasing. The biologic properties of Xe-133 and Xe-127 are identical, but their physical characteristics require that they be handled differently. Xenon-133 has a half-life of 5.3 days and gamma energy of 81 keV. These characteristics render shielding and disposal relatively easy. Xenon-127 has a 36.4-day half-life and gamma energies ranging from 58 to 375 keV. The long half-life and higher energies require heavier shielding and somewhat more careful handling than Xe-133. (The use of Kr-81m poses no environmental hazard in the concentrations encountered clinically because of its short half-life of 13 sec.)

Xenon-133 is supplied for medical use primarily in small, rubber-stoppered ampules containing 10 to 30 mCi (0.37 to 1.1 GBq). These ampules are easily stored in lead vials inside a fume hood. Xenon-133 is also supplied in curie amounts in crushable ampules that require a mechanical dispensing system. This system can develop leaks and must be stored in a fume hood or well-ventilated room. Transferring the gas into a glass syringe from the dispenser requires care and adequate ventilation to prevent the gas from escaping.

Xenon-127 is currently available only in crushable ampules. If a Xe-133 dispensing system is used, additional lead shielding must be used. There are two types of xenon disposal methods currently used. One method employs a hood that is placed over the patient and connected to a high volume exhaust fan. During the washout phase of the study, the radioxenon expired by the patient is exhausted to the outside atmosphere. Any xenon remaining in the shielded ventilator system is left for subsequent patients to utilize or is disposed of through the same exhaust system used for the patient.

The second disposal system employs a trapping system that contains activated charcoal as the collecting agent. Several commercial systems are available with up to 95% trapping efficiency.[19] The activated charcoal must be replaced periodically. Some commercial systems have a detector in the exhaust port of the trap to measure the concentration of xenon escaping from the charcoal filter. An alarm is meant to signal excessive exhaust concentrations, which presumably indicate the need for replacing the charcoal cartridge. For hospitals in which a high volume of lung scanning is performed, some sort of trapping system is required because of restrictions on exhausting to the outside.

The maximum permissible concentration of Xe-133 in air of a *restricted* area is 1×10^{-5} µCi/ml (0.37 Bq/ml). While xenon gas is heavier than air, it will remain uniformly distributed once it is dispersed. Because of the low MPC of radioxenon, adequate ventilation with high room air turnover is desirable. Nishiyama has shown that differences in room air ventilation can effect a hundredfold reduction in xenon that is inhaled by technicians performing ventilation scans.[20] Each laboratory should develop a system for monitoring ambient xenon levels. Commercial gas monitors are available for a variety of radioactive gases, including C-14 and H-3. Jacobstein has described a simple means of monitoring Xenon-133 by measuring the activity taken up by 10-ml vacutainer tubes.[21] These can be punctured with a 20-gage needle at the site to be monitored and measured in a well counter.

Protection of the Thyroid Against Effects of Radioiodine. In relatively few instances is prophylactic iodine administered to counteract inadvertent ingestion of radioiodine. This treatment has been recommended for technicians who radiolabel proteins with I-125 or I-131, thereby risking absorption of a significant burden of volatilized radioiodine through inhalation. The use of ventilated hoods, however, should be the first order of protection. Prophylactic iodine has also been recommended for physicians administering therapeutic doses of radioiodine; however, internal contamination in these instances has been greatly reduced by the addition of oxidizing agents to radioiodine solutions to impede volatilization of iodine.[15]

A potentially more serious problem is the treatment of workers and populations exposed to nuclear accidents. Certainly, the events of Three Mile Island have dramatized this subject. The operating core of a power nuclear reactor accumulates enormous quantities of radioiodine. Those with mass numbers 131 to 135 have sufficiently long half-lives to constitute a health hazard. A 2000-megawatt (thermal) reactor at saturation may contain each of these isotopes in quantities on the order of 10^7 Ci (3.7×10^{17} Bq). Even a minor leak may result in serious contamination, although of relatively short duration. One means of protecting the thyroid in exposed individuals is thyroid blockage. To block uptake, potassium iodide is an effective, and the least toxic, alternative. A dose of 100 mg iodine (130 mg KI) reduces thyroid uptake of radioiodine to less than 1%, and this dose given once daily maintains the blockade indefinitely.[22] This may be given as the saturated solution SSKI, which contains approximately 1 gm KI/ml, or as tablets containing 130 mg KI, which are commercially available.

There is little question about supplying reactor personnel with prophylactic KI, since they are at the highest risk and supply logistics are simple. Supplying prophylaxis to large populations, however, is a considerably larger problem, and the level of exposure that should trigger distribution is arguable. The NCRP has proposed administering prophylactic iodine when the potential for an exposure of 10 to 30 rads exists.[23] Robbins et al., however, argues that these levels may be unnecessarily low.[24] He proposes that the potential to receive 500 rads to the thyroid is a more reasonable circumstance for which iodine blockade on a large scale should be considered. This absorbed dose would be produced by about 330 µCi of I-131 in adults, 170 µCi at 10 years of age, 50 µCi at 1 year of age, and 30 µCi in newborn infants.[25] Robbins' reasoning contains the assumption that I-131 may be expected to cause one nodule per million per rad per year. A dose of 500 rads in a child is estimated to increase the incidence of thyroid nodules from about 0.1% per year (the rate in the general population) to 0.15% per year. If the death rate were to increase proportionately (by 1050 in the U.S. population in 1981), 2.5 additional deaths per million

persons per year might be expected. In adults, the risk would be much smaller.

Naturally, these considerations would not apply to a single individual, or even a few individuals; instead, they provide recommendations for prophylaxis to large populations. The situation is more complicated if the radioiodine has already accumulated in the gland. Clearly, thyroid blockade with KI is effective in limiting the reabsorption of radioiodine released by the metabolism of thyroid hormone. Thyroid-stimulating hormone (TSH) in doses of 10 units daily may be considered as a means to promote release of hormone from the gland, thereby decreasing the cumulative concentration within the thyroid. The benefit of this treatment, however, must be weighed against the risk of reaction to the TSH.

Control of External Contamination

Surface contamination may originate as gases, liquids, or solids. It may react with surfaces to become relatively fixed or may remain removable. In all cases, cleaning up any spilled radioactive material as soon as possible is important.

Detection of contaminated areas can be accomplished quickly by means of rate-meter surveys. Determination of removable activity can be made by wiping exposed surfaces with small pieces of filter paper (smearing) and measuring how much radioactivity is removed onto the smear. Routine surveys combining these methods provide good indications of the extent of laboratory contamination. Standards should be established for permissible levels of contamination in various work areas. Areas in which permissible levels are exceeded should be decontaminated to acceptable levels. Table 13–3 illustrates the range of values used in several laboratories.

Whenever areas of contamination are found, they should be clearly marked and the contamination promptly removed. It is important that contamination not be

TABLE 13–3. *Limits for Removable Surface Contamination in Medical Institutions**

	Type of radioactive material†		
Type of surface	Alpha emitters (μCi/cm^2)	Beta or x-ray emitters (μCi/cm^2)	Low-risk beta or x-ray emitters (μCi/cm^2)
1. Unrestricted areas	10^{-7}	10^{-6}	10^{-5}
2. Restricted areas	10^{-6}	10^{-5}	10^{-4}
3. Personal clothing worn outside restricted areas	10^{-7}	10^{-6}	10^{-5}
4. Protective clothing worn only in restricted areas	10^{-6}	10^{-5}	10^{-4}
5. Skin	10^{-6}	10^{-6}	10^{-5}

*Averaging is acceptable over inanimate areas of up to 300 cm^2, or for floors, walls, and ceiling, 100 cm^2. Averaging is also acceptable over 100 cm^2 for skin, or for the hands (over the whole area of the hand), nominally 300 cm^2.
†Beta or x-ray emitter values are applicable for all beta or x-ray emitters other than those considered low risk. Low risk nuclides include C-14, H-3, S-35, Tc-99m, and others whose beta energies are <0.2 MeV maximum, whose gamma or x-ray emission is less than 0.1 R/h at 1 meter per curie, and whose permissible concentration in air (see 10 CFR Part 20, Appendix B, Table 1[7]) is greater than 10^{-6} μCi/ml.
From NRC, 1981.[26]

allowed to spread to new surfaces or personnel during the course of the decontamination operation. Marking contaminated areas and posting warning signs help to minimize the spread of contamination in most cases. When large areas are affected or high radiation levels are present, it may be necessary to restrict access to the area by means of barricades. Personnel involved in decontamination activities should wear protective clothing, and appropriate personnel monitoring techniques should be applied. The degree of control and special precautions required depend on the extent and radiotoxicity of the contaminating event.

Generally, wet methods of decontamination reduce airborne radioactivity and are thus preferred to dry methods. Dusting, brushing, or sanding should especially be avoided. Vacuuming should be avoided unless the machine is equipped with absolute filters to prevent the exhaust from blowing radioactive dust into the air. Most contamination can be removed by gentle washing with soap and water. In the initial steps, scrubbing should be minimized and the primary effort directed toward removal of loose dirt and grease from the area. Commercial preparations of detergents and complexing agents are available for decontamination, but these have little value over soap and water. Care should be exercised to prevent the washing solution from moving the contamination into inaccessible areas. After each washing, the area should be surveyed to determine how much activity remains.

FACILITY DESIGN FOR RADIATION CONTROL

Well-designed working areas minimize the opportunity for error and allow operations to be conducted efficiently and safely. The design of radiation facilities should include provisions for control of external radiation hazards, storage of radiation sources, storage of radioactive waste, adequate ventilation, provisions for radiation monitoring and air sampling equipment, planning for easy decontamination, and efficient movement of personnel through the facility.

Specific design criteria are directly related to the operation being considered; however, certain general principles are applicable to most situations. The main object of radiation facility design is to provide maximum protection with minimal inconvenience to workers. In general, this goal involves making restrictions no more stringent than necessary to deal with all foreseeable hazards.

Access should be designed for flow of personnel from low- to high-activity areas, with restrictions increasing as the hazard increases. Such special areas as low-level counting rooms may require more control, to prevent measurement errors or losses of measurement sensitivity, than that required for personnel protection. The same considerations apply to areas in which low-level tracer studies are performed because of the possibility of cross-contamination. Model floor plans for nuclear medicine laboratories have been published by Frost and Jammet and by Sodd.[4,27]

Consideration of the flow of materials in an operation is also important. Radiopharmaceutical laboratories, for instance, should be designed to allow easy movement of radionuclides from storage areas to processing areas and easy transport of radioactive waste back to storage or disposal areas.

Ventilation is an important factor in limiting airborne radioactivity hazards to personnel. The need for ventilation can be reduced in small laboratories by the use of such containment devices as hoods or gloveboxes. In all cases, ventilation systems should be designed to prevent movement of contamination from controlled to uncontrolled areas. Air inlets should be located far enough away from outlets to prevent recirculation of contamination through the ventilation system.

Storage areas for either radiation sources or radioactive wastes should be designed to eliminate hazards from external exposure or leakage onto surfaces or into the air. In many cases, convenient access is also an important aspect in the design of storage areas. When possible, storage areas for radionuclides and sealed sources should be separate from but handy to the areas in which these materials are used. Shielding with lead or thick concrete walls should be used to reduce external exposure hazards, and the storage area should be adequately ventilated to prevent the accumulation of high concentrations of radioactivity in the air. Such substances as iodine, xenon, and radium are especially likely to constitute a hazard if stored in inadequately ventilated areas. In some cases, storage in a lead enclosure contained in a hood is adequate for small amounts of activity. Storage areas should be designed with smooth, unbroken, chemically inert surfaces to facilitate removal of contamination.

Areas for storage of radioactive waste have similar design requirements to those for other radiation sources, although consideration should also be given to storage of liquid wastes, requirements for processing, and access to disposal facilities. Specially marked waste containers for both liquid and solid waste should be provided in all working areas, and care should be taken to prevent accumulation of large amounts of activity in these containers.

Careful attention to the design and finishes of all surfaces in radiation areas decreases the hazard from surface contamination. In general, all surfaces should be smooth and nonporous. Dust catchers—such as ridges, sharp corners, and ledges—should be eliminated as much as possible. Porous surfaces should be permanently sealed with paint or plastic materials to make them smooth and easy to clean. Additional coatings of strippable lacquer or paint can be used in areas with a high probability of contamination.

Storage and Disposal of Radioactive Waste Products

Radioactive materials no longer required must be disposed of to avoid an environmental hazard. The basic principles of disposal as given in IAEA Publication No. 38 are listed on the next page.[28]

1. *Dilute and dispense* for low-level solid, liquid, and gaseous wastes.
2. *Delay and decay* for solid, liquid, and gaseous wastes that contain short-lived nuclides.
3. *Concentrate and contain* for intermediate and high-level solid, liquid, and gaseous wastes.

The design of waste disposal systems generally includes all of these methods, sometimes in combination.

In the laboratory or individual work area, emphasis should be placed on segregation of nonradioactive and radioactive waste. This segregation is generally accomplished by providing either specially marked containers for solid and liquid wastes or special drain lines to radioactive liquid waste holding tanks that can be monitored before release to sewers or processing operations designed to concentrate the material for disposal. Training programs play an important part in an effective waste management program.

Sanitary sewer systems are commonly used to dispose of small amounts of low-level liquid waste. Because the environment has limited capacity for removal of waste materials—in some cases, radionuclides actually concentrate during passage through food chains—this method should be applied cautiously with careful adherence to applicable regulations. Material should be diluted or decayed to low levels prior to release, and maximum permissible concentration (MPC) levels as established by the ICRP and national regulatory bodies should not be exceeded. Ensuring permissible levels requires measurement of the sewer effluent from the institution. Radioactivity may be released into the air as long as concentration levels outside controlled areas do not exceed applicable MPC levels. Measurements of both the total radioactivity to be released and the air capacity of the exhaust system are required. Incineration of radioactive waste, with release of radioactivity to the environment, is also possible. In some countries, however, such as the United States, special authorization is required from the regulatory body, and concentrations may not exceed MPC values.

Storage facilities for radioactive waste prevent the accumulation of hazardous levels of radioactivity in work areas and provide an opportunity to safely hold short-lived radionuclides until they have decayed to levels that are safe for conventional disposal. Storage facilities also may contain special handling equipment for concentration of liquid waste, compaction of solid waste, and packaging of waste into shipping containers. Containers for shipping radioactive wastes must meet standards established by agencies such as the U.S. Department of Transportation. Other regulations may apply to radioactive waste shipments. The details of transportation and disposal of radioactive wastes may be handled by companies specializing in this area.

PATIENTS AS RADIATION SOURCES

Whenever radionuclides are administered to patients or radiation sources are implanted in their bodies, they in turn become radiation sources and may constitute a radiation hazard. In general, doses in the microcurie range do not create serious hazards. When diagnostic and therapeutic procedures involving millicurie amounts of radionuclides are carried out, the radioactivity of the patient could be of concern. Two other factors should be considered in addition to the external exposure hazards: irradiation of the fetus, especially in early pregnancy, and transfer of radionuclides to young infants through breast milk.

The precautions that should be taken when dealing with radioactive patients are similar to those required for any radiation source but are complicated by the patient's mobility. The USNCRP has discussed many of the problems and procedures in

NCRP Report 37.[29] Four situations are treated in this report: patients receiving regular nursing care in a hospital, patients released from the hospital, emergency surgery on radioactive patients, and death of radioactive patients.

For the case of hospitalized patients, administered radioactivity must be documented in patient charts; radioactivity warnings must be attached to the patient's chart and room; patients must be monitored; isolation and routine care must be controlled for isolated patients; and exposures of hospital personnel must be regulated. Criteria for determining when patients should be released are based on limiting exposures to members of the general public with whom they may come in contact to less than 0.4 rem (4 mSv) per year and minimizing exposure to infants and small children.

In general, restriction of the number of visitors to therapy patients is unnecessary. The maximum permissible dose to an individual of this category is 0.5 rem (5 mSv) per year, and there is little likelihood of this dose being exceeded. Visitors should be advised to remain at least 6 feet from the patient, at which distance an absorbed dose of 0.1 rem (1 mSv) from a patient containing 100 mCi (3.7 GBq) would require 15 hours.

Emergency surgery is rarely required on patients containing high levels of radioactivity. In many cases involving administration of radionuclides, a delay of one to a few days results in a dramatic decrease in exposure to operating room personnel. When surgery is required, personnel should be aware of the hazards involved, especially of the possibility of large local doses to hands in direct contact with highly radioactive organs or tissues, and they should take steps to minimize exposures. When surgery involves areas remote from the sites of deposition or implant, the radiation hazard is much reduced, and the presence of radioactivity is of much less concern.

The death of a patient who contains therapeutic amounts of radioactivity poses several problems from the standpoint of radiation safety. If an autopsy is to be performed, the pathologist and other personnel may receive appreciable radiation exposure. During embalming procedures, both personnel exposure hazards and danger of contamination exist. If the body is disposed of by cremation, hazards include excessive release of radionuclides to the environment and inhalation of radioactive ashes by mortuary personnel. Because of the potential hazards involved, detailed procedures should be available to all persons who might be in contact with the patient. All procedures that might involve radiation risks to personnel or to members of the general public should be carried out under the supervision of a radiation protection specialist. Procedures are outlined in NCRP Report No. 37.[29]

REFERENCES

1. Morgan, K.Z., and Turner, J.E. (Eds.): Principles of Radiation Protection. New York, John Wiley & Sons, 1967.
2. Basic Radiation Protection Criteria, Report No. 39. Washington, D.C. National Council on Radiation Protection and Measurements, 1971.
3. Review of the Current State of Radiation Protection Philosophy, Report No. 43. Washington, D.C. National Council on Radiation Protection and Measurements, 1975.
4. Sodd, V.I. (Ed.): Radiation Safety in Nuclear Medicine: A Practical Guide. HHS Publication FDA 82–8180, November 1981.
5. Radiation Quantities and Units, Report No. 33. Washington, D.C. International Commission on Radiological Units and Measurements, 1980.
6. Branson, B.M., Sodd, V.I., Nishiyama, H., and Williams, C.C.: Use of syringe shields in clinical practice. J. Clin. Nucl. Med., *1*:56, 1976.
7. Code of Federal Regulations, Title 10-Energy (10 CFR). Office of the Federal Register, Washington, D.C. U.S. Government Printing Office, 1980.
8. Guide for the Preparation of Applications for Medical Programs, NRC Regulatory Guide 10.8. Washington, D.C. U.S. Nuclear Regulatory Commission, 1980.
9. Radiation Protection Instrumentation and Its Application, Report No. 20. Washington, D.C. International Commission on Radiological Units and Measurements, 1976.
10. General Principles of Monitoring for Radiation Protection of Workers. International Commis-

sion on Radiation Protection, Publication No. 12. London, Pergamon Press, 1969.

11. Recommendations of the International Commission on Radiological Protection. International Commission on Radiological Protection, Publication No. 2. London, Pergamon Press, 1959.

12. Recommendations of the International Commission on Radiological Protection. International Commission on Radiological Protection, Publication No. 6. London, Pergamon Press, 1962.

13. Limits for Intakes of Radionuclides by Workers, International Commission on Radiological Protection, Publication No. 30. London, Pergamon Press, 1979.

14. Radiation Protection. International Commission on Radiation Protection, Publication No. 26. London, Pergamon Press, 1977.

15. Luckett, L.W., and Stolter, R.E.: Radioiodine volatilization from reformulated sodium iodide I-131 oral solution. J. Nucl. Med., 21:477, 1980.

16. Evaluation of Radiation Doses to Body Tissues from Internal Contamination Due to Occupational Exposure. International Commission on Radiation Protection, Publication No. 10. London, Pergamon Press, 1968.

17. The Assessment of Internal Contamination Resulting from Recurrent or Prolonged Uptakes. International Commission on Radiological Protection, Publication No. 10A. London, Pergamon Press, 1971.

18. Applications of Bioassay for I-125 and I-131, NRC Regulatory Guide 8.20. Washington, D.C., U.S. Nuclear Regulatory Commission, September 1979.

19. McIlmoyle, G., Holman, B.L., Davis, M., and Chandler, H.L.: A portable radioxenon trap and patient ventilation system. Radiology, 127:544, 1978.

20. Nishiyama, H., and Lukes, S.J.: Exposure to xenon-133 in the nuclear medicine laboratory. Radiology, 143:243, 1982.

21. Jacobstein, J.: A simple method for the air monitoring of xenon-133. J. Nucl. Med., 20:159, 1979.

22. Blum, M., and Eisenbud, M.: Reduction of thyroid irradiation from I-131 by potassium iodide. J.A.M.A., 200:1036, 1967.

23. Protection of the Thyroid Gland in the Event of Releases of Radioiodine, Report No. 55. Washington, D.C. National Council on Radiation Protection and Measurements, 1977.

24. Robbins, J., Rall, J.E., and Gorder, P.: The thyroid and iodine metabolism. In Metabolic Control and Diseases. Edited by P.K. Bondy and L.E. Rosenberg. Philadelphia, W.B. Saunders, 1980.

25. Wellman, H.N., and Anger, R.T.: Radioiodine dosimetry and the use of radioiodines other than I-131 in thyroid diagnosis. Semin. Nucl. Med., 1:356, 1971.

26. Radiation Safety at Medical Institutions, NRC Regulatory Guide 8.23. Washington, D.C. U.S. Nuclear Regulatory Commission, 1981.

27. Frost, D., and Jammet, H.: Manual on Radiation Protection in Hospitals and General Practice. Vol. 2. Unsealed Sources. Geneva, World Health Organization, 1975.

28. Radiation Protection Procedures. Safety Series No. 38. Vienna, International Atomic Energy Agency, 1973.

29. Precautions in the Management of Patients Who Have Received Therapeutic Amounts of Radionuclides, Report No. 37. Washington, D.C. National Council on Radiation Protection and Measurements. 1970.

Chapter 14

RADIOIMMUNOASSAY AND COMPETITIVE BINDING ANALYSIS

JOHN HARBERT

Competitive binding analysis is the generic term for a type of radiochemical analysis that involves a progressive saturation of one reactive agent by another that one wishes to measure. *Radioimmunoassay* (RIA), one type of competitive binding analysis, is used in this chapter to illustrate the principles that govern this test. In the RIA, the reagents used are an antigen (Ag) and its specific antibody (Ab). Other types of saturation analysis employ various reactive agents, such as tissue receptors, carrier proteins, and enzymes. Thus one encounters several designations for the technique, such as receptor analysis, saturation analysis, radioimmunometric analysis, equilibrium analysis, radioimmunoanalysis and radioligand assay, but the general principles are identical.

RIA developed largely out of the pioneering work of Yalow and Berson, published in 1960.[1] The importance of this method lies, on the one hand, in permitting the quantitative measurement of extremely small fractions, on the order of nanograms (10^{-9}g) and picograms (10^{-12}g). On the other hand, the measurement is highly specific because of the immunologic character of the reagents. The application of this technique to the measurement of protein and peptide hormones has been an important advance in the biochemistry of hormones and endocrinology.

In RIA, a substance to be measured (Ag) is mixed with a radiolabeled substance (Ag*) to form a pool in which each element has an equal opportunity to bind to a *ligand* (Ab) to form a stable union. The ligand is usually present in a lesser concentration than the pool of Ag-Ag*, so that the net result is a group of bound and free fractions. These fractions are then separated, measured, and compared with known standards to determine the concentration of Ag in the original mixture.

If the competition between Ag and Ab continues until a mass equilibrium is reached, the assay is termed *equilibrium saturation.* If, on the other hand, saturation of the binder is divided into two consecutive steps (the first using the unlabeled ligand, the second using the labeled ligand) but the reaction is stopped before reaching equilibrium, the assay is termed *nonequilibrium analysis,* or *sequential saturation.*[2]

Radioassays are usually of the equilibrium type. The nonequilibrium analysis is used less frequently; it is specifically indicated when a large difference exists in the affinities of the labeled and unlabeled ligands for the binder.

For the equilibrium saturation analysis, both radioactively labeled and unlabeled ligands are assumed to have the same physicochemical properties and no allosteric effects are assumed to be present, the reaction will follow the first-order mass action law:

$$Ag + Ab \overset{k_1}{\underset{k_2}{\rightleftharpoons}} AgAb$$
$$Ag^* + Ab \overset{k_3}{\underset{k_4}{\rightleftharpoons}} Ag^*Ab$$

At equilibrium:

$$K = \frac{k_1}{k_2} = \frac{AgAb}{Ag \times Ab}$$

$$K^* = \frac{k_3}{k_4} = \frac{Ag^*Ab}{Ag^* \times Ab}$$

Both affinity constants, K and K^*, are assumed to be equal.

Because of the equilibrium established in this reaction, the addition of some quantity of unlabeled antigen Ag will compete with Ag^* for the binding sites on Ab, a process that yields AgAb and increases the concentration of Ag^* in the medium.

The ratio between the bound fraction B of labeled antigen Ag^*Ab and the free Ag^*, which is called F in this discussion, decreases with increasing concentration of the unlabeled antigen Ag. The ratio B/F can be determined by separating the bound and free fractions and measuring their activity.

The general form of the curve that relates B/F to the concentration of substance being determined, Ag, is shown in Figure 14–1. To obtain this "standard" curve, increasing quantities of Ag are added to constant quantities of Ag^* and Ab, and the corresponding B/F ratios are determined.

Unknown concentrations of antigen (substrate) are determined in the same way as the standard curve. A standard volume of sample containing the unknown quantity of substrate is added to the antibody and labeled antigen, and then the B/F is determined. The corresponding value of Ag then is read directly from the curve to give the antigen concentration (dotted line).

The standard curve can be obtained also by relating the antigen concentration to B/T, where T is the total radioactivity placed in the medium, or to B/B_0, where B_0 is the bound fraction at the zero point of the curve, i.e., when the concentration of Ag is zero.

$$\frac{B}{F} = \frac{[Ag^*Ab]}{[Ag^*]}$$

$$\frac{B}{T} = \frac{[Ag^*Ab]}{[Ag^*] + [Ag^*Ab]}$$

$$[Ab]_F = [Ab]_T - ([Ag^*Ab] + [AgAb])$$

Thus, $B/F = K ([B]_t - [Ag^*Ab])$

The last equation establishes a linear relationship between the B/F ratio and the concentration of the bound labeled ligand and is generally used to determine the affinity constant (K), as will be discussed later.

In every radioimmunoassay, the validity of the measurement depends upon the immunologic identity between the standard antigen and the antigen in the unknown samples. The identity between the labeled antigen Ag^* and the unknown antigen is of secondary importance.

ANTIGENS

Radiolabeling of Antigens

In general, the labeled antigen used as a tracer must be present in low concentrations, because the quantity of substance to be measured is usually small. *The concentration of Ag^* must not be greater than the least quantity of Ag to be measured.* It is necessary, therefore, to have labeled antigen of high specific activity, and once labeled, the antigen must maintain the

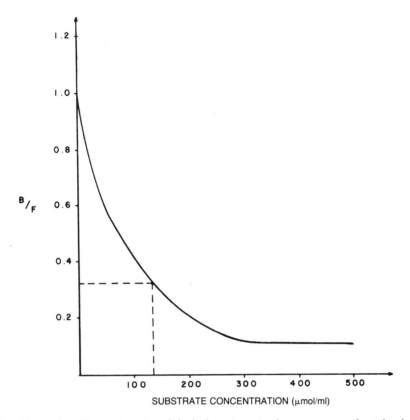

Fig. 14–1. The ratio of bound to free labeled antigen in the presence of antibody. At B/F = 1.0, there is no unlabeled antigen (substrate) in the sample, and half of the labeled antigen is bound, and half free. A value of B/F = 0.33 would occur when sufficient unlabeled antigen is added to displace half of the previously bound labeled antigen to the free state, i.e.,

$$B/F = \frac{4 \text{ Ag*Ab}}{4 \text{ Ag*}} + 8 \text{ Ag} \rightarrow \frac{2\text{Ag*Ab}}{6 \text{ Ag*}} + \frac{2\text{AgAb}}{6 \text{ Ag}} = 0.33$$

same characteristics of the unlabeled antigen to react qualitatively and quantitatively with the antibody. As radioactive labels, C-14 and H-3 have the principal drawback that their long half-lives (5740 yr and 12.3 yr respectively) require too much added label for the low concentration of substrate used in RIA systems, they are difficult to measure and require cumbersome liquid scintillation counting. Therefore, they are used almost exclusively in those systems in which the addition of a larger molecule alters the immunoreactivity of the system.

Radioiodine generally fulfills the label requirements; I-125 is preferred over I-131 because of its longer half-life, ease of handling, and higher counting efficiency. A method of producing radioiodinated proteins with high specific activity was found in 1962 by Hunter and Greenwood, using chloramine-T.[3] In this method, radioiodine is bound to the ring structure of tyrosine. Other methods have been developed, e.g., the use of iodine monochloride and electrolytic labeling, but chloramine-T continues to be most commonly used.[4]

Purification of Labeled Antigens

After labeling, the reaction medium contains labeled and unlabeled protein, denatured protein reactants, and unbound iodide. Purification is therefore essential and may be accomplished by a variety of techniques, including dialysis, gel filtration, adsorption chromatography, ion-exchange chromatography, and gel electrophoresis. Gel filtration, performed with a molecular sieve such as Sephadex, has been widely used because of the simplicity and efficiency it offers. The labeled antigen is filtered through a properly prepared column and several fractions are collected. The particular fraction that possesses both high specific activity and high immunoreactivity is chosen for the RIA.

Evaluation of Labeled Antigens

The sensitivity of RIA is related to the antigen-antibody reaction energy, and this energy in turn depends upon the antigen's affinity for binding with the antibody, i.e., its immunoreactivity. The causes of reduced immunoreactivity include the following:

1. The introduction of more than one iodine atom per molecule, which may alter the binding, especially in small antigen molecules.
2. The presence of iodine, substituting a hydrogen in the aromatic group of tyrosine.[5]
3. Protein degradation by excessive oxidation.
4. Presence of impurities in the radioiodine from commercial sources.
5. Incubation damage.

Generally, 5 to 10% of impurities reduce Ag* immunoreactivity sufficiently to limit its use to cases that do not require high precision (e.g., when there is a high Ag concentration). With greater than 10% impurities, prior purification is necessary.

Such alterations in the physicochemical properties of antigens as changes in electrophoretic mobility or in gel column filtration behavior may offer indirect evidence of antigen damage, but they do not measure the immunoreactivity directly.

The simplest and most direct test of immunoreactivity is performed by reacting a small amount of labeled antigen with excess antibody. If a significant amount of the label fails to bind to the antibody, the presence of nonimmunoreactive elements is assumed.

Storage and Stability

The useful life of products labeled with I-131 is largely limited by the half-life of the radionuclide. With both I-131 and I-125, other factors may affect stability:

1. Liberation of free iodine from the labeled antigen. In this case, repurification to remove the free radioiodine should be performed. Although some loss of specific activity occurs, it is not great, generally.
2. Decay catastrophe. Molecules labeled with more than one iodine atom can break when one of them decays and the remainder continues to be labeled. The protein fragment influences the counting rate but is no longer immunoreactive.
3. Gradual loss of immunoreactivity during storage, caused by chemical deterioration.

A labeled and purified antigen can usually be kept in solution for a week at 4°C without suffering appreciable loss in activity. It can be fractionated, rapidly frozen, and kept in a freezer at −23°C, or lyophilized and stored at 4°C, for a period of 60 to 90 days. Once thawed, the antigen should be used soon thereafter. Refreezing is generally not recommended.

Standards

In RIA as in any analysis where comparisons are made, reference standards are necessary, for interpolating the values of samples to be measured (Fig. 14–1). These standards allow comparisons of results obtained under different conditions and in different laboratories. There are several types of RIA standards: international standards distributed by the World Health Organization; such reference preparations as those distributed by the National Institute of Arthritis and Metabolic Disease; and laboratory preparations of restricted use, prepared by the investigator or a manufacturer and not having international validity.

In the case of RIA, international standards and reference preparations are not always available or do not exist in sufficient abundance for general distribution. In this case, reference materials must be prepared by the researcher or manufacturer and then tested against an international standard. Preparations used as references should maintain their character over long periods in storage conditions. They should also be available in sufficient supply to last several years. The reference standard must be immunologically, biologically, and chemically similar to the substance to be measured; that is, dilution curves of the standard and of the test substance should be parallel.

ANTIBODIES

The sensitivity and specificity of RIA depend on the affinity of the antigen-antibody reaction and the highly specific binding sites on the antibodies used. Consequently, the most important factor in establishing a satisfactory assay is the production of a good antiserum.

To produce a highly specific antiserum, the antigen should have a unique *antigenic determinant,* i.e., that portion of the molecule, usually a sequence of 4 to 8 amino acids, which confers its antigenic characteristics. It should possess a three-dimensional structure such that modification of a single amino acid would render union with the antibody impossible. Such small molecules as ACTH, with 30 amino acids, have only one or two antigenic determinants, while peptides like HGH, with 188 amino acid residues, may have several determinants in their structure. The anti-

genic determinant and the determinant of biologic activity may correspond to different portions of the molecule. Consequently, the treatment of antigenic substances may be quite different for RIA and for bioassays.

The immunogenicity of a substance depends directly on two main factors: its molecular size and its chemical structure. Some peptides of large molecular weight may be immunogenically poor. Other compounds, such as steroids, glycosides, and small peptides are not immunogenic in their native state and need to be linked to larger molecules to produce an immunologic response.

Antibody formation is generally augmented by adding an adjuvant to the antigen, which retards its absorption and increases the antigenic stimulus. These substances include aluminum hydroxide, gelatin, mineral oil, and Freund's adjuvant. The last item is used most often and consists of a neutral detergent, paraffin oil, and killed bacteria. By virtue of its hydrophilic properties, the detergent unites the aqueous phase, which contains the antigen, with the oil phase to form a stable emulsion, which thereby prevents absorption. The bacteria merely produce a nonspecific stimulant to the immune system. Such an adjuvant maintains a prolonged serum concentration of the antigen and prevents its breakdown by proteolytic enzymes. In the case of hormonal antigens, the adjuvant also minimizes other physiologic effects.

Some investigators prefer to use a semipurified antigen because the impurities act as an adjuvant to stimulate antibody production and because lesser grades of antigen are less expensive. The immunizing dose is not always easy to determine. There is a wide range between the minimum dose that is needed to stimulate the immune system and the maximum dose that causes an immunogenic overload or unwanted side effects in the animal injected, as with insulin, for example, which may induce hypoglycemia.

Choosing the type of animal to use is still a somewhat empirical process. Rabbits and guinea pigs are selected most often because they are small enough to be handled easily and large enough to withstand bleeding of up to 10 ml. Other animals such as sheep, fish, and birds may be used occasionally. A common immunization schedule for small animals includes serial immunization every 2 weeks for 3 to 5 doses and then boosting every 5 weeks. Various injection sites may be used, including intradermal, intramuscular, intraperitoneal, subcutaneous, and intravenous.

Figure 14–2 shows the change in antibody titer with successive antigen injections. In general, the antibody titer is maximal 10 to 14 days after the last injection. The antibody titer may be sufficiently high after only two injections, but usually, the affinity and specificity of the antiserum increase with time.

Properties of Antisera

Once harvested, the antisera is tested for antibody titer, sensitivity, and specificity to determine its suitability for RIA. The antibody titer must be high enough to perform a large number of tests. This requirement usually poses little problem because most antisera must be diluted several thousandfold, even millionfold, to achieve the appropriate concentration. To achieve a working solution, the antiserum is diluted until there is 50% binding of the labeled antigen (B/F = 1) in the absence of unlabeled antigen (Fig. 14–3). When this antibody dilution is used, the addition of unlabeled antigen (the substance to be tested) yields the curve in Figure 14–1. The dilution required depends on the specific activity of the antigen and on the specificity of the antibody. The higher the specific activity of the antigen, the greater the antiserum may be diluted. The more the antiserum can be diluted while maintaining antigen binding capacity, the greater the sensitivity of the assay system.

The sensitivity of the antiserum represents in practical terms its affinity for the antigen and must therefore be compatible with the concentration of the substance to be measured. The sensitivity of an antiserum used to measure picogram quan-

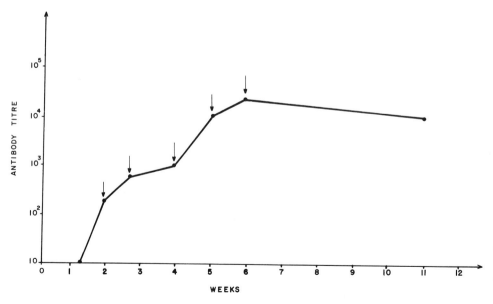

Fig. 14–2. Increase in antibody titer with successive injections of antigen.

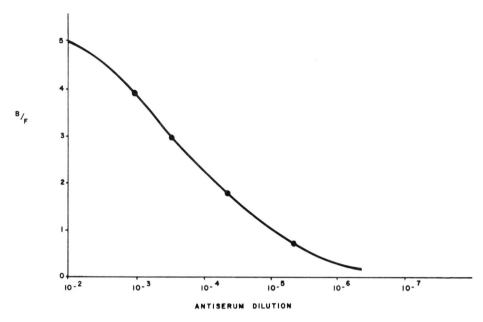

Fig. 14–3. Dilution of antiserum with labeled antigen. The dilution that gives B/F = 1 with the labeled antigen is the most appropriate working antibody titer.

tities of antigen must of necessity be greater than that required to bind to microgram quantities. Sensitivity is usually determined after the appropriate antiserum dilution has been made. Small amounts of unlabeled antigen are then incubated with the labeled antigen and the diluted antibody. That antiserum capable of distinguishing the smallest additions of added antigen is the most sensitive antibody, as determined from the steepness of the slope (Fig. 14–4).

As pointed out by Greenwood, this method is not always a rigorous test of sensitivity.[6] In 1968, Berson and Yalow proposed a more adequate test, in which titrations are made using varying quantities of labeled antigen.[7] The antiserum that is then capable of distinguishing the smallest difference in labeled antigen concentration is the most sensitive.

The specificity of the antisera is related to its capacity to bind only with the antigen to be measured and not with denatured antigen, its fragments, or antigens of similar chemical structure. A test of spec-ificity can be made by constructing dilution curves, not only with the antigen, but also with similar or cross-reacting substances or with drugs that may be present in the samples to be measured that may potentially interfere with the reaction.

Storage of Antisera

Once a suitable antiserum has been obtained, it must be stored so that it does not suffer alterations. The usual method is to draw off the serum, divide it into small aliquots, and store it at −23°C. The material, when ready for use, is thawed once and used immediately. An alternative method is to precipitate the gamma-globulin fraction, purify by dialysis, and lyophilize. The material can then be stored at −23°C for several years without alteration.

SEPARATION OF BOUND AND FREE COMPONENTS

One of the fundamental aspects of a satisfactory RIA is the final separation of the

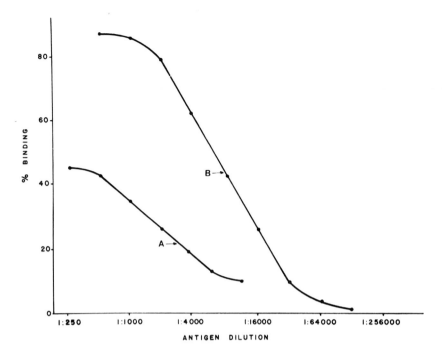

Fig. 14–4. Relationship between the percent binding of a labeled antigen in the presence of varying concentrations of unlabeled antigen for two antisera. Antiserum B has the greater sensitivity for detecting small changes in antigen concentration.

bound and free fractions after the incubation period. Among the methods from which the specific separation process can be selected, the following are well recognized.

Electrophoresis

Electrophoresis and chromoelectrophoresis have the advantage of being complete and specific with little or no interference from other hormones present. These two methods have the disadvantages of being time consuming and of using a very small volume, so that they are impractical for use with a large number of samples.

Filtration

Gel filtration in long chain dextrans (Sephadex) permits molecules larger than the largest pores of the swollen Sephadex to pass through in the first elutions. A clear separation is usually obtained; the method has been used primarily in research procedures.

Nonspecific Precipitation

Bound fractions can be precipitated using different reagents:

1. Organic solvents: ethanol, polyethylene glycol, dioxane, etc. In general, the procedure is inexpensive, rapid, and easy to automate. Additional advantages include no dissociation of the ligand-binder complexes without denaturation of protein, and even without rigid temperature control.
2. Inorganic salts: ammonium sulfate, sodium bisulfite; 50% ammonium sulfate is used in steroid assays after serum extraction (no protein interference).

Immunoprecipitation

In this technique, an antibody to the binding reagent is generated, usually in a larger animal (for example, goat antirabbit antibody), and added with a globulin carrier (from the same animal species in which the primary antibody was obtained). After centrifugation, the supernatant is aspirated or decanted and the precipitate is counted (the complex Ag-Ab-2nd Ab). The technique is widely used and offers both a clean separation without precipitation of free I-125 and almost universal applicability. Its main disadvantages are higher cost and the necessity of a second incubation period.

Adsorption

In this technique, the free ligand is adsorbed to a solid phase receptor. Because the adsorbent binds both free and bound ligand, the conditions of the reaction must be controlled to permit a selective adsorption of the free fraction, which leaves the complex ligand-binder in solution in the supernatant (which will be the fraction to count). The intensity of the adsorption depends on several conditions: pH, concentration of the adsorbent, nonspecific binding to the adsorbent, charge of the ligand, temperature, and incubation time between adsorbent and components of the reaction. Because of the insoluble nature of the adsorbents, they must be shaken or stirred during dispensing.

Dextran-coated and noncoated charcoal are the adsorbents used most frequently. Other adsorbents include talc, Florisil, magnesium silicate, magnesium carbonate, cellulose powder, zirconium phosphate, and anion exchange resins in the form of columns, sponges, tablets, and beads.

Solid-Phase Antibodies

This method introduces an insoluble antibody attached to a secondary insoluble structure. The primary goal of this technique is to simplify the assay by avoiding subsequent addition of a separating reagent. Antibodies used in the separation process may be bound to glass beads, Sephadex beads, para-aminocellulose, or polyacrylamide gels.

DOSE-RESPONSE CURVES AND DATA REDUCTION TECHNIQUES

In performing the radioimmunoassay, a set of standards is run first, followed by quality control standards and unknown samples. Data are usually recorded in terms of total counts measured for a fixed period of time.

The dose-response curve is established by the standards in a two-dimensional graphic representation in which the % B/T is plotted against antigen concentration. The concentration of antigen in unknown samples is found by relating raw data counts to the % B/T as shown in Figure 14–5. Then, a regression analysis technique is applied to define a functional relationship that can be extended to all the data.

The dose-response curves in radioassays are nonlinear; Figure 14–5 shows the hyperbola obtained in an androstenedione RIA, where hormone concentration is plotted against percentage B/T.

Several methods have been proposed for graphing these relationships to produce a linear curve. Linear dose-response curves make interpolation of values easier and are much more suitable for automated calculations. One method is to plot bound/total activity against the log of the dose (Fig. 14–6). This relationship tends to prolong the linear portion of the curve.

In 1944, Berkson introduced use of the *logistic function* (logit) as a method for linearization of sigmoid dose-response curves.[8] The logit function is defined as:

$$\text{logit } (y) = \ln(y/1 - y)$$

where y represents a measurable quantity

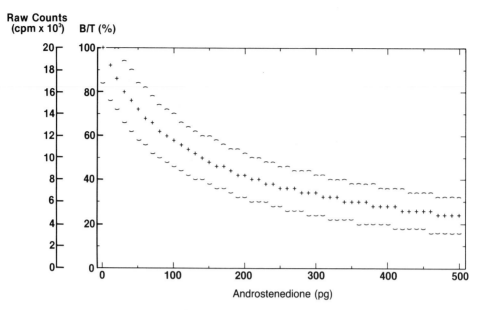

Fig. 14–5. Dose-response curve including 95% confidence limits for androstenedione RIA.

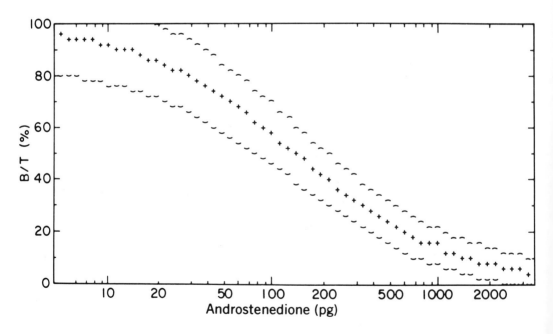

Fig. 14–6. Dose-response curve and 95% confidence limits for androstenedione RIA plotted as a log function.

of a response dependent on a variable dose (x).

When logit (y) is plotted against log (x), a linear dose-response curve is obtained.

Rodbard et al. showed that the logit transformation can be used for the linearization of the dose-response curves of competitive binding assays when percentage bound (B/B_0) is plotted against the log of the dose.[9,10,11]

$$\text{logit } (B/B_0) = \log_e[(B/B_0)/(1 - B/B_0)]$$

This may be symbolized as:

$$\text{logit } (y) = \log_e \left(\frac{1}{1 - y} \right)$$

where:

$$y = \frac{B - N}{B_0 - N}$$

and where B represents the bound activity; B_0 represents the counts bound in the absence of labeled antigen, and N represents counts bound in the absence of the receptor or antibody, i.e. the "plasma blank." The plot of y against the log of the dose usually yields a straight line. In assays where saturation levels of the binder change with the dose level of the ligand, logit plots become slightly sigmoid at both ends and approach a straight line in the midregion.

Figure 14–7 illustrates a logit-log plot for an androstenedione dose-response curve. The linear regression equation applicable to an estimation of the concentration of the unknown samples will be:

$$\text{logit } (B/B_0) = a + b \log (x)$$

CONTROL OF ASSAY CONDITIONS

It is not essential to a valid RIA system that labeled and unlabeled antigen be identical. It is sufficient that they behave similarly immunologically and that the plasma constituents do not affect the reaction. A necessary, although not suffi-cient condition, for a valid assay system is that the endogenous substrate on being diluted gives B/F curves that are also parallel with the standard curve.[12] Failure to obtain parallel curves on diluting samples may be due to a variety of causes.

Cross-Reaction of Antigens

More than one species of antigen may occur, as was the case with proinsulin in early insulin assays. Hormone fragments may also cause cross-reactivity.

Nonspecific Factors

This aspect includes variations in ionic concentration, pH, presence of anticoagulants, and denatured labeled antigen, all of which may reduce antigen-antibody binding.

Nonspecific factors are really specific chemical effects that can be avoided. In many assay systems, the energy of the antigen-antibody reaction can be greatly influenced by the buffer concentration or by the amount of mineral ions present in the plasma or urine samples. This fact becomes frequently evident when patients are treated with drugs that alter the serum or urine saline concentration. To reduce this interference, the sample can be diluted 1:5 or 1:10. Albumin can also be added to the reaction media, or better still, plasma from patients who are physiologically deficient in the hormone to be measured can be added.

The antigen-antibody complex frequently dissociates at extreme pH. It is therefore advisable to carefully maintain the pH between 7.4 and 8.6. Heparin also may affect certain hormone determinations because hormone concentrations in heparinized plasma appear greater than those in serum.[12] Thus each assay must be carefully examined for the factors that influence the antigen-antibody reaction.

RIA procedures must always contain a series of controls to evaluate the variability of results within the same assay, between successive assays, and between

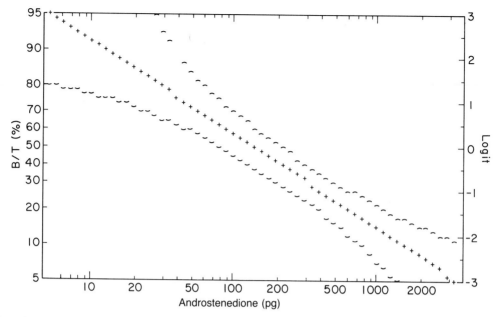

Fig. 14–7. Dose-response curve and 95% confidence limits for androstenedione RIA plotted as a log-logit function.

assays from different laboratories. Intra-assay controls are accomplished by running certain samples, and always the standards and control sera, in duplicate or triplicate. Statistical analysis of this variability helps establish the confidence limits of the particular run. Interassay control is accomplished by running pooled serum controls with high, intermediate, and low (or blank) concentrations of substrates with each assay run. Interlaboratory controls are obtained through the periodic analysis of international reference standards.

Pooled sera controls are measured with each assay and graphed on a running chart, with the standard deviations periodically determined. When one or more control determinations fall outside the limits of two standard deviations, the entire assay should be repeated.

In some countries, particularly in Europe and the United States, regional reference laboratories are established to check individual laboratory results by periodically supplying unknown test sam-ples. These same centers test commercial kits and reagents to prevent the sale and distribution of inadequate materials. In this manner, a high degree of standardization can be achieved while assuring a high quality of testing for the community.

EXTRACTION OF HORMONES FROM BIOLOGIC SOURCES

The hormones to be measured by RIA may come from macerated glands or organs, serum, plasma, urine, or other biologic sources. These samples may contain several factors that can influence the assay results, such as proteolytic enzymes, other hormones, or cross-reacting substances. In many cases, the hormone may exist in too low a concentration to be measured and thus must be concentrated after prior extraction. Generally, this is not necessary if the hormone to be measured exists in high concentration, if a highly specific antibody exists, or if the labeled hormone is of high specific activity.

The advantages of prior extraction are:

1. An increase in assay sensitivity by concentrating the hormone to be measured.
2. The removal of proteolytic enzymes and cross-reacting substances.
3. The dissociation of any pre-existing antigen-antibody complexes in patients who have been treated previously with the hormone to be measured.

Many extraction processes have been used, depending upon the demands of the given case. These include fractional precipitation by salts or organic solvents, electrophoresis gel filtration, chromatography, ultracentrifugation, and adsorption on solid media.

The criteria for selecting an extraction process are (1) ease, rapidity, and reproducibility; (2) specificity of the extraction; (3) preservation of immunoreactivity; and (4) expense.

LABELED ANTIBODIES

Immunoradiometric analysis (IRMA) is based on the same principle as RIA, except that the antibody is radioactively labeled:

$$[Ab^*] + [Ag] \leftrightharpoons [AbAg^*]$$

The same problems associated with RIA apply to IRMA, with additional problems related to labeling the antibody. Antibodies, as already shown, have at least two active sites, and the radioiodine is usually incorporated into one of these. One active site remains free because during the labeling process the antibody is adsorbed onto an immunoadsorbent, which protects some of the active sites. After labeling, the antibody is removed from the adsorber, freeing up the active site for fixation of the antigen.

There are certain advantages to labeling antibodies instead of antigens. When the antigen is highly contagious, as in the case of Australia antigen, working with standards and dilutions of the noncontagious labeled antibody is safer than working with the antigen. Another case is that in which one wishes to measure serum antibody, as in confirming previous exposure to a disease. In such a case, a labeled antibody provides a more specific assay system.

APPLICATIONS

The pace of new developments in RIA makes it impossible to create a "current" list of RIA applications that will remain current by the time of publication. Table 14–1 is a partial listing of applications, which gives an idea of the great range of usefulness of these procedures. The greatest activity in the sixties was directed toward endocrine hormones; thus, a whole new understanding as well as several new syndromes involving these organs was created. The applications in cardiology, rheumatology, gastroenterology, and gynecology soon followed with rapid advances. Many of these developments have been reviewed by Freeman and Blaufox and in an IAEA symposium.[13,14]

Drugs used in generally low concentrations or those that are difficult to measure chemically are increasingly being measured by RIA. Most drugs are relatively small molecules with molecular weights less than 1000 and are nonimmunogenic. Landsteiner showed that many small molecules (called *haptens*) could be covalently linked to such larger carrier molecules as proteins, polypeptides, and polysaccharides.[15] Antibodies formed to the larger substituted carrier molecules could react specifically with the smaller molecule alone. Butler and Chen used this technique to produce specific antibodies to digoxin, thus providing a means of assaying serum levels of digoxin, which often fluctuate widely and pose a serious threat of toxicity.[16,17]

Gentamicin and Tobramycin are antibiotics of the aminoglycoside group, both highly effective against *Pseudomonas*. They are, however, both potentially neu-

TABLE 14-1. *Some Substances Measured by Radioimmunoassay*

Peptide Hormones

Human growth hormone (HGH)
Insulin and proinsulin
Adrenocorticotropic hormone (ACTH)
Glucagon and Enteroglucagon
Thyroid-stimulating hormone (TSH)
Thyrotropin-releasing hormone (TRH)
Parathyroid hormone (PTH)
Calcitonin
Follicle-stimulating hormone (FSH)
Human chorionic gonadotropin (HCG)
Human chorionic somatomammotropin (HCS)
Substance P
Enkephalins
Endorphins
Melanocyte-stimulating hormone (MSH)

Lipotropin
Human Placental Lactogen (HPL)
Gastric inhibitory polypeptide (GIP)
Vasoactive intestinal polypeptide (VIP)
Gastrin
Secretin
Cholecystokinin
Pancreozymin
Angiotensin I
Bradykinins
Somatomedins
Oxytocin
Vasopressin
Prolactin
Luteinizing hormone

Steroid Hormones

Estrogen
Testosterone
Androsterone

Aldosterone
Cortisone
Progesterone

Other Hormones

Thyroxine
Serotonin
Melatonin
Ferritin

Triiodothyronine (T_3)
Thyroxine (T_4)
Reverse (T_3)

Nonhormonal Substances

Drugs
Digoxin
Digitoxin
Morphine and derivatives
Barbital and derivatives
LSD
Curare and derivatives
Vitamin A, B_{12}
Tobramycin
Gentamicin
Atropine
Netilmicin

Viral and Bacterial Substances
Australia Antigen (HAA)—{e, surface, core
Hepatitis antibody, A & B
Tetanus antibody
N. meningitidis antibodies
Vaccinia virus antibodies
Herpes virus antibodies
Enterotoxin
Staphylococcal antigen

Others
Folic acid
Thyroxine-binding globulin
Immunoglobulins A,E,G,M
Antihemophilic factor (AHG)
Intrinsic factor
Rheumatoid factor
Cyclic-AMP
Cyclic-GMP
Beta thromboglobulin
Myoglobin
Thyroglobulin
DNA
CK-MB
L-Dopa
Dopamine
Prostaglandins

Plasminogen, plasmin
Pancreatic esterase
Chymotrypsin, trypsin
Fibrinogen
Properdin
Hageman factor
Neurophysins
Carboxypeptidase
Aldose reductase
C_1-esterase
Carbonic anhydrase

Tumor Markers
Carcinoembryonic antigen (CEA)
α-fetoprotein
$α_1$-acid glycoprotein
Prostatic acid phosphatase

rotoxic and nephrotoxic if serum concentrations peak at too high levels. Therefore, it is prudent to measure both peak (to avoid toxicity) and trough (to assure adequate antibiotic effect) serum levels periodically during therapy. Peak concentrations in the range of 4 to 6 μg/ml at 30 to 60 min after injections are expected. Trough levels measured just prior to dosage should be adjusted so that levels in the range of 1.0 to 1.5 μg/ml are maintained. The toxic range lies above 12 μg/ml. RIA assays provide the ideal means of rapidly assaying these low levels of serum drug concentrations.

The search for specific tumor antibodies that would detect preclinical cancers and provide a means of following therapy and detecting recurrence is a challenging and worthy goal. Thus far, only relatively primitive and nonspecific tumor substances have been identified. Carcinoembryonic antigen, a glycoprotein with molecular weight of about 200,000, was first identified by Gold and Freedman.[18] This antigen is detectable in a high number of patients with cancers. In one collaborative study involving a large number of cancer patients and normal volunteers, abnormally elevated serum levels were found in 91% of patients with pancreatic carcinoma, 75% with lung cancer, 73% with colon and rectal carcinomas, and 61% with gastric carcinoma.[19] The two major problems with this test so far have been that it is nonspecific and that elevated levels are often not detected until the tumor volume is fairly large or until metastases have occurred. Nonspecificity would not be a hindrance necessarily if it were not also true that serum levels are elevated in some noncancer patients, such as smokers. Nevertheless, this assay has been useful in following the course of therapy and in detecting recurrence. Following total resection of gastrointestinal tumors, the serum levels usually return to normal.[20]

Another tumor substance, α-fetoprotein, which is normally present in fetal tissues

also has been found to be present in patients with hepatomas.[21] While this α-globulin is also useful in following the therapy of tumor patients, it occurs with such other diseases as hepatitis and cirrhosis; thus, its usefulness as a screening test is limited. The search for more sensitive tests to identify small tumor masses and for more specific agents will continue now that the tools for their discovery are at hand.

Recent developments in the radioimmunoassay of viral antigens and various human serum antibodies to hepatitis A and B have greatly increased our ability to detect these diseases and to understand the immune response to infection by these viruses. Figure 14–8 demonstrates the changing serum antibody titers that occur following injection with hepatitis A virus. Several serum antigens and antibodies are associated with hepatitis B infection (Fig. 14–9). Combinations of three tests, anti-hepatitis A virus (Anti-HAV-IgM), hepatitis B surface antigen (HBsAg), and hepatitis B core antigen (Anti-HBc) can be used in decision algorithms to make relatively secure diagnoses with wide-ranging significance (Table 14–2).[22]

NONIMMUNE COMPETITIVE BINDING ASSAYS

Competitive Protein Binding

Several different assay systems based upon saturation analysis have been and are being developed using nonimmune substances. The most widespread appli-

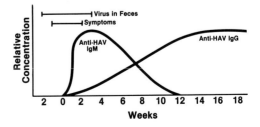

Fig. 14–8. Antibody response to hepatitis A virus.

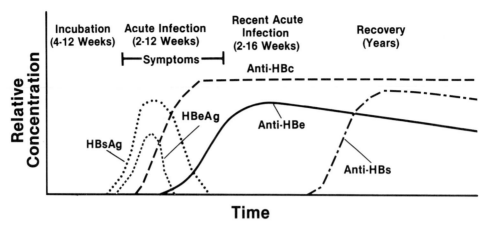

Fig. 14–9. Characteristic pattern of serologic markers to hepatitis B infection. HBsAg = hepatitis B surface antigen; HBeAg = hepatitis Be antigen; Anti-HBc = hepatitis B core antibody; Anti-HBe = hepatitis Be antibody; Anti-HBs = antibody to hepatitis B surface antigen.

TABLE 14–2. _Serodiagnosis of Acute Viral Hepatitis_

| | RIA Tests | | |
| | HBsAg | Anti-HAV Igm | Anti-HBc |
Interpretation			
Recent hepatitis A	−	+	−
Early acute hepatitis B	+	−	−
Acute hepatitis B	+	−	+
Possible recent acute hepatitis B	−	−	+
Possible non-A, non-B, hepatitis; other viral or toxic disease	−	−	−

After Soloway, H.B.[22]

TABLE 14–3. _Competitive Protein Binding Analyses_

Substrate	Specific protein binder
Thyroxine	Thyroxine-binding globulin (TBG)
Estrogens	Estrogen-binding protein of pregnancy
Androgens	Steroid-binding globulin
Cortisol	Cortisol-binding globulin
B_{12}	B_{12}-binding globulin
Folic acid	Folic acid reductase, lactoglobulin

cation has been the measurement of thyroxine using thyroxine-binding globulin (TBG) as the binder protein developed by Murphy et al.[23] When serum transport proteins are used as the ligand, the system is generally called _competitive protein binding_ (CPB) _analysis._ Several such assay systems have been developed, some of which are listed in Table 14–3. In general, these assays are less sensitive than RIA because of the lesser specificity of the binding proteins and near universal cross-reactivity with other plasma substances. Usually, steps must be taken to eliminate cross-reacting proteins by precipitation, filtration, or denaturation. Nevertheless, these assays are often useful because the binder substance is readily available and often quite stable.

Radioreceptor Assays

In the early 1960s, it became apparent that the action of many peptide hormones is exerted through the activation of cyclic AMP, which binds the hormones to globulins of the cell membranes of the target tissue. These globulins are called _receptors._ For example, the action of steroids is accomplished through its binding with intracellular receptors or transport globulins, which are very specific and which bind the hormone with a high equilibrium constant. This fact creates the possibility of an assay system based on binding with these biologic receptors.[24,25,26]

The method of saturation analysis using receptors has been applied with considerable success in the assay of FSH and LH, which almost invariably involves problems of cross-reactivity in RIA systems. The principle of the method is the same as RIA except that a biologic receptor is used in place of an antibody:

$$[S^*] + [S] + [R] \leftrightharpoons [SR] + [S^*R]$$

where S is the substance to be measured, S* is the radiolabeled substance, and R is the receptor.

Membrane receptor assays have several advantages. Because the membrane receptor sites normally extract circulating hormones, there is a high equilibrium constant for the association. In addition, because the receptor recognizes the active site of the hormone, tissues from various species may be used as receptors, and hormones from various species may also be used. This factor is especially useful when the human hormone is scarce, as is the case with TSH or prolactin. Finally, because the receptors usually are large molecules, separation of the bound fraction is facilitated.

Table 14–4 contains a list of hormones and their specific receptor tissues that have been used in assay systems.

Receptor assays present certain problems. The tissue receptors are often unstable. Because the receptors come from various tissues, they are not always soluble. They are also present in fairly low concentrations, and it is difficult to assure the same concentrations from assay to assay. Much progress in this field is required to develop dependable assay systems with a high degree of sensitivity and precision.

A still emerging assay system uses microorganisms (virus or bacterial) as the substrate and labeled immune complement as the binder substance. This kind of system can be used to detect either the presence of microorganisms or the titers of circulating immunoglobulins. Either the organisms or the protein can be labeled, and such a system has the advantage that the organism does not have to be kept living. Undoubtedly, the future literature will report many applications of this analysis system.

TABLE 14–4. *Radioreceptor Assay System*

Hormone	Tissue target
1. Releasing factors:	
CRF, TRF, GRF, LRF, FRF	Anterior pituitary
2. Anterior pituitary hormones:	
FSH	Seminiferous tubules
LH	Ovarian follicle
TSH	Leydig cells
HGH	Liver
ACTH	Mammary glands
MSH	Adrenal gland
Vasopressin	Toad skin
Oxytocin	Renal medulla
Angiotensin II	Adrenal cortex
Catecholamine	Uterus
Parathormone	Myocardium
Glucagon	Renal cortex
Secretin	Myocardium, liver tissue, adipose tissue
3. Other substances:	
Estrogens	Uterus, breast, vaginal tissues
Androgens	Prostate, seminal vesicle
ACTH	Adrenal cortex
TSH	Thyroid cell membrane
Insulin	Lymphocyte membrane sites

REFERENCES

1. Yalow, R.S., and Berson, S.A.: Immunoassay of plasma insulin in man. J. Clin. Invest., *39*:1157, 1960.
2. Zettner, A., and Duly, P.E.: Sequential saturation, a principle to increase sensitivity of competitive binding radioassays. Am. J. Clin. Pathol., *59*:145, 1973.
3. Hunter, W.M., and Greenwood, F.C.: Preparation of ^{131}I labeled growth hormone of high specific activity. Nature (Lond.), *194*:495, 1962.
4. Rosa, U., et al: Protein radioiodination by an

electrolytic technique. Strahlentherapie (Son-derb.), *60*:258, 1965.

5. Greenwood, F.C., Hunter, W.M., and Glover, J.S.: The preparation of ^{131}I labeled human growth hormone of high specific activity. Biochem. J., *89*:114, 1963.

6. Greenwood, F.C.: The radioimmunoassay of peptide hormones. Br. J. Hosp. Med., *2*:764, 1969.

7. Berson, S.A., and Yalow, R.S.: General principles of radioimmunoassay. Clin. Chim. Acta., *22*:51, 1968.

8. Berkson, J.: Application of the logistic function to bioassay. J. Am. Statist. Assoc., *39*:357, 1944.

9. Rodbard, D., et al.: Statistical quality control of radioimmunoassays. J. Clin. Endocrinol., *28*:1412, 1968.

10. Rodbard, D., Bridson, W., and Rayford, P.L.: Rapid calculations of radioimmunoassay results. J. Lab. Clin. Med., *74*:770, 1969.

11. Rodbard, D., and Hutt, D.M.: Statistical analysis of radioimmunoassays and immunoradiometric (labelled antibody) assay: a generalized, weighted, iterative, least-square method for logistic curve fitting. *In* Radioimmunoassay and Related Procedures in Medicine. Vol. 2. Vienna, IAEA, 1974.

12. Yalow, R.S., and Berson, S.A.: Introduction and general considerations. *In* Principles of Competitive Protein-Binding Assays. Edited by W.D. Odell and W.H. Daughaday. Philadelphia, J.B. Lippincott, 1971.

13. Freeman, L.M., and Blaufox, M.D. (Eds.): Radioimmunoassay. New York, Grune and Stratton, 1975.

14. International Atomic Energy Agency: Radioimmunoassay and Related Procedures in Medicine. Proceedings of the Symposium 31 October–4 November, 1977. IAEA and World Health Organization. STI/PUB/469, 1977.

15. Landsteiner, K.: The Specificity of Serological Reactions. Cambridge, Harvard University Press, 1945.

16. Butler, V.P., Jr., and Chen, J.P.: Digoxin-specific antibodies. Proc. Natl. Acad. Sci. U.S.A., *57*:71, 1967.

17. Smith, T.W., Butler, V.P., Jr., and Haber, E.: Determination of therapeutic and toxic serum digoxin concentrations by radioimmunoassay. N. Engl. J. Med., *281*:1212, 1969.

18. Gold, P., and Freedman, S.O.: Determination of tumor-specific antigens in human colonic carcinomata by immunologic tolerance and absorption techniques. J. Exp. Med., *121*:439, 1965.

19. Hansen, H.J., et al.: Carcinoembryonic antigen (CEA) assay. A laboratory adjunct in the diagnosis and management of cancer. Hum. Pathol., *5*:139, 1974.

20. Holyoke, E.D., Reynoso, G., and Chu, T.M.: Carcinoembryonic antigen (CEA) in patients with carcinoma of the digestive tract. Ann. Surg., *176*:559, 1972.

21. Tatarinov, T.S.: Presence of embryospecific-globulin in serum of patients with primary hepatocellular carcinoma. Vopr. Khim., *10*:90, 1964.

22. Soloway, H.B.: Diagnostic decision-making: Interpreting hepatitis profiles. Diagn. Med., Jan/Feb:29, 1980.

23. Murphy, B.E.P., Pattee, C.J., and Gold, A.: Clinical evaluation of a new method for the determination of serum thyroxine. J. Clin. Endocrinol. Metab., *26*:247, 1966.

24. Odell, W.D., and Daughaday, W.H. (Eds.): Principles of Competitive Protein-Binding Assays. Philadelphia, J.B. Lippincott, 1971.

25. Catt, K.J., Dufan, M.K., and Tsuruhara, T.: Radioligand-receptor assay of luteinizing hormone and chorionic gonadotropin. J. Clin. Endocrinol. Metab., *34*:123, 1972.

26. Berson, S.A., and Yalow, R.S. (Eds.): Methods in Investigative and Diagnostic Endocrinology. New York, American Elsevier, 1973.

Chapter 15

RADIOMICROBIOLOGY

EDWALDO E. CAMARGO AND
STEVEN M. LARSON

Radiometric detection of bacterial metabolism is based on the principle that bacterial action on C-14 substrates produces measurable amounts of $^{14}CO_2$. The use of radioisotopes for the detection of microorganisms was first reported by Levin and co-workers, who measured the $^{14}CO_2$ produced through oxidation of (1-^{14}C) lactose by *E. coli*.[1,2] Their method consisted of collecting the $^{14}CO_2$ by exhausting the test tube containing the bacilli and radioactive broth through a paper fiber pad moistened with a saturated solution of barium hydroxide. At selected intervals, the pad was removed, dried, and counted in a gas-flow proportional counter. With this method, it was possible to detect as few as 26 *E. coli* within 2 hr.

A natural consequence of the use of this method was the determination of antimicrobial activity, first described by Heim et al. in 1960.[3] The effect of various concentrations of several drugs on the metabolism of Staphylococcus, *E. coli,* and Proteus could be demonstrated within 2 to 6 hr after inoculation.

The system described by Levin and co-workers was further improved by using a mixture of equal parts of (U-^{14}C) glucose and C-14 formate.[4,5,6,7] Early detection of aerobes, anaerobes, facultative anaerobes, spore formers, and nonspore former organisms was then feasible. Such a system was used in the "Gulliver" project for detection of life on Mars.[8]

In the late 1960s, radiometric detection of bacterial growth was extended to clinical microbiology. DeLand and Wagner demonstrated the feasibility of using liquid scintillation counting for measuring $^{14}CO_2$ produced through bacterial oxidation of (U-^{14}C) glucose in a glucose-free thioglycollate medium.[9] In spite of the satisfactory results, automation of the system seemed difficult and the method's usefulness for clinical application was questionable. In 1969, an ion chamber prototype was substituted for the liquid scintillation system and was first tried in blood cultures with promising results.[10,11,12] This system has been improved, and fully automated models are available.

AUTOMATED RADIOMETRIC DETECTION SYSTEM

The gas evolved from the culture medium by bacterial action is usually $^{14}CO_2$; however, the evolution of $^{14}CH_4$ or C^3H_4 would also indicate bacterial metabolism.

The most important components of the radiometric detection instrument are shown in Figure 15–1: a culture gas tank (90 to 95% air and 5 to 10% CO_2), a set of two needles for culture gas exhaust and intake, a heat sterilizing unit for the needles, an ion chamber for measuring the radioactivity of the culture vial atmosphere, an electronic converter of the radioactivity into numbers, a circulating pump for removal of the atmosphere from the vial and from the ion chamber, a set of membrane pore filters (0.2 to 0.45 μm) between the gas tank and the needles, a droplet filter between the culture vial and the ion chamber, and a $^{14}CO_2$ trapping system that chemically converts CO_2 to a solid compound.

The reaction system consists of a sterile multidose serum vial containing a convenient culture medium, C-14 substrate, and bacteria. The rubber stopper of the culture vial should be sterilized prior to use. At the time of sampling, the sterilized set of needles of the measurement device penetrates the rubber stopper of the culture vial, and the cycle of the instrument begins: the ion chamber is exhausted, the culture gas is flushed through the culture vial into the ion chamber, the radioactivity is measured, and finally, clean air is drawn through the instrument to flush the radioactivity out of the chamber and into the CO_2 absorber. The entire cycle usually takes about 70 sec/sample.

Currently, there are different manual models with scales of 0 to 100, 0 to 1000, or 0 to 3000 "index units." These instruments are usually calibrated in such a way that 100 "index units" correspond to 0.025 μCi (0.92 kBq) of C-14 activity. More sophisticated and fully automated models exist also. Besides having all the components just described, they contain an incubator, a culture gas selector for both aerobic and anaerobic conditions, an automatic tray for changing samples, a display for sample selection, an automatic device for sterilizing the sample, a preset time display, and a printer. These models can be operated both manually and automatically. The automatic tray is designed to hold serum vials of different sizes.

The experimental vials should always be compared to controls for positivity. Control vials should contain the same reaction system, that is, the same amount of medium, C-14 substrate, and the same number of autoclaved bacteria added.

PLOTTING THE DATA

The data should be plotted in a manner that best illustrates numerical differences.

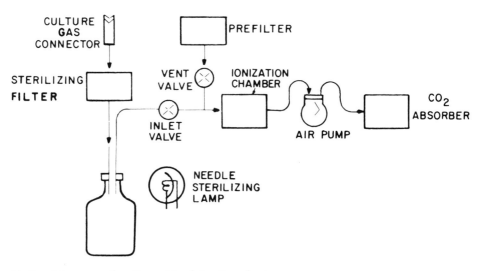

Fig. 15–1. Diagram of radiometric detection device.

Differential plotting is a convenient way to show changes in metabolic rates over the time course of an experiment. It represents the amount of $^{14}CO_2$ produced within a defined time interval (Fig. 15–2).

Cumulative plotting represents the total radioactivity obtained after any time interval. For example, Figure 15–3 represents a cumulative plot of the same data shown in Figure 15–2. One variation of this is plotting the cumulative as percent of control, which is particularly useful for studying the effects of drugs (Fig. 15–4).

Semilog plotting can be used to determine generation times or detection times,[13] as shown in Figure 15–5.

CLINICAL APPLICATIONS OF THE RADIOMETRIC SYSTEM

Bacteremia

Detection of bacteremia was the first clinical application of the radiometric system. Initially, (U-^{14}C) glucose alone was used as substrate for bacterial growth and 170 strains of 18 common pathogens were studied. Organisms from these strains were inoculated into sterile blood to simulate bacteremia. All of these organisms metabolized sufficient $^{14}CO_2$ to be detectable within a few hours in blood.[11] This study led to clinical comparisons of bacteremia detection by conventional and radiometric methods.[14,15,16,17,18,19]

The broad spectrum (Table 15–1) of the radiometric method has been well documented in over 10,000 blood cultures to date. Also, overwhelming evidence indicates that the radiometric method is more sensitive than routine methods for detecting bacteremia in general.[17,18,20,21,22,23,24] Being faster than the routine methods, the radiometric method permits earlier adjustment of antibiotic therapy and therefore plays an important role in the management of patients with serious infections. Today, the radiometric method is the procedure of choice for detecting bacteremia in over 900 hospitals in the United States.

Antibiotic Susceptibility Testing

Radiometric detection systems provide rapid and convenient assessment of bacterial susceptibility to antibiotics. The first clinical application of radiometric bacte-

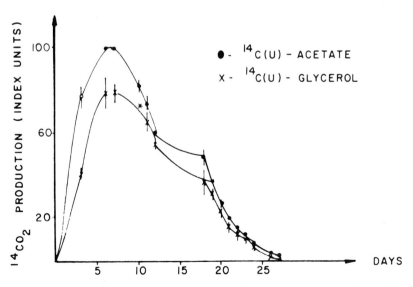

Fig. 15–2. Differential data plotting. Metabolism of (U-^{14}C) acetate and (U-^{14}C) glycerol by *M. lepraemurium.*

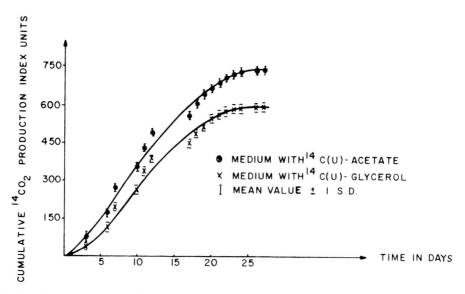

Fig. 15–3. Cumulative data plotting of results shown in Fig. 15–2.

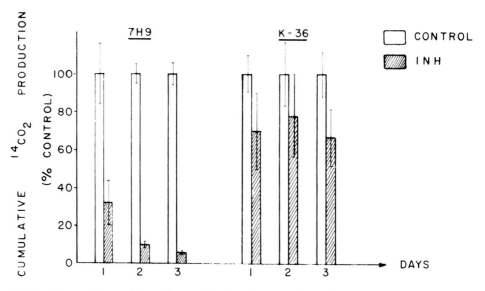

Fig. 15–4. Comparison of the effects of 1.0 μg isoniazid on the metabolism of C-14 formate by *M. tuberculosis* in 7H9 medium and K-36 buffer. Control vials contain no INH.

rial susceptibility testing was developed by DeBlanc et al.[25] Antibiotic effect on bacterial growth was evaluated by comparing the metabolism of a standard bacterial inoculum, with and without antibiotics, for 15 strains of organisms (5 species) and 17 antibiotics. Three hours was chosen as the reference time. The antibiotic concentration that reduced the amount of $^{14}CO_2$ by

at least 50% was chosen as the "radiometric inhibitory concentration." A standard tube dilution test was run in parallel with the radiometric study. A linear relationship over a wide range of concentrations existed between the tube dilution test and the radiometric 50% inhibition. Systematically higher concentrations of antibiotics were required to inhibit growth

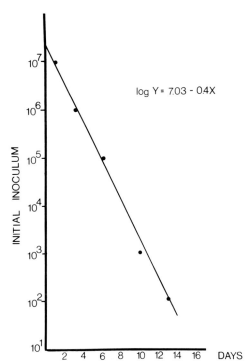

log Y = 7.03 - 0.4X

Fig. 15–5. Effect of inoculum size on detection times of *M. tuberculosis* using (1-^{14}C) lauric acid.

TABLE 15–1. *Organisms Detected by the Radiometric Method*

I) *Pyogenic Cocci*
  Staphylococcus aureus, S. epidermidis
  Micrococcus sp
  Streptococcus pyogenes, S. viridans, S.
    faecalis, S. durans, S. bovis, S. pneumoniae
  Neisseria meningitidis, N. gonorrhoeae, N.
    lactamicus, N. catarrhalis, N. sicca, N.
    flavescens, N. subflava

II) *Gram-Positive Bacilli*
  Clostridium perfringens
  Bacillus sp

III) *Enteric Gram-Negative Microorganisms*
  Escherichia coli
  Enterobacter aerogenes, E. cloacae
  Klebsiella pneumoniae
  Serratia marcescens
  Shigella flexneri
  Salmonella typhosa
  Proteus vulgaris, P. mirabilis, P. rettgeri, P.
    stuartii
  Pseudomonas aeruginosa, P. maltophilia
  Alcaligenes faecalis
  Citrobacter

IV) *Small Gram-Negative Rods*
  Hemophilus influenzae
  Moraxella sp

V) *Miscellaneous Microorganisms*
  Protoplasts
  Diphtheroids
  Bacteroides fragilis
  Herellea vaginicola
  Listeria
  Fusobacterium nucleatum
  Flavobacterium

VI) *Fungi*
  Candida albicans, C. krusei, C. parapsilosis,
    C. tropicalis
  Torulopsis glabrata
  Cryptococcus neoformans

VII) *Mycobacteria*
  M. tuberculosis (several strains), *M. bovis, M.*
    kansasii,
  M. intracellulare, M. chelonei, M. avium, M.
    lepraemurium

than were required to suppress metabolism to 50% at 3 hr, however. Thus this 3-hr test shows potential for application to drug susceptibility testing of conventional clinical pathogens.

DeLand also studied the effect of drug inhibition on bacterial metabolism and found a constant relationship between tube dilution and radiometric inhibition, for any particular bacteria.[26,27] The suppressive effect of antibiotics on metabolism has also been studied for the relatively fastidious organisms of the genus *Mycobacterium*. Camargo et al. showed the effect of 17 antibiotics on the metabolism of *M. lepraemurium*.[28] Kertcher et al. used C-14 formate to test the susceptibility of *M. tuberculosis* to isoniazid, streptomycin, rifampin, and ethambutol.[29] A 50% inhibition of $^{14}CO_2$ output at 48 hr was used as the radiometric inhibitory concentration. Dose-response curves obtained for these drugs compared the radiometric and the agar dilution methods. Except for ethambutol, the inhibitory concentrations were higher with the agar dilution method (Fig. 15–6). This may have resulted because formate oxidation can be blocked by a simple action on formate dehydrogenase, whereas the blockade of pro-

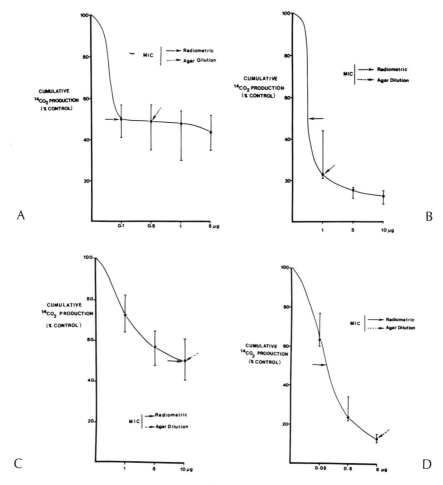

Fig. 15–6. Dose-response curves of *M. tuberculosis* isolates to isoniazid (*A*), Streptomycin (*B*), Ethambutol (*C*), and Rifampin (*D*).

tein synthesis (growth) and genetic function involves the action of the drug on more complex steps. Therefore, the radiometric method can be considered as a predictor of the outcome of the routine agar dilution method.

Yangco et al. have also reported good results with the radiometric test to determine the susceptibility of *M. avium-intracellulare* to drugs.[30] Beckwith and Guidon have reported their preliminary results on a 5-hr radiometric serum antibacterial assay for gram-positive cocci.[31] More recently, D'Antonio et al. have described a 4-hr radiometric serum test for antibiotic activity.[32] The test uses a mixture of (U-

^{14}C) glucose, (guanido-^{14}C) arginine, and (U-^{14}C) glycine to monitor the metabolic activity of both gram-positive and gram-negative organisms. When a >60% inhibition at 1:8 dilution was used, the method correctly predicted the outcome of the tube dilution method in 16 of 18 clinical samples.

Bacterial Speciation

Neisseria species are identified by their characteristic patterns of fermentation: glucose, maltose, sucrose, and lactose. *N. lactamicus* is the only organism capable of fermenting lactose. These fermentation reactions require from days to a week to allow certainty regarding the particular species of *Neisseria.* A radiometric test for speciation of *Neisseria* uses C-14 labeled glucose, maltose, and sucrose. Measurement is made after 3 hr of incubation at 37°C, and fermentation is assumed if $^{14}CO_2$ activity is more than two times background. Because C-14 labeled lactose is currently not available to measure β-galactosidase activity, a 3-hr enzyme test with the O-nitrophenyl-β-D-galactopyranoside (ONPG) disc is employed in conjunction with the radiometric reactions. In tests comparing classic fermentation reactions and the radiometric technique, perfect agreement was found between the two methods; however, the 3-hr radiometric technique offers a clear advantage in ease and rapidity.[33]

Strauss et al. also reported good results differentiating *N. flavescens, N. meningitidis, N. subflava,* and *N. lactamicus* with a *Neisseria* differentiation kit (Johnston Laboratories, Cockeysville, MD) containing C-14 labeled glucose, maltose, and fructose.[34] With the same kit, Appelbaum and Lawrence were able to identify 100% of *N. gonorrhoea* isolates and 100% of miscellaneous *Neisseria (lactamicus, sicca).*

Another approach with potential clinical application for speciating organisms is the immunologic inhibition technique. Type-specific antibodies inhibit bacterial metabolism in much the same way that antibiotics do (Fig. 15–7).[36] A series of simulated throat cultures showed that beta *streptococcus* could also be detected based on the specific inhibition of its metabolism by immune antisera.[37] Further extension of this method offers a potential means of detecting organisms in mixed culture within a few hours after inoculation.

Other Applications

Several products have been evaluated for sterility by the radiometric method. Of particular importance to nuclear medicine is an evaluation of the sterility of radiopharmaceuticals. Among 136 radiopharmaceutical samples studied by Chen et al., no false negatives with the radiometric method occurred.[38] A 4% false positive rate was observed, however, and was possibly related to gamma-ray background or contamination of the ionization chamber. The advantages of the system are the relative rapidity of detection and the possibility of automation.

Singh et al. have used a modification of the radiometric system described by Buddemeyer et al. to test antibiotic susceptibility in urinary tract infections.[39,40,41] This system consists of a two-component scintillation vial containing a sterile open glass metabolism vial surrounded by a cylinder of specially treated scintillating filter paper. The $^{14}CO_2$ produced by the organisms in the glass metabolism vial is trapped on the filter paper and quantitated automatically. With the system, results for clinical isolates of *E. coli, Proteus, Pseudomonas, Klebsiella,* and *S. epidermidis* were òbtained in 2 to 4 hr, a clear advantage over the disc diffusion method, which requires 48 hr for completion.

Another important application of the radiometric method consists of detection of viral infection in tissue cultures. The infected cells show a significant reduction of $^{14}CO_2$ production from $(1-^{14}C)$ glucose compared to control cells. Although the method has not yet reached clinical application, it promises a fast, simple, and objective means of studying viral effect on cell metabolism.[42]

A radiometric serum gentamicin assay has been described by Manos and Jacobs.[43] Although less precise than radioimmunoassays, it is considered acceptable for laboratories where radioimmunoassays are unavailable.

An interesting application of the radiometric method is the measurement of vitamin levels in food and body fluids. In essence, the method consists of using a suitable microorganism that does not grow

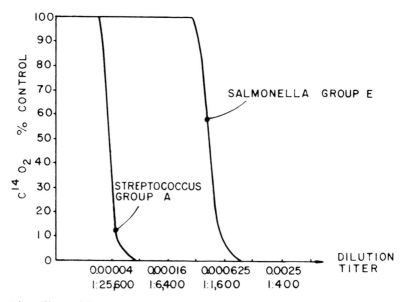

Fig. 15–7. The effect of *Streptococcus* A antisera on the metabolism of *Salmonella* group E and *Streptococcus* group A. (From Larson, S.M., et al.[36])

in the absence of the vitamin to be measured. A convenient C-14 substrate is also selected. Standard curves for known amounts of the vitamin in the medium are plotted; the test samples can then be measured. Chen et al. measured vitamin B_{12} levels in human serum using *L. leichmannii* and (guanido-^{14}C) arginine.[44] Chen et al. also measured folate levels in plasma and red blood cells, using L. *casei* and (1-^{14}C) gluconate.[45] Kertcher et al. were able to measure niacin levels in biologic fluids, using *L. plantarum* and (U-^{14}C) L-malic acid.[46] More recently, Guilarte et al. have described the use of *K. brevis* and (1-^{14}C) L-valine to measure vitamin B_6 levels in plasma and food samples.[47,48]

FACTORS AFFECTING RADIOMETRIC DETECTION OF BACTERIAL METABOLISM

Nature of Medium

Before a particular microorganism is studied radiometrically, the growth medium must be carefully chosen. This choice should be based on current microbiologic knowledge of optimum culture conditions performed to obtain the fastest and highest $^{14}CO_2$ output. In most studies performed with common clinical pathogens, glucose-free thioglycollate or trypticase soy broth has been used as a culture medium. For studying *M. tuberculosis,* Cummings et al. have used both the agar-free 7H10 medium and the 7H9 medium with albumin-dextrose complex.[49] Detection of metabolic activity of *M. lepraemurium,* an animal model of human leprosy, was feasible with both the K-36 buffer of Weiss and the complex NC-5 medium of Nakamura.[50,51,52,53] A complex medium, however, is likely to contain substrates to compete with the C-14 substrate for CO_2 production. Therefore, a simpler system may be preferable whenever a yes-or-no type of experiment is desired with a particular C-14 substrate.

pH of Medium

The pH of most culture media is 7.2. At this pH, the solubility of $^{14}CO_2$ in the medium is about 100%, so the release of

$^{14}CO_2$ into the experimental vial atmosphere is practically limited to surface exchange. Lowering the pH reduces the solubility of $^{14}CO_2$ in the medium and enhances the $^{14}CO_2$ release, but it also inactivates growth of microorganisms.[27] The presence of CO_2 in the culture gas is important for the exchange with $^{14}CO_2$ produced by bacterial metabolism.

Quality of Bacterial Suspension

For radiometric detection of most common clinical pathogens, it is unnecessary to take special precautions in the preparation of suspension. For such mycobacteria as *M. tuberculosis,* however, the quality of the bacterial suspension is essential, particularly in studying the effect of such drugs as isoniazid. When taken from the solid Lowenstein-Jensen medium and suspended in saline solution or buffer, *M. tuberculosis* invariably forms clumps, which makes difficult the interpretation of its metabolism in vitro. The best way to reduce the number and size of clumps is to grow the organisms in liquid 7H9 medium with albumin-dextrose complex in the presence of 0.05% Tween 80. With this procedure, the effect of isoniazid on susceptible strains can be demonstrated, whereas in the presence of clumps, inhibition may not be found.[54]

Inoculum Size

As a general rule, the fewer organisms in an experimental vial, the longer it takes for radiometric detection. Figure 15–5 illustrates the effect of inoculum size on detection time. For common clinical pathogens, the size of the inoculum is not a limiting factor; as few as 10 organisms can be easily detected within 2 to 4 hr.[11,14]

When studying slow-growing or uncultivable microorganisms, the number of bacteria per vial may be a decisive factor. Detection of 10^5 *M. tuberculosis* organisms is possible within 24 hr with (U-^{14}C) glycerol in glycerol-free 7H10 medium; however, detection of 10^2 to 10^3 organisms may take as long as 10 to 20 days (Fig. 15–5), depending on the strain. For *M. lepraemurium,* detection of inocula smaller than 10^9 organisms per vial has so far been impossible.[50]

C-14 Substrate

Clinical pathogens have been radiometrically detected using (U-^{14}C) glucose or a mixture of (U-^{14}C) glucose and C-14 formate. In addition, several other substrates have been employed.[55,56] Usually, 1 μCi of (U-^{14}C) glucose has been used in these studies, but activities as high as 10 μCi have been employed.[25] As the concentration of C-14 substrate in the medium increases, the $^{14}CO_2$ output increases, and the detection time decreases. This effect is particularly useful for studying slow-growing organisms.[51]

Because the amount of C-14 substrate is extremely small compared to unlabeled substances in the growth medium, the assimilation kinetics of the radioactive material by the microorganisms is markedly inhibited in the presence of the same stable substrate. For example, the presence of stable glycerol in NC-5 medium markedly inhibits the assimilation and oxidation of (U-^{14}C) glycerol by *M. lepraemurium.*[50] Both 7H10 and 7H9 media for growth of *M. tuberculosis* can be prepared with glycerol. For radiometric studies, however, glycerol should be omitted from the medium if C-14-glycerol is to be used for detection of these organisms.

The inhibitory effect of a stable substrate on the assimilation and oxidation of the C-14 substrate is not always structure-dependent, in the sense that competing substances may have different molecular structures. For example, stable oleic acid markedly inhibits the metabolism of (U-^{14}C) acetate by *M. lepraemurium.*[51]

If a particular microorganism is known to metabolize a stable substrate but fails to oxidize the same (U-^{14}C) substrate in a complex medium, the presence of competitors should be investigated. A yes-or-no type of experiment using the (U-^{14}C) substrate in a simple buffer system may be desirable. A positive test would then ensure that the organism is able to oxidize the substrate in vitro and would reaffirm the presence of competitors in the complex medium.

Incubation Temperature

Radiometric studies with common clinical pathogens have been performed at 37°C. For *M. lepraemurium* obtained from mice, the incubation temperature is 30°C. The $^{14}CO_2$ production from (U-^{14}C) acetate by *M. lepraemurium* at 30°C is about 60% higher than at 37°C.[51]

Species and Strain

The species of organism also influences the choice of the most suitable C-14 substrate. Examples of this are the speciations of *Neisseria* already described and the use of (1-^{14}C) fatty acids to speciate organisms of the genus *Mycobacterium*.[57,58]

Stress Environments

When a microorganism is placed in a hostile environment, there is a tendency to overcome the adverse condition, resulting in increased metabolism and $^{14}CO_2$ production. This initial higher $^{14}CO_2$ production is followed by a progressive decrease in the metabolism and death of the organism if the medium is not changed. When the environment is extremely hostile, the organism usually dies immediately, but the transition from an environment where metabolism is still possible to another where metabolism is totally inhibited is difficult to establish.

An example is *M. tuberculosis* metabolizing lauric acid in two different media, water and K-36 buffer. In the more hostile environment (water), there is initially a higher $^{14}CO_2$ output with an abrupt fall; in K-36 buffer, the initial $^{14}CO_2$ production is lower, but metabolism is maintained longer. It is probable that the radiometric detection of *M. lepraemurium* in vitro is feasible because of the early stimulatory effect caused by a stressing environment, the K-36 buffer.[50]

Presence of Drugs

The rapid detection of the effect of drugs on microorganisms is one of the most important uses of the radiometric method. Drugs usually depress the metabolism of microorganisms, which decreases $^{14}CO_2$ production (Figs. 15–4, 15–6). The nature of the medium is important when studying drugs because stressing environment may antagonize the effect of the drug (Fig. 15–4).

ASSIMILATION STUDIES

More information about bacterial metabolism can be obtained by combining oxidation ($^{14}CO_2$ production) and assimilation studies. With the combined studies, information regarding the fate of a particular substrate and its usefulness for energetic or structure purposes can be obtained. The study of assimilation of substrates involves the use of liquid scintillation counting techniques.

In general, at the end of the oxidation study ($^{14}CO_2$ production), all experimental vials containing the same C-14 substrate and live bacteria are pooled. The microorganisms are then removed from the medium by filtration of the suspension through membrane filters (0.2 to 0.45 μm pore size). The filter is then air dried and dissolved in ethyl acetate, scintillation fluid is added, and the radioactivity retained within the cells is counted. Aliquots of the washes are counted in the same manner.

As an extension of assimilation studies, radiochromatographic analysis of the metabolic products contained in the first wash can be performed. In this case, it is important to compare the radiochromatogram of the medium that contained live bacteria with radiochromatograms of the pure C-14 substrate and of the control vials.

REFERENCES

1. Levin, G.V., Harrison, V.R., and Hess, W.C.: Preliminary report on a one-hour presumptive test for coliform organisms. J. Am. Water Works Assoc., *48*:75, 1956.
2. Levin, G.V., Harrison, V.R., Hess, W.C., and Gurney, H.C.: A radioisotope technique for rapid detection of coliform organisms. Am. J. Public Health, *46*:1405, 1956.
3. Heim, A.H., Curtin, J.A., and Levin, G.V.: Determination of antimicrobial activity by a radioisotope method. Antimicrob. Agents Ann., *123*, 1960.
4. Levin, G.V., Harrison, V.R., Hess, W.C., et al.: Rapid radioactive test for coliform organisms. J. Am. Water Works Ass., *51*:1, 1959
5. Levin, G.V., Strauss, V.I., and Hess, W.C.: Rapid coliform organisms determination with ^{14}C. J. Water Pollu. Contr. Fed., *33*:1021, 1961.
6. Scott, R.M., Seiz, D., and Shaughnessy, H.J.: Rapid carbon-14 test for coliform bacteria in water. Am. J. Public Health, *54*:827, 1964.
7. Scott, R.M., Seiz, D., and Shaughnessy, J.H.: Rapid carbon-14 test for sewage bacteria. Am. J. Public Health, *54*:834, 1964.
8. Levin, G.V., Heim, A.H., Glendenning, J.R., and Thompson, M-F: "Gulliver"—a quest for life on Mars. Science, *138*:114, 1962.
9. DeLand, F.H., and Wagner, H.N., Jr.: Unpublished data, 1968.
10. DeLand, F.H., and Wagner, H.N., Jr.: Early detection of bacterial growth with carbon-14 labeled glucose. Radiology, *92*:154, 1969
11. DeLand, F.H., and Wagner, H.N., Jr.: Automated radiometric detection of bacterial growth in blood cultures. J. Lab. Clin. Med., *75*:529, 1970.
12. Schrot, J.E., Hess, W.C., and Levin, G.V.: Method for radiorespirometric detection of bacteria in pure culture and in blood. Appl. Microbiol., *26*:867, 1973.
13. Waters, J.R.: Sensitivity of the $^{14}CO_2$ radiometric method for bacterial detection. Appl. Microbiol., *23*:198, 1972.
14. DeBlanc, H.J., Jr., DeLand, F.H., and Wagner, H.N., Jr.: Automated radiometric detection of bacteria in 2,967 blood cultures. Appl. Microbiol., *22*:846, 1971.
15. Washington, J.A., and Yu, P.K.W.: Radiometric method for detection of bacteremia. Appl. Microbiol., *22*:100, 1971.
16. Caslow, M., Ellner, P.D., and Kiehn, T.E.: Comparison of the Bactec system with blind subculture for the detection of bacteremia. Appl. Microbiol., *28*:435, 1974.
17. Rosner, R.: Comparison of macroscopic, microscopic and radiometric examinations of clinical blood cultures in hypertonic media. Appl. Microbiol., *28*:644, 1974.
18. Strauss, R.R., Throm, R., and Friedman, H.: Radiometric detection of bacteremia: requirement for terminal subcultures. J. Clin. Microbiol., *5*:145, 1977.
19. LaScolea, L.J., Dryja, D., Sullivan, T.D., et al.: Diagnosis of bacteremia in children by quantitative direct plating and a radiometric procedure. J. Clin. Microbiol., *13*:478, 1981.
20. Renner, E.D., Gatheridge, L.A., and Washington, J.A.: Evaluation of radiometric system for detecting bacteremia. Appl. Microbiol., *26*:368, 1973.
21. Bannatyne, R.M., and Harnett, N.: Radiometric detection of bacteremia in neonates. Appl. Microbiol., *27*:1067, 1974.
22. Brooks, K., and Sodeman, T.: Rapid detection of bacteremia by a radiometric system. A clinical evaluation. Am. J. Clin. Pathol., *61*:859, 1974.
23. Thiemke, W.A., and Wicher, K.: Laboratory experience with a radiometric method for detecting bacteremia. J. Clin. Microbiol., *1*:302, 1975.
24. Hopfer, R.L., Mills, K., and Groschel, D.: Improved blood culture medium for radiometric detection of yeasts. J. Clin. Microbiol., *9*:448, 1979.
25. DeBlanc, H.J., Charache, P., and Wagner, H.N., Jr.: Automated radiometric measurement of antibiotic effect on bacterial growth. Antimicrob. Agent Chemother., *2*:360, 1972.
26. DeLand, F.H.: Metabolic inhibition as an index of bacterial susceptibility to drugs. Antimicrob. Agents Chemother., *2*:405, 1972.
27. DeLand, F.H., Bacteriologic cultures and sensitivities. *In* Nuclear Medicine In-Vitro. Edited by B. Rothfeld. Philadelphia, J.B. Lippincott, 1974.
28. Camargo, E.E., Larson, S.M., Tepper, B.S., and Wagner, H.N., Jr.: A radiometric method for predicting effectiveness of chemotherapeutic agents in murine leprosy. Int. J. Lepr., *43*:234, 1975.
29. Kertcher, J.A., Chen, M.F., Charache, P., et al.: Rapid radiometric susceptibility testing of *Mycobacterium tuberculosis*. Am. Rev. Resp. Dis., *117*:631, 1978.
30. Yangco, B.G., Eikman, E.A., Solomon, D.A., et al.: Rapid radiometric method for determining drug susceptibility of *Mycobacterium avium-intracellulare*. Antimicrob. Agents Chemother., *19*:534, 1981.
31. Beckwith, D.G., and Guidon, P.T., Jr.: Development of a five-hour radiometric serum antibacterial assay for gram-positive cocci. J. Nucl. Med., *22*:274, 1981.
32. D'Antonio, R.G., Camargo, E.E., Gedra, T., et al.: Rapid radiometric serum test for antibiotic activity. Antimicrob. Agents Chemother., *21*:236, 1982.
33. Camargo, E.E., Larson, S.M., Charache, P., et al: Radiometric assays in clinical microbiology. Clin. Res., *23*:301A, 1975.
34. Strauss, R.R., Holderback, J., and Friedman, H.: Comparison of a radiometric procedure with conventional methods for identification of *Neisseria*. J. Clin. Microbiol., *7*:419, 1978.
35. Reference deleted.
36. Larson, S.M., Charache, P., Chen, M., and Wagner, H.N., Jr.: Inhibition of the metabolism of

streptococcus and salmonella by type specific antisera. Appl. Microbiol., *27*:351, 1974.

37. Larson, S.M., Chen, M., Charache, P., and Wagner, H.N., Jr.: A radiometric identification of streptococcus Group A in throat cultures. J. Nucl. Med., *16*:1085, 1975.

38. Chen, M.F., Rhodes, B.A., Larson, S.M., and Wagner, H.N., Jr.: Sterility testing of radiopharmaceuticals. J. Nucl. Med., *15*:1142, 1974.

39. Singh, K.T., Ganatra, R.D., Shah, D.H., et al.: Radiorespirometric testing of antibiotic sensitivity in urinary tract infections. J. Nucl. Med., *21*:135, 1980.

40. Ganatra, R.D., Buddemeyer, E.U., Deodhar, M.N., et al.: Modifications in biphasic liquid-scintillation vial system for radiometry. J. Nucl. Med., *21*:480, 1980.

41. Buddemeyer, E.U., Wells, G.M., Hutchinson, R., et al.: Radiometric estimation of the replication time of bacteria in culture: an objective and precise approach to quantitative microbiology. J. Nucl. Med., *19*:619, 1978.

42. D'Antonio, N., Tsan, M-F, Charache, P., et al.: Simple radiometric techniques for rapid detection of herpes simplex virus type 1 in Wi-38 cell culture. J. Nucl. Med., *17*:503, 1976.

43. Manos, J.P., and Jacobs, P.F.: Evaluation of the Bactec serum gentamicin assay. Antimicrob. Agents Chemother., *16*:631, 1979.

44. Chen, M.F., McIntyre, P.A., and Wagner, H.N., Jr.: A radiometric microbiologic method for vitamin B_{12} assay. J. Nucl. Med., *18*:388, 1977.

45. Chen, M.F., McIntyre, P.A., and Kertcher, J.A.: Measurement of folates in human plasma and erythrocytes by a radiometric microbiologic method. J. Nucl. Med., *19*:906, 1978.

46. Kertcher, J.A., Guilarte, T.R., Chen, M.F., et al.: A radiometric microbiologic assay for the biologically active forms of niacin. J. Nucl. Med., *20*:419, 1979.

47. Guilarte, T.R., and McIntyre, P.A.: Radiometric microbiologic assay of vitamin B_6: Analysis of plasma samples. J. Nutr., *111*:1861, 1981.

48. Guilarte, T.R., Shane, B., and McIntyre, P.A.: Ra-diometric microbiologic assay of vitamin B_6: Application to food analysis. J. Nutr., *111*:1869, 1981.

49. Cummings, D.M., Ristroph, D., Camargo, E.E., et al.: Radiometric detection of the metabolic activity of *Mycobacterium tuberculosis*. J. Nucl. Med., *16*:1189, 1975.

50. Camargo, E.E., Larson, S.M., Tepper, B.S., and Wagner, H.N., Jr.: Radiometric measurement of metabolic activity of *M. lepraemurium*. Appl. Microbiol., *28*:452, 1974.

51. Camargo, E.E., Larson, S.M., Tepper, B.S., and Wagner, H.N., Jr.: Radiometric studies of *Mycobacterium lepraemurium*. Int. J. Lepr., *44*:294, 1976.

52. Weiss, E.: Adenosine triphosphate and other requirements for the utilization of glucose by agents of the psittacosis-trachoma group. J. Bacteriol., *90*:243, 1965.

53. Nakamura, M.: Multiplication of *Mycobacterium lepraemurium* in cell-free liquid medium containing α-ketoglutaric acid and cytochrome C. J. Gen. Microbiol., *73*:193, 1972.

54. Camargo, E.E., Charache, P., Larson, S.M., et al.: Radiometric testing of susceptibility of *M. tuberculosis* to drugs. 15th Interscience Conference on Antimicrobial Agents and Chemotherapy. Annals of the Society of Microbiology, 1975.

55. Camargo, E.E., Larson, S.M., Charache, P., et al.: Current status of radiometric detection of *M. tuberculosis* and *M. lepraemurium*. J. Nucl. Med., *16*:518, 1975.

56. Camargo, E.E., Kertcher, J.A., Larson, S.M., et al.: Radiometric measurement of differential metabolism of fatty acids by *Mycobacterium lepraemurium*. Int. J. Leprosy., *47*:126,1979.

57. Camargo, E.E., Kertcher, J.A., and Larson, S.M.: Radiorespirometry in identification of mycobacteria. *In* Frontiers in Nuclear Medicine. Edited by W. Horst, N.H. Wagner, Jr., and J.W. Buchanan. Heidelberg, Springer-Verlag, 1980, p. 286.

58. Camargo, E.E., Kertcher, J.A., Larson, S.M., et al.: Radiometric measurement of differential metabolism of fatty acid by mycobacteria. Int. J. Leprosy, *50*:200, 1982.

Chapter 16

LABELED CARBON BREATH ANALYSIS

WALTON W. SHREEVE

The principle of labeled CO_2 breath analysis is simple. A substrate labeled with radioactive or stable carbon that is metabolized to CO_2 is administered, and the labeled CO_2 exhaled in the breath is quantitated as a function of time. The methods of measurement may be simple or complex, depending upon the carbon isotope used, but some methods can be readily adapted for common usage in most nuclear medicine departments.

In tracer studies, C-11, C-14, and stable C-13 are all potentially useful. The short physical half-life of C-11 (20 min) poses formidable technical problems, requiring rapid chemical or biologic synthesis, and purification of organic compounds. Inhalation of $^{11}CO_2$, however, has been used to evaluate the number, sizes, and turnover rates of various CO_2-bicarbonate pools in the human body.[1]

The most commonly used isotope for CO_2 analysis has been C-14, the low-energy (150 keV) beta emitter with a half-life of approximately 5700 years. The long half-life has caused some concern about long-term radiation; however, the biologic half-lives of many labeled organic compounds (and of CO_2) are short enough that total whole-body radiation absorbed doses from common dosages (2 to 20 μCi) are usually not more than 20 to 200 mrads.[2,3,4,5] These modest exposures are well within the customary clinical diagnostic range and are mostly distributed over a period of many years because of the long-term retention of a small percentage of the administered dose.

Stable C-13, which has a natural abundance of about 1.1%, may be used with natural compounds, or with compounds artificially enriched with C-13, without radiation hazard. It is therefore acceptable for all patient groups, including pregnant women, children, and large populations in screening studies. The sensitivity and simplicity of C-13 assays, however, are not as great as those of C-11 or C-14.

METHODS
Carbon-14

Early techniques for capturing breath $^{14}CO_2$ from patients utilized rubber beach balls or Douglas bags with subsequent percolation of gas through NaOH solution. The CO_2 was then precipitated onto plates as $Ba^{14}CO_3$ and counted in gas flow or thin end-window Geiger-Müller counters.[2,6,7,8,9] This method is still feasible for laboratories equipped with such counters. Since all of the breath CO_2 can be collected, the total CO_2 production rate is known from the weight of $BaCO_3$. The plate preparation is time consuming, however, a self-absorption curve for $BaCO_3$ is required, and the counting is relatively insensitive.

The introduction by Tolbert et al. and by Le Roy et al. of continuous respiration pattern analyzers for $^{14}CO_2$ and total CO_2 afforded elegant but expensive devices.[10,11] The method of Tolbert et al. used an ionization chamber to analyze $^{14}CO_2$, while Le Roy et al. used continuous flow through a 4π G-M counter. Tolbert's device has been used in several clinical research studies.[4,12,13,14,15,16,17,18,19,20,21] In addition to providing total output of CO_2 the particular advantage of this device is the accurate determination of peak times, specific activity, and slopes. The device can be automated for prompt data display and can be programmed for computer readout of cumulative expiration of $^{14}CO_2$. The cost and maintenance requirements, however, tend to limit the availability of this instrument.

When liquid scintillation counting became available, $Ba^{14}CO_3$ could be counted in gel suspensions.[22] Other techniques involve transfer of $^{14}CO_2$ from NaOH solution,[23] or a gas manometric chamber,[24] into a vial where it is trapped by an organic base. Total CO_2 output can also be measured by these methods. Although the method of Abt and von Schuching does not permit measurement of total CO_2, it is convenient in that it allows the patient to breathe directly through tubing connected to a vial for $^{14}CO_2$ trapping preparatory to liquid scintillation counting.[25] With most apparatus, the breath is led through a drying trap and then into a vessel where $^{14}CO_2$ is captured by an organic amine (e.g., Hyamine) in ethanol solution.[26,27,28] In some cases, a one-way valve at the mouthpiece adds convenience and efficiency. Some workers omit a drying trap and use all-disposable parts.[29] A pH indicator such as phenolphthalein in the solution indicates the end-time (about 1 to 3 min) of collection of a known amount of

CO_2. This end-time is determined by the normality of the Hyamine. Multiple samples are obtained at various time intervals to construct an excretion curve. Collections are made directly into the scintillation counting vial, scintillator solution is added, and the vials are counted in a standard liquid scintillation counter (Fig. 16–1). Data are initially obtained as specific activity of $^{14}CO_2$, e.g., counts per minute per millimole CO_2. To normalize for body size, expression of the results in terms of $^{14}CO_2$ excretion per unit time and body surface area is desirable.[16]

A newer method described by Lorenz et al. utilizes plastic scintillator filaments for detecting C-14 in expired breath directly.[30] This system also measures total CO_2, has lower background variation than an ionization chamber, and is portable.

Carbon-11

Samples of $^{11}CO_2$ can be collected continuously in a Tolbert ionization chamber, or as described previously, in NaOH or Hyamine solution and then counted. Double-isotope studies with C-14 and C-11 are also possible. In this case, C-14 is counted after complete decay of the C-11 (4 to 5 hr). The use of C-11 requires direct access to a cyclotron and rapid synthesis of substrate compounds.

Carbon-13

In the past 15 years, techniques have been developed for measuring $^{13}CO_2$ using mass spectrometry.[31,32,33] Although mass spectrometers are not yet sufficiently available for common use in nuclear medicine departments, a few centers provide excellent service. Another technique for measuring C-13 enriched gases, including CO or CO_2, utilizes infrared spectroscopy.[34,35] Whereas mass spectrometry is much more sensitive than infrared spectroscopy, a practical limit is set by the variation in natural abundance of $^{13}CO_2$ in the breath due to varying C-13 content of foodstuffs and metabolic substrates. The gen-

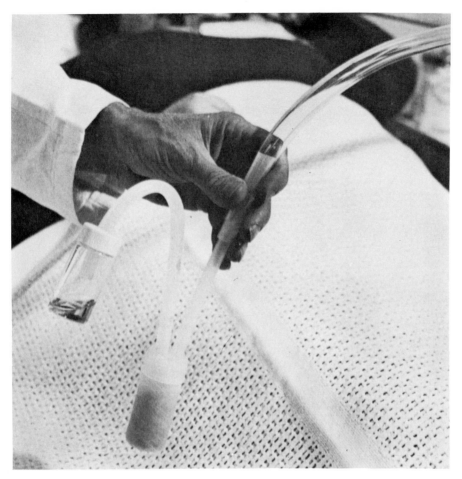

Fig. 16–1. Apparatus for direct trapping of expired $^{14}CO_2$ in ethanol-hyamine solution for liquid scintillation counting. Patient breathes through one-way valve and drying trap into counting vial, which is perforated for exit of breath.

eral technique requires prior analysis of this variation as "background" for each particular type and condition of study.[36]

APPLICATIONS

Malabsorption States

Among the earliest and still most useful tests of $^{14}CO_2$ excretion in the breath are those related to intestinal malabsorption. Schwabe et al. measured fat absorption by analyzing breath $^{14}CO_2$ following the oral administration of C-14 trioctanoin.[37] They found on the average fourfold lower rates

of oxidation in patients with steatorrhea than in control subjects. The results correlated with other measures of malabsorption, and the method was more convenient than measuring stool fat. Kaihara and Wagner used glyceryl-tripalmitate C-14 and measured $^{14}CO_2$ specific activity by liquid scintillation counting to verify the correlation with fecal fat content.[26] Chen et al. used C-14 tripalmitin and found a clear separation of patients with fat malabsorption from normal subjects (Fig. 16–2).[29] Further, they showed that administration of lipase with the C-14 tripalmitin restored oxidation to normal in patients with def-

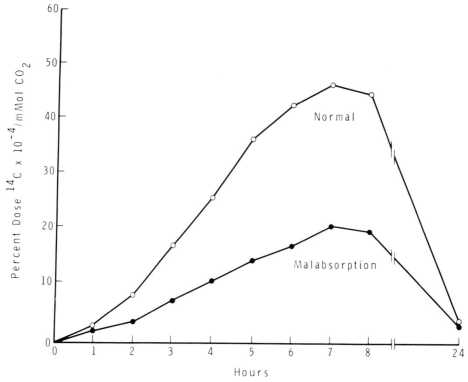

Fig. 16–2. Time course of specific activity of expired $^{14}CO_2$ after ingestion of C-14 tripalmitin by 10 normal subjects and 18 fat malabsorption patients. (From Chen, I.W., et al.[29])

inite pancreatic involvement, but not in those with other causes of fat malabsorption. Watkins et al. have used C-13 trioctanoin in children.[38] Carbon-14 triolein has proved superior to C-14 tripalmitin or C-14 trioctanoin to measure fat absorption.[39]

The C-14 triolein test can be performed in four hours with good discrimination.[40] A C-14 labeled, artificial mixed triglyceride, designed as a more specific test of pancreatic lipase activity, has given excellent results in patients with pancreatic disease or villus atrophy.[41] Some believe, however, that caution is indicated in accepting individual results of $^{14}CO_2$ or $^{13}CO_2$ production from any of the labeled triacylglycerols because of both overlap between steatorrheic and control subjects and wide variability in patients with diabetes, hyperlipemia, and obesity.[42] If findings with CO_2 are anomalous, the H-

3/C-14 ratio in serum lipids after administration of H-3 palmitic acid/C-14 tripalmitin mixture may be measured.[43]

Fish et al. showed that in malabsorption of vitamin B_{12} the rate of oxidation of C-14 propionic acid is slowed because B_{12} is required in the metabolism of methylmalonyl CoA to succinyl CoA.[44] Megaloblastic anemia due to B_{12} deficiency can be distinguished from that due to folic acid deficiency in that propionic acid is metabolized to CO_2 normally in the latter condition (Fig. 16–3). The same group observed that oxidation of C-14 histidine (2-ring) is depressed in folic acid-deficient anemia, whereas this oxidation is normal with B_{12} deficiency. Later, they showed that oxidation of the beta carbon of serine is also markedly depressed with folate deficiency and only moderately so with B_{12} deficiency.[45]

Intestinal "lactase deficiency" has been

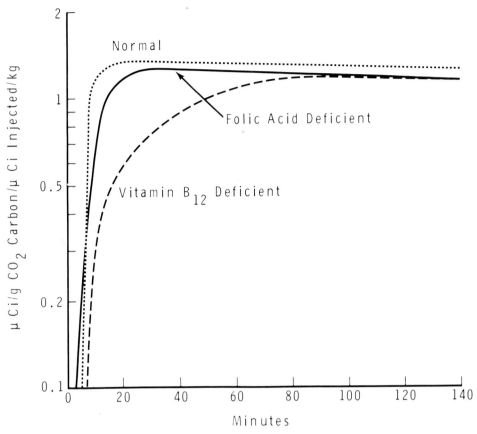

Fig. 16–3. Specific activity of $^{14}CO_2$ in a normal subject, a patient with folic-acid deficient anemia, and a patient with vitamin-B_{12} deficient megaloblastic anemia after intravenous injection of propionate-2-^{14}C. (From Fish, M.B., et al.[44])

studied by measuring the appearance of expired $^{14}CO_2$ after ingestion of C-14 lactose. Lactase deficiency is essentially a normal physiologic variant in a majority of individuals in certain races or ethnic groups, such as Orientals, American Indians, some Africans, and some Mediterraneans.[3] With widespread domestication of ruminants and extensive milk-drinking beyond weaning, man gradually developed greater amounts of intestinal lactase to enable digestion of milk products. In regions where milk-drinking beyond weaning was not practiced, a relative "deficiency" of intestinal lactase is found in the population. Individuals with this deficiency suffer symptoms from milk inges-

tion that may be confused with symptoms of other intestinal diseases. Although first explored by Cozzetto,[46] Sasaki et al. and Salmon et al. were better able to separate lactose-tolerant from lactose-intolerant groups by measuring $^{14}CO_2$ after administration of C-14 lactose (Fig. 16–4).[27,47]

The breath test with C-14 lactose (and possibly other labeled carbohydrates) can also be used to determine the nature and degree of damage to the small intestinal mucosa following pelvic radiotherapy.[48]

Some investigators have found that breath $^{14}CO_2$ analysis is less discriminating than measurement of serum galactose levels,[49,50] but the $^{14}CO_2$ test is simpler. On the other hand, the alternative H_2 breath

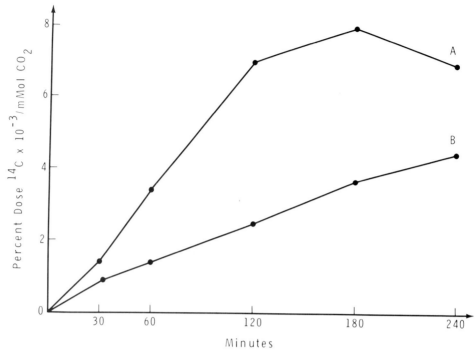

Fig. 16–4. $^{14}CO_2$ expired after oral administration of lactose-1-^{14}C. Curve A represents milk-tolerant subjects. Curve B represents patients with lactase deficiency. (From Sasaki, Y., et al.[27])

test was found to provide the best discrimination,[49] and it appears suitable for population screening.[42]

Normally, conjugated bile salts, which contain glycine, are reabsorbed in the enterohepatic circulation. Interference with this process, however, as by ileal resection, bypass operation, or abnormal bacterial colonization in the small bowel due to diverticulosis or "blind-loop" syndrome, causes excessive deconjugation and absorption of glycine. Glycine absorption can be measured by $^{14}CO_2$ breath analysis after oral administration of glycine-^{14}C-cholate or glycine-^{13}C-cholate.[51,52,53,54] The test with C-13 is not quite as sensitive as the test with C-14. Some surgical procedures, e.g., ileostomy and gastrectomy, may decrease rather than increase oxidation.[55] So also do such conditions as celiac disease and nontropical sprue, which are characterized by impaired glycine absorption. On the other hand, increased deconjugation with increased absorption and oxidation of glycine can occur in patients with cholecystectomy, radiation enteritis, or diabetes.[42,56,57] The use of antibiotics may normalize the test result if the problem is one of bacterial overgrowth. A distinction between the two major mechanisms of increased deconjugation and oxidation of absorbed glycine, i.e., small intestinal invasion by colonic bacteria vs. bile-acid malabsorption, can be made by fecal C-14 analysis or by the H_2 breath test.[42] The oral administration of Tc-99m colloid, or Tc-99m DTPA, along with the C-14 glycine-cholate provides a a marker for external monitoring of abnormal bowel transit patterns.[58] A recent challenge to the glycine-cholate breath test comes from a comparison with oxidation of D-^{14}C-xylose (a carbohydrate oxidized not by human tissues but by colonic bacteria).[59] The xylose test appeared to be more sensitive and specific for small intestinal bacterial overgrowth.

Liver Disease

The liver is a major site of such drug metabolic processes as oxidation by microsomal mixed-function oxidase, a reaction linked to demethylation. Following original experiments in rats, Bircher et al. found decreased oxidation of 4-dimethyl-^{14}C-amino-antipyrine (C-14 aminopyrine) in patients with alcoholic or primary biliary cirrhosis.[60] Hepner and Vesell demonstrated the value of a 2-hr breath analysis in which the oxidation was depressed up to 40% of normal in portal cirrhosis and hepatitis, 50% in malignancy, and 70% in fatty infiltration, but normal in cholestasis.[61] Others have made similar findings.[42] Schneider et al. and Suehiro et al. have validated the use of C-13 aminopyrine.[62,63] Greater sensitivity, specificity, and rapidity of testing with C-14 aminopyrine is achieved with intravenous administration in patients with cirrhosis or chronic active hepatitis.[64] Another labeled drug, C-14 phenacetin, is also metabolized by the liver and can be used to show major differences between normal and cirrhotic patients.[65]

Certain natural monosaccharides are metabolized almost entirely by the liver, and this forms the basis for the galactose tolerance test for liver function. Instead of repeated measurements of blood galactose levels, the tolerance can be more easily defined by breath analysis, using C-14 galactose or C-13 galactose.[4,28,66,67] Differences between normal and cirrhotic patients are shown in Figure 16–5. These differences are similar to those with the labeled aminopyrine breath test.[28,42] With "Indian childhood cirrhosis," there are more striking differences.[4] Although measurement of serum galactose affords better discrimination of liver disease than does the breath test with either oral C-14 galactose or C-14 aminopyrine,[42,66] the breath tests afford technical simplicity and patient comfort and are better suited for evaluating progression. Furthermore,

the intravenous test with C-14 aminopyrine,[64] or possibly with C-14 galactose, may provide superior discrimination. A feature of alcoholics with even mild liver disease is their relative lack of inhibition of galactose oxidation by an acute alcohol dose. Gregg et al. report that the breath test with C-13 galactose performed with and without ethanol in successive studies in the same patient may help evaluate minimal alcoholic liver disease.[67] Segal and Cuatrecasas demonstrated a profound deficiency of C-14 galactose oxidation in galactosemia.[68] The availability of chemical tests, however, favor their use over C-14 tracer tests.

Glaubitt has investigated the metabolism of some C-14 labeled amino acids in liver disease.[69] For reasons not yet known, oxidation of L-(methylene-^{14}C)-tryptophan is reduced, but oxidation of L-(1-^{14}C)-methionine and L-(U-^{14}C)-valine is increased in cirrhosis. Rabinowitz et al. found that oxidation of ingested C-14 octanoate to breath $^{14}CO_2$ reflects the decreased serum clearance that characterizes cirrhosis.[70]

Endocrine Diseases

The metabolism of glucose-U-^{14}C may be altered in diabetes.[7,9,14] When obese patients with abnormal glucose tolerance tests are given glucose-1-^{14}C orally with the glucose load, there is an inverse correlation between $^{14}CO_2$ production and the blood glucose level at 90 min.[32] Production of labeled CO_2 in the obese is lower than that of nonobese controls with a greater difference than is found in their blood glucose concentrations.[32,71,72] Nonobese, mildly diabetic subjects, however, have not shown significant differences from normal subjects in labeled CO_2 production after ingestion of glucose-1-^{14}C, glucose-6-^{14}C, or glucose-U-^{13}C.[32,73] When glucose tolerance is grossly abnormal, the appearance of $^{13}CO_2$ from ingested glucose-U-^{13}C is about half of normal. Nevertheless, the differences in $^{13}CO_2$ formation

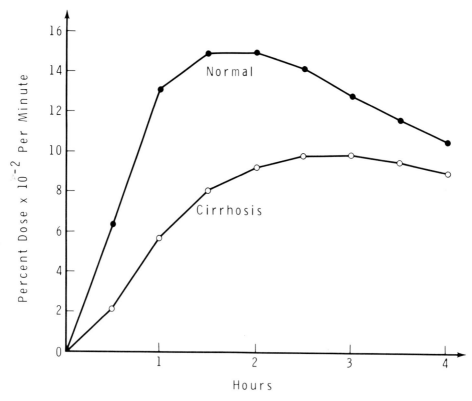

Fig. 16–5. Rate of $^{14}CO_2$ expiration after oral administration of galactose-U-^{14}C (10 g/m^2 body area) in normal subjects and patients with "cirrhosis." (From Shreeve, W.W., et al.[28])

between diabetic and nondiabetic subjects are not as great as the differences in blood glucose concentration.[32,71]

Various studies in rats and humans have suggested that oxidation of C-14 labeled lactate or pyruvate to $^{14}CO_2$ is depressed in diabetes.[32] An example of this effect is illustrated in Figure 16–6. Furthermore, insulin in the diabetic or glucose load in the nondiabetic has been shown to enhance the oxidation of lactate or pyruvate to CO_2.[15] There have been some indications that oxidation rates of labeled fatty acids, glucose, or glycine can be abnormal in thyroid disease.[18,69,74,75] None of these oxidation rates has been tried systematically as a diagnostic test, and none appears specific enough for diagnostic accuracy.

Special Metabolic Diseases

Several breath analysis tests have been proposed for the detection and study of amino acid abnormalities. They include C-14 or C-13 glycine in hyperglycinemia,[76] ^{14}C-5-hydroxytryptophan in depression,[77] and C-14 phenylalanine in phenylketonuria.[13] Although the oxidation rate for L-deoxyphenylalanine-1-^{14}C is not reduced per se in Parkinson's disease, its oxidation can be used to judge the adequacy of therapy designed to both depress L-dopa decarboxylase in extrahepatic tissues and maximize formation of dopamine in brain.[78]

Abnormal metabolism of asparagine in tumors is associated with deficient oxidation of L-U-^{14}C-asparagine to $^{14}CO_2$ and has led to trial of oxidation as a means for assessing therapy.[79] Oxidation of L-1-^{14}C-ornithine is increased in cancer. Changes may also reflect clinical response to therapy.[80]

Vitamin deficiencies may be readily

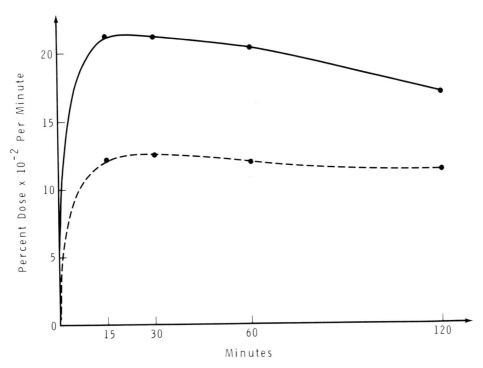

Fig. 16–6. Rate of $^{14}CO_2$ expiration in acromegalic patients (dashed line) following intravenous injection of pyruvate-2-^{14}C compared with normal rate (solid line). (From Shreeve, W.W., et al.[23])

evaluated by administration of specific labeled substrates. Thiamine deficiency causes a defect in intermediary carbohydrate metabolism that is expressed as decreased oxidation of C-14 ribose, C-14 pyruvate, or C-14 acetate in rats.[81,82] Pyridoxine deficiency can decrease the metabolism of L-tryptophan-carboxyl-^{14}C in rats.[83] In each of these cases, the possibility of a diagnostic test is suggested.

Some special disorders of carbohydrate metabolism besides galactosemia can be evaluated with labeled sugars. A common enzymatic abnormality among particular ethnic groups is glucose-6-phosphate dehydrogenase deficiency, which can cause serious anemia when sensitized by certain drugs or foodstuffs. The deficiency of G-6-PDH is frequently associated with glucose intolerance and low rates of oxidation of 1- or 6-^{14}C-labeled glucose.[84] Fructose intolerance can be recognized by meas-

uring the oxidation of C-14 fructose. Similarly, the congenital and rare intestinal disorder of sucrose intolerance or glucose-galactose intolerance could be evaluated, particularly with C-13, in these infant diseases.

This chapter has discussed several CO_2 breath analysis tests that have proved sensitive and simple to perform. These include tests of pancreatic function by hydrolysis and absorption of C-14 triglyceride, tests of bacterial overgrowth in intestinal diseases by hydrolysis and oxidation of C-14 glycine cholate or D-^{14}C-xylose, tests for lactase deficiency using C-14 lactose, studies of megaloblastic anemias with C-14 propionic acid and/or C-14 histidine, and evaluation of liver disease by oxidation of C-14 aminopyrine, C-14 phenacetin, or C-14 galactose. Some special amino acid abnormalities can also be recognized by this technique. Potential for diagnosis or evaluation of diabetes, obesity, thyroid disease, and other metabolic disorders also exist. Several of these tests have proved workable with stable C-13, which obviates the use of radioisotopes.

REFERENCES

1. Matthews, C.M.E., et al.: Exchange of $^{11}CO_2$ in arterial blood with body CO_2 pools. Respir. Physiol., 6:29, 1968.
2. Berlin, N.I., and Tolbert, B.M.: Metabolism of glycine-2-C^{14} in man. V. Further considerations of pulmonary excretion of $C^{14}O_2$. Proc. Soc. Exp. Biol. Med., 88:386, 1955.
3. Sasaki, Y.: Diagnostic applications of ^{14}C and ^{13}C compounds. In Nuclear Medicine in Japan. Edited by M. Iio. Tokyo, Japan Society of Nuclear Medicine, 1975, p. 249.
4. Da Costa, H., Shreeve, W.W., and Merchant, S.: Radiorespirometric study of carbohydrate metabolism in childhood liver disease. J. Nucl. Med., 17:218, 1976.
5. Pederson, N.T., and Marqverson, J.: Metabolism of ingested ^{14}C-triolein. Estimation of radiation dose in tests of lipid assimilation using ^{14}C- and ^3H-labeled fatty acids. Eur. J. Nucl. Med., 6:327, 1981.
6. Baker, N., et al: C^{14} studies in carbohydrate metabolism. I. The oxidation of glucose in normal human subjects. J. Biol. Chem., 211:575, 1954.
7. Shreeve, W.W., et al.: C^{14} studies in carbohydrate metabolism. II. the oxidation of glucose in diabetic human subjects. Metabolism, 5:22, 1956.
8. Shreeve, W.W., Hennes, A.R., and Schwartz, R.: Production of $C^{14}O_2$ from 1- and 2-C^{14}-acetate by human subjects in various metabolic states. Metabolism, 8:741, 1959.
9. Reichard, G.A., et al.: Blood glucose replacement rates in normal and diabetic humans. J. Appl. Physiol., 16:789, 1961.
10. Tolbert, B.M., Kirk, M., and Upham, F.: Carbon-14 respiration pattern analyzer for clinical studies. J. Appl. Physiol., 30:116, 1959.
11. Le Roy, G.V., et al.: Continuous measurement of specific activity of ^{14}C-labeled carbon dioxide in expired air. Int. J. Appl. Radiat., 7:273, 1960.
12. Fish, M.B., Pollycove, M., and Feichtmeir, T.V.: Differentiation between vitamin B_{12}-deficient and folic acid-deficient megaloblastic anemias with C-14 histidine. Blood, 21:447, 1963.
13. Fish, M.B., et al.: Effect of route and load of administered phenylalanine on human in vivo phenylalanine catabolism. J. Nucl. Med., 9:317, 1968.
14. Manougian, E., et al.: ^{14}C glucose kinetic studies in normal, diabetic and acromegalic subjects. J. Nucl. Med., 5:763, 1964.
15. Shreeve, W.W., DeMeutter, R.C., and Shigeta, Y.: Diabetes, insulin, tolbutamide and glucose load in the degradation of ^{14}C-labeled lactate and pyruvate. Diabetes, 13:615, 1964.
16. Shreeve, W.W., et al.: Formation of $^{14}CO_2$ and ^3HOH from glucose-1-^{14}C,-1-^3H during oral cortisone glucose tolerance tests in obese patients. Metabolism, 20:280, 1971.
17. Gordon, E.S.: New concepts of the biochemistry and physiology of obesity. Med. Clin. North Am., 48:1285, 1964.
18. Gordon, E.S., and Goldberg, M.: Carbon-14 studies of energy metabolism in various thyroid states. Metabolism, 13:591, 1964.
19. Shreeve, W.W.: Transfer of ^{14}C and ^3H from labeled substrates to CO_2, water and lipids in diabetic and obese subjects in vivo. Ann. N.Y. Acad. Sci., 131:464, 1965.
20. Bolinger, R.E., Schafer, M.E., and Kuske, T.T.: Effect of prolonged fasting on the expired $^{14}CO_2$ from palmitate and glucose in obese subjects. Metabolism, 15:394, 1966.
21. Rabinowitz, J.L., and Myerson, R.M.: The effects of triiodothyronine on some metabolic parameters of obese individuals. Blood glucose-^{14}C replacement rates, respiratory $^{14}CO_2$, the pentose cycle, the biological half-life of T_3 and the concentration of T_3 in adipose tissue. Metabolism, 16:68, 1967.
22. Frederickson, D.S., and Ono, K.: An improved technique for assay of $^{14}CO_2$ in expired air using the liquid scintillation counter. J. Lab. Clin. Med., 51:147, 1958.
23. Shreeve, W.W., Cerasi, E., and Luft, R.: Metabolism of pyruvate-2-^{14}C in normal, acromegalic and HGH-treated human subjects. Acta Endocrinol., 65:155, 1970.
24. Aronson, R.B., and Van Slyke, D.D.: Manometric determination of CO_2 combined with scintillation counting of ^{14}C. Anal. Biochem., 41:173, 1971.
25. Abt, A.F., and von Schuching, S.L.: Fat utilization test in disorders of fat metabolism. Bull. of the Johns Hopkins Hosp., 119:316, 1966.
26. Kaihara, S., and Wagner, H.N., Jr.: Measurement of intestinal fat absorption with carbon-14 labeled tracers. J. Lab. Clin. Med., 71:400, 1968.
27. Sasaki, Y., et al.: Measurement of ^{14}C-lactose absorption in the diagnosis of lactate deficiency. J. Lab. Clin. Med., 76:824, 1970.
28. Shreeve, W.W., et al.: Test for alcoholic cirrhosis by conversion of [^{14}C]- or [^{13}C]-galactose to expired CO_2. Gastroenterology, 71:98, 1976.
29. Chen, I.W., et al.: ^{14}C-tripalmitin breath test as a diagnostic aid for fat malabsorption due to pancreatic insufficiency. J. Nucl. Med., 15:1125, 1974.
30. Lorenz, E., et al: Plastic scintillation filament detector system for $^{14}CO_2$ breath-analysis tests. Med. Phys., 5:195, 1978.
31. Klein, P.D., Haumann, J.R., and Eisler, W.J.: Instrument design considerations and clinical applications of stable isotope analysis. Clin. Chem., 17:735, 1971.
32. Shreeve, W.W., et al: Evaluation of diabetes by oxidation of ^{14}C- or ^{13}C-labeled glucose to CO_2 in vivo. In Radiopharmaceuticals and Labeled

Compounds. Copenhagen, Symposium, International Atomic Energy Agency, 1973, p. 281.

33. Schoeller, D.A., and Klein, P.D.: A simplified technique for collecting breath CO_2 for isotope ratio mass spectrometry. Biomed. Mass Spectrom., 5:29, 1978.

34. McDowell, R.S.: Determination of carbon-13 by infrared spectrophotometry of carbon monoxide. Anal. Chem., 42:1192, 1970.

35. Hirano, S., et al.: A simple infrared spectroscopic method for the measurement of expired $^{13}CO_2$. Anal. Biochem., 96:64, 1979.

36. Schoeller, D.A., et al.: Clinical diagnosis with the stable isotope ^{13}C in CO_2 breath tests: methodology and fundamental considerations. J. Lab. Clin. Med., 90:412, 1977.

37. Schwabe, A.D., et al.: Estimation of fat absorption by monitoring of expired radioactive carbon dioxide after feeding a radioactive fat. Gastroenterology, 42:285, 1962.

38. Watkins, J.B., et al.: ^{13}C-trioctanoin: a nonradioactive breath test to detect fat malabsorption. J. Lab. Clin. Med., 90:422, 1977.

39. Newcomer, A.D., Thomas, P.H., and Hofmann, A.F.: Breath tests for detecting steatorrhea: comparison of labeled trioctanoin, triolein and tripalmitin. Gastroenterology, 70:923, 1976.

40. Butler, R.N., and Gehling, N.J.: Modification of the ^{14}C-triolein test. Clin. Chim. Acta, 112:371, 1981.

41. Ghoos, Y.F., et al.: A mixed-triglyceride breath test for intraluminal fat digestive activity. Digestion, 22:239, 1981.

42. Caspary, W.F.: Breath tests. Clin. Gastroenterol., 7:351, 1978.

43. Adlung, J., et al.: Über ein neues Verfahren in der Diagnostik der Maldigestion. Schweiz. Med. Wochenschr., 105:134, 1975.

44. Fish, M.B., Pollycove, M., and Wallerstein, R.O.: In vivo oxidative metabolism of propionic acid in human vitamin B_{12} deficiency. J. Lab. Clin. Med., 72:767, 1968.

45. De Grazia, J.A., et al.: The oxidation of the beta carbon of serine in human folate and vitamin B_{12} deficiency. J. Lab. Clin. Med., 80:395, 1972.

46. Cozzetto, F.J.: Radiocarbon estimates of intestinal absorption. Am. J. Dis. Child., 107:605, 1964.

47. Salmon, P.R., Read, A.E., and McCarthy, C.F.: An isotope technique for measuring lactose absorption. Gut, 10:685, 1969.

48. Weiss, R.G., and Stryker, J.A.: ^{14}C-lactose breath tests during pelvic radiotherapy: The effect of the amount of small bowel irradiated. Radiology, 142:507, 1982.

49. Newcomer, A.D., et al.: Prospective comparison of indirect methods for detecting lactase deficiency. N. Engl. J. Med., 293:1232, 1975.

50. Adlung, J., et al.: Diagnostik der Laktose-Malabsorption. Med. Klin., 71:2017, 1976.

51. Fromm, H., and Hofmann, A.F.: Breath test for altered bile-acid metabolism. Lancet, 1:621, 1971.

52. Sherr, H.P., et al.: Detection of bacterial deconjugation of bile salts by a convenient breath-analysis technique. N. Engl. J. Med., 285:656, 1971.

53. Sasaki, Y., et al.: Detection of bacterial deconjugation of bile salts using ^{13}C breath test. J. Nucl. Med., 18:636, 1977.

54. Solomons, N.W., Schoeller, D.A., and Wagonfeld, J.B.: Application of a stable isotope (^{13}C) labelled glycocholate breath test to diagnosis of bacterial overgrowth and ileal dysfunction. J. Lab. Clin. Med., 90:431, 1977.

55. Hirschowitz, B.I., et al.: Location of the site of bacterial bile-salt deconjugation by combining abdominal scintigraphy with expired C-14. J. Nucl. Med., 18:542, 1977.

56. Hepner, G.W., et al.: Increased bacterial degradation of bile acids in cholecystectomized patients. Gastroenterology, 66:556, 1974.

57. Scarpello, J.H.B., et al.: The ^{14}C-glycocholate test in diabetic diarrhea. Br. Med. J., 2:673, 1976.

58. Talbot, J.N., et al.: ^{14}C-glycocholate breath test and pathological digestive transit. J. Biophys. Med. Nucl., 6:59, 1982.

59. King, C.E., et al.: Comparison of the one-gram d-(^{14}C)-xylose breath test to the (^{14}C)-bile acid breath test in patients with small intestine bacterial overgrowth. Dig. Dis. Sci., 25:53, 1980.

60. Bircher, J., et al.: Aminopyrine demethylation measured by breath analysis in cirrhosis. Clin. Pharmacol. Ther., 20:484, 1976.

61. Hepner, G.W., and Vesell, E.S.: Quantitative assessment of hepatic function by breath analysis after oral administration of ^{14}C-aminopyrine. Ann. Intern. Med., 83:632, 1975.

62. Schneider, J.F., et al.: Validation of $^{13}CO_2$ breath analysis as a measurement of demethylation of stable isotope labeled aminopyrine in man. Clin. Chim. Acta, 84:153, 1978.

63. Suehiro, M., et al.: C-13-Aminopyrine breath test: A useful tool for evaluation of liver function. J. Nucl. Med., 23:P36, 1982.

64. Pauwels, S., et al.: Breath analysis after intravenous administration of ^{14}C-aminopyrine in liver disease. J. Nucl. Med., 21:P76, 1980.

65. Breen, K.J., et al.: A ^{14}C-phenacetin breath test in the assessment of hepatic function. Gastroenterology, 72:1033, 1977.

66. Caspary, W.F., and Schaeffer, J.: ^{14}C-D-Galactose breath test for evaluation of liver function in patients with chronic liver disease. Digestion, 17:410, 1978.

67. Gregg, C.T., et al.: Effect of ethanol on oxidation of galactose-carbon-13 to carbon dioxide in alcoholic liver disease. J. Nucl. Med., 19:679, 1978.

68. Segal, S., and Cuatrecasas, P.: The oxidation of C^{14} galactose by patients with congenital galactosemia. Evidence for a direct oxidative pathway. Am. J. Med., 44:340, 1968.

69. Glaubitt, D.M.H.: Predictive value of $^{14}CO_2$ breath tests for clinical use of $^{13}CO_2$ breath tests. *In* Proceedings of the Second International Conference on Stable Isotopes. Edited by E.R. Klein and P.D. Klein, Oak Brook, Ill, Argonne National Laboratories, 1975, p. 219.

70. Rabinowitz, J.L., et al.: Rate of (C-14)-octanoate

oxidation to (C-14) carbon dioxide as a test for cirrhosis. J. Nucl. Med., *19*:689, 1978.

71. Lefebvre, P., et al.: Naturally labeled ^{13}C-glucose. Metabolic studies in human diabetes and obesity. Diabetes, *24*:185, 1975.

72. Ravussin, E., et al.: Carbohydrate utilization in obese subjects after an oral load of 100 g. naturally-labelled ^{13}C-glucose. Br. J. Nutr., *43*:281, 1980.

73. Kallie, R.N., Shreeve, W.W., and Joubert, S.M.: Studies in primary hyperuricaemia III. The conversion of ^{14}C to breath $^{14}CO_2$ from glucose-1-^{14}C and glucose-6-^{14}C in hyperuricaemia and gout. S. Afr. Med. J., *42*:473, 1968.

74. Shames, D.M., Berman, M., and Segal, S.: Effects of thyroid disease on glucose oxidative metabolism in man. A compartmental model analysis. J. Clin. Invest., *50*:627, 1971.

75. Lütolf, U.M., et al.: Exhalationsstudien mit ^{14}C-markierten Substanzen. Radiol. Clin. Biol., *43*:348, 1974.

76. Sweetman, L., et al.: Glycine-1, 2-^{13}C in the investigation of children with inborn errors of metabolism. Proceedings of the First International Conference on Stable Isotopes. Edited by Klein and Paterson. Argonne, ILL, Argonne National Laboratories, 1973, p. 404.

77. Coppen, C., et al.: Changes in 5-hydroxytryptophan metabolism in depression. Br. J. Psychiat., *111*:105, 1965.

78. Mena, I., et al.: In vivo analysis of exhaled $^{14}CO_2$: a measurement of dopa decarboxylation in Parkinsonism and manganism. First World Congress of Nuclear Medicine, Tokyo and Kyoto. 1974, p. 606.

79. Chaudhuri, T.K., and Winchell, H.S.: Diminished oxidation of ^{14}C-UL-L-asparagine to $^{14}CO_2$ in mice and humans with tumors: a possible means for assessing efficacy of therapy? J. Nucl. Med., *11*:597, 1970.

80. Webber, M.M., et al.: Radiolabelled ornithine as a marker of cancer. J. Nucl. Med., *21*:32, 1980.

81. Brin, M.: The oxidation of ^{14}C-pyruvate and of ^{14}C-ribose in thiamine deficient intact rats. Isr. J. Med. Sci., *3*:792, 1967.

82. Ngo, T.M., et al.: Decreased $^{14}CO_2$ production in thiamine-deficient rats given pyruvate-1-^{14}C and acetate-1-^{14}C: a possible means for early diagnosis of beri-beri? J. Nucl. Med., *10*:676, 1969.

83. Tran, N., and La Plante, M.: The oxidation of L-tryptophan-carboxyl-^{14}C and DL-tryptophan (pyrrol-2-^{14}C) to $^{14}CO_2$ in vitamin B_6-deficient rats. Int. J. Biochem., *2*:307, 1971.

84. Eppes, R.B., et al.: Oral glucose tolerance in Negro men deficient in glucose-6-phosphate dehydrogense. N. Engl. J. Med., *275*:855, 1966.

Chapter 17

IN VIVO NEUTRON ACTIVATION ANALYSIS

STANTON H. COHN

Development of in vivo neutron activation analysis gave rise to an important approach to the analysis of elemental composition of human beings. Studies of body composition prior to this development were performed by means of isotope dilution, radiography, fluoroscopy, photon absorptiometry, biopsy, and whole-body counting. These studies yielded data on relative change in level but not on absolute quantities of the element. The one exception is total body potassium, which can be measured directly by means of whole-body counting of K-40. By means of total-body neutron activation analysis (TBNAA), calcium, phosphorus, sodium, and chlorine have been accurately measured, and with a refinement of TBNAA, levels of nitrogen and cadmium can be determined (Table 17–1). Not all elements of biologic interest, however, can be usefully detected by neutron activation. Analysis for iron, copper, and zinc, for example, is better performed by other techniques. Such elements as sulfur and phosphorus, though readily activated by thermal neutrons, yield isotopes that are pure beta emitters.

Neutron activation depends on nuclear rather than chemical rections; thus, measurements are independent of molecular structure. The essential physical parameters involved include the isotopic abundance, cross section, half-life, and energy emission of the product isotopes.

TBNAA systems, designed for in vivo studies, generate a moderated beam of fast neutrons to the total body of the subject. Neutron capture by atoms of the target elements creates unstable radionuclides that revert to a stable state by the emission of one or more gamma rays of characteristic energy. These energy levels identify the element, and the amount of radioactivity produced is proportional to its abundance. Radiation from the subject is measured in a highly shielded facility, and standard gamma spectrographic analysis is applied. Typical human gamma spectra resulting from exposure to two different neutron sources, 14-MeV neutrons and neutrons from a ^{238}Pu-Be source, are shown in Figure 17–1.

BASIC PRINCIPLES

The initial activity I_0 (in dps) present at the termination of irradiation of a target is given by:

$$I_0 = \frac{WN \, \phi \, \sigma \, m}{A} \left[1 - \exp\left(- \lambda \, t_1 \right) \right]$$

TABLE 17–1. Measurement of Body Elements by In Vivo Neutron Activation Analysis

Stable element	Amount in 70-kg standard man (g)	Proportion by weight in 70-kg standard man (%)	Induced nuclide	Neutron reaction	Gamma ray or x-ray to be measured
Oxygen	42,000	60	^{16}N	n, p (fast)	Delayed γ (6–7 MeV)
Hydrogen	7,000	10	^{2}H	n, γ (thermal)	Prompt γ (2.2 MeV)
Nitrogen	2,100	3	^{13}N	n, 2n (14 MeV)	Delayed γ (0.51 MeV)
				n, γ (thermal)	Prompt γ (10.8 MeV)
Calcium	1,050	1.5	^{49}Ca	n, γ (thermal)	Prompt γ (many); delayed γ (3.10 MeV)
Phosphorus	700	1	^{37}A	n, α (14 MeV)	Delayed X-ray (2.6 keV)
			^{28}Al	n, α (fast)	Delayed γ (1.78 MeV)
			^{32}P	n, γ (thermal)	Prompt γ (0.08 MeV)
Sodium	105	0.15	^{24}Na	n, γ (thermal)	Prompt γ (many); delayed γ (2.75 MeV)
Chlorine	105	0.15	^{38}Cl	n, γ (thermal)	Prompt γ (many); delayed γ (1.6, 2.2 MeV)
Magnesium	35	0.05	^{37}S	n, p (fast)	Delayed γ (3.10 MeV)
			^{27}Mg	n, γ (thermal)	Delayed γ (0.84 MeV)
			^{24}Na	n, p (fast)	Delayed γ (2.75 MeV)
Iron*	4.2	0.006	^{56}Mn	n, p (fast)	Delayed γ (0.84 MeV)
Iodine*	0.01 (in thyroid)	0.03 (in thyroid)	^{128}I	n, γ (thermal)	Delayed γ (0.45 MeV)
Manganese*	Trace	Trace	^{56}Mn	n, γ (thermal)	Delayed γ (0.84 MeV)
Copper*	Trace	Trace	^{64}Cu	n, γ (thermal)	Delayed γ (0.51 MeV)
Cadmium*	Trace	Trace	^{114}Cd	n, γ (thermal)	Prompt γ (0.559 MeV)

*Partial-body activation.
From Panel on In Vivo Neutron Activation Analysis, International Atomic Energy Agency, p. 224.[1]

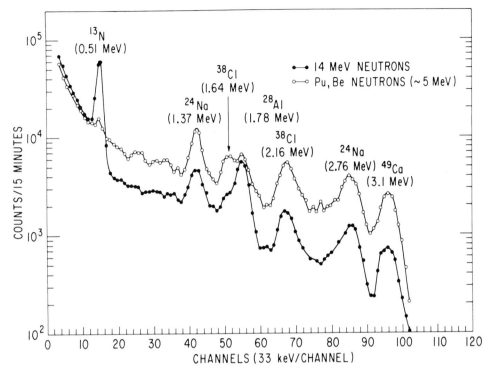

Fig. 17–1. Gamma spectra in human subject irradiated with 14-MeV neutrons and 5-MeV ²³⁸Pu-Be neutrons. (From Cohn, S.H., et al.[2])

where:

W = mass of element, g

N = Avogadro's number = 6.0225 × 10²³ atoms per gram atomic weight

A = atomic weight

φ = average neutron flux density, n/m²

σ = absorption cross section in barns (10⁻²⁸ m²)

m = fractional isotopic abundance

λ = decay constant $\dfrac{0.693}{T_{1/2}}$

t_1 = bombardment time (duration of irradiation)

The quantity in brackets is the *saturation factor;* it is a function of the length of bombardment time and the half-life of the nuclide formed. This expression is sometimes called the *growth factor.* When t = $T_{1/2}$, this factor has a value of 0.5; when t is large compared with $T_{1/2}$, it approaches unity. In practice, an irradiation time (t_1)

of about 6 half-lives induces a near maximum, or *saturation activity.*

The counting rate C(t) (cps) obtained after the initial activity has decayed for a time t_2 is given by:

$$C(t) = \psi I_0 \exp(-\lambda t_2)$$

where:

ψ = detector efficiency

t_2 = time between end of irradiation and measurement of activity

PARAMETERS AFFECTING SENSITIVITY

Sensitivity of neutron activation analysis procedures is a function of several factors: level of activity produced, detection efficiency, and background interference both in the form of "noise" in the detection system and from the presence of activity from competing nuclear reactions.

Activity

Given irradiation to saturation, the activity produced from a specific isotope is the product of the number of target atoms present, $\dfrac{WNm}{A}$; the absorption cross section, σ; and the neutron flux density, ϕ. Cross sections and the problems of neutron distribution through large biologic samples are discussed later. Flux densities of sufficient intensity are available from several sources, including accelerators, reactors, and portable (α,n) and fission sources.[3,4] Typical neutron energy spectra for these sources are shown in Figure 17–2. While activation is carried out predominantly with thermal neutrons (energy $\cong 0.025$ eV), the high-energy neutrons evident in the preceding spectra are of consequence for resonance and threshold reactions. In most cases, fast neutrons are used for irradiation because of the poor penetration of thermal neutrons in the human body. The fast neutrons are thermalized by the body mostly by elastic scattering with body hydrogen.

Detector Efficiency

Efficiency depends upon the solid angle subtended and the detector's inherent efficiency. Detector sizes range from a few millimeters to configurations subtending solid angles that approach 4π steradians. Sodium iodide detectors are used most often.

Background

The higher the measured counts are above background, the greater the possible precision. Accuracy of analysis deteriorates rapidly as C(t) approaches background levels.

PRACTICAL PROBLEMS

Interfering Nuclear Reactions

In activation analysis, interfering reactions occur when elements other than those being analyzed become radioactive and emit photons in the energy region being studied. They are of two types. Reaction interferences of type 1 are those in which the primary reaction leads to the same radionuclide as that from the element analyzed. For example, the reactions ^{23}Na (n,γ) ^{24}Na and ^{25}Mg (n,p) ^{24}Na both produce the same end-product. The seriousness of this type of interference depends on the reaction cross sections and relative abundance of the target nuclei. Reaction interferences of type 1 are those in which the primary reaction leads to the same radionuclide as that from the element analyzed. Reaction interferences of type 2 involve secondary reactions produced in the matrix by particles different from those of the primary beams. An example is the ^{16}O(p,α)^{13}N reaction, which occurs as a secondary reaction to the ^{14}N(n,2n)^{13}N reaction using fast neutrons.

Beam Attenuation

One major source of imprecision in activation analysis results from variation of the neutron flux density throughout large targets such as human subjects. Variation in flux density with depth for different neutron energies can be quite large. Various schemes for homogenizing the integrated flux have been designed to improve precision and accuracy. Use of moderators to prevent buildup of neutron flux densities in surface layers has proved quite effective.[5] Similarly, bilateral irradiation of large samples produces a more uniform flux throughout the tissue. In general, the neutron beam is monitored by some type of neutron detector, or by the concomitant activation of foils placed in the target field.

Flux density measurements must be made to determine absolute flux density and relative distribution throughout the human body. Examples of the measurement of neutron yield and flux density distributions in phantoms have been published.[6] Elements with low atomic numbers, such as those found in tissue,

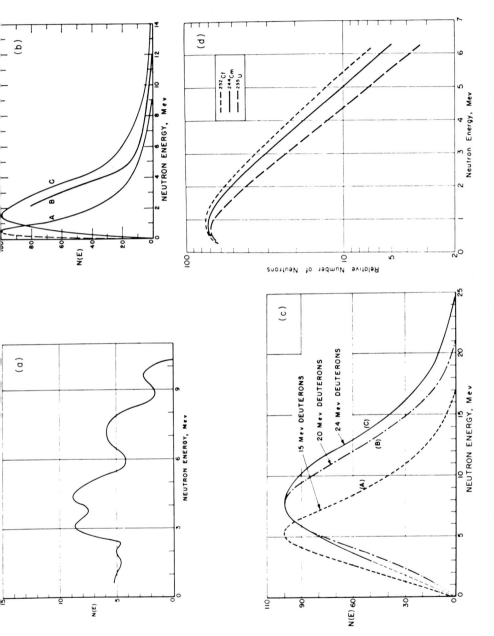

Fig. 17–2. Energy spectra of neutron sources: (a) ^{238}Pu(α,n) Be; (b) Accelerator neutron spectra: (A) 12-MeV protons on thick Be targets, (B) 6-MeV protons on thin Be targets, (C) 22-MeV protons on thick Be targets; (c) Accelerator deuterons on Be target. (d) Spontaneous fission of Cf-252, U-235, and Cm-244. (From Cohn, S.H., et al.[2])

have neutron absorption cross sections that vary with velocity in a way that allows accurate analysis utilizing thermal cross sections. Heavier elements, however, such as those sometimes used as neutron detectors (gold, indium) have cross sections with large resonances in the regions just above thermal energies and thus overreact to the higher energies in the neutron spectrum.

COMPARISON OF TECHNIQUES FOR TOTAL-BODY NEUTRON ACTIVATION

Neutron Sources and Patient Exposure Geometry

All of the initial neutron sources employed in human studies were designed for research in physics. Chamberlain et al. and Nelp and Palmer used neutrons produced by a 60-in. cyclotron, with peak energies of 3.5 and 8 MeV, respectively.[7,8,9,10] The spectra are continuous, and have wide energy ranges (see Fig. 17–2). Cohn originally used 14-MeV neutrons from a D,T neutron generator but has more recently employed α,n sources.[11,12,13] Characteristics of the various neutron sources used for TBNAA in man are listed in Table 17–2.

In Chamberlain's technique, the patient is irradiated lying on his side in a polypropylene chamber ($0.9 \times 0.9 \times 2$ m) to provide moderation of incident fast neutrons. In Nelp's technique, the patient is upright during irradiation, with the extremities placed in lucite containers of water, and the head encased in a plastic helmet for moderation. Cohn originally employed 14-MeV neutrons, with the patient standing upright, supported by crutches, and positioned tightly between two large sheets of 3.8-cm polyethylene moderator. In all three techniques, irradiation is performed with the patient facing first toward, and then away from, the source.

None of these procedures is particularly comfortable physically for the patient. For this reason, the Brookhaven group designed a portable α,n source that is installed in the hospital and permits simultaneous bilateral exposure of a patient resting supine on a bed.[14] The neutron source consists of a bank of 14 encapsulated 50-Ci (1.85-TBq) sources of ^{238}Pu-Be ($\bar{E} \sim 4.2$ MeV), positioned above and below the length of the patient.

Besides reduced dose to the patient, several other advantages derive from the use of α,n neutrons. The irradiation geometry is substantially improved, and significantly greater stability in neutron output is achieved; hence, the precision of measurement is enhanced. The operation of α,n neutron sources is much simpler than operation of neutron generators and cyclotrons, and the service of a trained operator is not required. Finally, the design of such a source for medical applications permits it to be located in a hospital environment. This is a significant advantage to both patients and investigators. If total-body neutron activation analysis is to have wide clinical application, the most likely direction for development to follow is in the application of "portable" α,n neutron sources.

The first body element to be studied intensively was calcium. Successful application of TBNAA to the measurement of total-body calcium content (particularly absolute levels) depends essentially on meeting two (in some cases, three) requirements:

1. A uniform distribution of thermal neutrons must be obtained to ensure uniform exposure.
2. A quantitative measure of the induced Ca-49 activity in the body must be obtained with a whole-body counter having uniform counting sensitivity.
3. When 14-MeV neutrons are employed, correction for interfering radionuclides produced from other

TABLE 17–2. Characteristics of Neutron Sources Used for Total-Body Neutron Activation Analysis in Man and Elements Measured

Sources and reactions	Neutron output (n/s)	Energy (MeV)	Irradiation time (min)	Premoderator thickness (cm)	SSD* (m)	Patient position	Elements measured
1. Cyclotron	8×10^{10}	*0.1–8 peak: 3.5	5	1.5	2	Lying on side	Ca, Na
^{7}Li(p,n)^{7}Be	5×10^{11}		10	Nil	3	Supine, motorized bed	N, Cd
2. Cyclotron ^{9}Be(d,n)^{10}B	5×10^{11}†	4–12 peak:8	1.3	0–few cm	3.7	Standing, turntable	Ca, Na, P
3. Cockcroft-Walton ^{3}T(d,n)^{4}He	1.5×10^{10}†	14 / 14	— / 3	3 / Various	1.1 / 1.0	Lying in arc / Lying on side, motorized bed	Na, Ca, Cl
4. Cockcroft-Walton ^{3}T(d,n)^{4}He	3×10^{10}	14	5	3.8	1.5	Standing, turntable	Ca, Na, Cl, P, N
5. ^{238}Pu(α,n)Be ^{9}Be(α,n)^{12}C	1.4×10^9	2–8 mean:4.5	5	2.9	0.3	Supine on bed	Ca, Na, Cl, P
^{241}Am-Be ^{9}Be(α,n)^{12}C	$2 \times (2 \times 10^4)$‡	2–8 mean: 4.5	33	None	~0.2	Supine, motorized bed	H
6. Sealed tube neutron-generator ^{3}T(d,n)^{4}He	$2 \times (3 \times 10^{10})$‡	14	1	4.0	0.72	Supine, motorized bed	Ca, Na, Cl, P, N

*SSD, Source-to-skin distance.
†Estimated value.
‡Two opposed sources.
From Panel on In Vivo Neutron Activation Analysis, International Atomic Energy Agency, p. 226.[1]

target elements present must be made. The reaction $^{38}Cl(n,p)^{37}S$ is of prime importance, because S-37 emits gamma rays of approximately the same energy as Ca-49.

Uniformity of Thermal Neutron Flux Density in the Irradiated Subject

The problem of obtaining uniform flux density of thermal neutrons in man is complicated by the nonuniform human shape. For the measurement of calcium, which is concentrated almost entirely in the skeleton, the problem of obtaining uniform flux to the target is even more difficult than that experienced with such homogeneously distributed elements as nitrogen, sodium, and chlorine. While much of the skeleton lies within a few centimeters of the skin, there are large differences in the amount of overlying tissue; this tissue serves to moderate the incident neutrons. To achieve greater uniformity of flux, investigators have found it necessary to utilize fast neutrons with moderators and bilateral exposure. For absolute measurements to be made, the degree of uniformity must be much higher than that required for relative measurements. It is highly desirable to activate as much of the skeleton as possible to obtain a high degree of precision.

In all three techniques used for total-body calcium measurement, the flux density profiles of thermal neutrons were estimated with the use of cubic phantoms of water or hydrogenous plastic of approximately the thickness of the human body.

Chamberlain, using cyclotron-produced neutrons ($\bar{E} \sim 3.5$ MeV) with a 20-cm thick polyethylene phantom, found a peak flux at 3 cm from the surface of the phantom when 1.5 cm of polypropylene moderator was used. The uniformity of neutron flux was $\pm 27\%$.

Nelp obtained a uniformity of $\pm 18\%$ in a cubic water phantom of 25.4 cm depth, with no moderator. The maximum flux occurred 4.5 cm from the surface. To assess the uniformity of flux in the human body more accurately, manganese capsules ($\frac{1}{2}$ in. $\times$ 1 in.) were placed at 1-in. intervals throughout the chest, thorax, extremities, and head of a cadaver. The variation in the activation of these capsules was $\pm 20\%$ of the median value. Manganese capsules located in individual bones of a cadaver revealed a standard deviation of 5.6%; the range of activation flux uniformity about the median value was $\pm 12\%$.

Cohn et al., using 14-MeV neutrons and a 5-cm moderator of paraffin against the front and back of the phantom, found that the uniformity of neutron flux over 23 cm was $\pm 5\%$.[15]

With ^{238}Pu-Be neutrons, Cohn found that the uniformity in a cubic water phantom 28 cm thick and with 2.5 cm of moderator was $\pm 15\%$. With a closely fitted 1.9-cm polyethylene moderator, a uniformity of $\pm 8\%$ was obtained in an Alderson phantom. This uniformity is due in part to the use of a 7.6-cm bismuth reflector lining the irradiation cell, which greatly increased the nondegraded reflectance of the generated neutrons.

Moderators

Both the thickness of the hydrogenous moderator and its position in relation to the body are critical in obtaining uniform flux. The goal of obtaining maximum buildup of the incident neutron flux in the moderator must be balanced against the decreased penetration of the neutrons in the body. With an air-space between the moderator and the skin, there is a divergence of the neutron beam, and a secondary buildup occurs when the neutrons hit the body.

The selection of a moderator to obtain the maximum activation of skeletal calcium is empirical for neutrons below 14 MeV. In the three studies described previously, however, the precision of activation is high—1 to 3%—although the accuracy of measurement is not nearly so good.

Measurement of Induced Activity

Because the principal gamma energy of Ca-49 is high (3.1 MeV), the attenuation and geometry corrections are not as large as for the measurement of N-13, Al-28 (phosphorus), Na-24, and Cl-38, but they cannot be ignored. In the Brookhaven technique, the whole-body counter-computer facility corrects for both geometry and attenuation effects for the individual patient being analyzed.

The counting efficiency varies with the volume of NaI detectors employed; volumes range from 4689 ml in Chamberlain's procedure to 50,000 ml in the Brookhaven counter.[5] Also, the Brookhaven counter has a further advantage in that it counts the entire body simultaneously. Nelp's counter scans the body with an annular array of four 4 × 9⅜-in. NaI detectors. These detectors move across the body at an exponential rate, synchronized to the $T_{1/2}$ of Ca-49. Chamberlain employs four 5 × 4-in. detectors in a fixed geometry. If the counts in the Ca-49 photopeak are divided by the rem dose to the patient, the ratio for Chamberlain, Nelp, Cohn (14 MeV), and Cohn (α,n) neutrons are 1:1.8:2.7:7.7 respectively.

Dosimetry

The radiation absorbed dose to the patient in the techniques reviewed here is generally measured with tissue-equivalent ionization chambers. The dose ranges from 0.3 rem (3.0 × 10⁻³ Sv) for ^{238}Pu-Be neutrons to approximately 2 rem. Comparisons of the measured doses with theoretic calculations have also been carried out for 14-MeV neutrons and for neutrons from various α,n sources. Clearly, 4.5-MeV neutrons have a considerable advantage over 14-MeV neutrons in reducing radiation absorbed dose to the patient. The factors responsible for reduction are:

1. Greater number of incident neutrons per rem.

2. Higher ratio of thermal neutrons per incident neutron.
3. Effect of simultaneous bilateral irradiation.
4. Effect of "broad-beam" source on ratio of thermal to fast neutron flux.

PARTIAL-BODY NEUTRON ACTIVATION

Partial-body activation has been used to measure calcium and phosphorus in localized areas of the body.[17,18] It has also been used to measure intrathyroidal iodine.[19,20] Isotopic neutron sources used were ^{238}Pu-Be and ^{241}Am-Be.[21,22,23,24] Californium-252 has also been investigated as a neutron source for partial-body activation.[25,26]

PROMPT GAMMA NEUTRON ACTIVATION ANALYSIS

The excess energy released in the binding of a neutron can be emitted as a prompt gamma (i.e., in less than 10⁻¹⁶ sec). The major difference between TBNAA and prompt gamma neutron activation analysis (PGNAA) is that in the latter technique, measurement of activity takes place simultaneously with the neutron exposure. Measurement of total-body hydrogen by prompt gamma analysis was first demonstrated in 1966 by Rundo and Bunce.[27] Although PGNAA can be used to measure most elements, it is particularly suitable for measuring such elements as cadmium and nitrogen. Cadmium locates preferentially in the liver and kidneys. The small size of the Ge(Li) detector used is well suited to the detection of activity in single organs. Cadmium also has a high radiative neutron-capture cross section at energies of up to 0.5 eV; above this value, the cross section drops sharply.

In vivo measurements of Cd by PGNAA were first demonstrated by Biggin et al.[28] Fast neutrons were produced in a pulsed mode by a cyclotron and counted between bursts. Fast neutrons require a finite time to slow down to thermal energies. During the major portion of the slowdown period, the analyzer does not accept any counts.

Improvements in both irradiation and detection were made by McLellan et al.[29] and by Harvey et al.[30] The performance of a portable system, utilizing a 10-Ci (370-GBq) ^{238}Pu-Be neutron source, was described by Harvey et al. and by Thomas et al.[31] Clinical studies have been published by Evans et al.,[32] Ellis et al.[33] and Vartsky et al.[34]

Palmer et al. were the first to demonstrate the feasibility of measuring total-body nitrogen (TBN) using TBNAA and the reaction ^{14}N(n,2n)^{13}N.[9] Cohn et al. measured absolute levels of TBN in cancer, renal, and osteoporotic patients with this technique.[13] Several groups currently use this n,2n method for measuring nitrogen.[35,36]

Two serious problems are associated with this technique. First, the n,2n reaction has a high neutron energy threshold. The product N-13 decays by positron emission to C-13; no gamma ray characteristic of N is emitted. The only radiations are the 511-keV annihilation photons. This lack of specificity creates problems of interference from positron emitters produced from body elements other than N.[37] For example, N-13 produced in the ^{16}O(p,α)^{13}N reaction contributes as much as 17% of the nitrogen counts detected. The protons in this reaction are generated by the collision of fast neutrons with protons in the body.

A second problem is the lack of uniformity of the fast-neutron fluence in the body.[38] Elliot et al. investigated the fast-neutron fluence uniformity with water phantoms.[39] Deviations from ± 7 to $\pm 22\%$ from the mean were reported for phantom thicknesses ranging from 15 to 30 cm.

Biggin et al., Harvey et al., and Ettinger et al. reported the use of PGNAA for in vivo measurement of TBN by the reaction ^{14}N(n,α) ^{15}N.[38,40,41] The excited nucleus of ^{15}N* has a life of approximately 10^{-15} sec.

It deexcites to the ground state by emission of a cascade of gamma rays, yielding stable N-15. Although the thermal neutron-capture cross section is relatively small, the production of a high-energy gamma ray (10.83 MeV) renders N readily measurable. Also, the neutron flux density in the body is more uniform with this technique.

Two problems are associated with the PGNAA technique. Thermal and epithermal neutrons are captured by iodine in the NaI(Tl) detecting crystal. Furthermore, a "pileup" of gamma rays occurs (the simultaneous arrival of two or more pulses) from lower-energy reactions or from the neutron source. The Birmingham group countered the pileup problem with the use of a pulsed neutron beam from a cyclotron and associated gated circuits.[40] By collimating the neutrons, pulsing the neutron beam, and shielding the detectors, the investigators achieved an accuracy of $\pm 2\%$ with an incident dose of 0.1 rem. Vartsky solved the problem of pileup with the use of fractional charge collection technique.[42] The overall signal-to-noise ratio was improved by a factor of 1.7. Vartsky also reported an improvement in the method for measuring absolute values of TBN, based on the use of total-body hydrogen as an internal standard.[42] Upon capture of slow neutrons, hydrogen emits a 2.23-MeV gamma ray with a yield of 100%.

The Brookhaven technique incorporates several recent technical improvements.[43] The neutron source is 85 Ci (3.1 TBq) ^{238}Pu-Be, designed to provide a rectangular beam 13 × 60 cm; the body is scanned by moving the bed over the beam. The entire facility is shielded with lead to reduce the intensity of the gamma rays emitted from both source and shielding. Two NaI(Tl) detectors are used for bilateral scanning. The total body dose equivalent to the subject is ~27 mrem (~2.7 × 10^{-4} Sv) for the bilateral irradiation. Precision, determined from phantom measurements, is ±2%; reproducibility, determined by sequential measurement of human subjects, is ~3%.[43]

Mernagh et al. were the first to report the feasibility of in vivo measurement of partial (truncal) body nitrogen.[44] Four collimated 5-Ci (185-GBq) ^{238}Pu-Be sources were arranged to deliver bilateral irradiation. Two heavily shielded NaI(Tl) detectors are used. The truncal irradiation delivers a dose of 50 mrem (5 × 10^{-4} Sv). The reproducibility is ±3%.[44]

CLINICAL APPLICATIONS

The first clinical applications of neutron activation analysis were studies of body calcium in patients with metabolic bone disorders. The study of changes in skeletal Ca in patients with these disorders requires normative data on the relation of Ca to sex, body habitus, and age. The noninvasive nature of neutron activation techniques and the low levels of radiation dose employed have made it possible to establish the baseline data through the study of normal subjects. Both TBNAA and PBNAA have been used to study bone mass.[23,45,46,47,48,49,50,51,52] Several studies have focused on osteoporosis, and various therapeutic regimens for the treatment of this condition have been evaluated.

In addition to studies based on total and partial body (truncal) irradiation, bone Ca concentrations have been determined by peripheral irradiation of the hand.[53] While the majority of investigations have been made on white patients, some studies have also been carried out with a black population.[47,48] The findings indicate that higher levels of Ca and K are normally found in black populations, hence, separate norms must be used.

Truncal PBNAA has been used to study adults with osteomalacia, hypophosphatemic rickets,[54] and osteomalacia resulting from anticonvulsant therapy.[55] Other studies have investigated Ca disturbances in

patients with renal osteodystrophy.[14,56,57,58,59,60,61,62,63,64] Measurement of Ca has also been useful in studying both patients with Paget's disease and patients with endocrine dysfunctions: thyroid and parathyroid disorders, Cushing's syndrome, acromegaly, osteoporosis in rheumatoid arthritis patients receiving corticosteroid therapy, osteogenesis imperfecta, myotonic dystrophy, thalassemia, and vitamin D rickets. Various therapeutic regimens for many of these conditions have been assessed through their effect on Ca levels in the body. Skeletal mass has been studied with TBNAA in chronic alcoholism with and without Laennec's cirrhosis. The effect of lithium carbonate has been investigated with the use of forearm PBNAA.

Sodium, chlorine, and phosphorus can be measured simultaneously with Ca from the spectra obtained. Baseline data have been obtained for total-body sodium and chlorine as a function of age, sex, and body habitus.[33]

Nitrogen and potassium measurements serve as indices of muscle mass, body protein content, and nutrition regimens.[65,66,67] Quantitative measurement has been made of body composition in normal subjects, and in patients with various forms of neoplastic disease.[65,68,69] Total-body nitrogen is determined with the use of PGNAA, total-body potassium is measured with the use of a whole-body counter.[15] Mass and protein content of the muscle compartment and of the nonmuscle lean tissue are determined by application of compartmental analysis techniques. Total-body water, determined simultaneously with the use of a tritium label, provides a measure of lean body mass. From these data, the body fat can be inferred. Baseline data on body composition of age- and sex-matched individuals, which have been obtained already in earlier studies, provide a basis for comparison and evaluation (see Vol. II, Chap. 22).

The internal accumulation of Cd, which deposits chiefly in the liver and kidney, is a potentially serious industrial health problem. It has been suggested that Cd poisoning is a causative factor in both hypertension and emphysema. Partial body PGNAA is currently used for in vivo studies of internally deposited Cd. Through use of transportable α,n sources, studies have been made of industrial workers at their plant sites in England, Belgium,[70] and the United States.[71] Studies of smokers show higher levels of internally deposited Cd than normal nonsmoking individuals.[72]

REFERENCES

1. In vivo Neutron Activation Analysis. Proc. Panel, Vienna, International Atomic Energy Agency, SC/PUB/322, 1973.
2. Cohn, S.H., Fairchild, R.G., and Shukla, K.K.: Theoretical considerations in the selection of neutron sources for total body neutron activation analysis. Phys. Med. Biol., 18:648, 1973.
3. International Commission on Radiological Units Report 13: Neutron fluence, neutron spectra and kerma. Washington, D.C., 1969.
4. NCRP Report 38, Protection Against Neutron Radiation. Washington, D.C., National Council on Radiation Protection, 1971.
5. Cohn, S.H., Fairchild, R.G., and Shukla, K.K.: Comparison of techniques for the total body neutron activation analysis of calcium in man. Panel on In Vivo Neutron Activation Analysis. Vienna, International Atomic Energy Agency, STI/PUB/322, 1973.
6. Guey, A.: Estimation of total body calcium. Panel on In vivo Neutron Activation Analysis. Vienna, International Atomic Energy Agency, STI/PUB/322, 1973.
7. Chamberlain, M.J., et al.: Total body calcium by whole body neutron activation: new technique for study of bone disease. Br. Med. J., 2:581, 1968.
8. Chamberlain, M.J., et al.: Use of cyclotron for whole body neutron activation analysis: theoretical and practical considerations. Int. J. Appl. Radiat. Isot., 21:725, 1970.
9. Palmer, H.E., et al.: The feasibility of in vivo neutron activation analysis of total body calcium and other elements of body composition. Phys. Med. Biol., 13:269, 1968.
10. Nelp, W.B., et al.: Measurements of total body calcium (bone mass) in vivo with the use of total body neutron activation analysis. J. Lab. Clin. Med., 76:151, 1970.
11. Cohn, S.H., et al.: Effect of porcine calcitonin on calcium metabolism in osteoporosis. J. Clin. Endocrinol. Metab., 33:719, 1971.
12. Cohn, S.H., et al.: Design and calibration on a "broad beam" ²³⁸Pu,Be neutron source for total body neutron activation analysis. J. Nucl. Med., 13:487, 1972.
13. Cohn, S.H., and Dombrowski, C.S.: Measurement of total body calcium, sodium chloride, nitrogen and phosphorus in man by in vivo neutron activation analysis. J. Nucl. Med., 12:499, 1971.
14. Cohn, S.H., et al.: Determination of body composition by neutron activation analysis in patients with renal failure. J. Lab. Clin. Med., 79:978, 1972.
15. Cohn, S.H., Dombrowski, C.S., and Fairchild, R.G., In vivo activation analysis of calcium in man. Int. J. Appl. Radiat. Isot., 21:127, 1970.
16. Cohn, S.H., et al.: Alterations in elemental body composition in thyroid disorders. J. Clin. Endocrinol., 36:742, 1973.
17. Boddy, K., and Glaros, D.: The measurement of phosphorus in human bone using radioactive sources—a technique for partial body in vivo activation analysis. Int. J. Appl. Radiat. Isot., 24:179, 1973.
18. Lenihan, J.M.A., et al.: Estimation of thyroid iodine in vivo by activation analysis. Nature, 214:1221, 1967.
19. Boddy, K., Harden, R.M.G., and Alexander, W.D.: In vivo measurement of intrathyroidal iodine concentration in man by activation analysis. J. Clin. Endocrinol. Metab., 28:294, 1968.
20. Lenihan, J.M.A., et al.: Estimating thyroid iodine by activation analysis in vivo. J. Nucl. Med., 9:111, 1967.
21. McNeill, K.G., et al.: In vivo neutron activation analysis for calcium in man. J. Nucl. Med., 14:502, 1973.
22. Appleby, D.B., et al.: Partial-body in vivo neutron activation of calcium in bone. Nuclear Activation Techniques in the Life Sciences. Proc. Symp., 1972. Vienna, International Atomic Energy Agency, 1972, p. 617.
23. Harrison, J.E., et al.: A bone calcium index based on partial body calcium measurements by in vivo activation analysis. J. Nucl. Med., 16:116, 1975.
24. Catto, G.R.D., McIntosh, J.A.R., and Macleod, M.: Partial body neutron activation analysis in vivo. Phys. Med. Biol., 18:508, 1973.
25. Maziere, B., Comar, D., and Kunz, D.: In vivo measurement of the Ca/P ratio by local activation. Proceedings International Conference on Modern Trends in Activation Analysis. Munich, 1:229, 1976.
26. Giarrantano, J.C.: Prompt gamma ray analysis of bone using Californium-252. Thesis, University of Texas, May 1974.
27. Rundo, J., and Bunce, L.J.: Estimation of total hydrogen content of the human body. Nature, 210:1023, 1966.
28. Biggin, H.C., Chen, N.S., Ettinger, K.V., et al.: Radioanalyt. Chem., 19:207, 1974.
29. McLellan, J.S., Thomas, B.J., Fremlin, J.H., and Harvey, T.C.: Cadmium—its in vivo detection in man. Phys. Med. Biol., 20:88, 1975.
30. Harvey, T.C., et al.: Measurement of liver cadmium in patients and industrial workers by neutron activation analysis. Lancet, 1:1209, 1975.

31. Thomas, B.J., Harvey, T.C., Chettle, D.R., et al.: A transportable system for the measurement of liver cadmium in vivo. Phys. Med. Biol., *23*:432, 1979.

32. Evans, C.J., Cummins, P., Dutton, J., et al.: A Californium-252 facility for the in vivo measurement of organ cadmium. Nuclear Activation Techniques in the Life Sciences, Proc. Symp., 1978. Vienna, International Atomic Energy Agency, 1979, p. 719.

33. Ellis, K.J., Vartsky, D., and Cohn, S.H.: A mobile prompt gamma neutron activation facility. Nuclear Activation Techniques in the Life Sciences. Proc. Symp., 1978. Vienna, International Atomic Energy Agency, 1979, p. 733.

34. Vartsky, D., Ellis, K.J., Chen, N.S., and Cohn, S.H.: A facility for in vivo measurement of kidney and liver cadmium by neutron capture prompt gamma analysis. Phys. Med. Biol., *22*:1985, 1977.

35. Spinks, T.J.: Measurement of body nitrogen by activation analysis. Int. J. Appl. Radiat. Isot., *29*:409, 1978.

36. Oxby, C.B., Appleby, D.B., Brooks, K., et al.: A technique for measuring total body nitrogen in clinical investigations using the $^{14}N(n,2n)^{13}N$ reaction. Int. J. Appl. Radiat. Isot., *29*:205, 1978.

37. Leach, M.O., Thomas, B.J., and Vartsky, D.: Total body nitrogen measured by the $^{14}N(n,2n)^{13}N$ method: a study of the interfering reactions and the variation of spatial sensitivity with depth. Int. J. Appl. Radiat. Isot., *28*:263, 1977.

38. Biggin, H.C., Chen, N.S., Ettinger, K.V., et al.: Determination of nitrogen in living subjects. Nature, *236*:187, 1972.

39. Elliot, A., Holloway, I., Boddy, K., et al.: Neutron uniformity studies related to clinical total body in vivo neutron activation analysis. Phys. Med. Biol., *23*:269, 1978.

40. Harvey, T.C., et al.: Measurement of whole body nitrogen by neutron activation analysis. Lancet, *1*:395, 1973.

41. Ettinger, K.V., Biggin, H.C., Chen, N.S., et al.: In vivo neutron activation analysis of nitrogen using capture gamma rays. Kerntechnik, *2*:89, 1975.

42. Vartsky, D.: Absolute measurement of whole body nitrogen by in vivo neutron activation analysis. Thesis, University of Birmingham, England, 1976.

43. Vartsky, D., Ellis, K.J., and Cohn, S.H.: In vivo measurement of body nitrogen by analysis of prompt gamma from neutron capture. J. Nucl. Med., *20*:1158, 1979.

44. Mernagh, J.R., Harrison, J.E., and McNeill, K.G.: In vivo determination of nitrogen using Pu-Be sources. Phys. Med. Biol., *5*:831, 1977.

45. Cohn, S.H., Vaswani, A.N., Zanzi, I., and Ellis, K.J.: Effect of aging on bone mass in adult women. Am. J. Physiol., *230*:143, 1976.

46. Cohn, S.H., Vaswani, A.N., Aloia, J.F., et al.: Changes in body chemical composition with age measured by total body neutron activation. Metab., *25*:89, 1976.

47. Cohn, S.H., Abesamis, C., Zanzi, I., et al.: Body elemental composition: Comparison between black and white adults. Am. J. Physiol., *232*:419, 1977.

48. Cohn, S.H., Abesamis, C., Yasumura, S., et al.: Comparative skeletal mass and bone density in black and white women. Metab. Clin. Exp., *26*:171, 1977.

49. Harrison, J.E., and McNeill, K.G.: Partial body calcium measurements by in vivo neutron activation analysis. Am. J. Roentgenol., *126*:1308, 1976.

50. Harrison, J.E., Meema, E., and McNeill, K.G.: A comparison of results from IVNAA of the trunk with results from X-ray densitometry of radium, Progress and Problems of In Vivo Activation Analysis. Proc. 2nd Symp. East Kilbride, Scotland. Edited by K. Boddy. Scottish Universities Research and Reactor Centre, 1976.

51. Harrison, J.E., McNeill, K.G., Hitchman, A.J., and Britt, B.A.: Bone mineral measurements of the central skeleton by in vivo neutron activation analysis for routine investigation of osteopenia. Invest. Radiol., *14*:27, 1979.

52. McNeill, K.G., and Harrison, J.E.: Measurement of the axial skeleton for the diagnosis of osteoporosis by neutron activation analysis. J. Nucl. Med., *18*:1136, 1977.

53. Maziere, B., Kuntz, D., Comar, D., and Ryckewaert, A.: In vivo analysis of bone calcium by local neutron activation of the hand: results in normal and osteoporotic subjects. J. Nucl. Med., *20*:85, 1979.

54. Harrison, J.E., Cumming, W.A., Fornasier, V., et al.: Increased bone mineral content in young adults with familial hypophosphatemic vitamin D refractory rickets. Metab. Clin. Exp., *25*:33, 1976.

55. Christiansen, C., and Robro, P.: Bone mineral content in anticonvulsant osteomalacia. Am. J. Roentgenol., *126*:1302, 1976.

56. Catto, G.R.D., and Macleod, M.: The investigation and treatment of renal bone disease. Am. J. Med., *61*:64, 1978.

57. Meema, H.E., Harrison, J.E., McNeill, K.G., and Oreopoulos, D.G.: Correlations between peripheral and central skeletal mineral content in chronic renal failure patients and in osteoporosis. Skelet. Radiol., *1*:169, 1977.

58. Harrison, J.E., McNeill, K.G., Meema, H.E., et al.: Partial body calcium measurements on patients with renal failure. Metab. Clin. Exp., *26*:255, 1977.

59. Winney, R., Robson, J.S., Tothill, P., et al.: Effect of dialysis calcium in 1α-hydroxyvitamin D3 on bone mineral loss and hyperparathyroidism in haemodialysis patients. Clinical Uses of 1α-hydroxyvitamin D3. Proc. Conf. New York, 1977.

60. Hoskins, D.J., and Chamberlain, M.J.: Calcium balance in chronic renal failure. Qtly. J. Med., *42*:467, 1973.

61. Denny, J.D., Sherrard, D.J., Nelp, W.B., et al.: Total body calcium and long term calcium balance in chronic renal disease. J. Lab. Clin. Med., *82*:226, 1973.

62. Cohn, S.H., Ellis, K.J., Caselnova, R.C., et al.: Cor-

relation of radial bone mineral content with total body calcium in chronic renal failure. J. Lab. Clin. Med., 86:216, 1976.

63. Asad, S., Ellis, K.J., Cohn, S.H., and Letteri, J.M.: Changes in total body calcium on prolonged maintenance hemodialysis with high and low dialysate calcium. Nephron, 23:223, 1979.

64. Cohn, S.H., et al.: Alterations in skeletal calcium and phosphorus in dysfunction of the parathyroid. J. Clin. Endocrinol. Metab., 36:750, 1973.

65. Cohn, S.H., Sawitsky, A., Vartsky, D., et al.: In Vivo quantification of body composition in normal subjects and in cancer patients. Nutr. Cancer, 2:67, 1980.

66. McNeill, K.G., Mernagh, J.R., Harrison, J.E., and Jeejeebhoy, K.N.: In vivo measurement of body protein based on the determination of nitrogen by prompt gamma neutron activation analysis. Am. J. Clin. Nutr., 32:1955, 1979.

67. Burkinshaw, L., Hill, G.L., and Morgan, D.B.: Assessment of the distribution of protein in the human body by in vivo neutron activation analysis. Nuclear Activation Techniques in the Life Sciences. Proc. Symp., 1978. Vienna, International Atomic Energy Agency, p. 787, 1979.

68. Cohn, S.H., Vartsky, D., Yasumura, S., et al.: Compartmental body composition based on total body nitrogen, potassium and calcium. Am. J. Physiol., 239:524, 1980.

69. Cohn, S.H., Gartenhaus, C., Sawitsky, A., et al.: Compartmental body composition of cancer patients by measurement of total body nitrogen, potassium and water. Metab., 30:222, 1980.

70. Roels, H., et al.: Critical concentrations of cadmium in renal cortex and urine. Lancet, p. 221, 1979.

71. Ellis, K.J., Morgan, W.D., Zanzi, I., et al.: Critical concentration of cadmium in human renal cortex (dose effect studies in cadmium smelter workers). J. Toxicol. Environ. Health, 7:691, 1981.

72. Ellis, K.J., Vartsky, D., Zanzi, I., et al.: Cadmium: In vivo measurement in smokers and non smokers. Science, 205:323, 1979.

Chapter 18

CEREBRAL BLOOD FLOW STUDIES USING XENON-133

JOHN A. CORREIA,
ROBERT H. ACKERMAN, AND
NATHANIEL M. ALPERT

Cerebral blood flow (CBF) is an important indicator of brain physiology, both in health and in disease. Although cerebral energy metabolism is more fundamental to brain function, the two processes are necessarily linked by the delivery of nutrients and oxygen. Many brain diseases, such as embolic stroke, are initiated by disruptions in blood flow. In a healthy brain and in many diseases, cerebral blood flow and energy metabolism are "coupled," that is, variations in blood flow show the same proportionate response to factors that alter regional metabolism. Measurements of cerebral blood flow therefore can be used in many clinical and research problems as an index of brain function.

Sequential CBF studies require a nontraumatic method that is practical to apply in complex clinical or investigational situations and that provides regional and hemispheric CBF estimates with good reproducibility between examinations under similar study conditions. The xenon-133 inhalation/IV injection method meets these criteria. Although it has a

number of specific limitations, it is sensitive to regional and hemispheric changes in CBF. Moreover, the reproducibility is sufficiently precise to permit meaningful comparisons of results obtained in response to normal aging, the natural history of disease, therapeutic trials, and neuropsychologic stimuli.

OVERVIEW

Figure 18–1 depicts a multidetector system for measuring regional CBF by either inhalation or IV injection of Xe-133. In the inhalation method, the subject inhales air mixed with 4 to 8 mCi ($\sim$150 to 300 MBq) per liter of Xe-133 from a shielded reservoir of 5 to 10 liter capacity for about 1 min and then breathes room air, which is exhausted to an activated charcoal trap or closed exhaust system for the remainder of the study. In the IV injection method, Xe-133 dissolved in saline (20 to 60 mCi) is injected, and the patient exhales into a collecting system during the entire study. In either case, some of the Xe-133 dis-

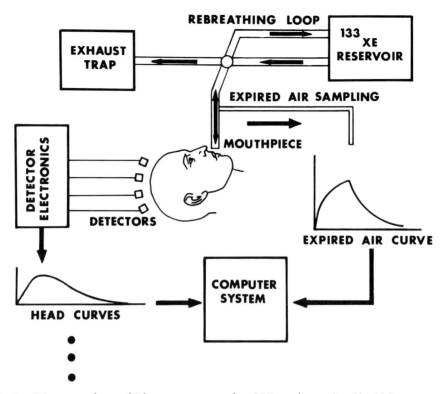

Fig. 18–1. Diagram of a multidetector system for CBF studies using Xe-133.

solved in blood is carried to the brain, where it diffuses across the blood-brain barrier into brain tissue. In the physiologic range of blood flow rates, xenon is freely diffusible, and its transport into the brain is flow-limited rather than diffusion-limited. Once deposited in tissue, xenon is cleared by blood flow only.

The buildup and clearance of radioactivity in the head is monitored by a set of discrete radiation detectors. Typically, data are collected for 11 to 16 min. The radioactivity in the expired air is monitored by a separate detector. From measured values in end tidal air, the arterial input concentration is determined to within a proportionality constant. The clearance data are fitted to a mathematical model to determine the flow rates of two types of tissue (i.e., fast and slow, or "gray" and "white" matter).

Detailed discussion of the various aspects of measurements and data analysis are given in this chapter.

THEORETIC CONSIDERATIONS

Measurements in animals obtained with diffusible tracers have shown that the distribution of blood flow in the brain is bimodal, that is, the various structures in the brain fall into either a high ("fast") flow category or a low ("slow") flow category.

A tracer introduced into this system mimics the behavior of flowing blood in both arteries and tissues but does not take part in any metabolic process. Xenon, because of its small molecular diameter and nonpolarity, is highly diffusible in brain tissue and yet is chemically inert. Radioactivity input to the brain is described by the arterial concentration of tracer as a function of time, $C_a(t)$. If the tracer is instantly and uniformly mixed in each compartment and the system is in a steady state—i.e., $F \neq F(t)$—and is constant over each compartment, the following differential equation can be derived for each compartment:

$$\frac{dQ_i(t)}{dt} = F_i C_A(t) - \gamma_i F_i Q_i(t) V_i \quad (1)$$

where:

  F_i = Steady state flow in compartment i.

  $Q_i(t)$ = Amount of tracer in compartment i at time t.

  V_i = Volume of distribution of tracer in compartment i.

  γ_i = Tissue: blood partition coefficient.

This equation can be solved by standard means to yield a solution for each compartment.[1] Since the two compartments are noninteracting (Fig. 18–2), separate solutions for each can be found and the results summed:

$$Q(t) = \sum_{i=1}^{2} A_i e^{-k_i t} \int_0^t C_A(t') e^{+k_i t'} \, dt' \quad (2)$$

where:

$$k_i = \gamma_i \frac{F_i}{V_i}$$

In the above equation, $Q(t)$ and $C_A(t')$ refer to instantaneous quantities. In an experimental situation, data are acquired as a set of points integrated over time (Fig.

18–3). The time intervals are typically on the order of 5 to 6 sec to characterize flows of 100 ml/100 g/min, which reasonably approximates the instantaneous value at this flow rate. The counting rate, $S(t)$, measured by an external detector is assumed to be proportional to the amount of activity within the detector field of view. Thus, $S(t) \sim Q(t)$. Such effects as photon attenuation and scatter cause some error.

This "model prediction" for a given set of values A_i, k_i can be compared to measured clearance data by the method of nonlinear least squares. This is a generalization of the familiar method of linear least squares, which deals with models (or functions) that are algebraically linear in parameters to be estimated.

Let $S(t_i)$ represent the measured head clearance data for a given detector and $S(t_i, A_j, k_j)$ represent the model prediction from equation (2) for a specific set of parameters (A_j, k_j).

$$\Phi = \sum_{i=1}^{n} [S(t_i) - \hat{S}(t_i, A_j, k_j)]^2 \quad (3)$$

The least squares criterion is that the values A_j, k_j, which minimize Φ, best characterize the measured data set $S(t_i)$. For linear least squares, this is simply a matter of computing derivatives of Φ for the A_j

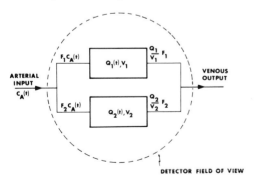

Fig. 18–2. Diagram of detector field of view subtending two parallel noninteracting compartments. One compartment represents cerebral gray matter, and the other, cerebral white matter.

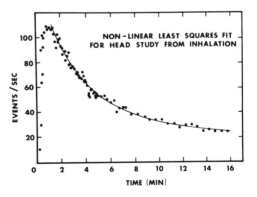

Fig. 18–3. Example of nonlinear least squares fit to a patient head curve. The fit begins at approximately 1.5 min and is represented by the solid line. Dots represent the measured data.

and k_j sets of values, setting them to zero, and solving the resulting linear equations.

When the model parameters are nonlinear, as is the case in inhalation studies, the minimization is no longer a simple matter. In this case, a scheme must be devised to search the space defined by the parameters (i.e., an *n*-dimensional space for *n* parameters) for a minimum. This is usually an iterative scheme in which an initial guess at the parameter values is made, a value of Φ is computed, a change in the parameters is made, and then a new Φ is computed and compared to the previous one. At each iteration, a new guess is generated and compared to the result of the previous iteration until *convergence* is achieved. Convergence is usually assumed to occur when the change in Φ from one iteration to the next is less than some specified value or when the change in any of the parameters from one iteration to the next is smaller than some specified value. Approaches to defining convergence criteria are described by Marquardt and by Fletcher.[2,3] Typical fit times for such nonlinear least square programs on a minicomputer are 15 to 45 sec per 100-point inhalation curve. An example of a typical head curve fit is shown in Figure 18–3. The fit is usually begun at a time between 1 and 2 min after the start of Xe-133 inhalation.

ESTIMATION OF THE ARTERIAL INPUT FUNCTION

To compute the model estimates $S(t,A_j,k_j)$ used in the parameter estimation, an independently measured estimate of the arterial input function $C_A(t)$ must be made. For both inhalation and IV injection studies, this is usually determined from measurements of Xe-133 concentration in the expired air. The assumptions are made that at end-tidal respiration the lung air is in equilibrium with lung arterial blood and that the Xe-133 concentrations in air and blood are equal at that time. This air

may be sampled with a constant volume pump, through a small diameter line at the patient's mouth. In most cases, a fixed lung-to-brain transit time is assumed (6 sec) and dispersion neglected, so that the lung arterial curve is assumed to be the input function to the brain at the carotid artery. Usually, measurements of counts per 0.2 to 0.3 sec are recorded by a shielded radiation detector that samples the subject's expired air. Figure 18–4A shows an example of such a curve, measured in a normal individual at a sampling interval of 0.3 sec. The variations of Xe-133 concentration with respiration are clearly seen. The buildup of activity during the first minute represents the equilibrium phase, during which the subject breathes from a reservoir of Xe-133. At 1 min, the subject is switched off the reservoir and breathes room air. The end-tidal points (dotted lines) are computed using the following derivative algorithm for determining maxima and minima:

$$\frac{dx_j}{dt} = \frac{1}{12\Delta t}\left[(x_{j-2} - x_{j+2}) - 8(x_{j-1} - x_{j+1})\right] \quad (4)$$

This algorithm is used to compute the derivatives of the measured curve as a function of time; the zero values in the derivative represent turning points. A computation of the second derivative identifies maxima and minima.

Several alternative ways of determining $C_A(t)$ have been proposed. A method suggested by Jagge and Obrist involves estimating the lung radioactivity with a radiation detector placed externally over the chest.[4] The measured lung activity is then assumed to be an estimate of the end-tidal arterial activity.

Refinements of the Inhalation Model

Scalp and Skull Activity. Some of the measured activity stems from blood flow to the scalp and skull. These are low-flow structures: 5 ml/100 g/min as opposed to 20 ml/100 g/min for cerebral white matter.

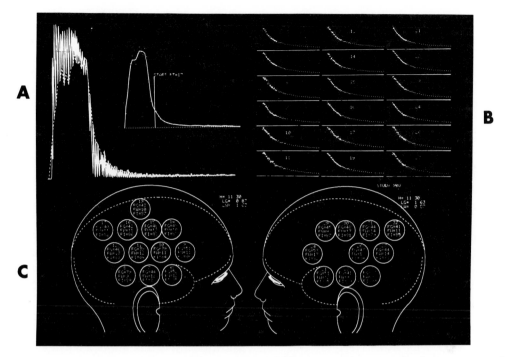

Fig. 18–4. *A.* Expired air curve and derived arterial input curve for normal subject. *B.* Sample head curves from 1.5 to 16 min after xenon administration for the same subject. *C.* Regional flow values computed for this subject in left and right hemispheres respectively.

The result of this extracerebral "contamination" is an underestimation of white matter flow. Obrist et al. have suggested that a third compartment be added to the inhalation model to account for scalp and skull blood flow.[5] In practice, this compartment is difficult to characterize because of the slow half-time clearance ($T_{1/2}$ = 28 min). To obtain a reliable estimate of the clearance rate constant, clearance measurements would require 30 to 40 min. In practice therefore, a two-compartment model is used for most patient studies with the recognition that the slow compartment is significantly influenced by contributions from the scalp and skull circulation.

Full-Curve Analysis. Although brain buildup and clearance curves can be measured from the beginning of the inhalation or IV injection, usually only the data from the time at which the air curve has decreased to 20% or less of its maximum

value are analyzed. The reason for this is that there is a significant contribution to the measured activity from photons scattered from the airways; this contribution decreases as the airway activity decreases. Several groups have proposed an extension to the two-compartment model to include effects due to airway scatter so that data from the entire measuring period can be utilized.[6,7,8] The assumption is made that the scatter contribution is proportional to the activity in expired air. In addition, several of these authors have proposed including the lung-to-brain transit time as a parameter rather than assigning it a fixed value.

With these generalizations, the model becomes:

$$S(t) = \sum_{i=1}^{2} A_i C^{-k_i t} \int_o^t C_A (t' + \delta) e^{k_i t'}\, dt'$$

$$+ m\overline{C}_A(t) \quad (5)$$

where:

$\overline{C}_A(t)$ = average concentration of the expired air data before end-tidal points are chosen.

m = a parameter to define the size of airway contribution.

δ = lung-to-brain transit time parameter.

The use of this extended model is being evaluated at several laboratories. The expected gain in statistical quality of parameter estimates appears initially to be offset by the increased uncertainty of a six-parameter fit, as opposed to a four-parameter fit. Also, some workers have suggested that a term be added to the model to account for the radioactivity in arterial blood during the early phase of the measurements.[6,7]

BLOOD FLOW INDICES

The computed parameters A_i, k_i often are combined in various ways to yield estimates or average flow and tissue compartment sizes that may be less susceptible to errors than the parameter values themselves. Some of these indices and their properties are given in Table 18–1. An index that reduces the four estimated parameters to a single number tends to be more precise (i.e., has less statistical noise) but also contains less information about the tissue volume viewed. For example, the mean flow provides an estimate of the average response of the tissue volume, but information about the response of individual fast and slow components is lost.

Several of these indices are computed so that dependence of the resulting number on tissue-to-blood partition coefficients is minimal. This is done because of evidence that these partition coefficients vary from normal to disease states. The ISI and $ISI_{2.5}$ are examples.

RADIATION DETECTOR SYSTEMS AND HARDWARE

The earliest inhalation CBF studies were made with one or two large scintil-lation detectors that viewed either an entire hemisphere or the whole brain.[13] Gradually, more and smaller detectors were added to these systems, so that modern systems have 16 to 32 detectors. Such a detector is shown in Figure 18–5A. Typically, the detector consists of a NaI(Tl) crystal, PM tube and associated electronics, and a collimator. The crystal is ½ in. to ¾ in. thick and ¾ in. in diameter. The thickness is chosen so that the detectors are 100% efficient for the 80-keV gamma rays from Xe-133. Since geometric detection efficiency increases as the square of the diameter of the detector, it is desirable to have the largest possible detectors consistent with the resolution requirements of the clinical or experimental problem to be studied. For systems with 16 to 32 detectors, the detector size—allowing for packaging and interdetector shielding—is about 1 in. outside diameter, which accommodates a ¾ in. diameter crystal.

Solid state detectors, including germanium and cadmium telluride, have been explored.[14,15] Germanium crystals have acceptable efficiency at 80 keV and good energy resolution (10 to 20 times better than NaI(Tl) detectors for this energy). They must be operated at cryogenic temperatures, however, to minimize detector noise, and they are relatively expensive. Cadmium telluride is a room temperature semiconductor with energy resolution properties similar to those of NaI(Tl) detectors and with good efficiency properties for 80-keV radiation. These detectors offer the potential for producing small portable arrays and perhaps will be widely used in the future.

Because of improvements in counting rate capability, scintillation cameras can now be used to collect Xe-133 CBF data.

The electronic circuitry in multidetector systems is of standard form. After pulse-height analysis, the data are scaled to reduce the number of events incident upon the computer interface. Data are then transferred to a digital computer for stor-

TABLE 18–1. *Blood Flow Indices Computed From Fitted Parameters*[5,9,10,11,12]

Name	Expression	Typical normal value	Properties
Weight gray	$\dfrac{A_1/F_1}{A_1/F_1 + A_2/F_2}$	0.40	Estimate of gray matter as fraction of tissue in field of view
Weight white	$\dfrac{A_2/F_2}{A_1/F_1 + A_2/F_2}$	0.60	Estimate of white matter as fraction of tissue in field of view
Mean flow	$\dfrac{A_1 + A_2}{A_1/k_1 + A_2/k_2}$	0.30	Index of average flow
Fast Flow Index (FFI)	$\dfrac{A_1}{A_1 + A_2}$	0.75	Index of gray-matter flow
CBF_1	$\dfrac{A_1 k_1 + A_2 k_2}{A_1 + A_2}$	0.70	Index of average flow
ISI	$\ln(A_1 e^{-2k_1} + A_2 e^{-2k_2})$ $- \ln(A_1 e^{-3k_1} + A_2 e^{-3k_2})$	0.32	Index of gray-matter flow. ln of slope of sum of two exponentials between 2 and 3 min.
$ISI_{2.5}$	$A_1 k_1 e^{-2.5k_1} + A_2 k_2 e^{-2.5k_2}$	0.36	Index of gray matter flow. Slope of sum of two exponentials at t = 2.5 min.

age and subsequent analysis. Several types of interfaces can be used. Data volume and data rates associated with xenon CBF measurements are not particularly challenging to modern computer technology. For example, maximum counting rates to be expected for a typical ¾-in. NaI(Tl) detector are on the order of 1000 events/sec; for the air-curve channel, they may be as high as 10,000 events/sec. Data can be encoded and stored in the computer memory on an event-by-event basis. Every event then produces an address and generates a computer interrupt. This approach is analogous to frame-mode acquisition. When a new time interval is begun, a new frame in memory is used as a collection buffer.

A second possibility, which makes fewer demands upon the computer, is a system in which a buffer that serves as a scaler is associated with each channel. Periodically, the computer reads out, stores,

and resets the buffer contents to zero. Typically, the air-curve buffer is scanned every 0.2 to 0.3 sec and the head-curve buffers are scanned every 5 to 6 sec. This scheme is readily adaptable to modern microprocessor technology and can be implemented by assembling commercially available components. Data for a completed study are usually stored on magnetic disk for subsequent analysis.

Collimators

Each detector in the CBF array is collimated to define its field of view. Usually, such collimators are 1- to 2-in. long, straight-bore cylinders of dense material, such as Pb, W, or Ta, chosen to maximize absorption. These have wide fields of view, as illustrated in Figure 18–5B. The collimator lengths shown here are chosen so that signals from tissue down to the first half-value layer of 80-keV photons (taking skull absorption into account) do not fall

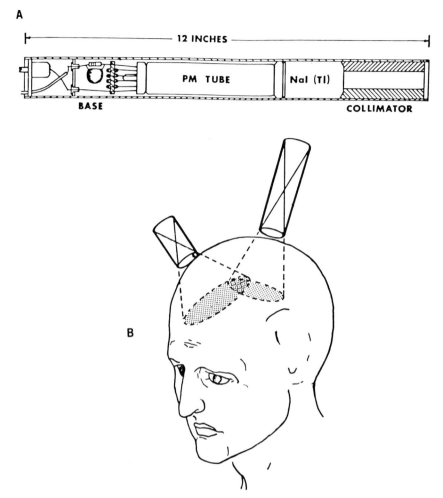

Fig. 18–5. *A.* Cross section of a NaI(Tl) detector for CBF with straight-bore collimator, PM tube, and preamplifier. *B.* Approximate fields of view for two different collimators (2½-cm and 5-cm straight bore) down to one half-value layer of 80-keV radiation in tissue. Note that the longer collimator provides a higher resolution sampling of the brain volume.

into the fields of view of adjacent detectors.

Detector Configurations

Several different detector geometries have been proposed for CBF studies. They include planar arrays and helmets with detectors arranged radially or elliptically (Fig. 18–6). Each of these geometries has its own particular strengths and weaknesses. The planar arrays, for example, are easy to construct and provide close packing of detectors with minimum overlap of detector fields, but detectors near the edges of the array tend to view large volumes of scalp and skull tissues. Also, repositioning detectors about the subject's head for repeat studies can be difficult. Helmet geometries, on the other hand, provide reasonably easy reproducibility, and detectors can be placed so that they view primarily brain tissue; however, their fields of view tend to overlap strongly, which reduces the amount of unique information obtained. Both types of detector arrays are widely used.

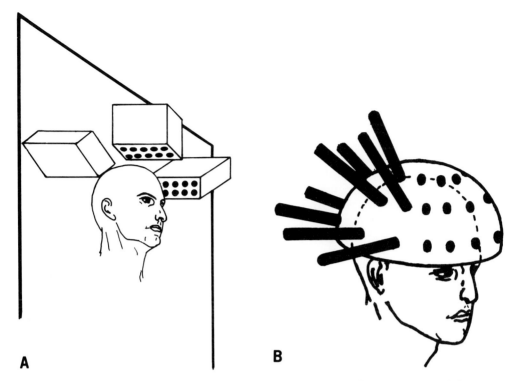

Fig. 18–6. *A.* Planar arrays of detectors. *B.* Helmet geometry for placement of detectors.

RADIATION DOSIMETRY

Estimates of radiation dose to various organs from typical Xe-133 inhalation and IV injection studies are shown in Table 18–2. Exposure of exhausted xenon gas to personnel and other individuals during a study is an additional source of concern. NRC regulations require that Xe-133 concentrations vented into the atmosphere be no higher than 3×10^{-7} mCi/l. Thus exhausted xenon must either be trapped in an activated charcoal trap and allowed to decay for six weeks (8 half-lives) or be sent through a dilution stack, which mixes the gas with large volumes of air before emission into the atmosphere.

TABLE 18–2. *Approximate Radiation Doses From Xe-133 Studies in Subjects With Normal Lung Function*

Organ	Inhalation (rad*)	IV Injection (rad†)
Lung	0.1	0.1
Airway Mucosa	1.0	0.7
Blood	0.005	0.15
Fat	0.035	0.05
Gonads	0.005	0.005
Whole Body	0.005	0.005

*1-min inhalation period at 5 mCi/l.
†IV injection of 40 mCi of Xe-133.
Derived from MIRD Dose Estimate Report No 9.[18]

LIMITATIONS OF THE XENON METHOD

There are several limitations to xenon CBF methods. One important experimental constraint is the need for the subject to maintain steady-state physiology during the entire measurement period, as required by the model. This requires that ambient conditions of lighting, noise level, and other environmental parameters be carefully controlled since transient changes in CBF caused by extrinsic stimuli must be minimized. The subject's level of consciousness must be kept constant. If the subject is awake at the start of the study, he must remain awake. Also, the subject's arterial level of CO_2 must be kept constant, and corrections for variations from normal must be performed in estimating CBF values.[19]

A second limitation arises from the partitioning of xenon between brain and blood. Estimates of tissue blood flow for the fast and slow compartments require estimated rate constants for brain-to-blood partition coefficients. Usually, fixed averaged values ($\gamma_g = 0.8$ and $\gamma_w = 1.5$) are assumed with corrections made for variations from the normal hematocrit. These are reasonable estimates for intact functioning tissue but are probably unacceptable for ischemic tissue or other disruptions. Several blood flow indices listed in Table 18–1 attempt to provide estimates that are less sensitive to variations in partition coefficients, but such variations remain unresolved problems.

The amount of isotope administered is limited by radiation dose considerations, so that typical peak counting rates are in the range of 250 to 1000 events/sec. Statistical counting errors are propagated through the curve-fitting procedure to give errors in the estimated flow parameters of 1 to 5% depending on peak counting rate and parameter values.[20] This problem, coupled with the physiologic variability of regional flow in normal populations, necessitates absolute changes in flow on the order of 10 to 20% for fast-flow estimates to be significant. Because of the relatively large volume viewed by a detector, large regions of decreased flow (e.g., 10 to 20 ml at 20% difference from surrounding gray matter) must be present to be detected.

A significant number of detected photons arise from low-flow extracerebral structures, resulting in an underestimation of cerebral white matter flow. Although several correction techniques have been proposed, none to date has proven successful. Scattering from either the same or the opposite hemisphere has the effect of enlarging the detector field of view and reducing resolution. Photon attenuation tends to moderate this effect, and the technique has sufficient spatial discrimination to identify uniquely the major arterial territories of the brain and is potentially useful in many clinical and research situations.

EXAMPLES OF HUMAN STUDIES

The Xe-133 inhalation/IV injection method has been applied to many differ-

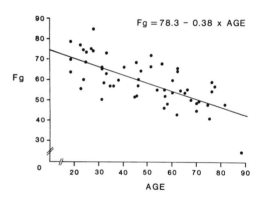

Fig. 18–7. Linear regression of hemispheric Flow-gray as a function of age for a group of 54 normal subjects, demonstrating a significant decrease in flow as age increases.

TABLE 18–3. *Mean Hemispheric CBF in Patients With TIA*

Type	No. of subjects	Mean Fg (ml/100/g/min)
Normals	48	66 ± 8
Transient Ischemic Attacks (TIA)— Total	32	48 ± 10
TIA—0 Tight Vessels	7	51 ± 11
TIA, 1–2 Tight Vessels	14	50 ± 9
TIA, 2+ Tight Vessels	11	42 ± 8

ent problems in medicine, including clinical research studies wherein populations of subjects are studied to establish clinical trends or to determine the relationships between CBF and other physiologic parameters. Several diagnostic studies of individual patients to determine cerebral status have been reported.[21-32] To date, applications of the latter type have been somewhat limited but they are evolving rapidly as the technique becomes more widely used.

Figure 18–4 shows the regional clearance curves and CBF estimates for a normal subject. The relative locations of the probes are indicated by circles and numerical values of F_g and F_w, and an initial slope index is indicated for each detector. This represents one study in a series of normal subjects ranging in age from 20 yrs to 88 yrs.[27] Figure 18–7 shows a linear regression of average hemispheric Flow-gray as a function of age, demonstrating a steady decline with increasing age. These

data are of value in determining deviations from normal CBF at different ages.

Table 18–3 summarizes the mean hemispheric F_g values in a group of subjects who had transient ischemic attacks. Flow values in the affected hemisphere for these individuals are related to carotid artery disease as determined by other diagnostic tests.[28] The data show a decrease in mean CBF as the severity of carotid artery disease increases.

Figure 18–8 shows maps of regional Flow-gray in the same subject during a hemiplegic migraine attack and between attacks. Note that CBF in the left temporal area decreases during migraine. This exemplifies the type of clinical information one might obtain in individual subjects.

To date, CBF studies have been used successfully in many clinical research studies and have the potential for routine use as a diagnostic tool. Despite its limitations, this technique can provide valuable information if used intelligently.

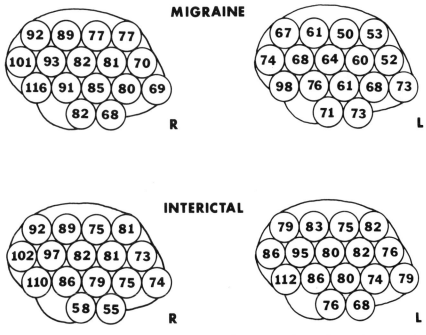

Fig. 18–8. Regional Flow-gray (cc./100g/min) values in a subject during hemiplegic migraine and between attacks. Note decreased regional Flow-gray in the left temporal area during the attack, which returns to normal between attacks.

Overinterpretation of results is perhaps the greatest danger. Several workers have begun to extend the use of this method to single photon tomography and x-ray CT, using inhalation of nonradioactive xenon gas.[33,34,35,36]

REFERENCES

1. Ince, E.L.: Ordinary Differential Equations, New York, Dover Publications, 1956.
2. Marquardt, D.W.: An Algorithm for Least Squares Estimation of Nonlinear Parameters. J. Soc. Indust. Appl. Math., *11*:431, 1963.
3. Fletcher, R.: An Approach to variable metric algorithms. The Computer Journal, *13*:317, 1970.
4. Jagge, J.L., and Obrist, W.D.: External monitoring of lung as a substitute for end tidal ^{133}Xe sampling in noninvasive CBF studies. rCBF Bulletin, *2*:25, 1981.
5. Obrist, W.D., Thompson, H.K., Wang, H.S., et al.: Regional cerebral blood flow estimated by ^{133}Xe inhalation. Stroke, *6*:245, 1975.
6. Jablonski, T., Prohovhik, I., Risberg, J., et al.: Fourier analysis of ^{133}Xe inhalation curves: accuracy and sensitivity. Acta Neurol. Scand., Suppl. 72, *60*:216, 1979.
7. Hazelrig, J.B., Katholi, C.R., Blauenstein, U.W., et al.: Total curve analysis of rCBF with ^{133}Xe inhalation: Description of the method and values obtained in normal volunteers. IEEE Trans. Biomed. Engl., *28*:609, 1981.
8. Obrist, W.D.: Department of Neurology, University of Pennsylvania, Private communication.
9. Waltz, A.G., Wanek, A.R., and Anderson, R.E.: Comparison of analytic methods for calculation of CBF. J. Nucl. Med., *13*:66, 1972.
10. Wyper, D.J., Lennox, G.A., and Rowan, J.O.: Two-minute slope inhalation technique for cerebral flow measurement in man. J. Neurol. Neurosurg. Psychiat., *39*:141, 1976.
11. Risberg, J., Ali, A.A., Wilson, E.M., et al.: rCBF by xenon inhalation—preliminary evaluation of an initial slope index in patients with unstable flow compartments. Stroke, *6*:142, 1975.
12. Heiss, W.D., Reisner, T., and Hoyer, J.: Changes in compartmental weight in the course of stroke. *In* Blood Flow and Metabolism in the Brain. Edited by M. Harper, B. Jennet, D. Miller, and J. Rowan. Edinburgh, Churchill Livingstone, 1975, p. 13.10.
13. Mallett, B.L., and Veall, N.: Measurement of regional cerebral clearance rates in man using xenon-133 inhalation and extracranial recording. Clin. Sci., *29*:179, 1965.
14. Reich, T., Rusinek, H., and Youdin, M.: Measurement of 3D distribution of CBF and partition coefficients with ^{133}Xe in humans. J. Cerebral Blood Flow Metab. Suppl. 1, *1*:133, 1981.
15. Correia, J.A., Ackerman, R.H., Buonanno, F., et al.: A portable device for the measurement of rCBF in the ICU and OR using CdTe detectors

and a Fourier transform based data analysis. IEEE Trans. Nucl. Sci., *28*:50, 1981.
16. Heiss, W.D., Podreka, I., and Roszuczky, A.: Regional cerebral blood flow measurement with a scintillation camera after intracarotid and IV injection of xenon. Cerebral Vascular Disease, Amsterdam Excerpta Medica, *2*:25, 1979.
17. Klassen, A.C., Myer, M.W., Werth, L.J., et al.: A single exponential index of rCBF for use with a gamma camera and inhaled [133]Xe. Cerebral Vascular Disease, Amsterdam Excerpta Medica, *2*:206, 1979.
18. MIRD Dose Estimate Report No. 9. J. Nucl. Med., *21*:459, 1980.
19. Ackerman, R.H.: The relationship of regional cerebrovascular CO_2 reactivity to blood pressure and regional resting flow. Stroke, *4*:725, 1973.
20. Correia, J.A., Chang, J.Y., Alpert, N.M., et al.: Simulation studies of statistical errors in inhalation and intracarotid injection studies. Acta Neurol. Scand. Suppl. 72, *60*:236, 1979.
21. Grotta, J., Ackerman, R.H., Correia, J.A., et al.: Whole blood viscosity parameters and cerebral blood flow. Stroke, *13*:296, 1982.
22. Norrving, B., Nilsson, B., and Risberg, J.: rCBF in patients with carotid occlusion: Resting and hypocapnic flow related to collateral pattern. Stroke, *15*:155, 1983.
23. Halsey, J., Morawetz, R., and Blauenstein, U.: The hemodynamic effect of STA-MCA bypass. Stroke, *13*:163, 1982.
24. Merory, J., Thomas, D.J., Humphrey, P.R., et al.: Cerebral blood flow after surgery for recent subarachnoid hemorrhage. J. Neurol. Neurosurg., Psychiatry, *43*:214, 1980.
25. Meyer, J.S., Sakai, F., Karacan, I., et al.: Regional cerebral hemodynamics during normal and abnormal human sleep. Acta Neurol. Scand. Suppl. 72, *60*:2, 1979.
26. Rao, N.S., Ali, M.D., Omar, H.M., et al.: Regional cerebral blood flow in acute stroke. Preliminary experience. Stroke, *5*:8, 1974.
27. Davis, S., Ackerman, R.H., Correia, J.A., et al.: Cerebral blood flow and reactivity in stroke age normal controls. J. Cereb. Blood-flow Metab. (Suppl.), *1*:547, 1981.
28. Ackerman, R.H., Gouliamos, A.D., Grotta, J., et al.: Extracranial vascular disease and cerebral blood flow in patients with TIA. Acta Neurol. Scand. Suppl. 72, *60*:442, 1979.
29. Little, J.R., Yamamoto, L.Y., Feindel, W., et al.: Superficial temporal artery to middle cerebral artery anastamosis: Interpretive evaluation by fluorescein angiography and xenon-133 clearance. J. Neurosurg., *50*:560, 1979.
30. Lazic, L., and Joronik, N.: rCBF patterns in schizophrenic patients. rCBF Bulletin, *3*:43, 1982.
31. Risberg, J., Gagstadius, S., and Gustarson, L.: Blood flow measurements in the study of drug effects. rCBF Bulletin, *3*:56, 1982.
32. Jenson, T.S., Voldby, B., Olivarous, F., et al.: Cerebral hemodynamics in familial migraine. rCBF Bulletin, *4*:71, 1982.
33. Stokely, E.M., Sveinsdottir, E., Lassen, N.A., et

al.: A single photon dynamic computer assisted tomograph (DCAT) for imaging brain function in multiple cross sections. J. Comp. Assist. Tomog., *4*:230, 1980.

34. Kanno, I., and Lassen, N.A.: Two methods for calculating regional cerebral blood flow from emission computed tomography of inert gas concentrations. J. Comput. Assist. Tomogr., *3*:71, 1979.

35. Drayer, B.P., Solfson, S.K., and Boehnke, M.: Physiologic changes in rCBF defined by xenon enhanced CT scanning. Neurol., *16*:220, 1978.

36. Drayer, B.P., Gur, D., Jones, H., et al.: Abnormality of the xenon brain/blood partition coefficient and blood flow in cerebral infarction using transmission CT. Radiology, *135*:349, 1980.

Chapter 19

ULTRASONOGRAPHY—RELATIONS TO NUCLEAR MEDICINE

MARTIN A. WINSTON

PHYSICAL PRINCIPLES

Ultrasound refers to sound frequencies above the audible range (greater than 20 kHz). Diagnostically useful frequencies range from 1 to 5 MHz, although for some applications, frequencies above 10 MHz are used.

Most diagnostic applications involve pulsed ultrasound, which is generated in short bursts, each lasting 1 μsec. In general, these pulses are emitted 1000 times/ sec, so that the device emits only 0.1% of the time and receives returning echoes the remainder of the time. Ultrasound is generated by a piezoelectric transducer made of synthetic crystal, such as lead-zirconate-titanate (PZT). The lattice within a piezoelectric crystal is polarized, so that electrical charges are aligned along the periphery. When the crystal is physically compressed or expanded even slightly, such as by the compactions and rarefactions in sound waves, electrical potential is generated across the surface of the crystal. This conversion of mechanical to electrical energy is termed the *piezoelectric effect* and forms the basis for ultrasound detection.

Conversely, when electrical potential is applied briefly to the crystal surface, rear-rangements in the crystal lattice cause it to contract and re-expand physically. This generates the outgoing pulse of sound and is termed the *reverse piezoelectric effect.* Other elements of the transducer include special backing material, which prevents transmission of the sound beam in the reverse direction and reduces the "ring-down" time of the crystal, thereby increasing *axial resolution.* This term refers to the ability to distinguish two objects aligned within the axis of the sound beam, one slightly distal to the other.

Each crystal has a characteristic resonance frequency, which depends upon its thickness and composition. The crystal both emits and responds to sound, however, in a band centered upon its resonance frequency. The width of this band is defined by its *Q-factor.*

$$Q = f_0/(f_2 - f_1)$$

where f_0 is the resonance frequency, and f_1 and f_2 are frequencies below and above the resonance at which amplitude is reduced by 3 dB. The lower the Q-value of the transducer, the wider the band. A low Q-value is, in fact, desirable, because a wider frequency range can be detected and the ring-down time is shorter. Transducers may also contain lenses located just in front of the crystal that serve, like optical lenses, to focus the beam of sound at a specific depth. Narrow beam width results in improved lateral resolution at focal depth, i.e., improved ability to resolve two objects aligned perpendicularly to the sound beam at the same distance.

The use of curved crystals avoids the need for an external lens and is referred to as *internal focusing.* Instead of a lens, coupling material is placed in front of the transducer to reduce the abrupt change in acoustic impedance between the crystal and the patient's skin. Less sound is reflected at the interface, leaving a stronger beam at depth.

A hemispheric beam of sound actually is generated from many points along the face of the crystal (Fig. 19–1). These points tend to reinforce directly in front of the crystal, thus producing a directional beam (Huygens' principle). The beam is initially as wide as the crystal itself and, in the absence of any focusing, gradually narrows over a distance termed the *near field,* or *Fresnel zone.* The length of the zone is

proportional to both the beam frequency and the diameter of the transducer, D.

Recurring maxima and minima of sound intensity occur within the near field, but the beam does not begin to decay until it transits from the near field into the *far field,* or Fraunhofer zone. At this point, the beam also begins to diverge, and the angle of divergence, θ, is inversely proportional to the beam frequency and crystal diameter. A usual practice is to balance the frequency and crystal diameter to produce optimal beam shape. Narrower transducers are desirable because they are more easily applied to the patient's body, but they require higher frequency than do wider transducers. Higher-frequency transducers, in addition to improved beam shape, have shorter ring-down time and improved sensitivity for small structures. One serious limitation to the application of higher frequencies, however, is attenuation. Aside from reflection, beams are attenuated in tissue by both scatter and absorption, and these effects increase proportionally with beam frequency. Crystals of 5 MHz and higher are generally restricted to the study of such superficial organs as the thyroid and eyes, or they may be used in infants.

INTERACTIONS OF ULTRASOUND IN TISSUE

The most diagnostically useful interaction is *reflection.* Part of the sound beam is reflected at the transition between materials of differing acoustic impedance. Acoustic impedance, Z, is the product of sound velocity in a medium, C, and the density of the medium, ρ:

$$Z = \rho C$$

The amount of incident beam intensity reflected, I_r, at an interface between two materials of impedances Z_2 and Z_1 is given by:

$$\frac{I_r}{I_i} = \left(\frac{Z_2 \cos\theta_i - Z_1 \cos\theta_r}{Z_2 \cos\theta_i + Z_1 \cos\theta_r} \right)^2$$

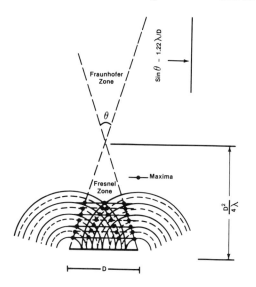

Fig. 19–1. Two waves arising from the transducer surface at two points reinforce each other at points where the waves are in phase (maxima). See text.

where the angles are as shown in Figure 19–2. When the interface is struck perpendicularly, i.e., $\theta_i = \theta_t = 0$, the equation simplifies to:

$$\frac{I_r}{I_i} = \left(\frac{Z_2 - Z_1}{Z_2 + Z_1}\right)^2$$

The intensity of the transmitted beam is:

$$\frac{I_t}{I_i} = \frac{4Z_1Z_2 \cos\theta_i \cos\theta_t}{(Z_2 \cos\theta_i + Z_1 \cos\theta_t)^2}$$

Most soft tissues differ only slightly in acoustic impedance, largely because they differ only slightly in density and inherent sound velocity, so that only a small fraction of the sound beam is reflected (the echo). Sound velocity increases markedly, however, upon transit from soft tissue to bone, resulting in a large reflection at this point. The speed of sound decreases greatly upon transition from soft tissue to air, causing nearly complete reflection of the beam. This process not only blocks further transmission of the beam but can also result in reverberation. This can occur because of the reflected beam striking the transducer and reflecting back to the soft tissue-air interface, a phenomenon that may be repeated several times. A characteristic reverberation artifact in the image is thus created (Fig. 19–3).

When an interface is considerably longer than the wavelength of the sound

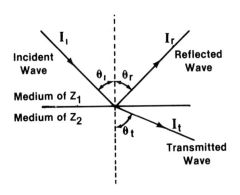

Fig. 19–2. The reflection and transmission of sound waves at the boundary between two media of different acoustic impedance Z.

beam, it acts like a mirror, causing *specular reflection,* in which the angle of reflection equals the angle of incidence. If such an interface is struck at an angle, the echo may be reflected away from the transducer and not be detected. This possibility is a major reason for *compound scanning,* i.e., scanning an organ from multiple angles, which increases the number of interfaces detected. The diaphragm is an example of a specular reflector. Tissue that is irregular, i.e., that has small interfaces relative to the sound wavelength, serves as a scatterer or nonspecular reflector. An example is the liver parenchyma, in which sound is reflected in many directions, so that some reaches the transducer and is recorded, regardless of the angle of incidence.

Another interaction that occurs at tissue interfaces is known as *refraction.* When the interface between tissues of differing acoustic impedance is struck at an angle of less than 90°, the sound transmitted into the next tissue is altered from its original path. Refraction follows Snell's law:

$$\sin\theta_t = \sin\theta_i \cdot \frac{C_2}{C_1}$$

This phenomenon is analogous to the apparent bending of a stick that extends from air under water.

When a specular interface is struck by a sound beam at a sufficiently acute angle, refraction may divert all distal reflections from the detector. This gives rise to a peculiar phenomenon when scanning through cystic structures, referred to as "edge shadowing." Through the center of the cyst, where the sound beam meets the far wall perpendicularly, there is enhanced echo detection beyond the cyst wall. This area is bounded on either side by a narrow band of reduced or absent echo content, where the beam has been reflected laterally from the cyst side wall (Fig. 19–4).

One of ultrasound's great strengths lies in tissue differentiation, particularly be-

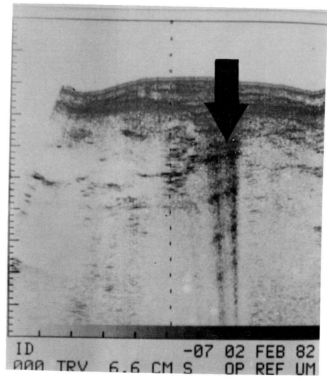

ID   -07 02 FEB 82
ΛΛΛ TRV 6.6 CM S   OP REF UM

Fig. 19–3. Reverberation artifact caused by abdominal gas.

tween fluid and solid structures. In a homogeneous tissue—fluid is the best example—there is no change in acoustic impedance to cause reflections. There are, however, some solid tissues, e.g., lymphomas, that are quite homogeneous and relatively free of internal echoes. The loss of beam intensity due to attenuation occurs much less rapidly in fluid than in solid tissue. Therefore, the beam intensity exiting from the far wall of the cyst is greater than from a solid mass of equal thickness. This so-called "through transmission sign" is felt to be the most reliable discriminator between cystic and solid tissue (Fig. 19–4).

SIGNAL PROCESSING AND DISPLAY

When the transducer is struck by an echo, it generates a voltage potential across its surface that is rectified, amplified, and finally displayed. Because echoes occurring more deeply within the body have undergone more attenuation, they require greater amplification than those from more superficial structures, to preserve uniformity of the image. Depth is determined by the time delay between the pulse and the echo. This progressive amplification is therefore referred to as *time gain compensation* (TGC), or *swept gain*. Much of the art of ultrasonography lies in the setting up of a TGC curve that results in uniform display intensity at all depths. When generating such a curve with digital equipment, the amplification should match the attenuation rate of sound in soft tissue, or approximately 1 db/cm/MHz. The speed of sound in soft tissue ranges from 1450 m/sec in fat to 1600 m/sec in muscle, which averages 1540 m/sec. Equipment is calibrated to convert time to distance, based on this average.[1]

A-Mode

The earliest display mode, still useful for certain applications, is *A-mode,* in

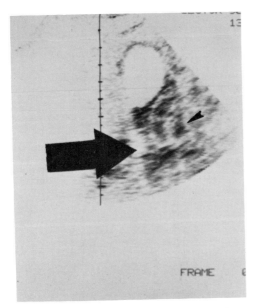

Fig. 19–4. Edge-shadowing artifact (large arrow) caused by refraction of beam from side wall of gallbladder. "Through transmission sign" (small arrowhead) produced by relatively less attenuated beam passing through fluid-filled structure.

which the echo signal is displayed as a vertical deflection from a horizontal baseline (Fig. 19–5). The depth of the echo's origin is represented by its distance from the transducer displayed to the left on the screen. The strength of each echo is represented by the *amplitude* of the vertical deflection—hence, the term A-mode. This mode may be useful in small organs, such as the eye. For example, the characteristic echo pattern of a small tumor may be sufficiently characteristic to identify that tumor with histologic accuracy.

B-Mode

In *B-mode*, or *brightness mode*, echoes are still displayed along the horizontal baseline, but in this case, as dots whose brightness is proportional to echo strength. *M-mode*, or *motion mode*, is a variant of B-mode, useful for studying the motion of oscillating structures, such as the heart and its valves. As a structure

moves toward the transducer, the dot representing its echo moves toward the left along the baseline and, when it moves away from the transducer, the dot moves toward the right. If the baseline is then shifted vertically across the screen, the dot from such a moving object describes a sort of sine-wave pattern. When this is photographed and the photo is rotated 90°, the typical echocardiographic display is shown (Fig. 19–6). This display is created by continuously moving a roll of optically sensitive paper across a light beam, which represents the moving echo pattern.

If the transducer is attached to an articulated arm whose motion and position in space can be recorded by sine-cosine potentiometers in each of three joints, the baseline can be rotated throughout 360° to correspond to the position and angle of the transducer at any given time (Fig. 19–7). Therefore, the dots representing echoes from internal structures can be joined together to form a two-dimensional image (sonogram). Originally, this was recorded on a CRT with retention phosphor or by an open shutter technique, in which the image from a rapidly decaying phosphor was integrated on film as the camera shutter remained open. These resulted in *bistable* images, in which all echoes above a certain intensity were recorded and those below were not. The stronger specular echoes from organ outlines could be recorded, but it was not possible to display at the same time the weaker nonspecular echoes from internal structures. Therefore, much anatomic detail went unrecorded.

Gray-Scale Display

With the advent of gray-scale imaging, the recording of echoes over a wide dynamic range, up to 60 db in many cases, became possible. In this display, ten shades of gray are assigned to various ranges of echo strength, the strongest being 60 dB more than the weakest (Figs. 19–3 and 19–4). Because sound intensities differ widely, their ratios are expressed on a

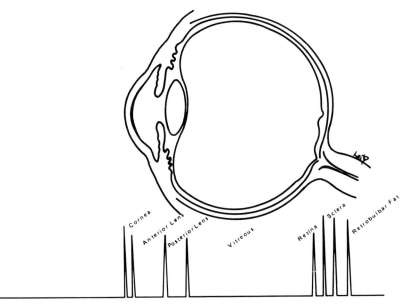

Fig. 19–5. Cross-sectional diagram of the eye with corresponding A-mode display showing signal spikes, which represent ocular structures.

logarithmic scale. The decibel notation employs this scale:

$$dB = 10 \times \log \frac{intensity\ 1}{intensity\ 2}$$

Thus, if the intensity of echo 1 is 1000 times greater than that of echo 2, the log of their ratio is 3 (1000 = 10^3) and dB = 30.

Gray-scale display was first based on the analog scan converter. This is a modified CRT, in which the incoming electron beam is directed, not onto a phosphor screen but onto an array of tiny silicon dioxide capacitors, 10 μm^2 usually arranged in a 1000 × 1000 matrix. These capacitors store the incoming information as positive charges that are then read nondestructively by an electron gun working in tandem with the electron gun on a TV screen, where the information is displayed in a typical TV raster of 512 horizontal lines. The gray level displayed is proportional to the capacitor charge. If an area is overwritten, i.e., scanned over several times, only the strongest echo from that area is retained on the corresponding capacitor; any lesser charge already residing there is displaced. If echoes of lesser strength are returned, the original charge remains undisturbed.

Digital Display

The principal disadvantage of analog scan convertors is instability. To correct this instability, microprocessor chips can be used to provide retention of incoming information in a random access memory (RAM). Depending on the number of bits allotted to each memory location, 16 or 32 gray levels can be assigned to each location of a 512 × 512 matrix. Digital processing allows great flexibility in assigning available gray levels in the display to match signal amplitude. Alterations can be made without disturbing the image in digital memory, e.g., available shades of gray can be expanded or contracted and shifted up or down to differentiate lower strength echoes or to emphasize various features of the image with echoes of greater strength. This is referred to as *post-scan processing*. Conversely, such assignments can also be made prior to performance of the scan *(pre-processing)*.

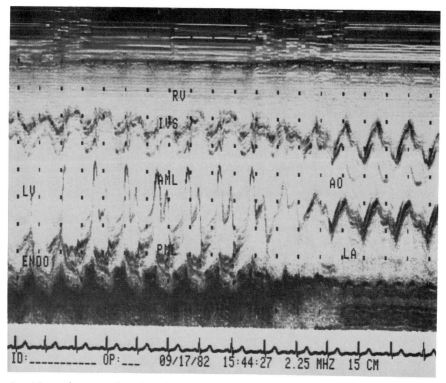

Fig. 19–6. M-mode scan showing the motions of several cardiac structures. The paper was advanced from left to right, so that the right-sided tracings were recorded earlier in time. AV = aortic valve; LA = left atrium; RV = right ventricle; AML = anterior mitral valve leaflet; PML = posterior mitral valve leaflet; LV = left ventricle; IVS = interventricular septum; ENDO = endocardium.

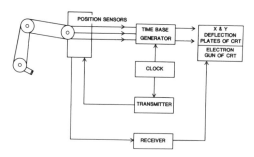

Fig. 19–7. Schematic of compound B-mode scanner.

Real-time Imaging

In *real-time display*, the CRT is refreshed sufficiently often to present a continuously moving field of view. Real-time display is effected using one of three types of transducers: a *linear array* of small transducers, a mechanically *sectored* single transducer, or a *phased array* in which multiple crystals are pulsed in sequence—literally, to steer a beam through a sector arc.

The linear array comprises a line of perhaps 32 crystals, each 5 mm in diameter, that are activated sequentially, typically in groups of four at a time, so that the beam behaves as if it were generated from a single larger crystal (Fig. 19–8). After the first group of crystals (1 through 4) is activated, delay lines allow the beam to travel to the furthest extent of the body and return before activating the next group of four (generally 2 through 5). Although such a system is rugged and relatively inexpensive to produce, it is clumsy in practice, because the large transducer surface cannot be applied in limited areas, such as the intercostal spaces.

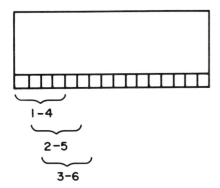

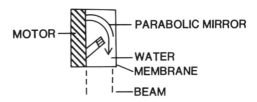

Fig. 19–10. Real-time sector scanner directed toward parabolic mirror. Note parallel beam.

Fig. 19–8. Linear array real-time scanner head. Note sequence of activation of crystals in groups.

PHASED ARRAY

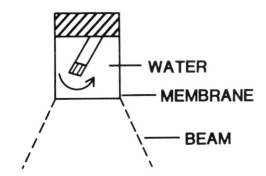

Fig. 19–9. Real-time mechanical sector scanner. Note diverging beam.

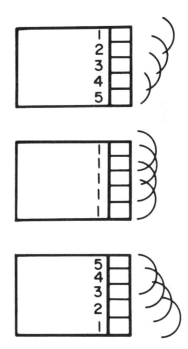

Fig. 19–11. Real-time phased array scanner. Note deviation of beam with changes in activation sequence.

The mechanical sector scanner overcomes this difficulty by permitting use of a much smaller transducer that oscillates within a water bath, which is bounded by a membrane in contact with the body through coupling gel (Fig. 19–9). This scanner may be rotated through an arc of up to 90°. A major disadvantage is that the arc is quite narrow close to the skin surface. Some attempt has been made to overcome this by moving transducers through an arc aimed not at the body but at a parabolic mirror within the water bath (Fig. 19–10). The sound is then reflected from this mirror in a parallel beam. Conversely, the transducer may remain fixed and the mirror may be oscillated. This construction, however, greatly increases the size and clumsiness of the head.

The phased array transducer is another

linear array, composed of very small crystals. A microprocessor controls the sequence of activation, which is continually changed (Fig. 19–11). Each crystal is activated whenever a pulse is emitted, but by changing the sequence, the beam can be steered through a 90° arc without motion of the transducer. If a wider crystal surface is used, lateral resolution is improved over mechanically sectored scanners, and the relatively small transducer is more easily positioned than is the typical linear array. For most clinical applications, however, current mechanical sector scanners provide the best combination of resolution at depth, maneuverability, and versatility.

Doppler Shift Detection

When striking a stationary structure, sound is reflected with the same frequency as when emitted. When reflected from a moving structure, however, with some component of its motion toward or away from the transducer, the echo frequency is shifted upward or downward respectively.

The frequency shift, Δf, depends upon the target velocity, V, and the frequency of the emitted pulse, f.

$$\Delta f \propto \frac{2fV}{c + V}$$

where c is the velocity of ultrasound in tissue. This equation neglects the angle of the transmitted and reflected beam but shows clearly that the Doppler shift is directly proportional to the frequency of ultrasound used. In fact, the Doppler shift is 1.3 Hz per MHz of beam frequency per mm/sec of target velocity.

Earlier instrumentation employed two transducers, one emitting continuously rather than in pulses and the other receiving the reflections. Emitted and returning sounds were compared, and their difference (the shift) became the output to a speaker because the difference was usually in the audible frequency range. More recently, "pulsed" Doppler has been employed so that elapsed time from emission to return can be used to determine the depth of the source of the shift. This, in turn, allows focus on a specific depth. Duplex instruments produce a two-dimensional realtime scan, e.g., of the carotid arteries, while allowing Doppler frequency shift measurements of blood velocity to be made at various points through the cross section of the vessels.

CLINICAL APPLICATIONS

Liver

Within the liver, the overall accuracy of both nuclear and ultrasonic techniques for detecting mass lesions is about equal at approximately 75% (Fig. 19–12).[2,3,4]

Nevertheless, some areas of the liver are inaccessible to ultrasound examination, particularly those obscured by overlying ribs. In any case, covering such a large organ minutely by what is basically a manual technique is technically difficult. In addition, not all solid masses have echo patterns sufficiently different from normal parenchyma to be easily visualized. Therefore, radionuclide scans are preferred to screen the liver for space-occupying disease. When a mass is discovered, ultrasound is useful in determining whether it is cystic or solid and as a guide for thin needle biopsy. With equivocal radionuclide scan patterns, particularly around the porta hepatitis, ultrasound is useful in clarification. Similarly, when lesions are not imaged but suggested clinically, a search of the deep hepatic parenchyma is indicated.

There are fewer signs characteristic of diffuse parenchymal disease in ultrasonography than in nuclear imaging, because the partition of blood flow to the various reticuloendothelial organs cannot be detected. Nevertheless, clues do exist, particularly in chronic hepatocellular diseases, such as cirrhosis or fatty infiltration, which typically cause increased echo density of the hepatic parenchyma. In cirrhosis, both increased reflectivity and attenuation occur, so that in comparison to the liver, the diaphragm and right kidney are less echogenic than usual. In one series of patients with cirrhosis, the sensitivity was 81%, but specificity only 76%.[5]

Spleen

The spleen is technically difficult to image by ultrasound because of overlying ribs. With real-time sector scanning trans-

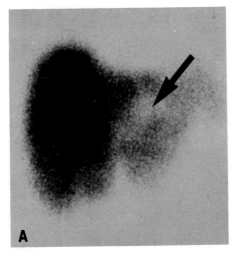
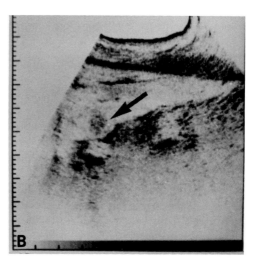

Fig. 19–12. *A.* Liver scan shows a defect (arrow) in the left lobe. *B.* This is confirmed as a solid mass on sonogram. Illustration is of longitudinal section several centimeters to the left of midline. Patient's head is toward the left. Focally increased echogenicity of the mass is seen deep in the left hepatic lobe (arrow).

ducers, the intercostal spaces can be used as windows to much of the organ. Nevertheless, nuclear scanning is more sensitive to trauma, infarction, and the presence of accessory spleens.

Pancreas

Computed tomography and ultrasonography have essentially replaced radionuclide scanning of the pancreas, at least until better tracers become available. As in all areas of the body, an air-free pathway must be found for transmission of sound from the skin to the organ of interest. Often, the left lobe of the liver serves this function; when it does not, filling the stomach with a fat solution such as Lipomul frequently proves satisfactory. Having the patient seated in a semi-erect position is also helpful.

Detection of pancreatic disease depends upon alterations in size, shape, and echo texture. Quantification of echo strength is still quite primitive, and the liver has been used as a standard of comparison. Normal pancreas is at least as echogenic as the liver at the same depth, and usually, slightly more so. Inflammation results in edema, which reduces the internal echogenicity and increases organ size (Fig. 19–13).

Other clues to the presence of disease are dense echoes, which suggest the presence of calcification. With modern equipment, it is often possible to visualize the pancreatic duct, which appears as a thin

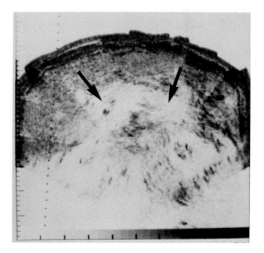

Fig. 19–13. Transverse sonogram shows enlarged, echolucent pancreas (arrows), which suggests pancreatitis.

line or small channel with an internal diameter less than 2 mm.[6] Larger diameters indicate pancreatic ductal dilatation and suggest inflammatory or malignant disease.

Biliary System

A good example of the complementary nature of nuclear and ultrasonic techniques is provided by biliary tract disease. Often, both anatomic and functional information are required to make a firm diagnosis. Ultrasonography is unsurpassed in detecting biliary calculi. Gallstones are recognized both by their sonic density, which results in distal shadowing and by their movement when the patient's position is changed (Fig. 19–14). One or both of these signs should be present before a stone is identified. Otherwise, the true diagnosis may be polyp or tumor of the gallbladder wall.

Ultrasonography is less useful, however, in determining whether stones are responsible for active disease. Rather, biliary scanning should be relied upon to detect patency of the cystic duct. Furthermore, cases of acalculous cholecystitis occur, in which the biliary scan shows cystic duct obstruction despite a normal ultrasonic study. Ultrasonic signs of gallbladder inflammation include thickening of the gallbladder wall, a nonspecific sign also found in the presence of chronic cholecystitis or ascites, or following contraction due to a meal. Occasionally, edema is seen in the tissues surrounding the gallbladder.[7]

Ultrasonography is quite sensitive in detecting biliary tract obstruction because it permits direct visualization and measurement of the extrahepatic biliary ducts (Fig. 19–15).[8] Ductal dilatation usually follows quite promptly the development of obstruction, although it may not occur for one or two days. On the other hand, dilatation often persists long after relief of obstruction; a functional study is then required to assess the meaning of this finding. Obstruction high in the porta hepatis can cause dilatation of small intrahepatic biliary ducts without involving the common duct or gallbladder.

Urinary Tract

Renal ultrasonography provides anatomic information independently of function and is therefore useful in renal failure in determining the size and shape of the kidneys, the presence of hydronephrosis, and the consistency of mass lesions. Statistically, cystic masses, particularly those with smooth walls and no internal echogenic foci, are likely to be benign cysts, and solid masses are likely to prove malignant (Fig. 19–16). Hydronephrosis and polycystic disease are detected even in the absence of renal function. Inflammatory processes and renal vein thrombosis may cause enlargement and reduced echogenicity of the renal parenchyma.[9]

Recent developments with high-resolution real-time scanning enable such structures as the renal pyramids, and occasionally the arcuate arteries, to be identified. In cases of renal transplants, these landmarks can be used to check for rejection; swelling of the renal pyramids is one of its earliest signs.[10] Later signs include increased echogenicity in the cortical zone, and finally, loss of demarcation between the cortex and collecting system.

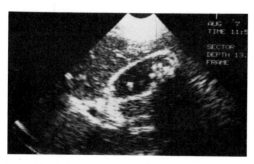

Fig. 19–14. Sector scan of gallbladder showing several small gallstones. Note the distal shadowing caused by the highly echogenic gallstones.

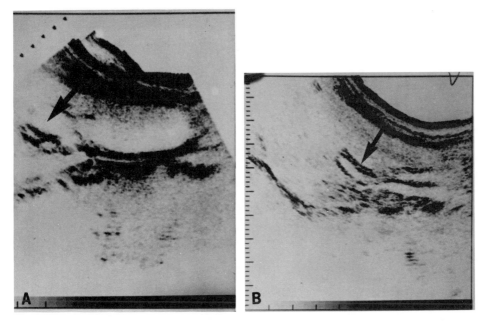

Fig. 19–15. *A.* Dilated extrahepatic bile duct is seen in this longitudinal section several centimeters to the right of midline. Duct is indicated by arrow, immediately anterior to the portal vein and cranial to the gallbladder. *B.* For comparison, a normal common duct.

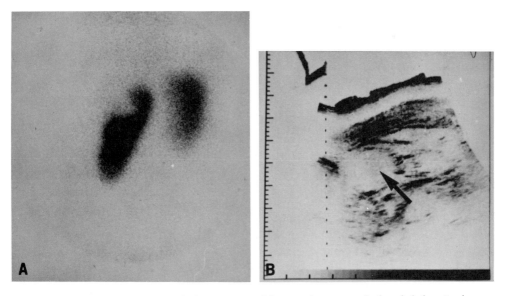

Fig. 19–16. *A.* Renal scintiscan, left posterior oblique view, reveals focal defect in the upper pole of left kidney. *B.* Longitudinal sonogram of the kidney shows the corresponding mass (arrow), which is solid in consistency despite relatively homogeneous internal structure that yields few internal echoes. Biopsy revealed metastasis.

Adrenal Glands

The adrenal glands can be recognized ultrasonically, but with some difficulty. In most series, CT provides the most accurate diagnosis.[11] Certain uncommon tumors, such as myelolipoma, are more easily recognized ultrasonically because of the densely echogenic appearance characteristic of fat in this particular lesion. In the newborn, in whom the adrenals are relatively large and hematomas common, ultrasonography is particularly effective.[12]

Bladder and Prostate

When the bladder is distended with fluid, mass lesions protruding into the lumen can be visualized. Recently, small transducers inserted through the urethra into the bladder have been introduced.[13] The prostate can be visualized through the filled bladder, or in more detail, transrectally. A rotating transducer encased in a water-filled balloon is inserted into the rectum and close inspection of the prostatic echo pattern often helps to distinguish between benign enlargement and malignant transformation.[14,15] The posterior pelvic compartment is well-demonstrated when both rectosigmoid colon and bladder are filled with fluid.[16]

Testes

Ultrasonography is most useful in demonstrating whether a palpable mass is intratesticular or extratesticular in origin, and in identifying intratesticular hematoma or extravasation of blood into the tunica albuginea.[17] Testicular torsion causes increased lucency within the testicular parenchymal echo pattern, probably because of swelling. In epididymitis, the testicular pattern remains unchanged, but frequently there is swelling of the epididymis.[18] Nevertheless, nuclear perfusion studies remain the definitive means of differentiating these two entities.

Thyroid

Ultrasonography is used in determining whether palpable thyroid masses are cystic or solid (Fig. 19–17). If a mass is found to be functional by radionuclide scanning, ultrasonography is not needed. If the mass is nonfunctional (cold), however, ultrasonography is recommended, because approximately 10% of cold nodules are cystic and require quite different management. Distinction must be made, however, between a wholly cystic nodule and a solid nodule in which a focus of cystic degeneration has occurred. No reliable ultrasonic criteria for the further differentiation of solid masses have yet been defined. Thin-needle aspiration of palpable nodules under ultrasonic guidance is used increasingly in this instance.[19] Inflammation of the thyroid gland, as with other tissues, changes the echo pattern of the parenchyma, making it more lucent. This phenomenon is seen, for example, in subacute thyroiditis. Changes in the overall size of the gland can be followed without repetitive nuclear scanning.

Parathyroid Gland

The thyroid provides a window to the parathyroid glands. When normal in size, they usually cannot be distinguished from tissue background. Enlargement in excess of 5 to 6 mm can be distinguished, and this includes between 50 and 70% of parathyroid adenomas. The parathyroids are identified by their typical location behind the thyroid lobe, immediately anterior to the prevertebral musculature.[20] Because they are located posterior to the lateral surface of the trachea, oblique scanning avoids the tracheal air shadow.

Central Nervous System

The earliest medical application of ultrasonography was A-mode scanning to detect midline shift from echoes generated in the area of the third ventricle. Echoencephalography has been largely supplanted by CT scanning. In adults, the calvarium prevents adequate two-dimensional ultrasonic visualization of the

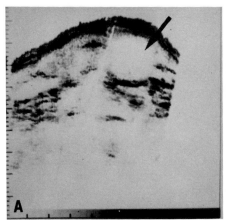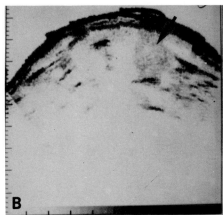

Fig. 19–17. *A.* Transverse sonogram of the thyroid reveals a large cystic mass in the left lobe (arrow). *B.* Thyroid adenoma (arrow) is shown for comparison.

brain. In the newborn and infant, however, the fontanels provide windows to the brain.[21] A sector scanner is well suited to imaging structures through a narrow aperture. Coronal and sagittal scans through the anterior fontanel identify much of the cerebral anatomy and are now widely applied in premature infants to identify intracerebral and intraventricular hemorrhage. Fresh hemorrhage produces echogenic material, within either the ventricle or the adjacent thalamus, and can be identified while the infant remains within its isolette.

Vascular System

Aortic aneurysms have long been imaged by ordinary B-scanning. Although occasionally obscured by overlying bowel gas, accurate measurement can generally be made of wall-to-wall distance independent of thrombus, which may shrink the lumen and thereby cause underestimation of aneurysm size by contrast studies or radionuclide perfusion scans.

Recently, the carotid bifurcation has been studied by high-resolution real-time scanners and gated Doppler ultrasound. The two-dimensional images detect hard plaques, particularly when there is some calcification.[22] They often miss so-called soft plaques or ulcerations, however, and most importantly, fail to identify the hemodynamic significance of any irregularities that are seen. The use of Doppler ultrasound, particularly when it is *range-gated* as previously described, is sensitive to hemodynamic disturbance. Normally, blood velocity is higher in the center of a vessel than near the wall. This variation is reflected by a change in the frequency of Doppler signals received from the vessel, but the range is normally rather narrow. Blood passing through a stenotic segment increases in velocity, which in turn increases the peak Doppler signal. The stenosis also results in a wider range of blood velocities; this occurrence is reflected in a broadened frequency range within the Doppler shift signal.[23] High-frequency real-time ultrasonography is also useful in evaluating stenotic, inflammatory, thrombotic, and aneurysmal complications of arterial grafts.[24]

Obstetrics and Gynecology

Much has been learned about intrauterine growth and development of the fetus through the application of two dimensional ultrasonic imaging. Growth curves have been described for the gestational sac and fetal crown-rump length during the first trimester, and fetal body parts during the last two trimesters.[25] Measurement of the biparietal diameter is used to gage intrauterine development, but measurement of fetal abdominal circumference best correlates with fetal weight.[26] Calculation of total intrauterine volume, including fetus, amniotic fluid, and placenta, is useful in certain forms of intrauterine growth retardation, in which the head continues to grow normally despite failure of the remainder of fetal growth.

Fetal malformations, including spina bifida, renal agenesis, bowel obstruction or reduplication, and hydrocephalus, are detected by the early second trimester. Gastroschisis, omphalocele, and meningomyelocele are detected as protrusions into the amniotic fluid space. Ascitic fluid within the fetal abdomen helps confirm the diagnosis of cytomegalovirus disease or erythroblastosis fetalis. Ultrasound is the best guide for amniotic fluid aspiration. In cases of multiple pregnancies, fluid can be aspirated from each fetal sac separately.

Ultrasonography has essentially replaced radionuclide scanning of the placenta. Placental localization and detection of intraplacental hematoma as a sign of placental abruption are widely used.[27]

Pelvic anatomy is visualized through the fluid-filled bladder in both sexes. Consistency and location of uterine and ovarian masses can be characterized. Cystic masses within the ovary do not have the benign significance attached to them elsewhere in the body, particularly in postmenopausal women. Adnexal cysts must be searched carefully for small amounts of solid tissue that suggest malignant foci. Cystic masses within the uterine musculature usually indicate necrotic fibromata.

Fluid in the cul-de-sac is associated with ruptured cyst, endometriosis, pelvic inflammatory disease, or ectopic pregnancy. The distinctions among these entities are not easily perceived through echographic criteria alone; in most instances, culdocentesis or culdoscopy is necessary.

Infection

Overall, ultrasonography, gallium scanning, and CT scanning each have about 75% reliability in detecting sites of abdominal and pelvic infection.[28] Nevertheless, some distinctions should be recognized. Ultrasonography can detect only frank abscess formation. Inflammation (phlegmon) alone cannot be detected with this method. Gallium localizes both types of inflammation but cannot distinguish between the two, so that the need for surgical drainage cannot be established solely by this test. The normal uptake of gallium by the liver makes detection of infection in the right upper quadrant difficult. The very presence of the liver as an acoustic window makes ultrasonic examination of this area quite easy (Fig. 19–18). Also, this method is probably superior in the pelvis when the bladder can be adequately filled. All three methods are more nearly equal in effectiveness in the midabdomen.

Invasive Procedures

Considerable experience has now been accumulated, particularly in Europe, in the use of ultrasound-guided thin-needle aspiration biopsy of various structures.[29] Biopsy transducers have been adapted to both B-mode and real-time scanners to guide placement of the needle. Special devices are now available to visualize exact alignment of the needle and give required depth, which greatly reduces the need for open biopsies (Fig. 19–19). Echography is an excellent guide for placing nephrostomy tubes, since this method does not depend on renal function.[30]

Breast

Dedicated breast scanning units incorporate a water bath in which the breast is suspended, highly focused transducers, and automated acquisition and sequential display of scan slices.[31,32] Besides the lack of ionizing radiation, this scanning method appears to have other definite ad-

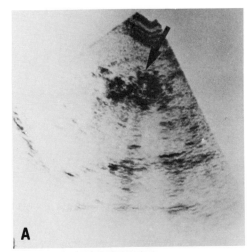

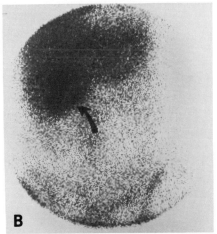

Fig. 19–18. *A.* Echogram reveals increased echogenicity within an abscess near the inferior margin of the liver. Although usually cystic in appearance, these abscesses occasionally show enhanced echogenicity with distal sonic shadowing, probably because of the presence of bacterially produced gas bubbles. *B.* Gallium-67 citrate scan.

vantages over mammography in young women with dense fibrous dysplastic breasts, in whom the x-ray pattern is frequently nondiagnostic. In older women with fatty replacement, x-ray remains a better screening technique, primarily because of its sensitivity for detecting microcalcifications.

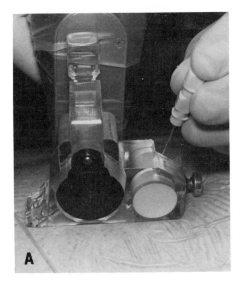

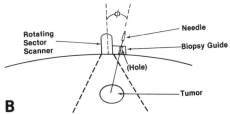

Fig. 19–19. Photograph (*A*) and schematic representation (*B*) of biopsy guide attached to a real-time transducer of the rotating sector scanner. As the needle is advanced, reflections determine the precise path of the needle. (Photo courtesy of Civco Medical Instrument Company, Inc.)

Eye

Echo-ophthalmology is most useful in studying the posterior globe when visualization by ophthalmoscopy is blocked by opaque lens or vitreous. Foreign bodies, retinal detachments, and tumors are well visualized. If the anterior chamber is to be studied, a water bath must be constructed between transducer and eye; otherwise, direct contact through the lid is adequate for most purposes.

Because of the change in velocity—and therefore refraction—of the sound beam as it enters and exits the lens, this structure is best avoided when studying the globe and orbit. During measurement of the axial length of the globe, the lens must be traversed, but the increase in sound velocity due to the greater density of this structure must be taken into account. Using the preset machine calibration of 1540 m/sec, rather than the actual 1641 m/sec, would result in underestimation of length.

Echocardiography

All of the heart valves can be evaluated by M-mode scanning. Recent developments of two-dimensional echocardiography have permitted improved orientation of these valvular structures and more extensive visualization of wall motion and chamber contents.

Ultrasonography is the best noninvasive means of investigating pericardial effusion, atrial myxoma, mural thrombi, and both global and asymmetric muscular hypertrophy. Regional thickening of the systolic wall can be used as an index of coronary disease.

The presence of abnormal interchamber connections can only be inferred from the size and motion of the heart chambers. Radionuclide flow studies reveal these abnormalities more directly. Evaluation of global ventricular function, particularly with exercise intervention, is better performed with radionuclide methods, although the use of ultrasonography is being actively investigated.[33,34,35]

REFERENCES

1. Dewey, G.B., and Wells, P.N.T.: Ultrasound in medical diagnosis. Sci. Am., *238*:98, 1978.
2. Bryan, P.J.: Correlation of computed tomography, gray scale ultrasound and radionuclide imaging of the liver in detecting space occupying processes. Radiology, *124*:387, 1977.
3. Taylor, K.J.W., Sullivan, D., Rosenfield, A.T., et al.: Gray scale ultrasound and isotope scanning: complementary techniques for imaging the liver. Am. J. Roentgenol., *128*:277, 1977.
4. Smith, T.J., Kemeny, M.M., Sugarbaker, P.H., et al.: A prospective study of hepatic imaging in the detection of metastatic disease. Ann. Surg., *195*:486, 1982.
5. Gosink, B.B., Lemon, S.K., Scheible, W., et al.: Accuracy of ultrasonography in diagnosis of he-

patocellular disease. Am. J. Roentgenol., *133*:19, 1979.
6. Ohto, M., Saotome, N. Saisho, H., et al.: Real time sonography of the pancreatic duct: application to percutaneous pancreatic ductography. Am. J. Roentgenol., *134*:647, 1980.
7. Finberg, H.J., and Birnholz, J.C.: Ultrasound evaluation of the gallbladder wall. Radiol., *133*:693, 1979.
8. Taylor, K.H., Rosenfield, A.T., and DeGraaff, C.S.: Anatomy and pathology of the biliary tree as demonstrated by ultrasound. Clin. Diagn. Ultrasound, *1*:103, 1979.
9. Rosenfield, A.T., Zeman, R.K., Cronan, J.J., et al.: Ultrasound in experimental renal vein thrombosis. Radiology, *137*:735, 1980.
10. Maklad, N.F., Wright, C.H., and Rosenthal, S.J.: Gray scale ultrasonic appearance of renal transplant rejection. Radiology, *131*:711, 1979.
11. Sample, W.F., and Sarti, D.A.: Computed tomography and gray scale ultrasonography of the adrenal gland: a comparative study. Radiology, *128*:377, 1978.
12. Mittelslaedt, C.A., Volberg, F.M., Merten, D.F., et al.: The sonographic diagnosis of neonatal adrenal hemorrhage. Radiology, *131*:453, 1979.
13. Nakamura, S., and Niijima, T.: Staging of bladder cancer by ultrasonography: a new technique by trans-urethral intravesical scanning. J. Urol., *124*:341, 1980.
14. Harado, K. Igari, D., and Tanahashi, Y.: Gray scale transrectal ultrasonography of the prostate. J. Clin. Ultrasound, *7*:45, 1979.
15. Greenberg, M., Neiman, H.L., Brandt, T.D., et al.: Ultrasound of the prostate. Radiology, *141*:757, 1981.
16. Kurtz, A.B., Rubin, C.S., Kramer, F.L., et al.: Ultrasound evaluation of the posterior pelvic compartment. Radiology, *132*:677, 1979.
17. Albert, N.E.: Testicular ultrasound for trauma. J. Urol., *124*:558, 1980.
18. Winston, M.A., Handler, S.J., and Pritchard, J.H.: Ultrasonography of the testis—correlation with radiotracer perfusion. J. Nucl. Med., *19*:615, 1978.
19. Van Herle, A.J., (moderator): The Thyroid Nodule (UCLA Conference). Ann. Int. Med., *96*:221, 1982.
20. Edis, A.J., and Evans, T.C.: High resolution, real-time ultrasonography in the preoperative location of parathyroid tumors. N. Engl. J. Med., *301*:532, 1979.
21. Dewbury, K.C., and Alwihare, A.P.: The anterior fontanelle as an ultrasound window for study of the brain: a preliminary report. Br. J. Radiol., *53*:81, 1980.
22. Cooperberg, P.L., Robertson, W.D., and Sweeney, V.: High resolution real time ultrasound of the carotid bifurcation. J. Clin. Ultrasound, *7*:13, 1979.
23. Crummy, A.B., Zwiebel, W.J., Barriga, P., et al.: Doppler evaluation of extracranial cerebrovascular disease. Am. J. Roentgenol., *132*:91, 1979.
24. Scheible, W., Skram, C., and Leopold, G.R.: High resolution real-time sonography of hemodialysis

vascular access complications. Am. J. Roentgenol., *134*:1173, 1980.

25. Green, B.: Pelvic ultrasonography. Med. Ultrasound, *4*:62, 1980.

26. Campbell, S., and Wilkin, D.: Ultrasonic measurement of the fetal abdomen circumference in the estimation of fetal weight. Br. J. Obstet. Gynaecol., *82*:689, 1975.

27. Jaffe, M.H., Schoen, W.C., Silver, T.M., et al.: Sonography of abruptio placentae. Am. J. Roentgenol., *137*:1049, 1981.

28. McNeil, B.J., Sanders, R. Alderson, P.O., et al.: A prospective study of computed tomography, ultrasound, and gallium imaging in patients with fever. Radiology, *139*:647, 1981.

29. Smith, E.H., Bartrum, R.J., Chang, Y.C., et al.: Percutaneous aspiration biopsy of the pancreas under ultrasonic guidance. N. Engl. J. Med., *292*:825, 1975.

30. Pedersen, J.R., Cowan, D.F., Kristensen, J.R., et al.: Ultrasonically guided percutaneous nephrostomy. Radiology, *119*:429, 1976.

31. Kobayashi, T.: Diagnostic ultrasound in breast cancer: analysis of retrotumorous echo patterns correlated with sonic attenuation by cancerous connective tissue. J. Clin. Ultrasound, *7*:471, 1979.

32. Maturao, V.G., Zusmer, N.R., Gilson, A.J., et al.: Ultrasound of the whole breast using a dedicated automatic breast scanner. Radiology, *137*:457, 1980.

33. Popp, R.L., Rubenson, D.S., Tucker, C.R., et al.: Echocardiography: M-mode and two-dimensional methods. Ann. Int. Med., *93*:844, 1980.

34. Quinones, M.A., Waggoner, A.D., Reduto, L.A., et al.: A new simplified and accurate method for determining ejection fraction with two-dimensional echocardiography. Circulation, *64*:744, 1981.

35. Parisi, A.F., Moynihan, P.F., and Folland, E.D.: Echocardiographic evaluation of left ventricular function. Med. Clin. North Am., *64*:61, 1980.

Chapter 20

COMPUTED TOMOGRAPHY— RELATIONS TO NUCLEAR MEDICINE

STUART G. MIRELL

Rarely has a technologic innovation received such rapid and widespread acceptance in medicine as has computed tomography (CT). Although the CT scanner is basically a highly sophisticated radiologic instrument, its impact has been so enormous in all diagnostic disciplines, including nuclear medicine, that its study is warranted here.

Various tomographic techniques have long been available in diagnostic radiography. Until the advent of CT scanners, however, these techniques were confined to focusing on a selected plane of interest and blurring the underlying and overlying regions. Subtle density variations on the plane in focus were obscured by superimposed structures and scattered radiation. Conventional radiographic tomography cannot adequately differentiate soft tissues. Consequently, much vital information is lost.

CT overcomes this deficiency by directing a highly collimated x-ray beam through the edge of an axial cross-sectional slice of the patient. The transmitted beam is intercepted and measured on the opposite side by one or more detectors. Several hundred thousand such measurements might be taken in the course of ac-

quiring data for a single cross-sectional view. Each measurement is made with the beam traversing the cross section at a unique angle and position. A computer then reconstructs a tomographic image from the transmission data.[1,2,3]

The principle of reconstructing tomographic images from a set of transmission measurements was described by Oldendorf in 1961.[4] Applying the same general principle, Hounsfield independently developed a clinically functional system at the Central Research Laboratories of EMI Limited.[5] Clinical studies were first presented in April of 1972.[6,7] The subsequent acceptance and commercial development was rapid; thousands of CT scanners are now in use.

PHYSICAL PRINCIPLES OF ATTENUATION

The attenuation of a beam of photons incident on an absorber of thickness Δx is described by the following exponential equation:

$$I = I_0 e^{-\mu \Delta x}$$

where I_0 and I are the incident and transmitted intensities respectively. The quantity μ is the linear attenuation coefficient, which depends upon the photon energy and the physical properties of the absorber.

The x-ray tube of CT scanners generally operates at 150 kV(p) or less. Photons in the primary energy range of the resultant polychromatic spectrum are attenuated by Compton scattering and, to a lesser extent, by photoelectric absorption. Compton scattering depends linearly upon the electron density, which is proportional to $\rho(Z/A)_{eff}$. Here ρ is the mass density (gm/cm^3) and $(Z/A)_{eff}$ is the effective ratio of atomic number and atomic weight for the constituent atoms of the target substance. Since most biologically prevalent atoms contain equal numbers of protons and neutrons (e.g., $^{12}_{6}C$, $^{16}_{8}O$, and $^{14}_{7}N$), their contribution to the effective ratio of Z (proton number) to A (mass number) is nearly a constant 0.5. As a result, the Compton scattering is essentially proportional to the mass density. The principal departure from this ratio arises from variations in the hydrogen content which, with its single proton structure, contributes 1.0 to the effective Z to A ratio. For example, $(Z/A)_{eff}$ for H_2O is $(1/1 + 1/1 + 8/16)/3 = 0.83$.

Photoelectric absorption has a much smaller effect on the attenuation coeffi-cient since Compton scattering predominates at energies above 30 keV for most tissues. Nevertheless, because photoelectric absorption is proportional to the effective value of Z^3, it depends strongly on the presence of relatively light (hydrogen) or heavy (calcium, iodine, iron) elements.

The linear attenuation coefficient μ for a specific photon energy spectrum is then the sum of the Compton scattering and photoelectric absorption linear attenuation coefficients:

$$\mu = \mu_c + \mu_p$$

with μ_c proportional to the electron density and the numerically smaller μ_p proportional to the effective value of Z^3 for the constituent atoms.

Gross variations in tissue density are reflected by nearly proportional variations in the associated value of μ. Referring to attenuation as directly dependent on the physical mass density is not entirely accurate, however, because of the effects noted previously.

The intravenous injection of iodinated contrast material in CT procedures provides a substantial enhancement between tissues taking up the contrast material and those not taking it up.[8,9,10,11] This enhancement is well out of proportion to the mi-

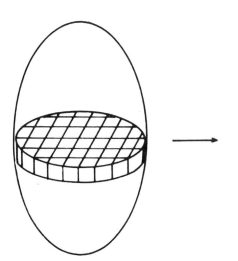
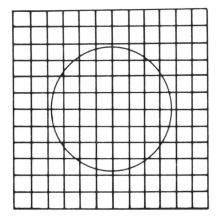

Fig. 20–1.   The computer matrix (at right) and the corresponding cells in the subject.

nute increase in physical mass density and is largely caused by strong photoelectric absorption in the presence of the high Z (53) iodine atoms.

MEASURING LINEAR ATTENUATION COEFFICIENTS

The image acquired by a CT scanner is a point-by-point representation of the x-ray attenuation in a cross-sectional slice of tissue. The scanner's computer divides the field of view into a grid, or matrix, of uniform cells, each of dimension ΔX by ΔX, as illustrated in Figure 20–1.

Each cell is actually a small rectangular volume, since the imaging process views a finite thickness of tissue at a given cross-sectional level. A narrow beam of x-rays penetrating the edge of a cross-sectional slice on one side and exiting on the edge of the other side traverses an entire row of cells, as illustrated in Figure 20–2. The x-ray beam of initial intensity I_0 is attenuated by the tissue in this row of cells.

The attenuation produced by a partic-

ular cell in the ith row and jth column is physically expressed by the associated linear attenuation coefficient μ_{ij} for that cell. In Figure 20–2 the x-ray intensity remaining after the first cell is traversed is given by $I_0 e^{-\mu_{41}\Delta x}$. After passing through the second cell, the intensity is further reduced to:

$$(I_0 e^{-\mu_{41}\Delta x}) e^{-\mu_{42}\Delta x}$$

and to:

$$((I_0 e^{-\mu_{41}\Delta x}) e^{-\mu_{42}\Delta x}) e^{-\mu_{43}\Delta x}$$

upon exiting the third cell. Mathematically, the beam intensity transmitted through the entire fourth row of cells may be expressed as:

$$I = I_0 e^{-(\mu_{41} + \mu_{42} + \mu_{43} + \ldots)\Delta x}$$
$$= I_0 e^{-\Sigma \mu \cdot \Delta x}$$

where the symbol $\Sigma\mu$ indicates the sum of μ_{ij} values in the cells through which the beam passes. I is the quantity actually

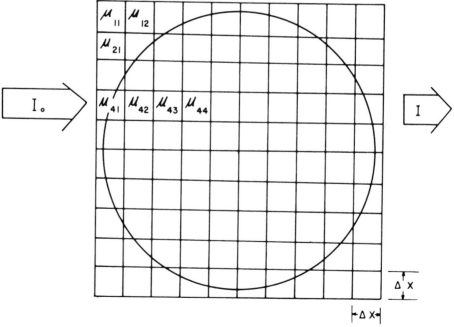

Fig. 20–2. X-ray beam traversing a row of cells.

measured by the scanner's detector. The ratio I/I_0 is called the *transmittance*, T. Thus $T = e^{-\Sigma\mu\cdot\Delta x}$. The value of T physically represents the fraction of the incident beam transmitted through the patient. After electronically generating the ratio T, a logarithmic value is computed:

$$\ln T = \ln e^{-\Sigma\mu\cdot\Delta x}$$
$$= -\Sigma\mu\cdot\Delta x$$

This processed signal for a single measurement is now proportional to the sum of the linear attenuation coefficients since $-\Delta x$ is a constant. For a beam traversing the fourth row, the processed signal would provide the following value:

$$\Sigma\mu = \mu_{41} + \mu_{42} + \mu_{43}\ldots.$$

A beam traversing the matrix at an oblique angle intersects fractional cells. Appropriate numeric factors are introduced by the computer to weigh the attenuation contribution of each intersected cell properly. For example, the processed detector signal arising from a beam oriented as in Figure 20–3 might provide the following value:

$$\Sigma\mu = 0.83\mu_{13} + 0.50\mu_{12} + 0.09\mu_{23}$$
$$+ 0.83\mu_{22} + 0.09\mu_{14} + 0.09\mu_{32}$$
$$+ 0.50\mu_{21} + 0.09\mu_{41} + 0.83\mu_{31}$$

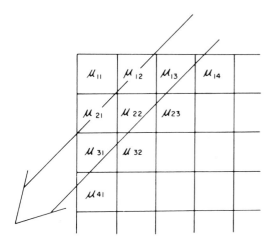

Fig. 20–3. X-ray beam traversing a matrix of cells at an oblique angle.

In either case, the numeric value of $\Sigma\mu$ is derived from the processed detector signal. Individual μ_{ij} values cannot be ascertained, however, from the single signal reading. Each such processed signal reading provides an equation with a numeric value appearing on the left and the appropriately weighted unknown μ_{ij} linear attenuation coefficients appearing on the right. For a single cross-sectional image, the scanning mechanism might acquire as many as several hundred thousand such readings (equations) to provide the computer with sufficient information to determine all individual μ_{ij} values. These readings are taken with the beam in a large number of different angular orientations, to interrelate all of the μ_{ij} linear attenuation coefficients.

RECONSTRUCTION ALGORITHMS

Operation of the mathematical reconstruction algorithm in deriving the μ_{ij} matrix values is most easily demonstrated by studying the profile projections.

A series of associated readings all taken with the beam traversing the patient at a given angle but at successively displaced positions constitutes a profile projection. Such a set of readings might be acquired by translating the x-ray tube in a linear motion as illustrated in Figure 20–4a. In practice, frequent sampling of the x-ray transmission might produce a profile consisting of several hundred separate readings per scan sweep. Each profile is the representation of attenuation readings on a series of adjacent narrow strips of tissue.

A small area of relatively diminished transmission, which appears on a single profile (Fig. 20–4a), merely indicates the presence of a region(s) of higher relative density somewhere along the corresponding strip. Taken by itself, the profile cannot establish the location of the attenuating region on the strip. The conventional radiologic solution is to take an additional view at a different angle. A similar ap-

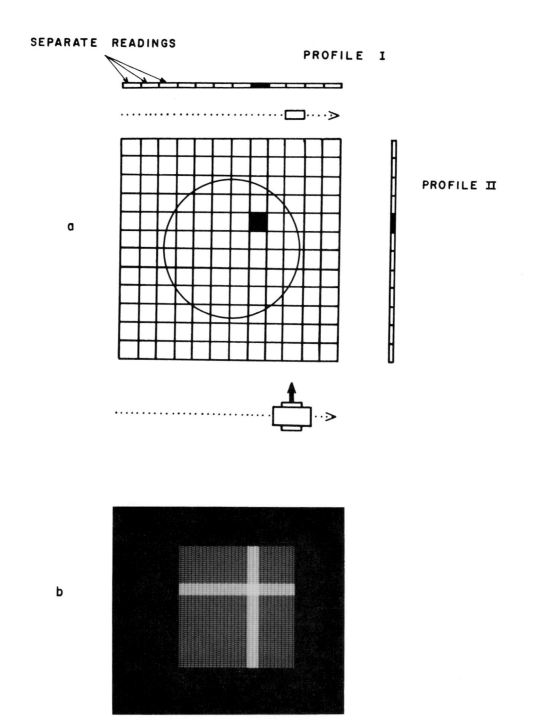

Fig. 20–4. Data acquisition and display: *a*, Linear sweep of x-ray tube and detector (dotted arrows); *b*, Back projection of the two profiles on a video screen.

proach is applied in CT scanning. Profile II taken 90° from profile I localizes the attenuating region. When back projected on a display screen, the attenuation spot appears, in the form of intermediate intensity bands. The intersection of these bands localizes the attenuating region on the display screen. This two-profile back projection is a simplification of the actual computer processing, but nevertheless illustrates the basic principle of the image reconstruction.

The high levels of density discrimination and spatial resolution of CT scanners require acquisition of many profiles taken in succession at small incremental angular positions as the x-ray tube rotates about the subject. The unsophisticated back-projection technique localizes the attenuating region on the display screen correctly but also introduces artifactual bands.

An image reconstruction algorithm based upon Fourier analysis is often utilized to remove the back-projection artifacts. A single attenuation spot on a given profile (Fig. 20–5a) is localized graphically as in Figure 20–5b. The algorithm represents this profile as a series of positive and negative components, as shown in Figure 20–5c. The principal effect upon the back-projected profile after the algorithm has been applied is the introduction of a negative band on either side of the intensified band. When the algorithm is applied to intersecting bands from two profiles, as in Figure 20–4a, the adjacent negative bands partially cancel the opposing artifactual bands but leave the region of their intersection intact, as illustrated in Figure 20–6A. The algorithm has in effect caused the artifactual bands to retreat from the region of true high density. By acquiring additional profiles at incremental angles about the subject and applying the algorithm, the true high-density region is further isolated (Fig. 20–6B), until ultimately, with sufficient profiles, the artifacts are effectively suppressed (Fig. 20–6C).

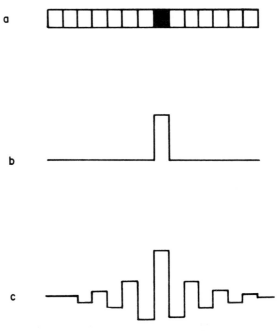

Fig. 20–5. Principle of Fourier algorithm: *a*, Original readings of a single profile; *b*, Graphic representation; *c*, Graphic representation after Fourier transformation.

Computation time for each image in CT computers employing Fourier analysis or related algorithms ranges from several seconds to several minutes.

Various alternative algorithms have been proposed and investigated. Perhaps the most obvious is the direct algebraic solution of the unknown μ_{ij} in the set of equations derived from the detector readings. In theory, a given number of unknowns can be solved from an equivalent number of independent equations. On a 200×200 matrix, however, this number would be 40,000. Even with a large computer, the time required for the direct algebraic solution of such a large set of equations is prohibitively long. The algebraic solution and related algorithms require the acquisition of all data before processing can begin, whereas the Fourier (and related filtered back-projection) algorithms permit processing of each profile as it is acquired during scanning.

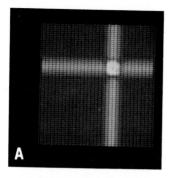

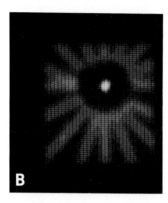

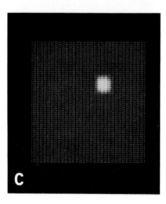

Fig. 20–6. Effect of increasing number of profiles in back projection following application of the Fourier-based algorithm: *A*, two profiles; *B*, eight profiles; *C*, multiple profiles.

SCANNER DESIGNS

The first commercially available scanner, which was developed and manufactured by EMI Limited, was restricted to head scanning.[5,7,12] In this system, an x-ray tube highly collimated to a "pencil" beam scanned the patient in a linear mo-

tion, as shown in Figure 20–7. A sodium iodide crystal detector on the opposite side of the patient moved in synchrony with the x-ray tube and intercepted the transmitted beam. The detector signal received during the linear sweep provided the scanner's computer with an attenuation profile of the irradiated cross section of the head. If imaged, this profile would resemble a single horizontal strip on a conventional skull x-ray film. The x-ray tube and detector apparatus then rotated by 1° and the scanning motion was repeated (in reverse), thereby providing a profile rotated by 1 degree from the previous profile. This process continued through 180 successive 1° rotations until the computer acquired 180 unique profiles. Because of the complicated repetitive mechanical motions, each complete sectional scan required 4.5 min. To reduce the lengthy scanning time, the x-rays were collimated so as to produce two pencil beams, each irradiating separate adjacent cross sections. Two scintillation detectors separately monitored the transmitted beam. In this manner, two adjacent cross sections were acquired in each 4.5-min scanning operation.

The first-generation EMI scanner required a water bag around the patient's head. The water-skull interface provided a much less abrupt density transition than that obtained with air surrounding the head. The computer image reconstruction process of this initial scanner system necessitated the reduction in density transitions obtained with the water bag. Data processing of subsequent scanners built by EMI and other manufacturers eliminated the need for the water bag. This modification permitted the introduction of total body scanning systems.[13,14]

Scanners of the second generation reduced the number of incremental angular rotations through use of a modified fan-beam design. Instead of irradiating each cross section with a single pencil beam, the x-ray output is collimated into multi-

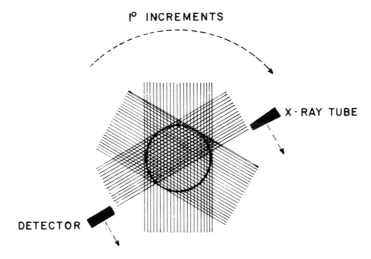

Fig. 20–7.   First-generation pencil-beam scanning.

ple pencil beams in a fan-shaped distribution. The modified fan-beam systems employ between 3 and 30 pencil beams, with a corresponding number of scintillation detectors on the opposite side of the patient. Each detector monitors a single pencil beam.

The reduction in the number of incremental rotations arises from the relative angulation of the multiple pencil beams (Fig. 20–8). A single linear sweep provides a different profile for each separate beam since each beam cuts across the section at its own unique angle. For example, a three-beam system would generate three separate profiles for each sweep. Such a system would then rotate 3° following each sweep, for a total of 60 incremental rotations. With systems using 30 separate beams and detectors, scanning time is reduced to slightly less than 30 sec. Some second-generation modified fan-beam systems acquire two slices per scan through use of dual sets of beams and detectors. The ultimate speed of second-generation systems is limited, because of the mechanical limitations associated with a complex rotate-sweep-rotate-sweep cycle. The reduction of scanning time to several seconds is primarily motivated by the objective of eliminating respiratory motion

in body scanning, which requires the patient to hold his breath.

Third-generation scanners achieve this objective easily by completely eliminating the sweep motion. Typical scanning times of 1 to 10 sec are achieved by smoothly rotating a continuous fan-shaped x-ray beam 360° about the patient, as depicted in Figure 20–9. An array of several hundred miniature ionization gas or solid state detectors on the opposite side of the patient follows the rotational motion. Each detector takes several hundred separate readings in the course of a single scan. The manner in which third-generation scanner computers must handle the detector data is necessarily different, in the sense that a conventional profile is not produced by each detector. However, the same basic information is being derived. During the course of a scan, whether it is with a first-, second-, or third-generation system, x-rays passing through any given point on a cross section are detected from many different angles. In the process, the relative attenuation of each point is interrelated with the attenuation of all other points on the cross section. The computer mathematically separates this interrelated data and displays it as a reconstructed image.

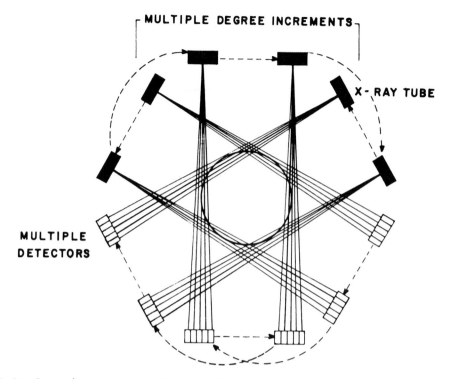

Fig. 20–8.   Second-generation multiple pencil-beam scanning.

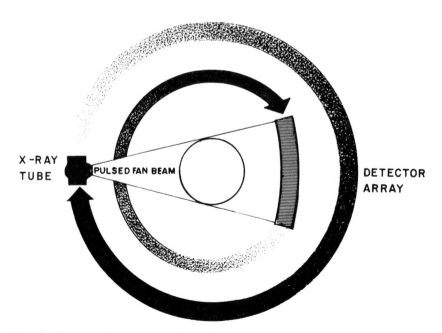

Fig. 20–9.   Third generation rotational fan-beam scanning.

A related scanner, which incorporates a further reduction in mechanical motion, may be regarded as a fourth-generation system. This scanner (Fig. 20–10) employs several hundred stationary detectors arranged in a circular array. An x-ray tube collimated to a fan-beam rotates on a track inside the circular detector array. At any given instant, an arc of the array intercepts the transmitted x-rays.

Scanning speed is important in any CT system because the image reconstruction process is extremely sensitive to motion. Such artifacts as obscuring streaks are produced by even slight patient movement. Acquisition of a complete scan while the patient holds his breath is essential, because unlike radionuclide imaging, the quality of the entire CT image may be reduced drastically as a consequence of motion in any part of the cross section.

Greater ease in constraining the head has resulted in the availability of multiple scanning speeds on most CT units. Slower speeds, which usually provide superior resolution, are reserved for head scanning, and faster speeds, particularly in newer-generation scanners, are utilized for total body scanning.

Second-, third-, and fourth-generation scanners are all still in commercial production since each offers specific advantages. Reconstruction of data with the sec-

ond-generation scanning sequence requires a less costly and lower-stability detector array than with subsequent generations of pure rotational scanning. Third-generation scan reconstruction demands high detector stability to avoid the circular artifacts to which it is susceptible, but scanning time is generally shorter than with second-generation scan reconstruction. Although fourth-generation systems eliminate mechanical rotation of the detector assembly, they require substantially more detectors, because only a fraction of the detectors subtend the x-ray fan beam at any given instant. These detectors, however, do not require the stability of the third-generation scanners. Aside from such factors as cost and scanning time, the second- to fourth-generation scanners all provide essentially equivalent image quality.

IMAGING STATISTICS

Matrix sizes of CT scanners vary from the 80×80 array of the earliest EMI system to 512×512 arrays on some of the more recent systems. Each point on the display matrix is referred to as a *pixel*. The displayed intensity of each pixel is a representation of the computed value of μ_{ij} for the corresponding cell of tissue in the cross-sectional slice. The initial EMI pixel displayed the measured attenuation of a 3×3 mm^2 area of the cross section. With a slice thickness of 13 mm, this pixel actually represented the average value of μ_{ij} in a 117 mm^3 volume of tissue. More recent developments in finer spatial data sampling have substantially improved the resolution of CT scanners. Detailed visualization of a structure as fine as the optic nerve is possible with these improvements. A 1×1 mm^2 area with 5-mm slice thickness is typical. In such a system, each pixel relates to a 5 mm^3 cell volume of tissue.

Larger matrix sizes do not necessarily imply a concurrent improvement in res-

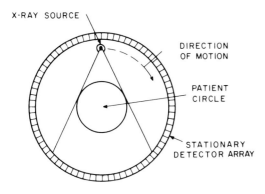

X-RAY SOURCE

DIRECTION OF MOTION

PATIENT CIRCLE

STATIONARY DETECTOR ARRAY

Fig. 20–10. Fourth-generation stationary detectors with pure rotational fan-beam scanning.

olution. The matrix size is an often-quoted system parameter that relates to the computer display. The x-ray transmission must be sampled with sufficient precision at a large number of points for the fineness of the display matrix to reflect accurately the resolving capability of the scanning mechanism.

In general, sufficient statistics are acquired to determine μ in each pixel to within 0.5% at one standard deviation. This calculation is necessary in view of the fact that μ differs by only several percent for nearly all soft tissues.[15,16,17] This level of attenuation resolution requires the detection of billions of photons for each CT image. The resultant radiation dose to the patient is typically several rads to the scanned sections.[18]

The numeric value of μ for any specified pixel can be displayed. Actually, a special scale of units is usually employed to express μ in terms of the linear attenuation coefficient for water, μ_w. The Hounsfield units extend from -1000 for air and 0 for water to $+1000$ for bone. Each 1% change in the calculated μ with respect to μ_w is given by 10 Hounsfield units. For example:

$$100\% \times \frac{\mu_m - \mu_w}{\mu_w} = 4.8\%$$

where μ_m is the measured attenuation coefficient for meningioma. The pixel value would be 48 Hounsfield units. An image consisting of those pixels falling within a selected window or range of units can be selected. The window can be set to display an enhanced image of a specific type of tissue.

CLINICAL RESULTS

CT has become an important diagnostic aid in the investigation of a wide range of systemic disorders. Neurologic scanning has demonstrated a clinical accuracy equal to or exceeding 90%. CT is now regarded as the most sensitive and least in-

vasive test in assessing many disorders of the brain (Figs. 20–11, 20–12, and 20–13). The full impact of intra-abdominal scanning on diagnostic imaging has become apparent as the newer and faster generation systems have come into widespread clinical use.

A number of investigations have compared the diagnostic accuracy of neurologic CT studies with that of radionuclide

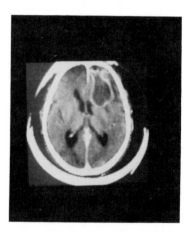

Fig. 20–11. Right frontal low-attenuation lesion with ring enhancement (after contrast infusion). Diagnostic possibilities include abscess or tumor.

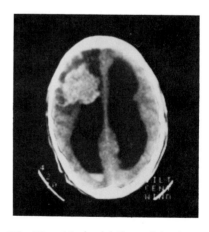

Fig. 20–12. Marked bilateral hydrocephalus and enhancing mass in left frontal area. Fluid levels are seen posteriorly in ventricles, with fluid attenuation number compatible with fresh blood. Diagnosis: tuberous sclerosis.

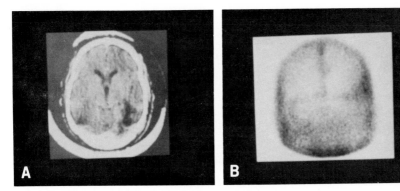

Fig. 20–13. *A.* CT scan shows low attenuation lesion consistent with old infarction. *B.* Radionuclide scan shows corresponding area of increased uptake in right occipital area.

studies. CT has demonstrated superiority in cerebral, cerebellar, and intraventricular hemorrhage. Comparable results for both techniques have been achieved in brain abscesses and supratentorial tumors. CT is quite specific in diagnosing acute subdural or epidural hematomas, although radionuclide static images, when accompanied by perfusion dynamics can also be definitive. The two techniques have been shown to be complementary in chronic subdural hematoma. CT demonstrates a definite superiority in diagnosing lesions of the brain stem, benign cysts, encephalomalacia, hydrocephalus, and porencephaly. In those neurologic cases studied with both techniques, the combined precision is equal to 95% or greater.

Many neurologic CT scans are repeated following the intravenous injection of contrast medium. A significant enhancement is believed to arise, in part, from the breakdown of the blood-brain barrier, which provides a mechanism of visualization analogous to that in radionuclide imaging.

The application of whole body scanning systems in imaging torso cross sections has been useful in diagnosing spinal, head and neck, lung, pleural, mediastinal, vascular, and intra-abdominal lesions. Among those regions most commonly studied are the liver, pancreas, retroperitoneum, and genitourinary tract.

CT scans of the normal liver show a somewhat higher density than that of other intra-abdominal organs.[19,20] The normal liver scan appears homogeneous. A CT study is indicated in evaluating jaundice, primary malignant tumor, metastatic disease, and inflammatory disease. Benign and malignant tumors in the liver usually show lower attenuation than the normal liver parenchyma. Intravenous administration of contrast medium typically improves the differentiation of the parenchyma with respect to tumor tissue. The uptake of contrast medium in highly vascular metastatic lesions may be sufficient, however, to decrease the relative differentiation.

Radionuclide imaging of the liver is useful in detecting liver masses; however, smaller deeper lesions are often missed. CT permits differentiation of solid from cystic lesions in addition to detecting many lesions not seen in radionuclide imaging.[12,21] In screening for liver metastases, Bryan et al. conclude that radionuclide imaging is preferred over CT, because the former offers a relatively low incidence of false-negative results.[22] Furthermore, isodense tumors are not well visualized on CT. Biello et al. and MacCarty et al. found that both techniques provided generally equivalent accuracy.[23,24] Hepatic tumors exceeding 3 cm in diameter are usually detected by radionuclide imaging, whereas CT detection extends to the 1-cm range (Fig. 20–14). Itai et al. compared the two methods in the diagnosis of hepatoma.[25] In 43 cases of liver metastases, they found equivalence in 35 cases, radionuclide imaging superior in 7 cases, and CT superior in 1 case. In judging the extent of tumor, however, both methods were equivalent in about half of the cases; in the remaining half, CT was superior to radionuclide imaging by a ratio of two to one.

CT studies have almost completely replaced Se-75 selenomethionine scans of the pancreas. Visualization of the pancreas is assisted by the presence of adjacent fat. Attenuation of carcinoma is not significantly lower than that of normal tissue. Consequently, morphologic changes are of diagnostic importance in pancreatic CT scanning.

The kidneys are well delineated in CT images as a consequence of the surrounding perinephric fat. Masses are evidenced by deformation of the kidney contour and deviations from normal parenchymal absorption. Renal carcinoma, which generally has a relatively lower absorption, may vary substantially with calcification, hemorrhage, and necrosis. Visualization of vascular tumors is generally aided by the intravenous injection of contrast material.

The application of CT scanning in the body appears to be most significant in observing abdominal masses, particularly those in the liver, pancreas, and retroperitoneal spaces. Alternative techniques tend to be overly invasive or insufficiently diagnostic, although in renal and chest diseases, this argument may be somewhat less valid.

CT has been compared to radionuclide gallium imaging in evaluating suspected abdominal abscess by several investigators.[26,27,28,29] These studies indicate that detection of the source of inflammation in febrile patients is usually equivalent for the two methods. McNeil et al. found no significant difference in sensitivity or specificity. Utilization of both techniques was shown to increase sensitivity to sepsis detection significantly, from approximately 60% to nearly 90% with a false-positive rate increase from 15% to 25%.

Levine et al. compared CT and radionuclide imaging in the evaluation of musculoskeletal tumors.[30] CT was found to be of diagnostic value for tumors in the bony pelvis, sacrum, and vertebral appendages (Fig. 20–15A). Bone involvement was reliably imaged by Tc-99m labeled phosphate; the principal value of radionuclide imaging was the detection of unsuspected skeletal involvement (Fig. 20–15B). CT was judged to be superior to radionuclide

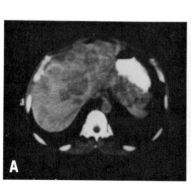
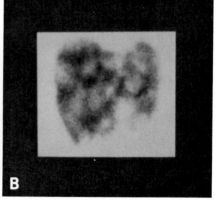

Fig. 20–14. *CT scan (A)* and Tc sulfur colloid scan *(B)* demonstrate multiple space occupying lesions throughout liver and spleen. Diagnosis: metastases from lung carcinoma.

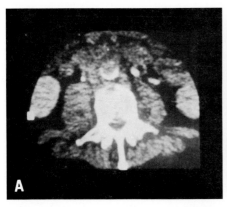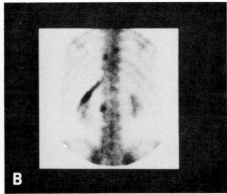

Fig. 20–15. *A.* CT scan demonstrates destruction of bony cortex and shows presence of soft tissue mass anteriorly. *B.* Comparative Tc MDP bone scan shows several areas of increased uptake, including the L-2 vertebra shown at left.

imaging in delineation of soft-tissue masses. In addition, Levine et al. found CT to be significantly more accurate than Ga-67 citrate in visualizing soft-tissue tumors and the soft-tissue components of bony tumors. Neither CT nor radionuclide imaging was found to be particularly useful in evaluating benign bone tumors.

DYNAMIC COMPUTED TOMOGRAPHY

Considerable emphasis is being placed upon the technologic development of dynamic CT systems that provide a time sequence of tomographic images, to permit visualization of dynamic processes within the body that are not readily discernible from static images. Conventional CT scanning is inherently restricted to static images because proper reconstruction of a cross section necessitates acquiring a large set of data samplings as the x-ray beam traverses the subject at multiple positions and angles. Subject movement during the scan acquisition time interferes with the interrelationship of the samplings and degrades the quality of the reconstructed image. Even such internal organ movement as the heart beating can impair reconstruction.

Nevertheless, a single cross section can be scanned repeatedly every several sec-onds with current CT systems, thereby providing a time sequence of static images.[31,32,33,34,35] Applications include brain circulatory abnormalities and the determination of bypass graft patency. The progressive flow of injected contrast media is monitored in this "slow" dynamic acquisition of the CT scanner.

Separation of phases of the cardiac cycle, however, is well beyond the capability of conventional CT scanners, which operate in the slow dynamic mode. To image the complete cardiac cycle, the time per image should be approximately 100 msec, i.e., a small fraction of the cycle duration. This "fast" dynamic capability has been achieved with conventional CT scanners by utilizing ECG gating, a process technically analogous to gated blood pool imaging in nuclear medicine (see Vol. II, Chap. 17).

Actual CT acquisition occurs over multiple cardiac cycles, and the data are reconstructed to give a single composite dynamic visualization of the cardiac cycle.[35,36,37,38,39] This dynamic visualization might consist of a progression of perhaps ten images, each corresponding to a successive phase through the complete cardiac cycle. If the entire progression of images is repeatedly displayed at the heart rate, a continuous (tomographic) cine of the heart motion is possible. The gated images can be used to quantitate infarct size and myocardial wall thickness, particularly with regard to variation during the cardiac cycle. Wall motion can be assessed with excellent spatial resolution because the images are tomographic, not projective as in x-ray angiography or conventional radionuclide blood-pool studies.

Gated CT affords a convenient means of achieving fast dynamic capability but is restricted to applications in which the physiologic function is repetitive, as with the heart. The conventional CT scanner could achieve fast dynamics simply by reducing the scan time from several seconds to perhaps 100 msec. Mechanical limitations of rapidly rotating an object as massive as an x-ray tube are prohibitive, however.

A unique imaging system known as the *dynamic spatial reconstructor* (DSR) circumvents this mechanical limitation by utilizing 28 sets of x-ray tubes and detectors in rotation.[40] The DSR, which was developed as a research instrument at the Mayo Clinic, can rotate every 4 sec, but because of the multiple imaging sets, sufficient angular samplings are acquired to reconstruct 60 sequential images per sec. In addition, the DSR detectors, which are analogous to fluoroscopic x-ray detectors, intercept a full two-dimensional projective image instead of the one-dimensional profile intercepted by conventional CT linear array detectors. As a result, up to 250 1-mm thick transverse sections of the subject can be reconstructed from each scan. The DSR is potentially capable of full three-dimensional fast dynamic imaging, at 60 times per sec, of a cylindric volume up to 30 cm in diameter and 25 cm in length.

An alternative approach to fast dynamic CT uses a scanning electron beam.[41,42] A focused electron beam is electromagnetically swept around a ring anode target in an annular vacuum bottle positioned coaxially to the subject. Associated ring collimation restricts the emitted x-rays to a fan beam directed at the subject. A stationary concentric circular detector array intercepts the fan beam after it passes through the subject. This configuration is analogous to the fourth-generation CT scanner (Fig. 20–10) except that there is no moving x-ray tube. Because no mechanical motion is involved, a scan can be completed in several microseconds. The scanning beam x-ray technology, however, still requires considerable developmental work in contrast to the well-established technology of conventional x-ray tubes utilized in virtually all other CT scanners.

REFERENCES

1. Brooks, R.A., and DiChiro, G.: Theory of image reconstruction in computed tomography. Radiology, *117*:561, 1975.
2. Cormack, A.M.: Reconstruction of densities from their projections with application in radiological physics. Phys. Med. Biol., *18*:195, 1973.
3. Goitein, M.: Three-dimensional density reconstruction from a series of two-dimensional projections. Nucl. Inst. Meth., *101*:509, 1972.
4. Oldendorf, W.H.: Isolated flying spot detection of radiodensity discontinuities: displaying the internal structural pattern of a complex object. I.R.E. Trans. Biomed. Electron., *8*:68, 1961.
5. Hounsfield, G.N.: Computerized transverse axial scanning. Part I. Br. J. Radiol., *46*:1016, 1973.
6. Ambrose, J.: Computerized Transverse Axial Scanning. Proceedings of the British Institute of Radiology, 32nd Annual Congress, 1972.
7. Ambrose, J.: Computerized transverse axial scanning. Part 2. Br. J. Radiol., *46*:1023, 1973.
8. Alfidi, R.J., et al.: Experimental studies to determine application of CAT scanning to the human body. Am. J. Roentgenol., *124*:199, 1975.
9. Gado, M.H., Phelps, M.E., and Coleman, R.E.: An extravascular component of contrast enhancement in cranial computed tomography. Part I: The tissue-blood ratio of contrast enhancement. Radiology, *117*:589, 1975.
10. Gado, M.H., Phelps, M.E., and Coleman, R.E.: An extravascular component of contrast enhancement in cranial computed tomography. Part II: Contrast enhancement and the blood-tissue barrier. Radiology, *117*:595, 1975.
11. New, P.F.J., et al.: Computed Tomographic Aspects of Intra- and Extra-Vascular Blood. Presented at the International Conference on Computerized Axial Tomography, Montreal Neurological Institute, May 1974.
12. Sheedy, P.F., et al.: Computed tomography of the body: initial clinical trial with the EMI prototype. Am. J. Roentgenol., *127*:23, 1976.

13. Ledley, R.S., et al.: Computerized transaxial x-ray tomography of the human body. Science, *186*:207, 1974.

14. Stanley, R.J., Sagel, S.S., and Levitt, R.G.: Computed tomography of the body: early trends in applications and accuracy of the method. Am. J. Roentgenol., *127*:53, 1976.

15. Phelps, M.E., Hoffman, E.J., and Ter-Pogossian, M.M.: Attenuation coefficients of various body tissues, fluids, and lesions at photon energies of 18 to 136 keV. Radiology, *117*:573, 1975.

16. Rao, P.S., and Gregg, E.C.: Attenuation of monoenergetic gamma rays in tissues. Am. J. Roentgenol. Radium Ther. Nucl. Med., *123*:631, 1975.

17. Ter-Pogossian, M.M., et al.: The extraction of the yet-unused wealth of information in diagnostic radiology. Radiology, *113*:515, 1974.

18. McCullough, E.C., et al.: An evaluation of the quantitative and radiation features of a scanning x-ray transverse axial tomography: the EMI scanner. Radiology, *111*:709, 1974.

19. Alfidi, R.J., et al.: Computed tomography of the liver. Am. J. Roentgenol., *127*:69, 1976.

20. Philips, R.L., and Stephens, D.H.: Computed tomography of liver specimens. Radiology, *115*:43, 1975.

21. Stephens, D.H., Sheedy, P.F., Hattery, R.R., and MacCarty, R.L.: Computed tomography of the liver. Am. J. Roentgenol., *128*:579, 1977.

22. Bryan, P.J., Dinn, W.M., Grossman, Z.D., et al.: Correlation of computed tomography, gray scale ultrasonography, and radionuclide imaging of the liver in detecting space-occupying processes. Radiology, *124*:387, 1977.

23. Biello, D.R., Levitt, R.G., Siegel, B.A., et al.: Computed tomography and radionuclide imaging of the liver: A comparative evaluation. Radiology, *127*:159, 1978.

24. MacCarty, R.L., Wahner, H.W., Stephens, D.H., et al.: Retrospective comparison of radionuclide scans and computed tomography of the liver and pancreas. Am. J. Roentgenol., *129*:23, 1977.

25. Itai, Y., Nishikawa, J., and Tasaka, A.: Computed tomography in the evaluation of hepatocellular carcinoma. Radiology, *131*:165, 1979.

26. Shimshak, R.R., Korobkin, M., Hoffer, P.B., et al.: The complementary role of gallium citrate imaging and computed tomography in the evaluation of suspected abdominal infection. J. Nucl. Med., *19*:262, 1978.

27. Korobkin, M., Callen, P.W., Filly, R.A., et al.: Comparison of computed tomography, ultrasonography, and gallium-67 scanning in the evaluation of suspected abdominal abscess. Radiology, *129*:89, 1978.

28. Levitt, R.G., Biello, D.R., Sagel, S.S., et al.: Computed tomography and [67]citrate radionuclide imaging for evaluating suspected abdominal abscess. Am. J. Roentgenol., *132*:529, 1979.

29. McNeil, B.J., Sanders, R., Alderson, P.O., et al.: A prospective study of computed tomography, ultrasound, and gallium imaging in patients with fever. Radiology, *139*:647, 1981.

30. Levine, E., Lee, K.R., Neff, J.R., et al.: Comparison of computed tomography and other imaging modalities in the evaluation of musculoskeletal tumors. Radiology, *131*:431, 1979.

31. Dobben, G., Valvassori, G., Mafee, M., and Berninger, W.: Evaluation of brain circulation by rapid rotational computed tomography. Radiology, *133*:105, 1979.

32. Heinz, E.R., Dubois, P., Osborne, D., et al.: Dynamic computed tomography study of the brain. J. Comput. Assist. Tomogr., *3*:641, 1979.

33. Traupe, H., Heiss, W., Hoeffken, W., and Zulch, K.: Hyperperfusion and enhancement in dynamic computed tomography of ischemic stroke patients. J. Comput. Assist. Tomogr., *3*:627, 1979.

34. Brundage, B., Lipton, M., Herfkens, R., et al.: Detection of patent coronary bypass grafts by computed tomography: A preliminary report. Circulation, *61*:826, 1980.

35. Berninger, W., Redington, R., Lene, W., et al.: Technical aspects and clinical applications of CT/X, a dynamic CT scanner. J. Comput. Assist. Tomogr., *5*:206, 1981.

36. Sagel, S., Weiss, E., Gillard, R., et al.: Gated computed tomography of the human heart. Invest. Radiol., *12*:563, 1977.

37. Harell, G., Guthaner, D., Breiman, R., et al.: Stop action computed tomography. Radiology, *123*:515, 1977.

38. Alfidi, R.J., Haaga, J.R., MacIntyre, W.J., et al.: Gated computed tomography of the heart. Comput. Tomogr., *1*:51, 1977.

39. Berninger, W., Redington, R., Doherty, P., et al.: Gated cardiac scanning: Canine studies. J. Comput. Assist. Tomogr., *3*:155, 1979.

40. Ritman, E.L., Kinsey, J.H., Robb, R.A., et al.: Physics and technical considerations in the design of the DSR: A high temporal resolution volume scanner. Am. J. Roentgenol., *134*:369, 1980.

41. Haimson, J.: X-ray source without moving parts for ultra-high-speed tomography. IEEE Trans. Nucl. Sci., *26*:2857, 1979.

42. Boyd, D.P., Gould, R.G., Quinn, J.R., et al.: A proposed dynamic cardiac 3-D densitometer for early detection and evaluation of heart disease. IEEE Trans. Nucl. Sci., *26*:2724, 1979.

Chapter 21

MAGNETIC RESONANCE—RELATIONS TO NUCLEAR MEDICINE

VAL M. RUNGE,
C. LEON PARTAIN, AND
A. EVERETTE JAMES, JR.

Since Lauterbur produced the first anatomic images in 1972,[1] the field of *nuclear magnetic resonance* (NMR), now generally referred to as *magnetic resonance* (MR), has progressed rapidly. MR has become a powerful tool of the organic chemist for determining chemical structure and molecular interactions that cannot be determined by other techniques. Its application to clinical medicine, however, required the ability to resolve signals spatially from within a sample. Within a year of Lauterbur's initial work, several investigators had developed MR imaging techniques, and the series of rapid technologic advances needed to realize MR body imaging systems had begun.[2,3] Interest in MR imaging as a diagnostic tool in medicine stems from three factors: 1) the use of non-ionizing energy, 2) increased soft-tissue contrast, and 3) the ability to select and image anatomic planes electronically in any orientation.

PHYSICAL PRINCIPLES

MR depends upon the ability of certain nuclei to act as magnetic dipoles (or more simply, as small bar magnets) in the presence of a magnetic field. Nuclei with odd numbers of protons or neutrons, which possess both charge and spin, have this property; their intrinsic angular momentum ("spin") interacts with the electric charge distribution of the nucleus, leading to the generation of a small magnetic field. Such nuclei as $^{1}_{1}H$, $^{13}_{6}C$, $^{19}_{9}F$, and $^{31}_{15}P$ have an odd number of protons or neutrons. Consequently, they have a net spin and magnetic moment and may be studied by MR techniques (Fig. 21–1a,b). Such nuclei as $^{24}_{12}Mg$, $^{32}_{16}S$, and $^{40}_{20}Ca$, with even numbers of protons and neutrons, have no net spin, lack magnetic moment, and do not figure in MR imaging. When nuclei that possess magnetic moment e.g., hydrogen (protons), are placed in an externally applied magnetic field, they attempt to align themselves with the magnetic field lines.

According to classic electromagnetic theory, this process also results in *precession* of the magnetic moment about the magnetic field, as shown in Figure 21–1c. A common analogy is the precession, or wobble, of a spinning top in the earth's

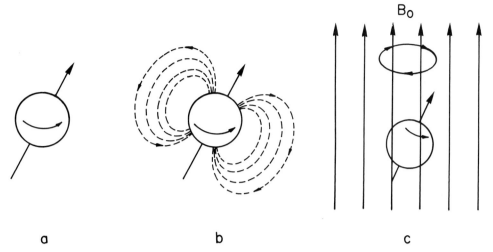

Fig. 21–1. Magnetic resonance. *a.* The hydrogen nucleus (proton) has a charge of +1 and a spin of ½, which results in a nuclear magnetic moment. *b.* The magnetic moment generates magnetic force fields. *c.* When an external magnetic field B_0 is applied, the magnetic moment rotates (precesses) about the lines of magnetic force.

gravitational field. The spin of each nucleus is often characterized by its angular frequency, ω_0 (radians/sec), rather than by its cyclical (resonant) frequency, f_0 (hertz, or cycles/sec). The two are related by the following equation:

$$f_0 = \omega_0/2\pi \qquad (1)$$

The characteristic angular frequency is called the *Larmor frequency* and depends on both the strength of the magnetic field, B_0, and the *gyromagnetic ratio*, γ, specific for each nuclear species, so that:

$$\omega_0 = \gamma\, B_0 \qquad (2)$$

The resonant frequency (hertz) is given by:

$$f_0 = (\gamma/2\pi)B_0 \qquad (3)$$

Nuclear resonant frequencies are in the same range as radiowave frequencies in the electromagnetic spectrum, i.e., $\sim 10^3$ to 10^8 Hz. This corresponds to quantum energies of $\sim 10^{-11}$ to 10^{-6} eV.

The magnetic field strengths characteristically used in MR imaging are on the order of 0.1 to 1.5 tesla, (T), which is equivalent to 1,000 to 15,000 gauss (G) in the cgs system. The earth's magnetic field strength equals approximately 0.5 G. Large magnets require large energies to maintain a uniform field of 0.1 to 1.5 T throughout the body.

T_1 and T_2

Before application of an external magnetic field, the magnetic moments of all nuclei making up the tissue or object are randomly aligned. When a magnetic field is applied, the individual magnetic moments tend to align with the direction of the magnetic field (Fig. 21–1c).

Conventional descriptions of the coordinates of the magnetic field utilize a three-dimensional coordinate system with the z axis parallel to the lines of force. The nuclear magnetic moments are summed to produce a net magnetic *moment*, M_0, a vector, symbolized by the heavy arrow in Fig. 21–2. The constantly changing x and y components caused by precession and thermal interaction of individual nuclei are random with respect to one another and thus cancel out. If the object is irradiated in the x-y plane by a radiofrequency (RF) transmitter at the same frequency as the nuclear resonant frequency, the mag-

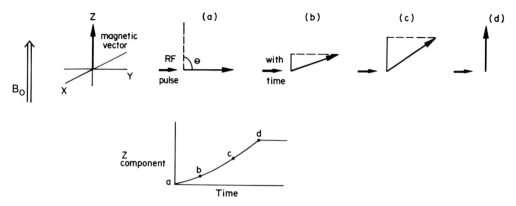

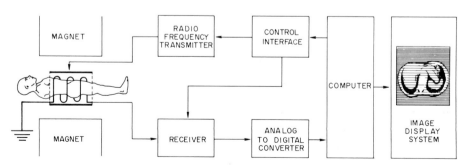

Fig. 21–2. T_1 describes the return of the z component of the magnetic vector to its original equilibrium value M_0 following application of a radiofrequency (RF) pulse perpendicular to the Z axis. In this case, a 90° RF pulse ($\theta = 90°$) was given to displace the magnetic vector 90° into the x-y plane, resulting initially in a value of zero for the z component of the magnetic vector. B_0 is the strength of the externally applied magnetic field. (a) Magnetic vector orientation after $\pi/2$ RF pulse. (b) Magnetic field orientation after delay time, τ_1. (c) Magnetic field orientation after longer delay time, τ_2. (d) Magnetic vector orientation after return to original equilibrium position.

netic vector becomes displaced away from the z axis, as shown in Figure 21–2a. The angle of displacement, θ, is related to the amplitude and duration, τ_p, of the RF pulse. The net momentum M_2 now precesses with the same characteristic frequency ω_0 because each individual nucleus is in phase with the radiofrequency of the excitation pulse. As in an electric generator, charged rotating objects within a magnetic field induce an electric current in a surrounding coil. If the object irradiated is positioned inside a coil oriented perpendicularly to the magnetic force B_0, as shown in Figure 21–3, the precessing

nuclei induce a current within the coil. The measurement of this signal and its characterization are central to defining the spatial distribution of the excited nuclei and to producing the MR image.

Following the RF pulse, the net magnetic vector returns (relaxes) to the original vector, M_0, as shown in Figures 21–2b through 21–2d. The return of the magnetization vector, M, (thus, the decay of the signal amplitude within the coil) is exponential with time and is analogous to radioactive decay. The decay of the MR signal can be described by two time (relaxation) constants, which are analogous

Fig. 21–3. Schematic representation of an MR imaging system. (From Partain, C.L., et al.[4])

to λ, the radioactive decay constant. The return of the magnetization vector M_z to equilibrium M_0 following termination of the RF stimulation is characterized by a rate constant $1/T_1$, known as the *spin-lattice relaxation rate*. The process is given this name because it characterizes the interaction and exchange of energy between the perturbed nuclei and the existing lattice structure of the material irradiated.

Simultaneously, the magnetic vector returns to equilibrium in the longitudinal direction, and the individual nuclei begin to dephase with respect to one another in the transverse plane (Fig. 21–4). The time required for dephasing is also exponential and is described by a second rate constant, $1/T_2$, where T_2 is the average decay time for the process. In this respect, T_2 is analogous to λ, the decay constant. Recall that $\overline{T}$, the *average* radioactive decay time, is equal to $1/\lambda$. The amplitude of the initial MR signal A_0 decays in the x-y plane exponentially with time t:

$$A = A_0 e^{-t/T_2{}^*} \qquad (4)$$

where T_2^* is the time constant that characterizes the decay of a single free induction decay signal. T_2 is called the *spin-spin relaxation constant* or the *transverse relaxation time.* In all materials, $T_1 \geqq T_2 \geqq T_2^*$, and in most materials, $T_1 >> T_2$.

The recorded MR signal following a single excitation pulse at the resonant frequency describes an oscillating sine wave, as shown in Figure 21–5. The amplitude of this signal decays according to equation (4) and is referred to as *free induction decay.* If the Fourier transform of this signal is taken, the lower curve is generated. This curve describes the distribution of spin frequencies within the sample. Its full width at half-maximum can be used to approximate T_2^*.

Three signals may thus be obtained from the sample by MR: T_1 and T_2, the two relaxation times, and ρ, the nuclear spin density (Table 21–1). T_1 and T_2 are markedly sensitive to molecular motion. In solids, T_1 may be several seconds while T_2 is only microseconds. In liquids, T_2 begins to approximate T_1. In pure water, both pa-

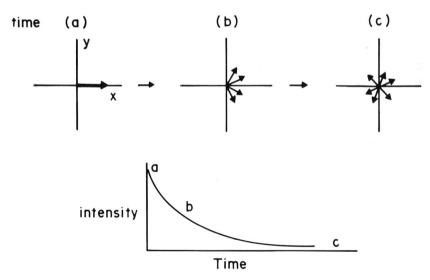

Fig. 21–4. With the application of an RF pulse of resonant frequency to the measured sample, all affected nuclei spin in synchrony (a). After cessation of the RF pulse, the x-y vectors of individual nuclei begin to dephase with respect to one another (b). This leads to a cancellation of that portion of the MR signal with a time referred to as the T_2 relaxation time (c). Points a, b, and c on the intensity graph correspond to points a, b, and d in Fig. 21–2.

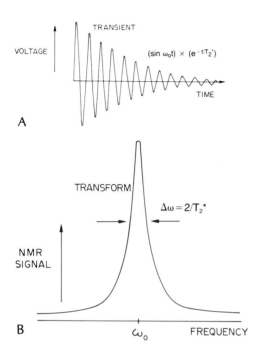

TABLE 21–1. *Definition of Basic MR Parameters*

Parameter	Definition
ρ	Spin density. ρ is the observed *signal strength* of the RF pulse emitted from the sample following excitation.
T_1	Spin-lattice relaxation time. T_1 is the rate constant describing the return of the z component of the magnetic vector M to its original value M_0 following application of a radiofrequency pulse to the sample (see Fig. 21–1).
T_2	Spin-spin relaxation time. The change in the x-y (transverse) component of the magnetic vector (following excitation by a RF pulse) with time due to local differences in magnetic field strength. If this change were due entirely to sample-induced local differences in magnetic field strength (without any contribution from inhomogeneities in the applied magnetic field), the rate constant describing this decay would equal T_2 (see Fig. 21–2).

Fig. 21–5. *A.* The recorded MR signal on the receiver coil, following a single RF pulse, describes a sine wave that decays exponentially with time, e^{-t/T_2^*}. *B.* The Fourier transform of the signal produces a Lorentzian line whose FWHM is equal to T_2.

rameters are on the order of 2 sec. MR signals are not, however, observed from rigidly bound nuclei because of the short T_2; hence, the signal from bone is negligible and appears black on MR images.

IMAGING SYSTEMS

Magnets

At present, three basic magnet designs—air-core resistive magnets, superconducting magnets, and permanent magnets—are used in MR imaging systems. Resistive magnets are costly in terms of electrical energy consumption. Typically, they generate magnetic fields on the order of 0.1 T, and power consumption rises steeply with increasing magnetic fields. Superconducting magnets have superior magnetic field strength, homogeneity, and stability. Typical magnetic fields are 0.5 to 2.0 T. Initial investment costs and cooling requirements for superconducting magnets are substantial, however. Permanent magnet systems have a different set of advantages and disadvantages. Advantages include low initial cost and lower operating costs. Disadvantages include thermal instability, inferior uniformity, and weight.

The signal-to-noise ratio can be increased by using higher magnetic fields. As B_0 increases, however, higher frequencies are required to produce changes in the magnetic vector, and this in turn results in increased attenuation of RF signals by tissue.

RF Transmitter and Receiver

The RF transmitter is connected to the sample coil, which serves as the antenna for both transmission of the excitation pulse and reception of the MR signal (Fig. 21–3). After an excitation pulse of some duration t_d, the radioreceiver, tuned to the resonant frequency of the sample, is switched on during the RF emission period. The pulsing sequence may be simple, as in *free induction decay,* or complex, as in *inversion-recovery pulsing.*

RF Pulse Sequences

The simplest RF pulsing sequence consists of a brief pulse at the resonant frequency of duration τ, which rotates the M_0 vector out of the z direction. When the pulse is turned off, the excited atoms return to the alignment parallel to M_0, emitting an oscillating sine wave signal that decays with time e^{-t/T_2}, as shown in Fig. 21–4. This is observed with the application of a 180° RF pulse. This process is known as *spin-echo pulsing* and provides a measure of T_2 (Table 21–2). The maximum MR signal is obtained when the RF emission rotates M through 90°. A typical value of T_2 for water at 4 MHz radiofrequency is 2700 msec.

Current medical MR imaging techniques depict the location and behavior of protons in terms of T_1, T_2, and ρ. The extent to which any of these signals contributes to image contrast depends upon the RF pulse sequence used (Table 21–2).[5] One common pulse sequence uses pulse spacing based on the relaxation times and is known as a *steady-state-free-precession* (SSFP) pulse technique, with pulse intervals much smaller than the relaxation times. Two other pulse techniques are the *saturation-recovery* and *inversion-recovery* sequences. With saturation-recovery pulsing, equally spaced 90° pulses are applied, and both T_1 and spin-density maps can be constructed from these pulses. The inversion-recovery technique utilizes an inverted 180° pulse followed by a 90° pulse (with a substantial time delay between pulse pairs) to highlight T_1 values. The image intensity with SSFP pulsing is a complex function of ρ, T_1, and T_2. Spin-echo techniques are used to determine T_2 values.

Clinical data from patients can be obtained by point,[6,7] line,[8] or planar-volume scanning techniques.[9,10,11] The greater sensitivity of planar- and whole-volume techniques has directed research toward development in these areas. To image the plane of interest, a magnetic field gradient is applied orthogonally to the plane. Selective irradiation with a narrow frequency band RF pulse or with an oscillating magnetic field gradient (two common approaches among the many available) achieve further planar definition.[8,12] Filtered backprojection, two-dimensional Fourier transformation, or similar reconstruction techniques are then used to create an anatomic image, a process analogous to computed tomography.

To date, medical imaging with MR by excitation of hydrogen atoms has been satisfactory only because of the relative abundance of hydrogen atoms in the body and their relatively high MR signal per nucleus. MR measurements of other biologically important nuclei, especially $^{13}_{6}C$, $^{19}_{9}F$, $^{23}_{11}Na$, $^{31}_{15}P$, and $^{39}_{19}K$ are possible; however, the lower inherent MR sensitivity for these nuclei and their lower physiologic concentrations limit the image resolution.

Of particular interest is the potential for studying cellular energy metabolism and enzyme kinetics by the excitation of P-31

TABLE 21–2. *Basic MR Pulse Sequences*

Method	Pulse sequence	Parameter measured
saturation-recovery	90°, τ, 90°: repeated n times for various values of τ	T_1
inversion-recovery	180°, τ, 90°: repeated n times for various values of τ	T_1*
steady-state-free-precession	time interval between pulse sequences $<<$ T_1 or T_2	ρ, T_1, T_2
spin-echo	90°, τ, $[180°, \tau]_k$: repeated n times for various values of τ	T_2

*The inversion-recovery method highlights T_1 more strongly than the saturation-recovery method.
Adapted from Partain, C.L., et al.[5]

in ATP and phosphocreatine.[13] Potential clinical applications lie in detecting metabolic alterations in malignant tissues and in understanding such musculoskeletal diseases as McArdle's syndrome.[14,15] Nonimaging topical instrumentation is being used to study in vivo phosphate metabolism. Because phosphorus is present in low concentration in tissues (0.4% of hydrogen abundance), however, and is 2.5 times less sensitive to resonance than hydrogen, the resolution achievable with present instrumentation is poor.

In terms of safety, there are no known biologic hazards associated with the magnetic fields and radiofrequency wavelengths used in medical MR imaging. Preliminary studies with bacteria, human erythrocytes, and cell cultures have demonstrated no deleterious effects.[16,17,18]

CLINICAL APPLICATIONS

Soft-tissue contrast is greatly increased with MR compared with x-ray CT. Unlike CT, the MR signals from fluids, soft tissue, and fat are much stronger than those from bone. Preliminary work indicates that MR may be useful in differentiating benign from malignant tissues. Results from serum studies remain unresolved;[19,20] however, some tumors have highly abnormal T_1 values.[21,22] MR shares with radionuclide imaging the property of being a functional, physiologic imaging technique.

MR may be applicable to measuring large-vessel blood flow. As mentioned, T_1 and T_2 are quite sensitive to molecular motion. Various scanning methods depict the signal from blood and cerebrospinal fluid (CSF) in different manners, because of the relative weight given to T_1, T_2, and ρ.[23,24,25]

Contrast agents may be necessary in MR, as in CT, to study certain regions of the body. Stable paramagnetic complexes may be given orally or intravenously to enhance tissue differences or metabolic changes. Paramagnetic agents decrease the T_1 signal of tissues when present in sufficient concentration. Compounds may also be labeled with nitroxide radicals for use as tissue-specific scanning agents.[26,27] Such flexibility is not present with CT or ultrasound. Design of agents may parallel the development of compounds for nuclear medicine and may enable functional imaging of such tissues as the pancreas.

Brain

In the brain, MR imaging easily identifies such space-occupying lesions as hematoma, abscess, and neoplasm, which are detected routinely by CT and radionuclide imaging (Fig. 21–6). T_1 images reveal striking gray-white matter differentiation, permitting visualization of basal ganglia and thalamus, and thus opening a new field for the diagnosis and classification of white matter diseases. For example, preliminary work has identified demyelinated plaques in patients with multiple sclerosis and normal CT scans.[28] MR may be useful in studying metabolic diseases and diffuse infectious diseases of brain parenchyma, two areas in which CT and radionuclide scanning have been of limited use.

Because of the absence of artifacts from surrounding bone, MR images clearly visualize the spinal cord, brainstem, and cerebellum, including their internal structure (Figs. 21–7 and 21–8). The major blood vessels can also be identified.

Heart

Gated cardiac imaging can be performed with MR, and anatomic resolution is sufficient to determine ventricular wall thickness, volume, cardiac motion, and ejection fraction (Fig. 21–9). Development of a paramagnetic contrast agent with properties similar to thallium would render the diagnosis of ischemia and infarction possible. Preliminary studies with intravenous Mn^{2+} demonstrate increased uptake of this agent by infarcted myocardial tissue

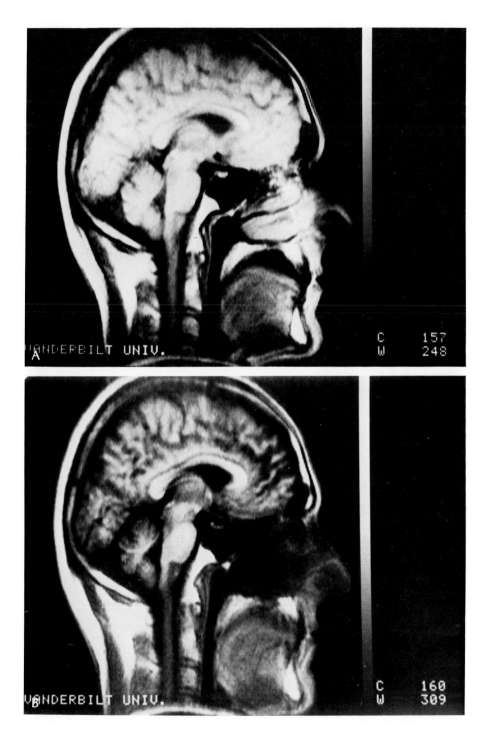

Fig. 21–6. Midline sagittal MR images of the head obtained using the Vanderbilt University 5000 Gauss Technicare superconducting imaging system. *A.* Spin echo pulse sequence, 2.3 min scan time. *B.* Inversion recovery pulse sequence, 6.7 min scan time. Note striking gray-white matter differentiation achieved in the brain image with strong T_1 dependence.

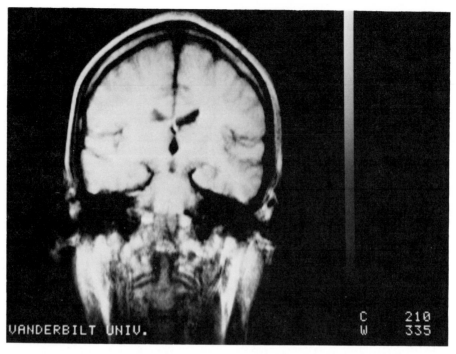

Fig. 21–7. Coronal MR image of the head obtained using 5000 Gauss superconducting system—spin echo pulse sequence, 2.3 min scan time. Note the excellent anatomic spatial resolution as well as the soft-tissue contrast resolution.

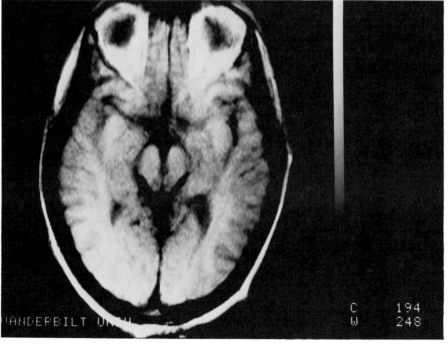

Fig. 21–8. Transverse MR image of the head, spin echo pulse sequence, 2.3 min scan time.

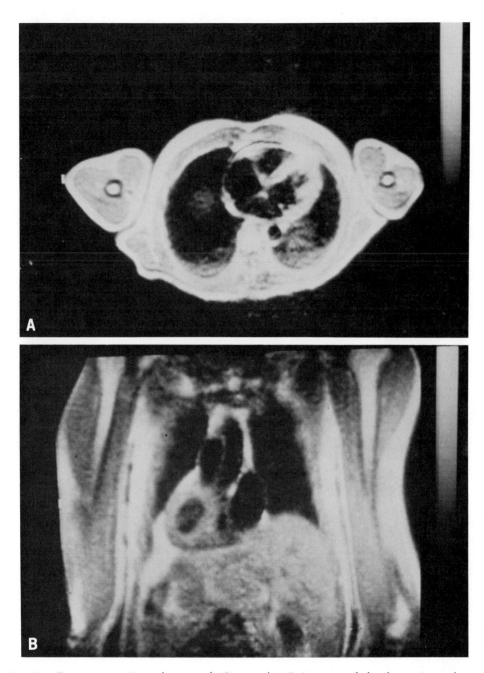

Fig. 21–9. Transverse (*A*) and coronal (*B*) gated MR images of the heart in end systole. (Courtesy, Technicare, Inc., Solon, Ohio)

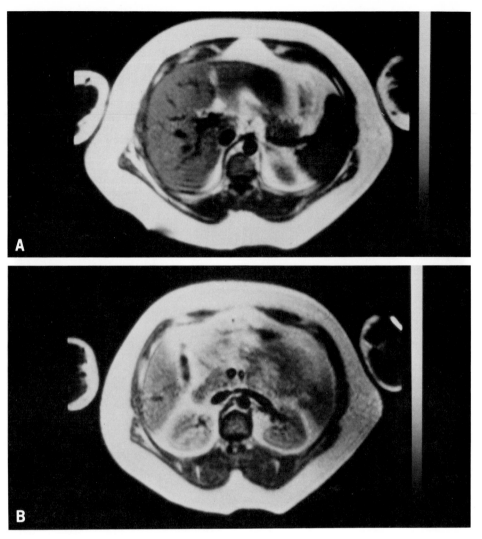

Fig. 21–10. Transverse images of the abdomen by MR. (*A*) Upper abdomen. (*B*) Midabdomen. (Courtesy, Technicare, Inc., Solon, Ohio)

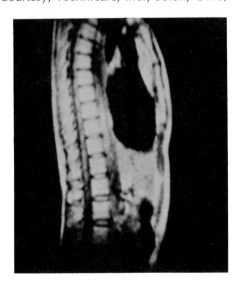

Fig. 21–11. Sagittal MR image of the spine and spinal cord. (Courtesy, Technicare, Inc., Solon, Ohio)

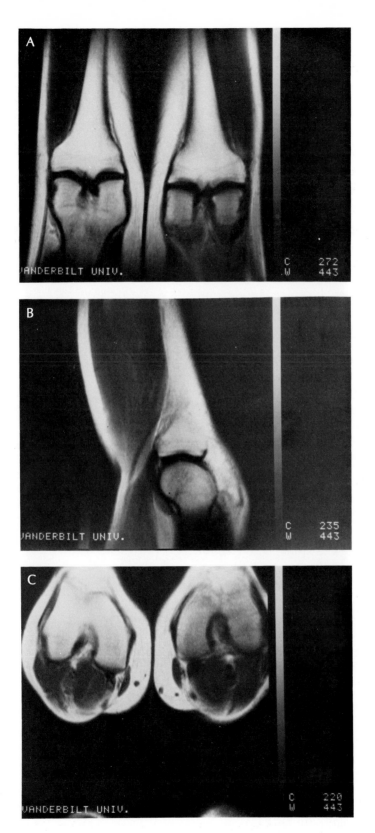

Fig. 21–12. MR images of the knee using a 5000 Gauss superconducting system—spin echo, 2.3 min scan time. (*A*) Coronal view; (*B*) Sagittal view; (*C*) Transverse view.

435

and thus selective enhancement of these areas in MR images.[29]

Abdominal Viscera

Such paramagnetic ions as iron and copper in sufficient concentration decrease the T_1 values of tissue. Liver diseases with increased concentrations of these ions include hemochromatosis, Wilson's disease, primary biliary cirrhosis, and certain states of alcoholic cirrhosis. Such measurements have not yet been proven clinically valuable.

Imaging by the inversion-recovery technique can distinguish renal cortex from medulla (Fig. 21–10). With the addition of an intravenously administered and renally excreted contrast agent, MR may prove useful in evaluating renal disease.[26] Assessment of renal blood supply and function is theoretically possible; however, the prospect of MR being able to compete in cost effectiveness or simplicity (even in terms of diagnostic information) with comparable radionuclide studies is doubtful.

Spine

Because of the absence of bone artifacts and the high soft-tissue resolution, MR imaging of the spine and spinal cord (1-mm-thick slice at any angle) is potentially useful as an alternative to myelography (Fig. 21–11). The gray and white matter of the cord can be differentiated, and the cauda equina identified. Neurologic diagnoses, which were previously possible only by histologic examination, may be feasible with MR.

Extremities

The major joints, including ligaments and tendons, can be identified in addition to the joint space (Fig. 21–12).

Recent symposia transactions and a comprehensive MR textbook are available that describe the historical perspectives, physics, technology, initial clinical results, correlation with other imaging techniques, economics, legal considerations, and current areas of investigation in MR imaging and diagnostic chemistry.[28,30,31,32]

REFERENCES

1. Lauterbur, P.C.: Image formation by induced local interactions: examples employing NMR. Nature, *242*:190, 1973.
2. Hutchison, J.M.S., Mallard, J.R., and Goll, C.: In vivo imaging of body structures using proton resonance. *In* Proc. 18th Ampere Congress, Nottingham, 1974. Edited by P.S. Allen, E.R. Andrew, and C.A. Bates. Amsterdam, North Holland, 1974, p. 283.
3. Mansfield, P., Grannell, P.K., and Maudsley, A.A.: "Diffraction" and microscopy in solids and liquids by NMR. *In* Proc. 18th Ampere Congress, Nottingham, 1974. Edited by P.S. Allen, E.R. Andrew, and C.A. Bates. Amsterdam, North Holland, 1974, p. 431.
4. Partain, C.L., James, A.E., Watston, J.T., et al.: Nuclear magnetic resonance and computed tomography. Radiology, *136*:767, 1980.
5. Partain, C.L., Price, R.R., Patton, J.A., et al.: Nuclear magnetic resonance imaging: An overview of the physical principles, clinical potential, and interrelationship with radionuclide imaging. *In* Nuclear Medicine Annual 1983. Edited by L. Freeman and H.S. Weissmann. New York, Raven Press, 1983.
6. Damadian, R.: Field-focusing nuclear magnetic resonance (FONAR) and the formation of chemical scans in man. Philos. Trans. R. Soc. Lond., *289*:489, 1980.
7. Hinshaw, W.S.: Image formation by nuclear magnetic resonance: the sensitive point method. J. Appl. Phys., *47*:3709, 1976.
8. Mansfield, P., Maudsley, A.A., and Baines, T.: Fast scan proton density imaging by NMR. J. Phys. (E.), *9*:271, 1976.
9. Mallard, J., Hutchison, J.M.S., Edelstein, W. et al.: Imaging by nuclear magnetic resonance and its bio-medical implications. J. Biomed. Eng., *1*:159, 1979.
10. Holland, G.N., Hawkes, R.C., and Moore, W.S.: Nuclear magnetic resonance (NMR) tomography of the brain: coronal and sagittal sections. J. Comput. Tomog., *4*:429, 1980.
11. Andrew, E.R.: Nuclear magnetic resonance imaging: the multiple sensitive point method. IEEE Trans. Nucl. Sci., *27*:1232, 1980.
12. Brooker, H.R., and Hinshaw, W.S.: Thin-section NMR imaging. J. Mag. Res., *30*:129, 1978.
13. Burt, C.T., Cohen, S.M., and Barany, M.: Analysis of intact tissue with ^{31}P NMR. Annu. Rev. Biophys. Bioeng., *8*:1, 1979.
14. Koutcher, J.A., and Damadian, R.: Spectral differences in the ^{31}P NMR of normal and malignant tissue. Physiol. Chem. Phys., *9*:181, 1977.
15. Ross, B.D., Radda, G.K., Gadian, D.G., et al.: Examination of a case of suspected McArdle's syn-

drome by ³¹P nuclear magnetic resonance. N. Engl. J. Med., *304*:1338, 1981.

16. Thomas, A., and Morris, P.G.: The effects of NMR exposure on living organisms. I: A microbial assay. Br. J. Radiol., *54*:615, 1981.

17. Cooke, P., and Morris, P.G.: The effects of NMR exposure on living organisms. II: A genetic study of human lymphocytes. Br. J. Radiol., *54*:622, 1981.

18. Wolff, S., Crooks, L.E., Brown, P., et al.: Tests for DNA and chromosomal damage induced by nuclear magnetic resonance imaging. Radiology, *136*:707, 1980.

19. Ekstrand, K.E., Dixon, R.L., Raker, M., and Ferree, C.F.: Proton NMR relaxation in the peripheral blood of cancer patients. Phys. Med. Biol., *22*:925, 1977.

20. Hazelwood, C.E., Cleveland, G., and Medina, D.: Relationship between hydration and proton nuclear magnetic resonance relaxation times in tissues of tumor bearing mice: Implications for cancer detection. J. Natl. Cancer Inst., *52*:1849, 1974.

21. Goldsmith, M., Koutcher, J., and Damadian, R.: NMR in cancer. XI. Application of NMR malignancy index to human gastro-intestinal tumors. Cancer, *41*:174, 1978.

22. Koutcher, J.A., Goldsmith, M., and Damadian, R.: NMR in cancer. X. A malignancy index to discriminate normal and cancerous tissue. Cancer, *41*:174, 1978.

23. Singer, J.R.: Blood flow measurements by NMR of the intact body. *In* Nuclear Magnetic Resonance (NMR) Imaging. Edited by C.L. Partain, A.E. James, F.D. Rollo, and R.R. Price. Philadelphia, W.B. Saunders, 1983.

24. Bergmann, W.H.: A new approach to NMR flow imaging and analysis. *In* Nuclear Magnetic Resonance (NMR) Imaging. Edited by C.L. Partain, A.E. James, F.D. Rollo, and R.R. Price. Philadelphia, W.B. Saunders, 1983.

25. Singer, J.R.: Blood flow rates by nuclear magnetic resonance measurements. Science, *130*:1652, 1979.

26. Runge, V.M., Clanton, J.A., Jones, M.M., et al.: Paramagnetic NMR contrast agents: Development and evaluation of oral and intravenous agents. Radiology, *147*:789, 1983.

27. Brasch, R.C., Nitecki, E.D., Brant-Zowadzki, M.N., et al.: "NSFR": NMR contrast agent for the CNS. (Abstract) XII Symposium Neuroradiologicum, Washington, D.C., 1982.

28. Partain, C.L., James, A.E., Rollo, F.D., and Price, R.R. (Eds.): Nuclear Magnetic Resonance (NMR) Imaging. Philadelphia, W.B. Saunders, 1983.

29. Gore, J.C., Doyle, F.H., and Pennock, J.M.: Relaxation rate enhancement observed in vivo by NMR imaging. *In* Nuclear Magnetic Resonance (NMR) Imaging. Edited by C.L. Partain, A.E. James, F.D. Rollo, and R.R. Price. Philadelphia, W.B. Saunders, 1982.

30. James, A.E., and Partain, C.L.: Proc., Vanderbilt Nuclear Magnetic Resonance (NMR) Imaging Symposium. J. Comp. Tomog., *5*:285, 1981.

31. Witcofski, R.L., Karstaedt, N., and Partain, C.L.: NMR Imaging Proceedings, International Symposium on Nuclear Magnetic Resonance Imaging. Bowman Gray School of Medicine of Wake Forest University, 1982.

32. Lauterbur, P.C., Pohost, G., et al.: Proc. Soc. Magnetic Resonance in Medicine, Boston, August 1982.

Chapter 22

DIGITAL SUBTRACTION ANGIOGRAPHY—RELATIONS TO NUCLEAR MEDICINE

DENNIS D. PATTON AND
GERALD D. POND

Digital subtraction angiography (DSA) is a branch of the broader imaging technology known as *photoelectronic radiology.* This technology relies upon advanced large-memory, high-speed computer techniques to present a highly processed and manipulated image of the original object, with the characteristics of greatest interest to the observer accentuated. These images, whether reproductions of chest radiographs, bony structures, or vascular anatomy, are viewed on a CRT on which the images can be actively manipulated. The needs and preferences of different viewers can be satisfied, and the object can be imaged with emphasis on different details and features.

Photoelectronic radiology includes a wide variety of techniques for processing radiographic images; digital subtraction angiography is one subspecialty area within this field.[1,2,3,4,5] Also known as *intravenous angiography* (IVA), as *digital video subtraction angiography* (DVSA), and by other terms, DSA is one of the most advanced and developed forms of photoelectronic radiology in that subtraction techniques, which first made diagnostic DSA images possible, are best suited to examination of the vascular system. The basic technique for producing subtraction radiographs has been available since 1935.[6] Further development of the original subtraction technique was desirable because of the high toxicity of the original radiographic contrast agents, which could be used safely only at low concentrations. Conventional radiographic subtraction using photographic techniques has been widely available, but its use is limited by the technical difficulties involved in accurate registration of films and in achieving optimal exposure. The advent of the computer gave rise to a completely new range of image manipulation techniques, especially control of exposure and registration. Image subtraction still involves some trial and error, but the trials are computer operations requiring only a few seconds, and the images are presented to the viewer instantly.

Therefore, digital subtraction angiography is an idea whose timing is remarkable, but not coincidental: only in recent years has the computer technology needed for DSA become accessible. Techniques of image manipulation have developed rapidly, largely because of the development of CT scanners, although DSA image reconstruction is based on a different principle. Also, much has been learned about the relationships between X-ray absorption coefficients and film density, and between contrast and conspicuity. Thus the technological background of DSA rests largely upon the prior development of other imaging methods.

Until recently radiologists were accustomed to viewing radiographs that represented x-ray transmission through organ structures recorded on film, with no manipulation other than ordinary film processing. Largely because of the development of CT, radiologists are now more experienced with images that represent more than simple, two-dimensional reproductions of the original object. They can interpret images that have been filtered, smoothed, subtracted, enhanced, and otherwise manipulated to bring out certain details.[7] As a rule, interpretation of DSA images is made from the cathode-ray display unless logistic factors prevent it. Active manipulation of the image is simplest when using computer-CRT interaction. Usually, final record on film is made to produce a "hard copy" for the patient's file.

The advantages of using DSA are many. Patients do not require any special preparation and usually do not need premedication. The procedure is ordinarily done on an outpatient basis since arterial puncture is unnecessary and close postprocedural observation of the patient is not required. Because digital subtraction studies are less expensive than conventional angiography, the savings to the patient, including the avoidance of hospitalization, are impressive. Ordinarily, the cost of DSA is about one third that of conventional angiography.[8,9] DSA studies usually require only 30 to 45 min, depending on the area of the body being examined. Whereas intra-arterial injections are often painful,[10] intravenous studies are associated only with a sensation of flushing, or with occasional transient nausea; more severe complications are rare. Overall, DSA causes the patient little discomfort and gains excellent patient acceptance.

Safety is an essential advantage of DSA since the complications of conventional angiography can be serious.[11] These complications include arterial extravasation, arterial embolization, arterial spasm leading to tissue ischemia, and hematoma, in addition to the hazards of the contrast agent itself, which are often greater in arterial than in intravenous injections. Although DSA is occasionally performed with intra-arterial injections (with the advantages of lower contrast dose administration than with conventional angiography and virtually instantaneous subtraction), the majority of examinations involve injections into the central venous system. This approach has proved to be remarkably safe.[12,13,14,15,16]

TECHNICAL DESCRIPTION

The basic equipment required for DSA consists of a high-resolution x-ray machine combined with a large-memory, high-speed computer. The system and a block diagram are shown in Figures 22–1 and 22–2. Sufficient exposure at the image intensifier face is mandatory for satisfactory imaging, and a one-milliroentgen exposure at the intensifier is usually required. Therefore, the x-ray tube must be a high-flux, high-heat-capacity tube that allows for multiple relatively short exposures. This condition is especially important at such rapid imaging rates as with cardiac examinations, which may require image acquisition at frame rates of up to 30/sec. A typical contemporary video system might use an Amperex frogs-head Plumbicon incorporated into a Sierra

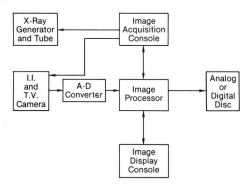

Fig. 22–1. Block diagram of digital subtraction angiography system. The configuration of this prototype system has been altered several times, but the basic system design remains the same. I.I. = image intensifier.

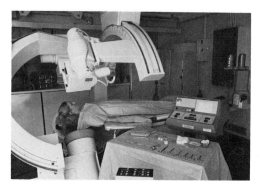

Fig. 22–2. DSA facility with double C-arm for biplane compatibility. Both 9-in. and 16-in. image intensifiers are located beneath patient's head. Power contrast injector is at right.

video camera that is optically coupled to the image intensifier. The signal-to-noise ratio of this high-resolution system is approximately 1000:1, compared with approximately 300:1 in a typical fluoroscopic system.

Another feature of the DSA system is the image stability from one exposure to the next. This feature is important because subtraction images cannot be successfully obtained if comparable exposure levels are not made in each image frame, especially at rapid filming rates. The video camera can operate in either an *interlaced* or a *noninterlaced* mode. Noninterlaced image acquisition is analogous to a "snapshot" in which 256 to 1024 lines of information can be obtained in a single exposure. In the interlaced mode of operation, two sequential frames of information are displayed simultaneously, so that the interlaced scan lines provide twice the number of lines of information per unit area on the display. This method probably is used most effectively with rapid frame rates because sequential images may contain virtually the same information. At slower frame rates, motion precludes using the interlaced mode.

Analog-to-digital converters must have a high-speed capacity. Digitization of a 512 × 512 pixel matrix must be made with 8-bit precision (256 gray levels) in real time. The digitized image is sent to an image processor, which is essentially the image storage and manipulation device. The image processor can then transfer bidirectionally to and from the disk for storage (although it can access this stored information nearly instantaneously). The image processor also interacts directly with the image-acquisition console and with the image-display console.

Several mathematical manipulations are performed on the image signal at different stages, including logarithmic amplification, windowing, temporal smoothing, and scaling. Even rapid computers, in evaluating complex algebraic, logarithmic, or trigonometric functions, usually use more computer time when evaluating the function analytically than when using lookup tables to find the output value corresponding to a given set of input values. Since in this application the final image has only a limited number of gray levels (typically 256), assigning a gray level to a given signal by using a lookup table is faster than calculating the gray level analytically. Lookup tables greatly speed image processing and make real-time digital subtraction imaging possible, providing what amounts to a fluoroscopic study.

The image intensifier used for DSA must provide very high resolution. At present, most intensifiers have a maximum diameter of 9 in., which limits the field of view. Newer image intensifiers (Thompson, Inc.) have a nominal 16-in. maximum diameter (with a usable field of approximately 14.5 in.). These intensifiers make examinations of the thorax, viscera, and peripheral "run-off" feasible. This tube also offers 10-in. and 6-in. modes.

The intensifier is scanned by a 512 × 512 television system that limits resolution to approximately two line pairs/mm. Because contrast injections given on the venous side may be as dilute as 0.5% by the time they reach the arterial side, high-signal amplification is required. For this reason, the system is designed so that as little electronic noise as possible is added to the x-ray image. To preserve image quality, the television camera system used with the image intensifier should have a signal-to-noise ratio better than that of the image intensifier, i.e., better than 300:1, and ideally over 1000:1.

Among the factors influencing resolution is size of the focal spot in the x-ray tube. In general, focal spots are 0.5 to 2 mm in diameter, but focal spots as small as 0.05 mm are available. Small focal spots provide high resolution, but cannot be obtained using a high flux of electrons, because the x-ray output must be limited. Large focal spots are compatible with high output, but they limit resolution.

In the detector portion of the image intensifier, x-rays are converted to light by a phosphor, which emits visible light of a wavelength suitable for the image intensifier system. The light output of the phosphor has a flux much higher than that of the incoming x-ray beam. In other words, several light photons are produced for each x-ray photon striking the phosphor. The multiplication of photons (from x-ray to light) does not improve the signal-to-noise ratio, and in fact, the excess light places a burden on the intensifier system. To limit the amount of light that the image intensifier has to handle, a diaphragm is positioned between the detector and the intensifier. (Decreasing x-ray exposure decreases the signal-to-noise ratio; decreasing the number of light photons does not appreciably affect the ratio, because many of the light photons are redundant.)

Currently available resolutions are on the order of two line pairs per millimeter under optimum conditions (lead bars separated by air and no scatter medium). In current systems, the image intensifier itself limits resolution. Quantum mottle and scatter of light within the optics of the image intensifier (*veiling glare*) reduce contrast and limit resolution. The crystal grain size of the phosphor does not appear to limit resolution.

Once the image has been digitized and stored (in 256 shades of gray), the dynamic range of video intensity is selected. Because the video display can handle only 12 shades of gray, the window (typically selected to correspond to the contrast established by iodine in Renografin 76 by Squibb) can be narrowed electronically so that subtle changes in x-ray attenuation are spread out over the entire window to accentuate small differences between structures. This manipulation is virtually identical to that used for CT interpretation.

Window

In the original subtraction image, there is a distribution of brightness levels as shown in Figure 22–3A. Features of anatomic interest within a brightness range can be enhanced as follows. In the unsubtracted image, a brightness range is selected (B_1 to B_2). This image is convoluted with a function having a variable amplification factor in different brightness regions (Figure 22–3B). The amplification factor is low in regions outside the window, but is high within the window B_1 to

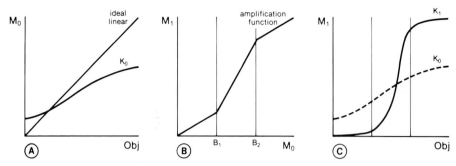

Fig. 22–3. Windowing and differential amplification; see text for details. All axes indicate brightness level. Obj = object (in this case, the image intensifier screen). M_0 = unprocessed image. M_1 = processed image. K_0 = relationship of image to object brightness in unprocessed image. K_1 = same, in processed image.

B_2. The convoluted image is shown in Figure 22–3C, in which regions outside the window have low contrast, but the regions within the window have greatly enhanced contrast. The narrower the window, the greater the contrast within a more limited range of pixel brightness. The slope of the amplification curve at any point is analogous to the gamma function of ordinary film. The amplification function can be modified in many ways: the slopes can be altered at will, the slopes can be inverted (reversing whites and blacks), or the function can be repeated periodically over the entire brightness range, giving a "folded" image.

In the clinical setting, an image frame is recorded prior to contrast injection. This image frame is used as a "mask" for subtraction purposes. The contrast is then injected, and when the peak concentration within the vascular area of interest is reached, this raw data frame is recorded, and the two images are electronically subtracted in the image processor. The image initially produced after subtraction, if perfect, shows only faint contrast within the arterial structures of interest and no other structures. Subtraction images are often less than perfect, however: patients breathe, move involuntarily, or swallow (especially troublesome on cervical vessel studies). Peristaltic motion is difficult to overcome in some patients during abdom-

inal studies, although using abdominal compression and intravenous glucagon may help to minimize this motion. In cardiopulmonary studies, vessel and cardiac pulsation make it difficult to obtain high-quality subtraction images. ECG gating or image acquisition at higher frame rates may increase the probability of a good match between the *raw data* and *mask* frames.

Following the initial computer subtraction, the window level is selected and the window width is compressed to accentuate contrast. Figure 22–4 shows a typical example of mask and raw data frames, electronic subtraction, and contrast enhancement. Contrast can be reversed to white on black, if desired.

Contrast Injection

The contrast agent can be delivered by several means. Peripheral injections can be made through short 16-gauge angiocatheters introduced into a large antecubital vein. This technique is more convenient than a central catheter but is also associated with occasional contrast extravasation. A centrally placed 5, 6 or 7 French pigtail catheter can be introduced over a guidewire passed after venipuncture using a thin-walled needle. This requires only a few minutes more than peripheral introduction of the catheter and has the advantage of preventing local ex-

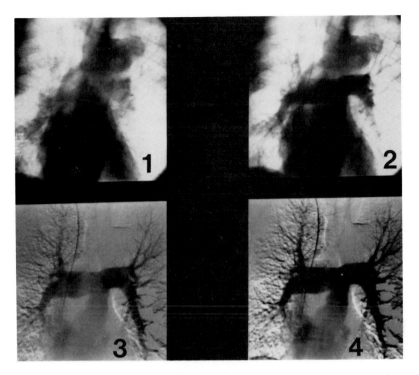

Fig. 22–4.   Sequence of images in pulmonary DSA: (1) "Scout" image, prior to contrast arrival. (2) "Raw data" frame, at peak arterial contrast. (3) Initial nonenhanced subtraction. (4) Contrast enhancement after video density slope is increased.

travasation at the venipuncture site. In addition, the central bolus of contrast appears to be delivered more compactly, with improved visualization of the arteries. Most contrast injections, however, are made into the superior vena cava, or preferably the right atrium, with apparently no increased risk to the patient. In patients injected intra-atrially, no contrast extravasation has been observed. Premature atrial contractions are noted in approximately 5% of patients injected through either the superior vena cava or the right atrium. Previous studies of electrocardiographic response during intravenous urography have shown that arrhythmias are not rare, regardless of the injection site of the contrast agent.[17,18] Ventricular tachycardia and other serious arrhythmias have been reported in conjunction with routine urography but are rare.

Intra-atrial injections deliver an observ-

ably better bolus of contrast for several reasons. First, the right atrium is a distensible structure, unlike the superior or inferior vena cava, and as a consequence, the power-injected contrast agent distends the atrium rather than refluxing up and down the vena cava. At the same time, the rapid distension of the atrium causes a positive inotropic effect (Starling's law), which results in a stronger atrial contraction. This in turn increases right ventricular end diastolic volume, and the same mechanism produces a stronger ventricular systole.

The amount of contrast agent injected varies depending on both the region examined and the clinical circumstances of the study. This amount ranges from 10 to 25 ml/sec for a total of 20 to 50 ml. Image acquisition rates also vary considerably. For some patients with severe peripheral vascular disease, frame rates of 1 film/3 sec for a total of 1 min would not be unusual.

Cardiac cases require up to 30 frames/sec. Ordinarily, an intracranial or visceral study requires from 1 to 6 frames/sec.

Conventional angiography requires an intra-arterial concentration of radiographic contrast agent of at least 40 to 50% for reliable detection. With conventional photographic subtraction, this lower limit ranges from 4 to 5%. With DSA, however, the lower limit of concentration can range from 0.4 to 2%.[3,14] The DSA technique increases apparent contrast resolution at the expense of spatial resolution,[19] an advantage nonetheless, since many clinical decisions do not require the exquisite anatomic detail obtainable with conventional angiography. MacIntyre et al. have studied the imaging capabilities of DSA systems.[3] For very small objects (less than 0.3 mm), DSA requires higher contrast for reliable detection than that required by conventional film systems, although less contrast is needed for objects over 2 mm partly because of the greater number of photons detected in the region of interest. The threshold detection in the contrast sensitivity range is basically noise-limited. But image contrast and signal-to-noise ratio do not adequately describe the detection process, nor do they explain why DSA images seem to allow the features of interest to "jump out." The concept of *conspicuity* was developed to gain a better understanding of detection. Revesz et al. define conspicuity as the ratio of contrast to complexity, i.e., the contrast in a region of the image in relationship to the complexity of its surroundings.[20] The subtraction process of a mask image from a raw data image results in both enhancement of the contrast in the structures whose x-ray absorption changed, and reduction of the nontarget background that did not change, which in turn result in greatly enhanced conspicuity (Fig. 22–4). In general, the signal-to-noise ratio in the subtracted image is lower than that in the unsubtracted image, so DSA does not improve signal over noise.

It does improve conspicuity and thereby the ability of the observer to detect image features that represent change.

Dual-Energy Subtraction

The conspicuity of the iodine-containing contrast agent in the image can be enhanced by a dual-energy technique described by Mistretta et al.[21] Recall that photon energies below the binding energy of the K-shell electrons are incapable of ejecting these electrons from the atom by the photoelectric effect, and that photons above this energy can. Thus a sharp discontinuity in the absorption coefficient for iodine occurs in the region of the K-shell binding energy, which is approximately 33 keV (see Fig. 3–15). Atomic numbers of most other elements in the body are much lower, with lower K-shell binding energies. Thus, for photons in the 33 keV range, only iodine would be expected to show a substantially higher absorption coefficient for photon energies slightly exceeding the 33-keV discontinuity.

To enhance the iodine content of the image, two images are taken—one using photons of energy slightly lower than 33 keV, the other using photons of slightly higher energy. One image is subtracted from the other. Since tissue that does not contain iodine has about the same absorption with each of the two energies, differences in the two images should be ascribable to iodine.

This technique involves several major problems that have limited its development. The nearly monoenergetic x-rays required for this technique are difficult to generate. Conventional filters can be used but result in significant loss of intensity. Using iodine and cerium filters, Mistretta et al. generated two photon beams with peaks above and below the iodine K-edge.[21] The differential absorption by iodine was approximately 40% of that expected for monoenergetic beams—a 15-fold loss of beam intensity occurred. The second problem is that even with monochromatic x-rays the differential absorption signal is only 2.5% for each mg/cm^2 of iodine, and only 1% using a nearly monoenergetic beam.[21] This low contrast can be handled by current video imaging techniques, temporal smoothing, and computer manipulation.

A further limitation is the high absorption of 33-keV photons in tissue, which limits the body thickness that can be effectively imaged with this technique. Quantum mottle significantly degrades images of bodies thicker than approximately 15 cm, and to date, no computer program has been written that effectively removes this type of image degradation. Dual-energy subtraction can be used in real-time.[22] Iodine and cerium filters are used to filter alternate frames of pulsed 50-kVp x-rays. The iodine image is isolated by weighted subtraction of successive video fields.

CLINICAL APPLICATIONS

Digital subtraction angiography is replacing conventional angiography in many areas because diagnostically adequate images can be produced with DSA more quickly, less expensively, and with less risk to the patient than with conventional techniques. The need for arteriotomy is averted, as is the need for arterial catheterization, which can produce significant complications. The safety aspect of DSA has opened a new area of vascular investigation: screening angiography. Screening patients for any type of asymptomatic or subclinical disease using routine arteriography is considered too risky. Now, however, screening for carotid occlusive disease, renovascular hypertension, peripheral vascular lesions, and even coronary artery disease is possible with DSA.

Studies of the Central Nervous System

Digital subtraction angiography permits adequate visualization of the carotid arteries and branches down to the third order.[23] DSA can be used to demonstrate stenoses, occlusions, atheromatous ulcers, and abnormal vascular patterns. It can be used routinely to assess the carotid artery following endarterectomy. Although the detail of the intima is not nearly as clear with DSA as with conventional angiography, it is adequate for almost all clinical applications (Fig. 22–5). The internal carotid artery can be well visualized in the petrous, cavernous, and supraclinoid segments. Such techniques for determining carotid patency as Doppler, real-time, and duplex ultrasound (which combines real-time and Doppler capabilities) are excellent noninvasive techniques, reasonably sensitive for high-grade stenosis, but less reliable when stenoses are less severe. Ulcerations within plaques cannot be routinely detected by these noninvasive techniques, and the technique is less sensitive after endarterectomy.

Images of the intracranial vasculature provide valuable information about flow patterns and identify many aneurysms (both intracranial and extracranial), arteriovenous malformations, thrombosis of the superior sagittal sinus, subdural hematoma, intracranial tumors, and stroke patterns (Figures 22–5 through 22–7). Luxury perfusion patterns as well as areas of reduced blood flow are readily demonstrated. The characteristic "flip-flop" pattern of stroke with delayed perfusion via collaterals can be demonstrated by the DSA study in the same manner as it is demonstrated by the conventional radionuclide dynamic blood flow study.[2,13,14,24,25,26,27,28,29,30]

In CNS examinations using DSA, motion is the most common problem and results in a nondiagnostic study. Low cardiac output, with consequent failure to deliver a compact arterial bolus, and technical difficulties account for some failed studies.

Pulmonary Studies

The main pulmonary artery and branches down to the third order can be

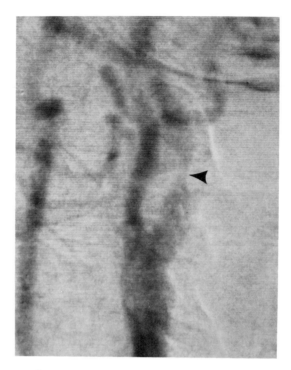

Fig. 22–5. DSA image showing a stenotic lesion at the proximal internal carotid artery (arrowhead). Note filling of vertebral artery. Oblique projection is used to avoid superimposition of vertebral and carotid arteries.

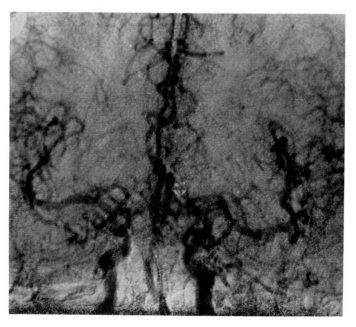

Fig. 22–6. Normal intracranial vessels (arterial phase) in anterior projection. Note distribution of internal carotid, anterior cerebral, and middle cerebral arteries.

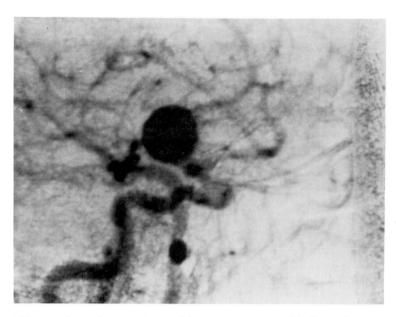

Fig. 22–7. Oblique view of internal carotid artery aneurysm (dark area).

readily demonstrated by DSA. In most patients, unless large image intensifiers are used, the entire lung cannot be examined at one time. The DSA study is useful in demonstrating pulmonary emboli in patients whose perfusion lung scans demonstrate nonspecific perfusion defects. Patient cooperation is necessary for this study: the patient must hold his breath for several seconds during passage of the contrast bolus. Breath holding is difficult for many patients with pulmonary disease, including pulmonary embolism, and as a result, not all DSA studies yield the desired information.

The perfusion lung scan is important for selecting patients for pulmonary DSA studies. Prior to performing any pulmonary intravenous angiography, except in the most emergent situations (as in the case of anticipated emergency pulmonary embolectomy), a perfusion lung scan is obtained. This scan serves to exclude patients who have no convincing evidence for pulmonary embolism, and also serves as a "road map" to the area of highest probability of emboli.

Limited-field-of-view image intensifiers

permit greater resolution. Radiographic contrast agent is injected directly into the right atrium to provide a compact, undiluted bolus. Films are obtained at the rate of 2 per sec, usually for 10 to 15 sec. Subtraction images are available from the computer display almost immediately, and these initial views are analyzed. The combination of the perfusion lung scan and the pulmonary DSA study (if the lung scan suggests pulmonary emboli) can give definitive diagnostic information in a short time, and at relatively little risk or discomfort to the patient.[31] Figure 22–8 shows a representative case of a patient with pulmonary embolism in whom chest x-ray, lung scan, pulmonary DSA, and conventional pulmonary angiography were performed.

Cardiac Studies

By appropriately manipulating the sequence of images taken during transit of the bolus of contrast agent through the heart, images of the heart in end diastole, end systole, or any other stage can be obtained. Both the atria and the ventricles can be shown clearly, though not reliably

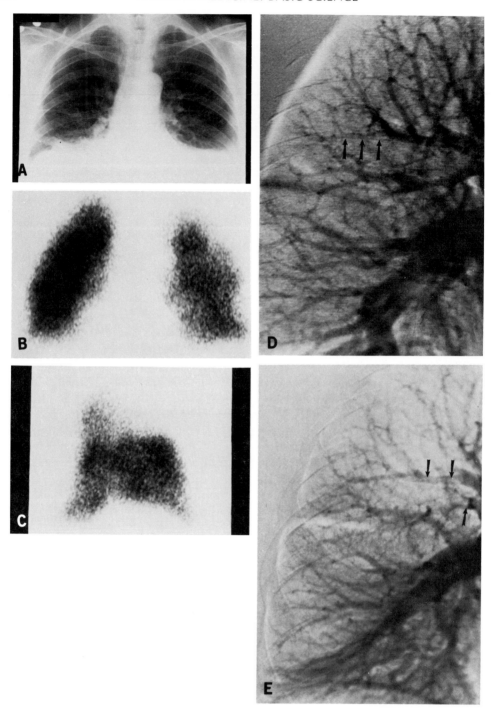

Fig. 22–8. Pulmonary embolism. *A*, chest x-ray; *B*, perfusion lung scan (posterior view); *C*, perfusion lung scan (right lateral view); *D*, DSA image (catheter in right atrium) showing intraluminal defect in anterior segmental branch of right upper lobe (note raster lines in this older image); *E*, conventional pulmonary arteriogram with subtraction (catheter in right main pulmonary artery), confirming the DSA finding. Note superior resolution on the conventional angiogram. Perfusion lung scans showed the lesion and possibly others; angiograms established the diagnosis.

in all cases. Myocardial contractility can be assessed on a regional basis, and areas of abnormal wall motion can be identified. DSA can be used to estimate left ventricular ejection fraction and wall motion; the techniques are analogous to those used in radionuclide studies of the heart.[16] Carey et al. measured cardiac output in dogs by using DSA techniques and found excellent correlation with thermodilution techniques.[32] Left ventricular volume was measured using area-length methods. The so-called time-interval difference (TID) mode is a form of DSA and has been used by Crummy et al. and Kruger et al. at the Cleveland Clinic to evaluate myocardial contractility.[1,33]

Usually, the valve plane is easier to locate in cardiac images than in radionuclide images. Furthermore, subtraction of end systole from end diastole yields functional images that contain considerably more detail than corresponding radionuclide images. Paradoxical motion is often clearly shown. With appropriate projections, the valve planes and cardiac chambers can be imaged (Figure 22–9). The pulmonary, mitral and aortic valves are often seen to good advantage on the DSA images. Simple superimposition of the end-diastolic and end-systolic images, with computer subtraction, yields images in which dyskinetic and akinetic segments of the myocardial wall can be easily identified. Figure 22–9C shows a canine model in which the left anterior descending coronary artery has been ligated, producing an anterior wall myocardial infarction. The ventricular aneurysm that occurs in most instances after coronary ligation can be readily demonstrated. The occlusion of the left anterior descending artery is identifiable, as are the remaining normal branches.

The intravenous technique for visualizing the coronary arteries, however, is beset with problems that need to be resolved. Because of the rapid cardiac motion, good subtraction studies are often difficult to obtain. Dual-energy techniques can be used to obtain images almost simultaneously but at different energies, so that iodine is emphasized in one frame and de-emphasized in the other. Theoretically, use of these techniques can result in nearly perfect subtraction.

Quantitative studies of cardiac function, such as calculation of left ventricular ejection fraction, depend on accurate determination of blood volume within a defined region. Left ventricular ejection fraction, for example, could be calculated by assuming a relationship between volume and radiographic density within the left ventricle. This relationship is complex, and as of this writing, no completely satisfactory densitometric measurements of left ventricular ejection fraction have been achieved, although considerable work is progressing in this direction.[34,35,36] The densitometric approach to the determination of left ventricular volume is analogous to the use of count-density information in radionuclide determination. A more common approach to measuring left ventricular volume is a geometric one based on the conventional area-length method. This approach requires accurate determination of ventricular major axis and area, preferably in two projections. The resolution of DSA (on the order of 1 mm) is much better than that of radionuclide imaging (on the order of 1 cm), so that cardiac chamber edges, valve planes, and other anatomic landmarks are defined more easily.

Several constraints, however, limit the accuracy of DSA in quantitative studies of left ventricular performance: (1) The subtraction process requires accurate registration of images, which means that there should be no patient motion, although in practice there is often involuntary motion through respiration, body movement, or the ballistocardiographic effect. (2) Cardiac motion is a complex combination of rotation and translation that defies simple analysis by subtraction of images obtained

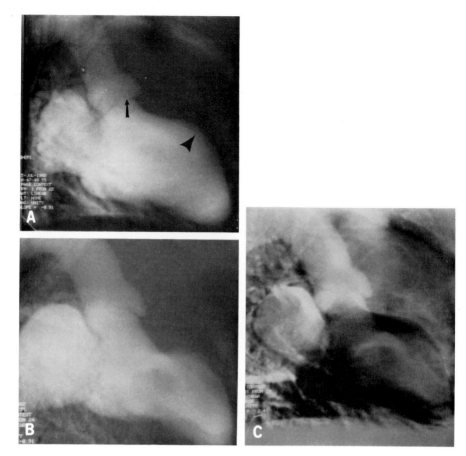

Fig. 22–9. Right anterior oblique view of canine heart one week after ligation of the left anterior descending branch of the left main coronary artery. *A*, end-diastolic image. Note aneurysm along anterior wall of left ventricle (arrowhead), and definition of aortic valve cusps (arrow). *B*, end-systolic image. The atrium is in end diastole, the ventricle at end systole. Note akinesia at the aneurysm site. *C*, subtraction image (of another canine heart study); end diastole minus end systole. Ejection fraction can be estimated from this analysis.

at different points in the cardiac cycle. (3) The major axis of the left ventricle may change between systole and diastole and be difficult to track, especially in patients with regional wall motion abnormalities. (4) Even at low concentrations in DSA studies, the contrast agent may still have some effect on myocardial contractility.[37]

There is hope that DSA can ultimately be used as a substitute for invasive selective coronary arteriography by serving as a screening procedure to allow direct evaluation of the coronary arteries.[32,38] At present, however, injections are made into

the aortic root, which is a nonselective but still invasive method. The nonselective coronary artery study is safer than selective catheter placement, as it overcomes the problems of introducing small emboli, raising intimal flaps, or producing coronary artery spasm from catheter introduction. Figure 22–10 demonstrates nonselective injection into the aortic root to visualize the coronary arteries in a canine model.

Pediatric congenital heart disease with pulmonary atresia, aortic arch anomalies, and coarctation has also been studied, and

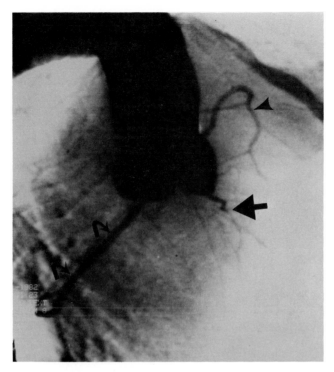

Fig. 22–10. Coronary arteries (canine) after aortic injection. (Same dog as in Figs. 22–8A,B.) Note circumflex branch of left coronary artery (arrowhead), as well as the ligated proximal left anterior descending artery (arrow) and right coronary artery (curved arrows).

has shown good correlation with conventional cine studies, two-dimensional echo, and respiration-gated images.[39]

The superior resolution of DSA images offers competition to radionuclide studies of the heart, especially those involving cardiac output, ejection fraction, and wall motion. The contrast studies are analogs of labeled blood pool studies, and they convey much of the same information, though in a different format. The complementary roles of DSA and radionuclide studies of the heart have yet to be determined.

Renal Studies

The abdominal aorta, renal arteries, and branches down to the third order are demonstrated by DSA. Renal conditions that can be elucidated by visualizing the vascularity can be expected to be of intense interest in the development of DSA. Un-

fortunately, vessel overlap and patient motion are critical problems in this area. One major difficulty in visualizing the renal and other visceral arteries is peristalsis, which can be only partially remedied by intravenous administration of glucagon and application of abdominal compression to displace overlying bowel gas. In many cases, the artifact caused by peristalsis creates technical problems in interpretation, and usually as a result, multiple views are needed to arrive at a reliable diagnosis. Overlap of the myriad vessels in the abdomen is the other major difficulty, especially overlap of the superior mesenteric artery and its branches. In spite of these limitations, the DSA technique has proved valuable.

For the first time, a noninvasive technique that allows direct visualization of the renal arteries has been made available. This technique enables safe screening of a patient population suspected of having renovascular hypertension potentially correctable by surgery.[15,40,41] If in screening for renovascular hypertension a renal arterial lesion is found (Fig. 22–11), the venous catheter can simply be advanced selectively into the renal veins to obtain selective renin samples in the same sitting.

An important application is found in screening potential renal donors. The number, size, and position of the renal arteries can be evaluated easily. The problem of vascular overlap, however, and the tragic surgical complications that can result from failure to recognize an accessory renal artery, mean that DSA will probably not replace conventional arteriograms in every case.

In patients who have undergone renal allograft transplants, intravenous angiography of the transplanted kidney has been extremely helpful in differentiating occlu-

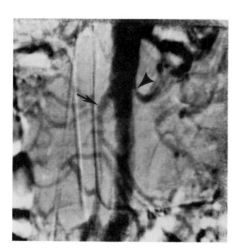

Fig. 22–11. High-grade stenosis of left renal artery (arrowhead) in patient with hypertension. Note diffuse atheromatous disease in distal abdominal aorta. Right renal artery is not well seen in this projection due to superimposition of superior mesenteric artery (arrow): at least one other projection would be necessary to visualize artery in this case. Note also the peristaltic artifact interfering with accurate subtraction, especially in the right side of the abdomen.

sion of arterial inflow from acute tubular necrosis, obstruction, renal rejection, and other causes of decreased function.[15]

Peripheral Vascular Studies

A principal application of digital subtraction angiography is in the study of the major vessels of the trunk and extremities. DSA can be used to evaluate flow patterns in the aorta and major vessels and can demonstrate occlusion, stenosis, aneurysm, shunts, and graft patency. The results of percutaneous angioplasty can be readily evaluated. Patients with peripheral vascular disease are somewhat difficult to study with conventional arteriography, largely because of the risks of the catheter itself, such as intimal tears, hematoma, and arterial spasm. In addition, the procedure is painful.[10] The intravenous technique allows the physician to examine peripheral arteries with acceptably low risk,[1] and it is nearly pain-free. Although anatomic detail with DSA is not as clear as with conventional angiography, it is usually adequate for clinical decisions (Fig. 22–12). The DSA technique has been used to evaluate patients with atherosclerosis obliterans, Buerger's disease, diabetes mellitus, and similar peripheral vascular pathology.

Blood Flow Measurement

The term "blood flow" as it is used in the medical literature often seems to confuse two distinct concepts: flow through a vessel (units: ml/min), and tissue perfusion (units: ml/min/gm or equivalent). The latter is most readily measured by techniques involving the washout of diffusible indicators and is not further discussed in this section. Blood flow through a vessel is not readily measurable by conventional angiographic techniques because (1) the volume containing the contrast material is not well defined, (2) the relationship between concentration of contrast agent and resulting film density is not well defined and certainly is not linear in the range of

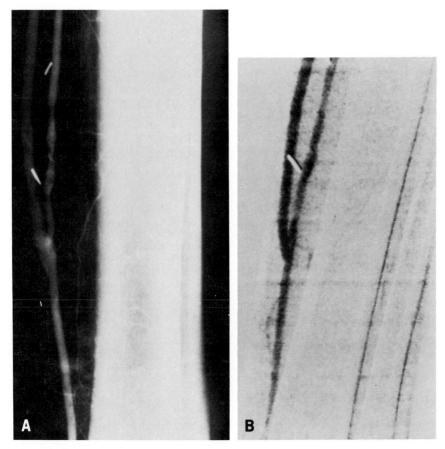

Fig. 22–12.   *A,* Intraoperative (conventional) arteriogram showing distal anastomosis of femoroposterior tibial arterial graft. *B,* when patient's symptoms worsened, an intravenous study was performed, confirming continued graft patency.

concentration needed for conventional angiography, and (3) at the concentrations of contrast agent needed, the agent itself would affect blood flow. The DSA technique avoids the latter two limitations.

At the low concentrations of contrast agent used in DSA, the relationship between iodine concentration and x-ray attenuation coefficient is nearly linear.[3,42] The measured attenuation coefficient depends on beam energy, detector energy dependence, scatter, and fidelity of the logarithmic amplifier. The "density" (in conventional film terms) can be used to estimate the concentration of contrast agent, opening the way for quantitative measurement of blood flow by digital videodensitometry.

Link et al. have reported a video dilution technique for estimating peripheral blood flow.[36] Although the technique is not directly related to DSA, its concept is readily applicable. Blood flow in an artery is compared with flow in a reference artery, in terms of fraction of total cardiac output. Erikson et al. have used videodensitometry to determine myocardial blood flow.[35] Some inherent limitations of DSA, however, may impede progress in this direction. These limitations include the effects of scatter, veiling glare (spreading of light within the image intensifier), geometric distortion due to uncertainties or irregularities in tissue thickness, and noise in the image processing system.[19]

REFERENCES

1. Crummy, A.B., Strother, C.M., Liebermann, R.P., et al.: Digital video subtraction angiography for evaluation of peripheral vascular disease. Radiology, *141*:33, 1981.
2. Crummy, A.B., Strother, C.M., Sackett, J.F., et al.: Computerized fluoroscopy: A digital subtraction technique for intravenous angiocardiography and arteriography. Am. J. Roentgenol., *135*:1131, 1980.
3. MacIntyre, W.J., Pavlicek, W., Gallagher, J.H., et al.: Imaging capability of an experimental digital subtraction angiography unit. Radiology, *139*:307, 1981.
4. Ovitt, T.W., Capp, M.P., Fisher, H.D., et al.: The development of digital video subtraction system for intravenous arteriography. *In* Noninvasive Cardiovascular Measurements. Edited by H.A. Miller, E.V. Schmidt, and P.C. Harrison. Society of Photo-Optical Instrumentation Engineering, *167*:61, 1978.
5. Ovitt, T.W., Christenson, P.C., Fisher, H.D. et al.: Intravenous angiography using digital video subtraction: X-ray imaging system. Am. J. Roentgenol., *135*:1141, 1980.
6. Ziedses des Plantes, B.G.: Subtraktion: Roentgenographische Methode zur separaten Abbildung bestimmter Teile des Objekts. Fortschr. Rontgenstr., *52*:69, 1935.
7. Drew, P.G.: The coming revolution in digital radiography. Diagn. Imaging, *3*:10, 1981.
8. Detmer, D.E., Fryback, D.G., and Strother, C.M.: Digital subtraction arteriography cost-effectiveness. *In* Digital Subtraction Arteriography. Edited by C.A. Mistretta, A.B. Crummy, C.M. Strothers, et al. Chicago, Year Book Medical Publishers, 1982.
9. Freedman, G.S.: Economic analysis of outpatient digital angiography. Appl. Radiol., *11*:29, 1982.
10. Guthaner, D.E., Silverman, J.F., Hayden, W.G., and Wexler, L.: Intraarterial analgesia in peripheral arteriography. Am. J. Roentgenol., *128*:737, 1977.
11. Sigstedt, B., and Lunderquist, A.: Complications of angiographic examinations. Am. J. Roentgenol., *130*:455, 1978.
12. Buonocore, E., Meaney, T.F., Borkowski, G.P. et al.: Digital subtraction angiography of the abdominal aorta and renal arteries. Radiology, *139:*281, 1981.
13. Chilcote, W.A., Modic, M.T., Pavlicek, W.A., et al.: Digital subtraction angiography of the carotid arteries: a comparative study in 100 patients. Radiology, *139*:287, 1981.
14. Christenson, P.C., Ovitt, T.W., Fisher, H.D., et al.: Intravenous angiography using digital video subtraction: Intravenous cervicocerebrovascular angiography. Am. J. Roentgenol., *135*:1145, 1980.
15. Hillman, B.J., Ovitt, T.W., Nudelman, S., et al.: Digital video subtraction angiography of renal vascular abnormalities. Radiology, *139*:227, 1981.
16. Meaney, T.F., Weinstein, M.A., Buonocore, E., et al.: Digital subtraction angiography of the human cardiovascular system. Am. J. Roentgenol., *135*:1153, 1980.
17. Owens, A., and Ennis, M.: Arrhythmias occurring during intravenous urography. Clin. Radiol., *31*:291, 1980.
18. Stadalnik, R.C., Vera, Z., DaSilva, O., et al.: Electrocardiographic response to intravenous urography: Prospective evaluation of 275 patients. Am. J. Roentgenol., *129*:825, 1977.
19. Mistretta, C.A., Crummy, A.B., and Strother, C.M.: Digital angiography: A perspective. Radiology, *139*:273, 1981.
20. Revesz, G., Kundel, H.I., and Graber, M.A.: The influence of structured noise on the detection of radiologic abnormalities. Invest. Radiol., *9*:479, 1974.
21. Mistretta, C.A., Ort, M.G., Kelcz, F., et al.: Absorption edge fluoroscopy using quasi-monoenergetic X-ray beams. Invest. Radiol., *88*:402, 1973.
22. Houk, T.L., Kruger, R.A., Mistretta, C.A., et al.: Real-time digital K-edge subtraction fluoroscopy. Invest. Radiol., *14*:270, 1979.
23. Pond, G.D., Osborne, R.W., Capp, M.P., et al.: Digital subtraction angiography of peripheral vascular bypass procedures. Am. J. Roentgenol., *138*:279, 1982.
24. De Lahitte, M.D., Marc-Vergnes, J.P., Rascol,, A., et al.: Intravenous angiography of the extracranial cerebral arteries. Radiology, *137*:705, 1980.
25. Little, J.R., Furlan, A.J., Modic, M.T., et al.: Intravenous digital subtraction angiography in brain ischemia. J.A.M.A., *247*:3213, 1982.
26. Modic, M.T., Weinstein, M.A., Chilcote, W.A., et al.: Digital subtraction angiography of the intracranial vascular system: Comparative study in 55 patients. A.J.N.R., *2*:527, 1981.
27. Pond, G.D., Cook, G.C., Woolfenden, J.M., and Dodge, R.R.: Pulmonary thromboembolism: evaluation by digital intravenous angiography. SPIE, *314*:256, 1981.
28. Seeger, J.F., Weinstein, P.R., Carmody, R.F., et al.: Digital video subtraction angiography of the cervical and cerebral vasculature. J. Neurosurg., *56*:173, 1982.
29. Strother, C.M., Sackett, J.F., Crummy, A.B., et al.: Clinical applications of computerized fluoroscopy. The extracranial carotid arteries. Radiology, *136*:781, 1980.
30. Turnipseed, W.D.: Potential clinical applications of digital subtraction angiography. Appl. Radiol., *11*:83, 1982.
31. Pond, G.D., Smith, J.R.L., Hillman, B.J., et al.: Current clinical applications of digital subtraction angiography. Appl. Radiol., *10*:71, 1981.
32. Carey, P.H., Slutsky, R.A., Ashburn, W.L., and Higgins, C.B.: Validation of cardiac output estimates by digital video subtraction angiography in dogs. Radiology, *143*:623, 1982.
33. Kruger, R.A., Mistretta, C.A., Houk, T.L., et al.:

Computerized fluoroscopy techniques for intravenous study of cardiac chamber dynamics. Invest. Radiol., *14*:279, 1979.

34. Buersch, J.H., Hahne, H.J., Brennecke, R., et al.: Assessment of arterial blood flow measurements by digital angiography. Radiology, *141*:39, 1981.

35. Erikson, U., Helmius, G., Hennis, K., et al.: Determination of myocardial blood flow by videodensitometry. Fortschr. Rontgenstr., *135*:404, 1981.

36. Link, D.P., Foerster, J.M., Lantz, B.M.T., and Holcroft, J.W.: Assessment of peripheral blood flow in man by video dilution technique: A preliminary report. Invest. Radiol., *16*:298, 1981.

37. Higgins, C.R., Norris, S.L., Gerber, K.H., et al.: Quantitation of left ventricular dimensions and function by digital video subtraction angiography. Radiology, *144*:461, 1982.

38. Weinstein, M.A., Modic, M.T., Buonocore, E., et al.: Digital subtraction angiography: Experience at the Cleveland Clinic Foundation. Appl. Radiol., *10*:53, 1981.

39. Sahn, D.J., Pond, G.D., Allen, H.D., et al.: Evaluation of aortic arch abnormalities and pulmonary artery anatomy by intravenous digital subtraction angiography and 2D echo. Presented at the 55th Annual Meeting of the American Heart Association. Dallas, TX, November 1982.

40. Hillman, B.J., Ovitt, T.W., Capp, M.P., et al.: The potential impact of digital video subtraction angiography on screening for renovascular hypertension. Radiology, *142*:577, 1982.

41. Osborne, R.W., Jr., Goldstone, J., Hillman, B.J., et al.: Digital video subtraction angiography: Screening technique for renovascular hypertension. Surgery, *90*:932, 1981.

42. Kruger, R.A., Anderson, R.E., Koehler, R., et al.: A method for the noninvasive evaluation of cardiovascular dynamics using a digital radiographic device. Radiology, *139*:301, 1981.

Chapter 23

PERCEPTION PARAMETERS IN MEDICAL IMAGES

JAMES C. CARLSON

Scan images have often been characterized as the *man/machine interface,* representing the link between physical detector and human understanding. Great effort has been dedicated to perfecting the techniques, materials, and instrumentation for collecting images. Parallel efforts should be made to optimize conditions for perceiving the information obtained from the imaging device. Producing such optimal conditions requires understanding both the machine output and human perception.

Human perception is a complex process that has been extensively studied yet is far from being perfectly understood. Optical illusions illustrate one of the problems in understanding perception. Under certain circumstances, the eye receives seemingly conflicting information. For example, is the image in Figure 23–1A a vase or two people facing each other? Is the image in Figure 23–1B a triangle superimposed over other objects, or are the objects fortuitously placed to suggest the triangle? At the end of this chapter is a discussion of Ginsburg's recently proposed unified theory of perception to explain optical illusions.

This chapter discusses many of the physical parameters of perception—not the psychology of pattern interpretation. Following an introduction to some basic ideas about perception, certain perception parameters are discussed in detail, and their relation to nuclear medicine is considered. Some characteristics of cathode-ray tubes, multiformaters and films used in creating images are presented.

ELEMENTS OF HUMAN PERCEPTION

Basic Concepts

Hecht et al., Rose, and deVries developed a description of perception phenomena in the early 1940s.[1,2,3,4] They regarded the eye as an instrument of photon detection. In this theory, statistical fluctuation in photon reception by the retina is the basic limiting factor in image perception. A more recent version of the equation developed by Rose in 1948 to express the operating characteristics of an ideal photon detector was given by Schnitzler in 1973:[3,5]

$$Q \propto \frac{5 \ k^2 \times 10^{-3}}{EC^2\alpha^2D^2 \ t} \tag{1}$$

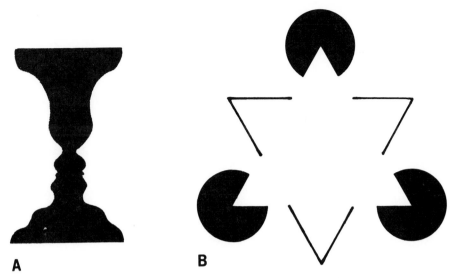

Fig. 23–1. Sometimes paradoxical images are easily recognized. *A.* Do you see a vase or two people facing each other? *B.* Pac-men aligned with three angles create the impression of a nonexistent white triangle.

where:

Q = photon yield required for a given accuracy of target detection,

k = signal-to-noise ratio (SNR),

C = contrast,

α = angular size of the target in min,

E = background luminance* in foot-lamberts,

D = detector aperture diameter in cm,

t = exposure time in sec

Although this formula relates the fundamental factors for any detection system (human or physical), it does not completely describe the human visual system. For example, exposure time t in a physical system has no limits and could approach infinity. The human eye, however, has narrow limits of photon integration time, varying from about 0.05 sec at 1000 foot-lamberts to about 0.2 sec at 10 foot-lamberts. When precise information is not available, many authors arbitrarily set t equal to 0.1 sec. On the other hand, a time-luminance reciprocity feature of the human visual system, known as the *Bunsen-Roscoe law,* states that for times less than 0.1 sec, the product of time and contrast is constant for a given threshold response.

Equation (1) implies that contrast for a given set of parameters must increase as the angle subtended by the target α decreases. Experiments confirm this for humans, but only over a limited range. In the human visual system, this relationship fails at very small angles (small targets) and at very large angles (large targets). The minimum SNR for target detection depends upon illumination, which varies from a minimum of about 1.9 at middle luminance values to 19 at high luminance values. A more complete list of factors affecting image perception includes patterns, scene context, Mach effects, observer search patterns, motion, system resolution, gestalt-stimulated perception, color, and contouring.

Some of the following data, taken from a variety of reports, appear inconsistent. These inconsistencies arise from the large number of parameters affecting perception and the lack of standardized testing environments. Various investigators have

_____

*Luminance is a precise term for the characteristic commonly referred to as brightness. Luminance is discussed in detail by Akin and Hood.[6]

used different viewing distances, luminance levels, target shapes, target placement, and display format. Despite inconsistencies in details, general trends are consistent with equation (1).

Contrast

Contrast as used in equation (1) is defined as the regional change in photons in the target area, $N_t - N_b$, divided by the photons in the background area, N_b:

$$C = \frac{|N_t - N_b|}{N_b} \qquad (2)$$

This equation uses the absolute value of the change in photons, so that a positive value always results. If this convention is not obeyed, negative values result when the target is an area of decreased photons, as with liver lesions in colloid scans. To express contrast as a percentage, multiply the number obtained in equation (2) by 100.

Equation (1) requires no minimum contrast for detection, but a limit does occur in human experience. The minimum contrast required for perception of a difference is called the *contrast sensitivity*. Reported values of contrast sensitivity for the human eye vary greatly. Green found a contrast sensitivity of 20% for detecting differences in densities of dot patterns placed in adjacent fields.[7] Using black disks on a white background—a suprathreshold condition—Mallard found an average contrast of 10% was required for detecting a change in average density.[8] According to calculations by Whitehead, targets in nuclear medicine images require a contrast of about 8% when SO-179 film is used and about 17% when Polaroid film is used.[9] The generalized curve of observer response shown in Figure 23–2 indicates that objects with contrast as low as 2% should be detectable. Figure 23–3, which relates contrast sensitivity of the eye to

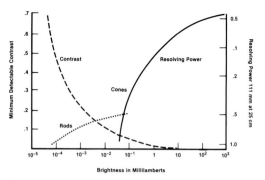

Fig. 23–2. Generalized curves showing increasing contrast sensitivity and resolving power with increasing luminance. (Adapted from Henny, G.C., and Chamberlain, W.E.[10])

target frequency,* illustrates that with optimum target size, contrast sensitivity is as low as 0.5%.

The data from Figure 23–2 are replotted in Figure 23–4 to show that as luminance increases, the required contrast percentage decreases for a given target size. For example, when the graph is read vertically at a reciprocal angle of 0.1 min, the contrast sensitivity is 2% at 10 foot-lamberts approximately 7% at 0.1 foot-lamberts. Also, Figure 23–4 implies that at constant illumination, the contrast sensitivity increases as target size decreases, i.e., greater contrast is required to distinguish smaller targets.

Border sharpness is another factor affecting contrast sensitivity: sharp borders are more easily detected than blurred borders. Gregg described an experiment in

---

*This use of the word *frequency* should not be confused with the description of frequency distributions in an image described in Fourier space. Here, target frequency refers to the size of the target in terms of the angle subtended by the target. For example, a target, together with an equal background space occupying a visual angle of 0.1 degrees, has a frequency of 10 cycles per degree. In Fourier space, images with sharp borders and small objects require large values for the high-frequency coefficients in the Fourier transforms. Such images are said to contain high frequencies. The reader who is unfamiliar with the use of Fourier space as a means of describing images can review the section "Fourier Transforms," which appears later this chapter.

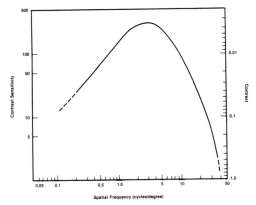

Fig. 23–3. The relationship between contrast sensitivity of the human eye and target size. The eye is most sensitive to target contrast when the target subtends 1.5 to 5.0 cycles per degree of visual angle. See footnote appearing in "Contrast" in this chapter. (From Ginsburg, A.P.[11] Reproduced by permission of the Technical Information Service.)

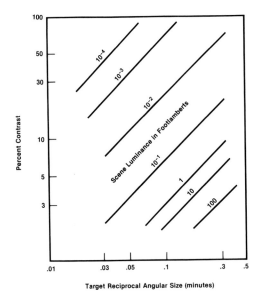

Fig. 23–4. At a given luminance, the contrast required for lesion detection increases as the angle subtended by the lesion decreases. As luminance increases, the contrast required for lesion detection decreases.

which density changed gradually across a film; a 25% density difference from one film edge to the other was required to describe the orientation of the density gradient correctly. When displayed on a large screen in an auditorium, luminance differences of 100% or greater from one edge to another were required for detection.[13]

Targets with sharp borders are more easily detected than targets with blurred borders because of the *Mach band effect*, a phenomenon in which the eye enhances a sharp border by darkening the dark side of the border and brightening the light side. This effect can be observed in the step wedge of Figure 23–5, where the printing in each step is a constant gray. Many investigators of perception phenomena use targets with sharp borders, consequently incorporating the Mach band effect in their results. Although this effect changes the absolute value of the data, it does not alter the general trend. In general, with ideal viewing conditions and a good signal-to-noise ratio, a sharply defined edge can be seen with a contrast of less than 2%; however, if the edge change is gradual, greater target contrast is required for detection.

Signal-to-Noise Ratio

DeVries postulated that the absorption of light by the retina is somehow quantified, and that the sensory signals generated obey the Poisson probability law for random discrete events.[4] Poisson statistics are familiar in scintillation counting, in which they are used to estimate counting errors. DeVries used Poisson distributions to develop an indicator of image quality, which he labeled the *signal-to-noise ratio* (SNR).

$$k = \frac{|N_t - N_b|}{\sqrt{N_b}} = \frac{\Delta N}{\sqrt{N_b}} \qquad (3)$$

where k is the SNR expressed as a positive number.

Unlike equations (1) and (3), which are based on the number of photons reaching

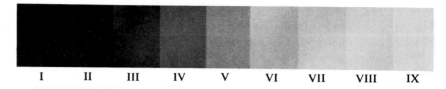

I	II	III	IV	V	VI	VII	VIII	IX

Fig. 23–5. Because of the Mach band effect, these uniform steps of gray appear nonuniform to the observer.

the detector (retina), analysis of the SNR in medical images is based on the photons used to create the image. Usually in medical imaging, image quality is not limited by the number of photons reaching the retina from light transmitted by the film, because the film illuminator is photon-rich. Instead, limitations in image parameters are related to the number of photons collected by the imaging device. Signal-to-noise ratio, which is probably the most fundamental limitation in nuclear medicine imaging, is discussed in relation to other parameters in the next section.

Target Size and Visual Angle Subtended

Visual acuity is the reciprocal of the visual angle (in minutes) subtended by the minimum pair of lines that can be resolved. (A pair consists of a dark line and a white line in a test pattern composed of multiple, equal-width dark and white lines.) For a test object of high contrast under good illumination, the eye has a visual acuity of about 1.0; i.e., the minimum angle subtended by a line pair is 1 min of arc. At 45 cm from the eye, this measurement corresponds to 0.013 cm. Under poor lighting and low contrast, visual acuity drops to about 0.1 (i.e., minimum angle of 10 min, or about 0.13 cm at 45 cm). Visual acuity is not a limiting factor in nuclear medicine imaging, because the resolution of imaging devices is low in comparison with human visual acuity.

For test patterns larger than the limits of visual acuity and of low contrast, the eye is found to be most sensitive to targets representing a frequency of approximately 3 cycles per degree of visual angle (Fig.

23–3). (Ginsburg uses this curve as an early indication of amblyopia.[11])

As can be expected from this frequency dependence, target detection depends on target size, and larger targets are not necessarily observed more readily than smaller ones. As shown by the data of Rosell and Willson (Fig. 23–6), larger targets require a larger SNR for detection.[14] Data from medical imaging agrees with this data. Using television-produced square test patterns, Mosley and Kelsey experimented with the detection of 10-mm nodules on radiographs. They found that optimal detection occurred at a viewer distance of 91 cm rather than 45 cm.[15] At

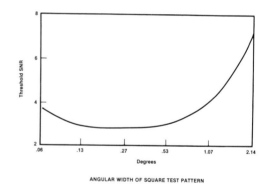

ANGULAR WIDTH OF SQUARE TEST PATTERN

Fig. 23–6. The minimum SNR required for square test pattern detection as a function of the visual angle subtended by the test squares. The SNR reaches a minimum value of approximately 3 over a range of 0.1 to 0.5 degrees angular subtense. (After Rosell, F.A., and Willson, R.H.: Recent psychological experiments and the display signal-to-noise ratio concept. In Perception of Displayed Information. Edited by L.M. Biberman. New York, Plenum Press, 1973.)

91 cm, the lesion subtends 0.63 degrees visual angle, and at 45 cm, it subtends 1.27 degrees. Note in Figure 23–6 that the SNR required for a target of 1.27 degrees visual angle is approximately 4.6, whereas for 0.63 degrees, the required SNR is approximately 3.0. The lesion requiring the smaller SNR for detection is seen more easily, and is the one viewed from 91 cm. These relationships are further discussed in the following sections.

Contouring

Contouring develops when computer-generated images are produced with an inadequate number of gray levels. In contoured images, each level of gray is clearly distinguished from the next (Fig. 23–7). Contoured images are undesirable for several reasons: they introduce high-frequency components that detract from the structures of interest, they create confusion and constitute added noise by enhancing features of no interest, and they hide significant data by compressing all variations within a range to a single display value.

Reports suggest that at least 64, and perhaps as many as 256, gray levels should be employed in computer-displayed images to prevent contouring.[16] Experienced radiologists can distinguish between films produced with 127 and those produced with 255 gray levels.

Color

Humans can distinguish more than 1500 colors. Because changes in color are observed more easily than changes in gray levels, a color image might be assumed to reflect the count distribution more accurately if a different color is assigned to very narrow pixel count ranges. Also, lesion visibility might be expected to increase using color coding of count density. These assumptions are incorrect, however. Investigators of image perception tend to ignore color as a factor in target detection. Lesions seen in radiographs, radionuclide

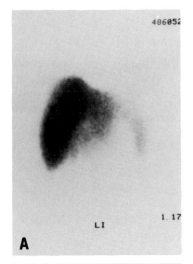

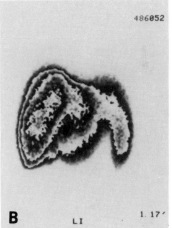

Fig. 23–7. Unprocessed (*A*) and gray-level processed (*B*) liver scans. In the contoured image, the entire count range has been divided into eight levels.

images, and ultrasound images represent transmission, absorption, emission, or reflection properties shared equally by many other tissues. If a value of one of these properties is assigned a color, other tissues having the same value must be assigned the same color. In this case, color assignment may confuse, not enhance, lesion detection.

Color in routine static images creates problems similar to those in contoured gray-scale images. The display, and hence lesion detection, depends on the operator. The target (lesion) may be buried in a color contour or may be dramatically displayed, depending on the contour levels selected by the operator. Most available color display systems use only 8 to 20 of the thousands of colors available. Thus the displayed images contain contours even more highly accentuated than gray-level contours. The remaining noise problems in the images are dramatized, and the high-frequency components are disturbing.

Wagner and others have advocated color as a coding mechanism for defining physiologic parameters in "functional images."[18] Functional images lend themselves to color displays because they represent calculated functional or parametric characteristics (see "Quantifying Images," Chap. 7). For situations in which these functional characteristics can be easily separated, e.g., during the phase of a cardiac cycle, the colored functional image is a superior mode of presentation. Color provides an excellent coding mechanism.

Patterns

Humans are highly sensitive to patterns.[19] The same contour selection process that might produce an orange tumor in a blue brain, for example, can be used to produce a cross-hatched tumor in a field of dots; inexpensive black and white monitors and film can be used instead of expensive color display systems and film. Although patterned displays are applied extensively in graphic materials, they are seldom used in image presentation because the dazzling patterned images are difficult to interpret.

Television displays, in which raster lines are often visible, are commonly used in imaging departments. Visibility of raster lines, however, is not an inherent property of either the television camera or its display. In well-designed and well-adjusted television systems, the raster lines can and should be invisible, even at close viewing distances.[20] Proper adjustment should be made because the raster pattern is an interfering signal; like noise, it prevents detection of small detail. For the same reason, computer images displayed in recognizable matrix patterns can confuse image perception, making low- and medium-frequency patterns of interest difficult to perceive.

CLINICAL APPLICATIONS

The importance of SNR in target detection within an image and its relationship to target size are observed in the determination of the count density required for adequate imaging. The frequently suggested optimum density of 800 counts/cm^2 for thyroid imaging is examined using the following calculations. Assume a 1-cm diameter lesion in a 3-cm diameter thyroid lobe. Also assume that the count density in the lesion area is uniformly 80% of the normal surrounding thyroid. From equation (3):

$$N_t = counts/cm^2 \times area \times concentration$$
$$= 800 \times \pi \times (0.5)^2 \times 0.80$$
$$= 502$$

$$N_b = counts/cm^2 \times area \times concentration$$
$$= 800 \times \pi \times (0.5)^2 \times 1.0$$
$$= 628$$

$$SNR = \frac{|N_t - N_b|}{\sqrt{N_b}}$$

$$= \frac{628 - 502}{\sqrt{628}} = \frac{126}{25.1} = 5.0$$

On a life size display (1:1) the angular subtense of this 1-cm diameter lesion observed at 45 cm is 1.27 degrees. Compare this calculated SNR of 5.0, which is based on the requirement of 800 counts/cm^2 to the SNR of 4.6 obtained from Figure 23–6 for a pattern of 1.27 degrees angular subtense. Under similar assumptions, a lesion of 1.5 cm diameter would have a SNR of 7.5, although Figure 23–6 indicates that it should be about 7. Although not identical, these numbers agree closely and support the evidence that larger lesions require a larger SNR for detection. Although the curve in Figure 23–6 is derived from experimental data from the field of perception, the results correspond with empiric experience gained in nuclear medicine imaging.

The data of Figure 23–6 were used to create Table 23–1, which provides estimates of the tumor sizes expected to fall within what might be considered the optimum bounds of visual angle, i.e., between 0.1 and 0.5 degrees. Table 23–1 states that an image containing a 1.4-cm diameter tumor acquired on a small field-of-view camera and displayed as a format of 4 occupies a visual angle of 0.5 degrees when observed at a distance of 45 cm. From Figure 23–6, at an angular subtense of 0.5 degrees, a SNR of at least 3.0 is required to distinguish the lesion. A 4.2-cm diameter tumor in this same image would occupy a visual angle three times as great, or 1.5 degrees. A 4.2-cm tumor, using the data of Figure 23–6, requires a SNR of 5.7 or almost twice that required for the smaller tumor.

A simple calculation based on equations (2) and (3) shows that doubling the SNR while maintaining the contrast constant requires acquisition of four times as many counts.:

$$k_1 = C_1\sqrt{N_1} \text{ and } k_2 = C_2\sqrt{N_2}$$

for $k_1/k_2 = 2$:

$$C_1\sqrt{N_1} = 2\,C_2\sqrt{N_2}$$

Square both sides and note that initial conditions require that $C_1 = C_2$. Then:

$$N_1 = 4\,N_2$$

This increase in counts can be achieved either by increasing the patient dose by a factor of 4 or by increasing the counting time by a factor of 4.

The suggestion that changing observer distance can change the SNR required for detection is supported by additional evidence from Rosell and Willson.[14] They showed that when observer viewing distance increased from 28 to 56 in., the SNR required for detection changed exactly as predicted on the basis of visual angle subtended. Consequently, instead of increasing the patient dose or the imaging time by a factor of 4, in this example the observer can reduce the SNR required for perception by moving his chair back an additional 90 cm, where the large tumor subtends 0.5 degrees. This solution is viable when the target size exceeds 0.5 degrees. When it is less than 0.1 degree, some means of magnification is needed. Variable viewing distance and minification techniques are commonly used in radiology today. In general, every medical image must be viewed from several distances to optimize the probability that the defect

TABLE 23–1. *Tumor Size Subtending 0.1 to 0.5 Degrees for an Observer at 45 cm From an 8 × 10-in. Film*

Multi-image format	Camera 25 cm diam. field of view		Camera 38 cm diam. field of view	
	0.1 degrees	0.5 degrees	0.1 degrees	0.5 degrees
1	0.14 cm	0.70 cm	0.21 cm	1.05 cm
4	0.28 cm	1.4 cm	0.42 cm	2.1 cm
16	0.56 cm	2.8 cm	0.84 cm	4.2 cm

Calculations in this table are given with the assumption that a single image has a 14.2-cm diameter, i.e., 70% of the 8-in. dimension. For formats of 4 and 16, the image size is assumed to be reduced by ½ and ¼ that of the single image, which results in image diameters of 7.1 and 3.55 cm.

will fall within the target visual angle size requiring the minimum SNR.

The size and character of the dots that form the image are also important. A dot size that permits both overlap and integration of gray dots produces an image with lower-frequency noise than one produced with dark nonoverlapping dots. An image with less noise is more acceptable to the viewer. Although the viewer is capable of integrating some of the area represented by separated dots, contrast sensitivity becomes worse and lesion detection becomes more difficult when such integration is required (Fig. 23–8).

Contrast sensitivity is related to the number of gray levels that can be observed on a film. Transparencies that have a maximum density of about 1.6 are best received by the viewer. (See the section "Types of Film" for a definition of density.) If a contrast of 15% between each step of a step wedge is required for step detection, the total number of gray levels on a film with a maximum density of 1.6 is 25.* When a contrast sensitivity of 8% is used, the total number of gray levels is 45, and when 25% sensitivity is used, it becomes 15 or 16. A consistent solution to the number of gray levels visible on a film cannot be expected as long as different values for contrast sensitivity are obtained; different values are obtained under different experimental conditions.

INSTRUMENTATION

Image Recording Systems

Images may be recorded on transparent film, on such nontransparent media as Polaroid film or paper, by persistence or memory CRT, and in computer memory.

Photographic film

Of the many characteristics that serve to describe a photographic film, only those of interest to or controllable by medical imaging personnel are addressed here.

The fundamental light-sensitive element of film is a silver halide, which is immersed in a gelatinous coating on a plastic base. The base may be coated on both sides to form a double-emulsion film (generally used in radiography) or on only one side to create single-emulsion film. Negative emulsions use various proportions of silver bromide and silver iodide, whereas positive emulsions contain silver chloride and silver bromide. These halides are sensitive to the blue region of the spectrum. Film is made sensitive to the green and red light by the addition of suitable dyes to the emulsion. The dyes absorb the photons with longer wavelengths (green to red) and transfer the energy absorbed to the silver halides, reducing them to free silver. Films with dyes that sensitize them to blue and yellow are labeled *orthochromatic*. Films made sensitive to the entire visible spectrum are called *panchromatic*. Films without dyes are insensitive to red light; hence, red light can be used in the darkroom without affecting the film.

Film development is basically a chemical amplification process whereby any silver halide crystal that has been partially reduced to free silver is completely reduced. Shades of gray are created by the number of crystals so changed, not by the amount of change occurring in each crystal. If allowed to proceed long enough, the development process is sufficiently active to change all film crystals to silver. For this reason, overdevelopment produces an even gray density called *fog*. Development at excessively high temperatures also produces fog, because high temperatures speed the development process. Fixing so-

---

*This value is calculated as follows. Assume the minimum density of the film is 0.10; the difference, then, between the maximum density of 1.6 and the minimum is 1.5. A density range of 1.5 represents a contrast range, or ratio, of $10^{1.5}$, or 31.6. The number of 15% steps in this range is determined by the expression $1.15^k = 31.6$. Solving for k yields 24.7, or approximately 25.

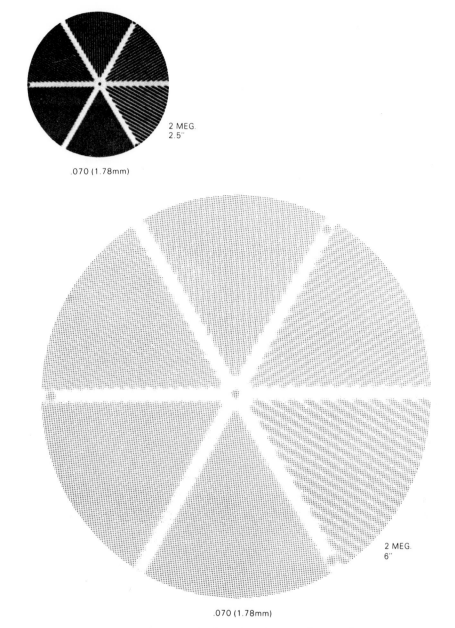

Fig. 23–8. Superior images are obtained when the dots producing the image are contiguous, as in the smaller diagram. (From Enos, G.[21])

lutions are used in these situations to stop the developing process and to clear away undeveloped silver halide.

Sensitometry

Sensitometry, a common method of describing the relationship between light ex-posure and density, was developed by Hurter and Driffield. The curve shown in Figure 23–9 is traditionally called an *H and D curve*, after these investigators. Some authors prefer to use the term "D-log-E" or "D versus log E" curves because the parameters plotted are density (D) ver-

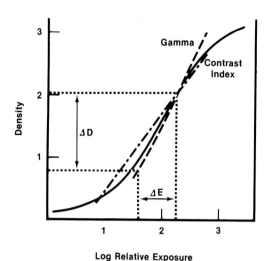

Fig. 23–9. Film gamma and contrast indexes are similar but possess slightly different parameters. Calculation of gamma—the slope of the midportion of the curve—from D/E is illustrated.

sus the logarithm of exposure (E). *Density* is best explained in terms of *transmittance.* Transmittance is the ratio of the light transmitted through the film to the light incident on the film. *Opacity* is the reciprocal of transmittance, and density is the logarithm to the base 10 of the opacity:

Transmittance (T)

$$= \frac{\text{transmitted luminance}}{\text{incident luminance}} \quad (4)$$

$$\text{Opacity} = \frac{1}{T} \quad (5)$$

$$\text{Density (D)} = \log \frac{1}{T} \quad (6)$$

These relationships are illustrated in Figure 23–10. The following examples serve to illustrate the meaning of density. A film density of 1.4 indicates that the incident luminance is 25 times the transmitted luminance, i.e., $10^{1.4} = 25$. A film density of 0.3 indicates a transmitted luminance 50% of the incident luminance. Likewise, a change in film density from

0.8 to 1.1, a net density change of 0.3, indicates a 50% decrease in luminance from the area of 0.8 density to the area of 1.1 density. Note that a density increase of 0.3 results for a reduction in transmitted luminance of 50%. In terms of radiation absorption, this value corresponds to a "half-value layer," i.e., that thickness of material reducing photon transmission by 50%. In absorption phenomena, a fixed change in material thickness results in a fixed percentage change in transmission. In film sensitometry, a fixed change in density values represents a fixed percentage of change in light transmission.

Most radiographic films have a base density of about 0.2 and a maximum density ranging from 2.0 to 3.5. With normal viewbox lighting, film density changes that occur above approximately 2.0 are difficult to discern. Density changes above this level can be discerned only with more intense lighting. Interestingly, a normal outdoor scene contains luminance levels in the range of 130:1, i.e., the brightest area has a luminance 130 times that of the shaded area; these levels correspond to those in films with densities ranging from 0.2 to 2.3.

Film Gamma

The slope of the straight line portion of the sensitometric curve is known as the *film gamma.*:

$$\text{gamma} = \frac{D_2 - D_1}{\log E_2 - \log E_1} \quad (7)$$

where D_1 and D_2 are the density values corresponding to exposure values E_1 and E_2.

Because this descriptive parameter of the midportion of the film characteristic curve does not always yield consistent results for the photographer making paper prints from film, a descriptive parameter called the *contrast index* is sometimes used. As can be seen in Figure 23–9, the contrast index is the slope of the straight line drawn between the points of mini-

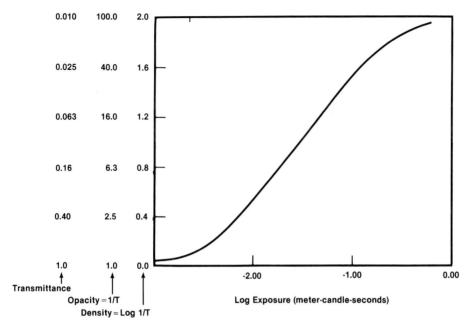

Fig. 23–10. Transmittance, opacity, and density use different mathematical operations in describing a common parameter; the amount of light transmitted by a film.

mum and maximum useful densities; it differs only slightly from film gamma.

Contrast was described in equation (2) as being linearly related to photon flux, but contrast is also a measure of the density difference between two points on the film. In comparing two points A and B whose densities are respectively 0.75 and 1.00, the contrast between them can be correctly stated as 0.25. But because film densities are based on logarithmic values of luminance (photon flux), contrast measured in this way does not agree with contrast as described in equation (2), according to which the contrast between A and B of this example is 0.78, or 78%. In addition to these two well-established meanings of contrast, others are in common use. Therefore, when describing the slope of the H and D curve, the terms film gamma, gradient, slope, and contrast index are all preferred to "contrast," a term that is already ambiguous.

When the film gamma value is high (steep H and D curve), small changes in subject luminance produce large changes in film density. High-gamma films are essential in radiography and nuclear medicine, fields in which most lesions result in only slight changes in film exposure. Theoretically, low-gamma film could be used for CRT-displayed images, for which contrast and exposure can be controlled electronically or by computer; however, overcoming the limitations of CRT contrast, as discussed in the next section, requires a high-gamma film for imaging from the CRT.

Development Conditions

Sensitometric curves are modified by the following development conditions: time, temperature, type of developer, and age of developer. Figure 23–11 shows that the contrast index of Kodak Plus-x film can be changed from a value of 0.3 for a 4-min development to a value of 0.85 for a 15-min development. When a constant development time of 4 min is used, the contrast index can vary from 0.30 for Microdol-X developer to 0.55 for DK 50. Although these phenomena are illustrated

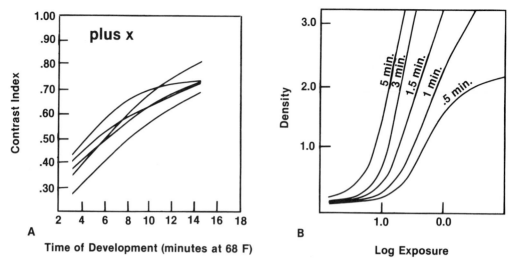

Fig. 23–11. Development time and type of developer have a significant influence on the value of the contrast index of a film. *A.* The contrast index for Kodak Plus-x is plotted for five different developers. Its sensitivity to temperature of the developer is not illustrated. *B.* Specific sensitometric curves for a single film type, Kodak SO-392, illustrate the significant changes resulting from a change in development time.

with data for Plus-x film, a film commonly used in photography, similar results can be expected using various x-ray and nuclear imaging films and developers.

Types of Film

Film contrast characteristics for scintillation camera imaging depend on many factors not normally encountered with photon-rich imaging (photography in normal room light or of television displays). In addition, film contrast characteristics for photon-rich sources do not apply strictly to nuclear medicine images. These characteristics vary with total counts collected, image size, and CRT spot size. In blood flow studies, in which the total count per frame is low, all film types exhibit similar contrast characteristics because the films are being used in a bipolar manner, i.e., the display intensity is increased to the extent that there are no gray dots, only black ones. In this case, gray scale is created only by dot density. With high-count static images, films approach the photon-rich sensitometric characteristics because the CRT is adjusted to pro-

duce gray dots that overlap to produce gray levels.

Recognition of the importance of dot size and character is essential for proper film selection for nuclear medicine images, especially for those taken from random access CRTs.[22] The individual dots of light produce a more diffused dot when double emulsion film is used, because of image parallax on two separate emulsions. Whereas this "soft" dot has an effect similar to defocusing, which gives the impression of reduced resolution, the high-frequency "textural noise" is reduced. In general, double-emulsion films have higher gamma, which results in increased contrast for a given change in count density. Single-emulsion films usually exhibit low contrast. They produce sharp, "hard" dots, which give the impression of increased resolution but also increase textural noise, reducing the observer's ability to perceive small differences in activity (Fig. 23–12).

Polaroid films 107 and 667, favored for scintiphotography, are thought of as high-

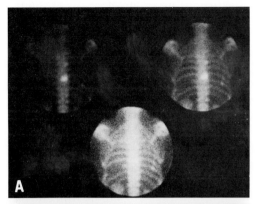

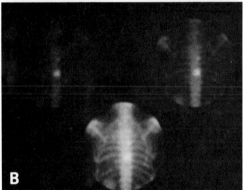

Fig. 23–12. The effects of dot structure detail are shown as applied to static imaging. The "hard" dot image (*A*) exhibits increased "textural noise" and a lack of data integration. The "soft" dot image (*B*) exhibits reduced "textural noise" and improved data integration, resulting in better contrast and image perception.

contrast films having insufficient density* range. These films therefore require the use of a camera with three lenses, each with a different aperture or neutral filter. Polaroid film, however, has a dense black and a clear white, and its useful luminance range is excellent for normal scene viewing. The limitations of Polaroid film, or any printed image, are related to limitations in reflectance and in the media

gamma. Reflected images, such as Polaroid or paper prints, have a limited range of reflectance. If the white area is arbitrarily assigned a reflectance of 100, the reflectance of the black portions can be as low as 4. The ratio of these two reflectance values is 25. In general, the ratio of the maximum to minimum reflectance of any printed image does not exceed 25.[23] This ratio corresponds to a maximum density range of 1.4—a value close to data published by Polaroid wherein the density ranges of films 107, 611, and 667 are given as 1.54 to 1.57.[24] Any transparency having a maximum density range greater than 1.57 has a greater contrast range; consequently the range of count densities or the ultrasound signal strength variations visible on the display are greater.

Another parameter involved in this comparison is the gamma of the film itself. Polaroid films 107, 611, and 117 have gamma values of 1.40, 1.0, and 1.45 respectively. For a given change in count density, a transparency film with a gamma greater than 1.45 produces a greater contrast. Transparencies appear to be better, because if properly selected, they have not only a greater overall density range but also a higher gamma. These two parameters result in greater sensitivity to count density variations and in a greater range of observable counts. Improper film selection or improper matching of computer or CRT display parameters to the film characteristics may negate these advantages, which apply only when comparing Polaroid films obtained with a single-lens camera. When a triple-lens Polaroid camera with different f stops in each lens is used, the count range displayed on Polaroid film can exceed the range on any transparency film obtained with a single-lens camera.

At the machine/man interface, data is often displayed on a TV monitor or CRT, where it is observed by an operator (soft copy) or recorded on film (hard copy). The contrast ratio criteria for hard copy is quite different from that required for soft copy.

---

*For reflected images, density is the log of the reciprocal of reflectance; for transparencies, density is the log of the reciprocal of transmittance.

As receptors, the eye and film have different characteristics. Under proper adaptation, the eye can detect as few as two photons and distinguish features in a flux exceeding 10^{15} photons/sec, which is a range greater than 10^{14}. On the other hand, the usual working luminance range of the eye is approximately only 100 to 150, with adjustments and accommodations occurring as the scene luminance shifts. This range is long compared with the contrast range of 13 to 35 accommodated by high-gamma film.[25] When the CRT contrast is adjusted to satisfy the needs of the operator, it is found to be too great for film; hence, a CRT adjusted for the operator produces inferior hard-copy images. This type of error occurs frequently in systems in which a Polaroid camera is used to obtain hard-copy images from the same CRT used by the operator. These experiences, which are actually operator errors, have been erroneously attributed to the characteristics of Polaroid film. To avoid this conflict, the use of two separate CRT displays is advised: one adjusted to the needs of the operator, and one adjusted to the film used to create hard copy. In a properly adjusted hard-copy image with a computer-produced gray step wedge, the step wedge should extend from clear at one end to maximum black at the other end with all intermediate steps distinct.

Cathode-Ray Tubes

Most nuclear medicine images are displayed on cathode-ray tubes (CRTs) of either the analog or the television type. A television tube is a CRT operated under specific standardized conditions. In television tubes, an image is formed on the tube phosphor by sweeping the beam across the tube face in regular line patterns called *raster lines.* This pattern starts in the upper left corner. Voltages applied to the beam deflection electrodes drive the beam across the tube face to the right. As the beam sweeps, the intensity is modulated according to the strength of the television signal. After reaching the right border, the beam is reset to the left edge and continues on its slight downward drift, giving the appearance of a new line.

Schade suggested the use of raster scan wobble to reduce the effect of raster lines, which introduce undesirable high-frequency noise.[26] One manufacturer of multiformatting systems uses a technique of slightly shifting the raster up or down with each frame displayed, thereby filling in the interraster spacing on the film and creating a final image free of the raster lines.

Display oscilloscopes in scintillation cameras operate differently. In the random mode, the CRT imitates the pattern that would be observable if the scintillation camera crystal could be observed directly. The X and Y positioning signals, which represent the location of a photon interaction, adjust the electron beam of the CRT to the proper X,Y coordinates. The CRT beam is then turned on for a short time by the Z pulse, or unblanking signal. In this analog mode, the beam is unblanked only at those coordinates corresponding to the gamma camera's reception of photons, and at a rate corresponding to the counting rate at which the camera is operating.

CRT Contrast Ratio

The *CRT contrast ratio* is defined as the ratio of the maximum luminance to the minimum luminance in the display. The contrast ratio obtained on a CRT is limited in comparison with that obtained on film unless specific measures are taken. CRT contrast ratios are reduced by light scattering in the glass screen, reflections from tube walls, screen curvature, scattered electrons, ambient room light, and reflections from the screen face. Under common conditions in which 30% of the phosphor is in contact with the glass face and no optical filter is used on the face, the contrast ratio is only 9. (A film with a maximum density of 2.0 has a contrast ratio near 100.) Some of these problems can be obviated by the use of screen filters. A filter on the CRT face that reduces the luminance by only 20% increases the contrast ratio by a factor of approximately 7 when ambient lighting is insignificant. In strong ambient lighting, however, a filter with 40% transmission increases the contrast ratio by a factor of only 3. When photographing the CRT directly, many of these adverse effects can be overcome by careful selection of high-gamma film. Of course, ambient lighting is not a factor in a closed photographic system.

Phosphors

Multiformat systems have used a P4 phosphor composed of two separate phosphors, one emitting blue light and the other emitting yellow light. Combined, these lights appear white to the observer, but films can differentiate them. A blue-sensitive film registers only the blue light. Orthochromatic film is sensitive to some yellow light, also. Creation of a P4 phosphor involves mixing the blue- and yellow-emitting phosphors and spreading them uniformly over the CRT face. Any nonuniformity in the phosphor coating results in nonuniform image densities. One solution is to use a P45 phosphor, which emits many different wavelengths. This solution eliminates nonuniformity of response caused by poor mixing of the two components in the phosphor; however, nonuniform deposition of phosphor remains a problem.

CRT Resolution

The resolution obtainable on CRT systems depends on many factors, one of which is raster lines per picture height. Home television sets operating on EIA RS170 standards have 525 raster lines per picture height. (Actually, only 490 are observed, because 35 are used for interframe flyback.) Other standards permit 675, 729, 875, 945, or 1023 raster lines. The greater the number of raster lines per picture height, the finer the possible image resolution. Raster lines per picture height, however, represent only one of many parameters controlling resolution. For example, increasing the number of raster lines to "improve resolution" without appropriately adjusting the bandwidth decreases the SNR and degrades target detection.

The size of the luminous spot is a major factor in resolution. Spot size depends on controlling voltages in the electron gun, focusing mode, deflection yoke, phosphor grain size, signal strength, and beam offset. Because the focal plane of the electron beam sweeps out a spherical segment, the scanning spot cannot be in focus on all parts of the screen unless the tube face is congruent with the spherical plane. In practice, a CRT system is adjusted for optimum focus at some area between the center and the edge except when dynamic focusing tubes are used. These tubes use electronic circuits to modify the focusing voltages in accordance with the beam's position across the tube face.

The luminous spot of optimum size is not necessarily the smallest spot on the screen. If the spot is too small, the luminance may be inadequate, and the raster lines may become pronounced. On the other hand, excessively large spots may overlap adjoining raster lines, resulting in loss of resolution in both directions.

Computer Storage of Images

The cardiac images in Figure 23–13 can serve as a departure for analyzing the techniques of generating images from computer memory. Note that a matrix of 32 × 32 pixels presents a poor image of the heart. Also note the distortion of the cardiac border imposed by the large pixel size. A better image results from expanding the matrix size to 64 × 64, and even better, to 128 × 128. At 256 × 256, however, little improvement in image quality is observed, although the number of bytes of memory used show a fourfold increase (65,535 versus 16,383). (In digital radiog-

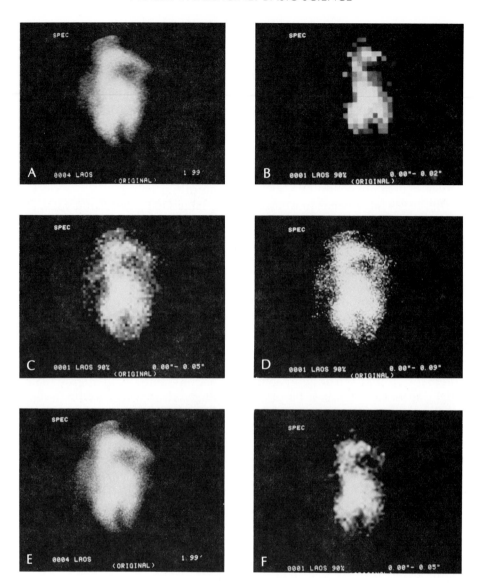

Fig. 23–13. Gated radionuclide ventriculogram in LAO view. Each image contains 400k counts. *A.* The unprocessed image from the scintillation camera. *B.* The same data digitized to a 32 × 32 matrix. *C.* 64 × 64 matrix. *D.* 128 × 128 matrix. *E.* 256 × 256 matrix. *F.* The 64 × 64 matrix data interpolated to 512 × 512.

raphy, however, which involves sufficient available photons and equipment resolution capabilities, matrix sizes of 256 × 256 are minimal, 512 × 512 are desired, and in some cases, 1024 × 1024 are required.) To conserve memory, an attempt is made in some systems to create a more pleasing image with less high-frequency noise by interpolating between matrix data points to display an image with pixels four times as numerous as elements in the stored matrix. Even though this method may create a "better" image, it does not increase information content.

In a report on the relative importance of sampling elements (pixels) and shades of gray, Gaven found that if an image is limited by the total number of bits available, optimum utility is achieved with fewer sampling elements and more encoding bits per sampling element.[28] That is, whenever the higher number of sampling elements results in fewer than three encoding bits per element, fewer rather than more sampling elements should be used. In terms of nuclear medicine studies, this finding suggests that if the total count per pixel becomes less than eight, the matrix size should be reduced to increase the counts per pixel.

FOURIER TRANSFORMS

Image contents are frequently described in terms of their value in frequency space. Techniques of image manipulation and description in Fourier space are used because of their completeness, simplicity, and universal application. Fourier (1768–1830) demonstrated that a mathematical function could be represented by a power series of sine and cosine functions. This mathematical operation has many applications, among them are those in imaging system analysis. Without derivation from the general to the specific, a specific imaging system example (after

work by Rossman[29]) is used to illustrate this concept.

The image parameter to be described by the Fourier series is a sharp edge, as shown in Figure 23–14A. This graph could represent a plot of density versus linear distance over one small area of an image. Expressed as a Fourier series, it is:

$$f(X) = \frac{\pi}{2} + 2 \sin X + \frac{2}{3} \sin 3X$$

$$+ \frac{2}{5} \sin 5X + \dots \dots \quad (8)$$

The result of plotting these terms is illustrated in Figure 23–15A and 23–15B. In part A, the first term, $\pi/2$, is the straight line labeled 1. The sum of the first two terms—i.e., the constant, $\pi/2$, and the largest sinusoidal term—is labeled 2. The sum of the first three terms is labeled 3. The sum of the first four terms is plotted separately in Figure 23–15B for clarity. Notice that as each new term is added, reproduction of the step function of Figure 23–14A becomes more accurate.

Equation 8 is a specific form of the general Fourier series, which is:

$$f(x) = A_0 + \sum_{n=1}^{\infty} A_n \cos nkx$$

$$+ \sum_{n=1}^{\infty} B_n \sin nkx \quad (9)$$

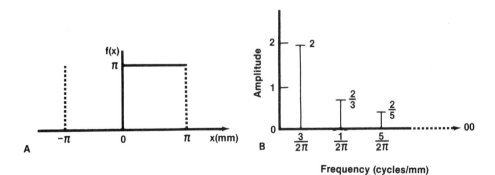

Fig. 23–14. *A.* The edge of a sharp border in an image may show a density change as represented by this plot of a mathematical function that has a y value of 0 for x between $-\pi$ and 0 and a y value of π for x between 0 and π. *B.* The amplitude of the coefficient corresponding to a given frequency term in the Fourier series has been plotted.

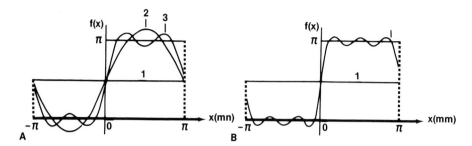

Fig. 23–15. *A.* The straight line (labeled 1) is a plot of the first term of the Fourier series. Curve 2 is the sum of the first two terms, and curve 3, the first three terms. *B.* The sum of the first four terms is plotted separately to demonstrate clearly that the Fourier series approaches the original step function.

Since the purpose of presenting equation (9) is to illustrate the use of coefficients for each sine or cosine term, the specific meaning of nkx is not discussed here beyond saying that n represents the integers from 1 to infinity. The coefficients A_1, A_2, A_3 ... and B_1, B_2, B_3 ... are coefficients that determine the magnitude of each succeeding term. Each succeeding term represents a higher frequency. In the specific example of equation (8), the coefficients for the cosine terms are zero.

In some applications, a generalized description of the image is given by describing the distribution of coefficients for various frequencies. The coefficients A_1, A_2, etc. of the Fourier transform describe the maximum amplitude of the particular frequency in the series. Low frequencies are needed to describe large objects. High frequencies are required to describe small objects and to modify the low frequencies, so that rapidly changing densities and edges are represented. An image with small objects or sharp edges has large Fourier coefficients for high frequencies. Consequently, such an image is said to have many high-frequency signals.

To create the Fourier transform of an image, the total image is represented by a series of lines in the X direction and a series of lines in the Y direction. Each line is then transformed into its equivalent Fourier series. The entire set of transforms constitutes the new image described in Fourier space. (With a television system, reasonable results can be achieved by doing this only in the X direction, since density changes are described only by variations in time, which correspond with the X direction in the display.)

After the coefficients are calculated, the image density values can be described by the sine terms and their coefficients instead of by X and Y coordinates. Image densities described by the Fourier series are said to be described in *Fourier space,* or *frequency space.* A graph of the magnitude of each term versus the X value for this example is shown in Figure 23–14B. This graph describes the magnitude of the coefficients of the frequency components of the Fourier series; therefore, it is a plot in frequency (or Fourier) space of the sharp density change shown in Figure 23–14A. When images are manipulated in frequency space, these magnitude coefficients are being manipulated. Mathematically, using a Fourier description to operate on an image is easier than using Cartesian coordinates.

Because the modulation transfer function (MTF) describes a system's image transfer characteristics in frequency space, description of the image itself in frequency space becomes essential and extremely useful. To determine the appearance of an output image after degradation or enhancement by computer operations, an optical system, or any instrumentation, the input image is expressed in frequency space and multiplied by the MTF of the system. The output image in frequency space is then transformed back to coordinate space by inverse Fourier transformation. This technique is used widely in image analysis and processing.

UNIFIED THEORY OF PERCEPTION

Why does the observer fill in the blank areas of Figure 23–1B to perceive a triangle when none is present? In Ginsburg's theory of perception,[11] image analysis is based on the brain's ability to sort the image into frequency components, similar to the Fourier components just described. The image received by the eye is divided (presumably by the brain) into seven frequency channels, each two octaves wide and having center-channel frequencies of 1, 2, 4, 8, 16, 32, and 64 cycles per visual degree. The brain examines low-frequency channels first, and if time and interest permit, it then examines the information in higher-frequency channels. Within Figure 23–1B, a white triangle is perceived because a low-frequency channel describes a triangular area. Subsequent review of higher-frequency channels shows the first impression to be imprecise. As the high-frequency channels are reviewed, the details of individual objects of the image do not support the first impression of a white triangle. Changes in response can be made at this point.

Rapid examination of gross features, as given in the low-frequency channels, allows the observer to identify objects rapidly, leaving consideration of details to a time when speed is less essential. It promotes survival in a primitive world, where man must quickly decide if the object in his field of vision merits flight or fight. Ginsberg's theory helps explain why a simple cartoon drawing of only 10 pen strokes allows an observer to identify Bob Hope or Winston Churchill, and why certain objects or people in poor lighting or in relief are recognized even when represented by an image in only two levels of gray (white and black). Recognition occurs because the brain finds a match to previously learned patterns of fundamental frequencies.

REFERENCES

1. Hecht, S., Shaler, S., and Pirenne, M.H.: Energy quanta and vision. J. Gen. Physiol., *25*:819, 1942.
2. Rose, A.: The relative sensitivities of television pickup tubes: photographic film and the human eye. Proc. IRE, *30*:295, 1942.
3. Rose, A.: The sensitivity performance of the human eye on an absolute scale. J. Opt. Soc. Am., *38*:196, 1948.
4. DeVries, H.: The quantum character of light and its bearing upon threshold of vision, the differential sensitivity and visual acuity of the eye. Physica, *10*:553, 1943.
5. Schnitzler, A.D.: Analysis of noise-required contrast and modulation in image-detecting and display systems. *In* Perception of Displayed Information. Edited by L.M. Biberman. New York, Plenum Press, 1973.
6. Akin, R.H., and Hood, J.M.: Photometry. *In* Display Systems Engineering. Edited by H.R. Luxenberg and R.L. Kuehn. New York, McGraw-Hill, 1968.
7. Green, B.A.F., Wolf, A.K., and White, B.W.: The detection of statistically defined patterns in a matrix of dots. Am. J. Psychol., *72*:503, 1959.
8. Mallard, J.R.: A statistical model for the visualization of changes in the count density of radioisotope scanning displays. Br. J. Radiol., *42*:530, 1969.
9. Whitehead, F.R.: Minimum detectable gray-scale differences in nuclear medicine images. J. Nucl. Med., *19*:87, 1978.
10. Henny, G.C., and Chamberlain, W.E.: Roentgenography: fluoroscopy. *In* Medical Physics. Vol. 1. Edited by O. Glasser. Chicago, Year Book Publishers, 1944.
11. Ginsburg, A.P.: Visual information processing based on spatial filters constrained by biological data. Vols. 1 and 2. AMRL-TR-78-129. Springfield, VA, National Technical Information Service, 1978.
12. Gregg, E.C.: Image manipulation in radiology. *In* Physics of Diagnostic Radiology. Proceedings of a Summer School Held at Trinity University, San Antonio, TX, July 12–17, 1971. Edited by D.J. Wright. USDHEW Publication No. (FDA) 74-8006. Rockville, MD, U.S. Dept. of Health, Education and Welfare, 1971.
13. Luxenberg, H.R.: Recording media. *In* Display Systems Engineering. Edited by H.R. Luxenberg and R.L. Kuehn. New York, McGraw-Hill, 1968.

14. Rosell, F.A., and Willson, R.H.: Recent psychological experiments and the display signal-to-noise ratio concept. *In* Perception of Displayed Information. Edited by L.M. Biberman. New York, Plenum Press, 1973.

15. Moseley, R.D., and Kelsey, C.A.: Observer performance testing in clinical radiology. *In* Second International Visual Psychophysics and Medical Imaging Conference. Edited by C.C. Jaffee. IEEE Catalog No. 81CH 1676-6. New York, Institute of Electrical and Electronic Engineers, 1981.

16. Prewitt, J.M.S.: Object enhancement and extraction. *In* Picture Processing and Psychopictorics. Edited by B.S. Lipkin and A. Rosenfeld. New York, Academic Press, 1970.

17. Dunn, J.F.: Cathode ray tube (CRT) film recording of video based medical images. *In* Picture Archiving and Communication Systems (PACS) for Medical Applications. Edited by A.J. Duerinckx, Billingham, The Society of Photo-Optical Instrumentation Engineers. 1982.

18. Wagner, H.N.: Color: Contributions or camouflage? *In* Nuclear Medicine. Edited by H.N. Wagner. New York, HP, 1975.

19. Rosenfeld, A., and Lipkin, B.S.: Texture synthesis. *In* Picture Processing and Psychopictorics. Edited by B.S. Lipkin and A. Rosenfeld. New York, Academic Press, 1970.

20. Biberman, L.M.: Image quality. *In* Perception of Displayed Information. Edited by L.M. Biberman. New York, Plenum Press, 1973.

21. Enos, G.: Factors affecting imaging performance and perception. Picker Journal, *2*:15, 1981.

22. Schwenker, R.P.: Film performance in analog nuclear medicine imaging. *In* The Physics of Medical Imaging: Recording System Measurements and Techniques. Edited by A.G. Haus. New York, The American Institute of Physics, 1979.

23. Vlahos, P.: Film-based projection systems. *In* Display systems Engineering. Edited by H.R. Luxenberg and R.L. Kuehn. New York, McGraw-Hill, 1968.

24. Polaroid Black & White Land Films: For Professional, Industrial, Medical, Scientific and General Use. Polaroid publication P1810 AC/AC 5/80. Cambridge, MA, Polaroid Corporation, 1980.

25. Carlson, J.C.: Matching gray scale display programs to various film types. *In* Proceedings of the Second Symposium on Sharing Computer Programs and Technology in Nuclear Medicine. April 21–22, 1972. AEC CONF-720430. Oak Ridge, TN, U.S. Technical Information Center, 1972.

26. Schade, O.H.: Image reproduction by a line raster process. *In* Perception of Displayed Information. Edited by L.M. Biberman. New York, Plenum Press, 1973.

27. Asher, R.W., and Martin, H.: Cathode-ray devices. *In* Display Systems Engineering. Edited by H.R. Luxenberg and R.L. Kuehn. New York, McGraw-Hill, 1968.

28. Gaven, J.V., Tavitian, J., and Harabedian, A.: The informative value of sampled images as a function of the number of gray levels used in encoding the images. Photo. Sci. Engng., *14*:16, 1970.

29. Rossman, K.: Image quality. *In* Physics of Diagnostic Radiology. Proceedings of a Summer School Held at Trinity University, San Antonio, TX, July 12–17, 1971. Edited by D.J. Wright. US-DHEW Publication No. (FDA) 74-8006. Rockville, MD, U.S. Dept. of Health, Education and Welfare, 1971.

APPENDIX A

TABLE A–1. *SI Base and Supplementary Units*

Quantity	Name	Symbol
SI base units		
length	meter	m
mass	kilogram	kg
time	second	s
electric current	ampere	A
thermodynamic temperature	kelvin	K
amount of substance	mole	mol
luminous intensity	candela	cd
SI supplementary units		
plane angle	radian	rad
solid angle	steradian	sr

From Radiation Quantities and Units, International Commission on Radiological Units and Measurements Report No. 33, Washington, D.C., ICRU, 1980.

TABLE A–2. *SI Derived Units with Special Names*

| Quantity | SI unit | | | |
	Name	Symbol	Expression in terms of other units	Expression in terms of SI base units
frequency	hertz	Hz		s^{-1}
force	newton	N		$m \cdot kg \cdot s^{-2}$
pressure, stress	pascal	Pa	N/m^2	$m^{-1} \cdot kg \cdot s^{-2}$
energy, work, quantity of heat	joule	J	$N \cdot m$	$m^2 \cdot kg \cdot s^{-2}$
power, radiant flux	watt	W	J/s	$m^2 \cdot kg \cdot s^{-3}$
quantity of electricity, electric charge	coulomb	C	$A \cdot s$	$s \cdot A$
electric potential, potential difference, electromotive force	volt	V	W/A	$m^2 \cdot kg \cdot s^{-3} \cdot A^{-1}$
capacitance	farad	F	C/V	$m^{-2} \cdot kg^{-1} \cdot s^4 \cdot A^2$
electric resistance	ohm	Ω	V/A	$m^2 \cdot kg \cdot s^{-3} \cdot A^{-2}$
conductance	siemens	S	A/V	$m^{-2} \cdot kg^{-1} \cdot s^3 \cdot A^2$
magnetic flux	weber	Wb	$V \cdot s$	$m^2 \cdot kg \cdot s^{-2} \cdot A^{-1}$
magnetic flux density	tesla	T	Wb/m^2	$kg \cdot s^{-2} \cdot A^{-1}$
inductance	henry	H	Wb/A	$m^2 \cdot kg \cdot s^{-2} \cdot A^{-2}$
Celsius temperature*	degree Celsius	°C		K
luminous flux	lumen	lm		$cd \cdot sr$
illuminance	lux	lx	lm/m^2	$m^{-2} \cdot cd \cdot sr$
activity (of a radionuclide)	becquerel	Bq		s^{-1}
absorbed dose, specific energy imparted, kerma, absorbed dose index	gray	Gy	J/kg	$m^2 \cdot s^{-2}$

*In addition to the thermodynamic temperature (symbol T), expressed in kelvins (see table A–1), use is also made of Celsius temperature (symbol t) defined by the equation

$$t = T - T_0$$

where $T_0 = 273.15$ K by definition. The unit "degree Celsius" is equal to the unit "kelvin," but "degree Celsius" is a special name in place of "kelvin," for expressing Celsius temperature. A temperature interval or a Celsius temperature difference can be expressed in degrees Celsius as well as in kelvins.

From Radiation Quantities and Units, International Commission on Radiological Units and Measurements Report No. 33, Washington, D.C., ICRU, 1980.

TABLE A–3. *SI Prefixes*

Factor	Prefix	Symbol
10^{18}	exa	E
10^{15}	peta	P
10^{12}	tera	T
10^{9}	giga	G
10^{6}	mega	M
10^{3}	kilo	k
10^{2}	hecto	h
10^{1}	deka	da
10^{-1}	deci	d
10^{-2}	centi	c
10^{-3}	milli	m
10^{-6}	micro	μ
10^{-9}	nano	n
10^{-12}	pico	p
10^{-15}	femto	f
10^{-18}	atto	a

From Radiation Quantities and Units, International Commission on Radiological Units and Measurements Report No. 33, Washington, D.C., ICRU, 1980.

Certain units which are not part of the SI are used so widely that it is impractical to abandon them. The units that are accepted for continued use in the United States with the International System are listed in Table A–4.

TABLE A–4. *Units in Use with the International System**

Name	Symbol	Value in SI unit
minute (time)	min	1 min = 60 s
hour	h	1 h = 60 min = 3600 s
day	d	1 d = 24 h = 86400 s
degree (angle)	°	$1° = (\pi/180)$ rad
minute (angle)	'	$1' = (1/60)°$
		$= (\pi/10800)$ rad
second (angle)	"	$1'' = (1/60)'$
		$= (\pi/648000)$ rad
liter	L*	$1\ L = 1\ dm^3 = 10^{-3}\ m^3$
metric ton	t	$1\ t = 10^3\ kg$
hectare (land area)	ha	$1\ ha = 10^4\ m^2$

*The international symbol for liter is the lowercase "l," which can easily be confused with the numeral "1." Accordingly, the symbol "L" is recommended for United States use.

From Radiation Quantities and Units, International Commission on Radiological Units and Measurements Report No. 33, Washington, D.C., ICRU, 1980.

TABLE A–5. *Quantities and Units for Use in Radiation Protection*

Quantity Name	Symbol	SI	SI restricted name*	Special†
Dose equivalent	H	$J\ kg^{-1}$	Sv	rem
Dose equivalent rate‡	$\dot{H}$	$J\ kg^{-1}s^{-1}$	Sv s⁻¹	rem s⁻¹
Absorbed dose index	D_I	$J\ kg^{-1}$	Gy	rad
Absorbed dose index rate‡	$\dot{D}_I$	$J\ kg^{-1}s^{-1}$	Gy s⁻¹	rad s⁻¹
Dose equivalent index	H_I	$J\ kg^{-1}$	Sv	rem
Dose equivalent index rate‡	$\dot{H}_I$	$J\ kg^{-1}s^{-1}$	Sv s⁻¹	rem s⁻¹
Shallow dose equivalent index	$H_{I,s}$	$J\ kg^{-1}$	Sv	rem
Deep dose equivalent index	$H_{I,d}$	$J\ kg^{-1}$	Sv	rem

*The symbol for the special name of the SI unit restricted to specified quantities.

†One should not infer that the size of a unit given in this column is equal to the size of a unit on the same line in the other columns.

‡Day (d), hour (h), and minute (min) may be used instead of second (s).

Adapted from Radiation Quantities and Units, International Commission on Radiological Units and Measurements Report No. 33, Washington, D.C., ICRU, 1980.

TABLE A–6. *Other Units and Conversion Factors*

Physical quantity	Unit	Symbol	Definition or conversion factor
Length	inch	in.	2.54×10^{-2} m
	foot	ft	0.305 m
	angstrom	Å	10^{-10} m
Mass	pound (avoirdupois)	lb	0.453 592 kg
Force	kilogram-force	kgf	9.806 65 N
Area	barn	b	10^{-28} m^2
	square centimeter	cm^2	0.155 in.^{2}
Pressure	atmosphere	atm	101 325 Pa
	torr	Torr	133.322 Pa
	bar	bar	10^5 Pa
Stress	pound-force per sq. inch	lbf/in.^{2}	6894.757 Pa
Energy	electron volt	eV	3.336×10^{-10} C
			1.602×10^{-12} erg
			1.602×10^{-19} J
	watt	W	1 J/s
	kilowatt hour	kWh	3.6×10^6 J
	erg	erg	10^{-7} J
			6.24×10^5 MeV
			2.39×10^{-8} cal
	calorie	cal	4.184 J
			2.62×10^{13} MeV
			4.184×10^7 erg
Radioactivity	Curie	Ci	3.7×10^{10} Bq
	millicurie	mCi	37 MBq
	microcurie	μCi	37 kBq
Radiation Dose	roentgen	R	2.58×10^{-4} C/kg std air
			2.082×10^9 ion pairs/ml std air
			7.02×10^4 MeV/ml std air
			8.38×10^{-6} J/gram air
	rad	r	100 ergs/gram
			10^{-2} J/kg
			0.01 Gy
	rem	r	10^{-2} J/kg
			10^{-2} Sv
	sievert	Sv	1 J/kg
			100 rem

TABLE A–7.   *Physical Constants*

Constant	Value
mass of C^{12} atom	12.0000 amu
atomic mass unit (amu)	1.661×10^{-27} kg
	931.501 MeV
	1.49×10^{-3} erg
elementary charge (e)	1.6022×10^{-19} C
electron charge	-4.803×10^{-10} esu
	-1.6022×10^{-19} C
proton rest mass (m_p)	1.0073 amu
	1.6726×10^{-27} kg
neutron rest mass (m_n)	1.0087 amu
	1.6749×10^{-27} kg
mass of hydrogen atom (m_H)	1.007825 amu
	1.6743×10^{-27} kg
Avogadro's number (N_A)	6.0220×10^{23} mol^{-1}
electron rest energy ($m_e c^2$)	.51101 MeV
electron rest mass (m_e)	9.1091×10^{-31} kg
	5.486×10^{-4} amu
speed of light in vacuum (c)	2.9979×10^8 m/s
Planck's constant (h)	6.6262×10^{-34} J·s

APPENDIX B

DECAY SCHEMES AND NUCLEAR PARAMETERS OF SOME MEDICALLY IMPORTANT RADIONUCLIDES

The following nuclear decay schemes and emission parameters are taken from MIRD Pamphlet No. 10, The Society of Nuclear Medicine, by permission. The symbols referring to various transitions are as follows:

K ALPHA-1 X-RAY $\equiv$ K $-$ L_{III} transition.

K ALPHA-2 X-RAY $\equiv$ K $-$ L_{II} transition.

K BETA-1 X-RAY $\equiv$ K $-$ M_{III} transition.

K BETA-2 X-RAY $\equiv$ K $-$ N_{II} transition.

L ALPHA X-RAYS $\equiv$ $L_{\alpha1}$ (L_{III} $-$ M_V transition) and $L_{\alpha2}$ (L_{III} $-$ M_{IV} transition). A weighted average energy is determined.

L BETA X-RAYS $\equiv$ $L_{\beta1}$ (L_{II} $-$ M_{IV} transition), $L_{\beta2}$ (L_{III} $-$ N_V transition), $L_{\beta3}$ (L_I $-$ M_{III} transition), and $L_{\beta4}$ (L_I $-$ M_{II} transition) x-rays. A weighted average energy is determined.

L GAMMA X-RAYS $\equiv$ $L_{\gamma1}$ (L_{II} $-$ N_{IV} transition), $L_{\gamma2}$ (L_I $-$ N_{II} transition), $L_{\gamma3}$ (L_I $-$ N_{III} transition), and $L_{\gamma4}$ (L_I $-$ O_{III} transition) x-rays. These all have similar energy, and the $L_{\gamma1}$ energy is used because it is considerably more intense than the other L_γ x-rays.

L X-RAYS $\equiv$ x-rays that arise because of a vacancy in the L shell. For atomic numbers <70 the computer calculates an average energy associated with the L x-rays. For $Z \geq 70$, a breakdown of the various L x-rays is given.

KLL AUGER ELECT $\equiv$ an Auger electron emitted from the L shell as a result of the transition of another L-shell electron to a vacancy in the K shell. Because there are three L subshells of slightly different energy, a weighted average energy is associated with these Auger electrons.

KLX AUGER ELECT ≡ an Auger electron emitted from the X shell, in which X stands for any shell higher than the L shell, as a result of the transition of an L-shell electron to a vacancy in the K shell. Because of the presence of subshells of slightly different energy in the L and X shells, a weighted average energy is associated with these Auger electrons.

KXY AUGER ELECT ≡ an Auger electron emitted from the Y shell as a result of the transition of an X-shell electron to a vacancy in the K shell, where X and Y each stand for any shell higher than the L shell. Because of the presence of subshells of slightly different energy in the X and Y shells, an average energy is associated with these Auger electrons.

LMM AUGER ELECT ≡ an Auger electron emitted from the M shell as a result of the transition of another M-shell electron to a vacancy in the L shell. Because of the presence of subshells of slightly different energy in the L and M shells, an average energy is associated with these Auger electrons.

MXY AUGER ELECT ≡ an Auger electron emitted from the Y shell as a result of the transition of an X-shell electron to a vacancy in the M shell, where X and Y each stand for any shell higher than the M shell. The average M-shell binding energy is associated with these Auger electrons.

HYDROGEN-3
BETA-MINUS DECAY

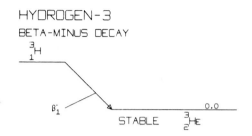

```
         3
         H
         1
  _____
             \
              \
               \
  β⁻₁           \                              0.0
                 _____
                    STABLE        3
                                  ₂HE
```

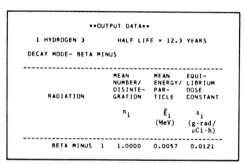

```
                        ••OUTPUT DATA••

          1 HYDROGEN 3        HALF LIFE = 12.3 YEARS
     DECAY MODE- BETA MINUS
     ----------------------------------------------
                        MEAN       MEAN      EQUI-
                        NUMBER/    ENERGY/   LIBRIUM
                        DISINTE-   PAR-      DOSE
          RADIATION     GRATION    TICLE     CONSTANT

                          nᵢ        Ēᵢ         Δᵢ
                                   (MeV)    (g-rad/
                                             μCi-h)
     ----------------------------------------------
          BETA MINUS  1   1.0000    0.0057    0.0121
```

CARBON-14
BETA-MINUS DECAY

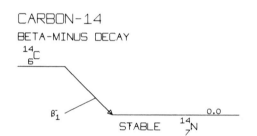

```
         14
         C
         6
  _____
             \
              \
               \
  β⁻₁           \                              0.0
                 _____
                    STABLE       14
                                 ₇N
```

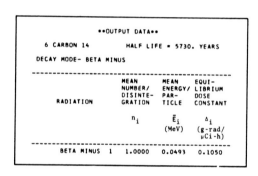

```
                        ••OUTPUT DATA••

          6 CARBON 14        HALF LIFE = 5730. YEARS
     DECAY MODE- BETA MINUS
     ----------------------------------------------
                        MEAN       MEAN      EQUI-
                        NUMBER/    ENERGY/   LIBRIUM
                        DISINTE-   PAR-      DOSE
          RADIATION     GRATION    TICLE     CONSTANT

                          nᵢ        Ēᵢ         Δᵢ
                                   (MeV)    (g-rad/
                                             μCi-h)
     ----------------------------------------------
          BETA MINUS  1   1.0000    0.0493    0.1050
```

FLUORINE-18
ELECTRON CAPTURE AND
BETA-PLUS DECAY

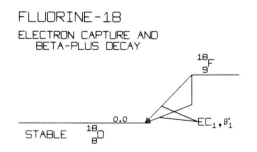

```
                                   18
                                   F
                                   9
                            _____
                           /|
                          //|
                         ///|
              0.0       ////|
  _____\▲////     EC₁,β⁺₁
     STABLE    18
               ₈O
```

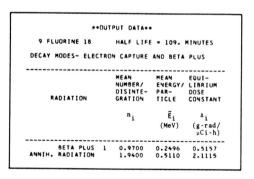

```
                        ••OUTPUT DATA••

          9 FLUORINE 18       HALF LIFE = 109. MINUTES
     DECAY MODES- ELECTRON CAPTURE AND BETA PLUS
     ----------------------------------------------
                        MEAN       MEAN      EQUI-
                        NUMBER/    ENERGY/   LIBRIUM
                        DISINTE-   PAR-      DOSE
          RADIATION     GRATION    TICLE     CONSTANT

                          nᵢ        Ēᵢ         Δᵢ
                                   (MeV)    (g-rad/
                                             μCi-h)
     ----------------------------------------------
                BETA PLUS  1   0.9700    0.2496    0.5157
     ANNIH. RADIATION      1.9400    0.5110    2.1115
```

SODIUM-24
BETA-MINUS DECAY

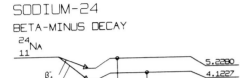

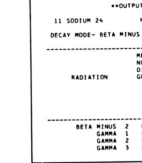

```
                    **OUTPUT DATA**

      11 SODIUM 24          HALF LIFE = 15.0 HOURS

      DECAY MODE- BETA MINUS
```

RADIATION	MEAN NUMBER/ DISINTE- GRATION n_i	MEAN ENERGY/ PAR- TICLE $\bar{E}_i$ (MeV)	EQUI- LIBRIUM DOSE CONSTANT Δ_i (g-rad/ μCi-h)
BETA MINUS 2	0.9992	0.5547	1.1805
GAMMA 1	0.9999	1.3685	2.9149
GAMMA 2	0.9991	2.7539	5.8610
GAMMA 3	0.0008	3.8595	0.0065

PHOSPHORUS-32
BETA-MINUS DECAY

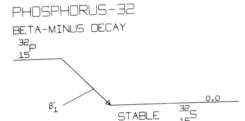

```
                    **OUTPUT DATA**

      15 PHOSPHORUS 32      HALF LIFE = 14.3 DAYS

      DECAY MODE- BETA MINUS
```

RADIATION	MEAN NUMBER/ DISINTE- GRATION n_i	MEAN ENERGY/ PAR- TICLE $\bar{E}_i$ (MeV)	EQUI- LIBRIUM DOSE CONSTANT Δ_i (g-rad/ μCi-h)
BETA MINUS 1	1.0000	0.6948	1.4799

CHROMIUM-51
ELECTRON CAPTURE DECAY

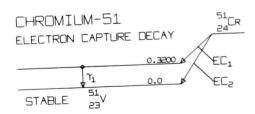

```
                    **OUTPUT DATA**

      24 CHROMIUM 51        HALF LIFE = 27.7 DAYS

      DECAY MODE- ELECTRON CAPTURE
```

RADIATION	MEAN NUMBER/ DISINTE- GRATION n_i	MEAN ENERGY/ PAR- TICLE $\bar{E}_i$ (MeV)	EQUI- LIBRIUM DOSE CONSTANT Δ_i (g-rad/ μCi-h)
GAMMA 1	0.1018	0.3200	0.0694
K ALPHA-1 X-RAY	0.1289	0.0049	0.0013
K ALPHA-2 X-RAY	0.0659	0.0049	0.0006
K BETA-1 X-RAY	0.0224	0.0054	0.0002
KLL AUGER ELECT	0.5614	0.0044	0.0052
KLX AUGER ELECT	0.1240	0.0048	0.0012
LMM AUGER ELECT	1.5323	0.0004	0.0014
MXY AUGER ELECT	3.2177	0.0000	0.0002

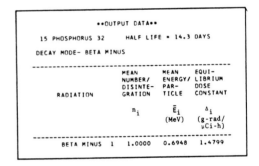

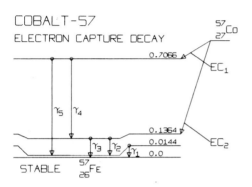

COBALT-57
ELECTRON CAPTURE DECAY

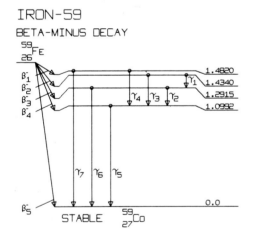

IRON-59
BETA-MINUS DECAY

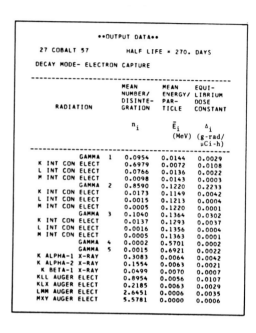

••OUTPUT DATA••

27 COBALT 57   HALF LIFE = 270. DAYS

DECAY MODE- ELECTRON CAPTURE

RADIATION		MEAN NUMBER/ DISINTE- GRATION n_i	MEAN ENERGY/ PAR- TICLE $\bar{E}_i$ (MeV)	EQUI- LIBRIUM DOSE CONSTANT Δ_i (g-rad/ μCi-h)
GAMMA	1	0.0954	0.0144	0.0029
K INT CON ELECT		0.6979	0.0072	0.0108
L INT CON ELECT		0.0766	0.0136	0.0022
M INT CON ELECT		0.0098	0.0143	0.0003
GAMMA	2	0.8590	0.1220	0.2233
K INT CON ELECT		0.0173	0.1149	0.0042
L INT CON ELECT		0.0015	0.1213	0.0004
M INT CON ELECT		0.0005	0.1220	0.0001
GAMMA	3	0.1040	0.1364	0.0302
K INT CON ELECT		0.0137	0.1293	0.0037
L INT CON ELECT		0.0016	0.1356	0.0004
M INT CON ELECT		0.0005	0.1363	0.0001
GAMMA	4	0.0002	0.5701	0.0002
GAMMA	5	0.0015	0.6921	0.0022
K ALPHA-1 X-RAY		0.3083	0.0064	0.0042
K ALPHA-2 X-RAY		0.1554	0.0063	0.0021
K BETA-1 X-RAY		0.0499	0.0070	0.0007
KLL AUGER ELECT		0.8954	0.0056	0.0107
KLX AUGER ELECT		0.2185	0.0063	0.0029
LMM AUGER ELECT		2.6451	0.0006	0.0035
MXY AUGER ELECT		5.5781	0.0000	0.0006

••OUTPUT DATA••

26 IRON 59   HALF LIFE = 45.0 DAYS

DECAY MODE- BETA MINUS

RADIATION		MEAN NUMBER/ DISINTE- GRATION n_i	MEAN ENERGY/ PAR- TICLE $\bar{E}_i$ (MeV)	EQUI- LIBRIUM DOSE CONSTANT Δ_i (g-rad/ μCi-h)
BETA MINUS	2	0.0122	0.0381	0.0009
BETA MINUS	3	0.4609	0.0808	0.0793
BETA MINUS	4	0.5228	0.1496	0.1666
BETA MINUS	5	0.0030	0.6396	0.0040
GAMMA	1	0.0096	0.1420	0.0029
GAMMA	2	0.0292	0.1922	0.0119
GAMMA	3	0.0023	0.3347	0.0017
GAMMA	4	0.0002	0.3810	0.0001
GAMMA	5	0.5548	1.0990	1.2987
K INT CON ELECT		0.0000	1.0912	0.0002
GAMMA	6	0.4411	1.2920	1.2140
K INT CON ELECT		0.0000	1.2842	0.0001
GAMMA	7	0.0009	1.4810	0.0028

COBALT-60
BETA-MINUS DECAY

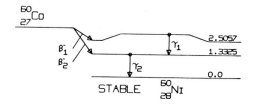

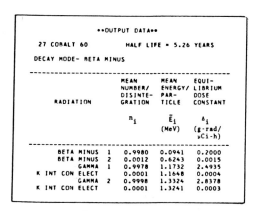

```
                    **OUTPUT DATA**

    27 COBALT 60           HALF LIFE = 5.26 YEARS

    DECAY MODE- BETA MINUS
    ----------------------------------------------------
                          MEAN      MEAN     EQUI-
                          NUMBER/   ENERGY/  LIBRIUM
                          DISINTE-  PAR-     DOSE
           RADIATION      GRATION   TICLE    CONSTANT

                          n_i       Ē_i      Δ_i
                                    (MeV)    (g-rad/
                                             μCi-h)
    ----------------------------------------------------
        BETA MINUS   1    0.9980    0.0941   0.2000
        BETA MINUS   2    0.0012    0.6243   0.0015
           GAMMA     1    0.9978    1.1732   2.4935
    K INT CON ELECT       0.0001    1.1648   0.0004
           GAMMA     2    0.9998    1.3324   2.8378
    K INT CON ELECT       0.0001    1.3241   0.0003
```

GALLIUM-67
ELECTRON CAPTURE DECAY

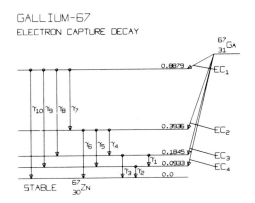

```
                    **OUTPUT DATA**

    31 GALLIUM 67          HALF LIFE = 78.1 HOURS

    DECAY MODE- ELECTRON CAPTURE
    ----------------------------------------------------
                          MEAN      MEAN     EQUI-
                          NUMBER/   ENERGY/  LIBRIUM
                          DISINTE-  PAR-     DOSE
           RADIATION      GRATION   TICLE    CONSTANT

                          n_i       Ē_i      Δ_i
                                    (MeV)    (g-rad/
                                             μCi-h)
    ----------------------------------------------------
           GAMMA     1    0.0326    0.0913   0.0063
    K INT CON ELECT       0.0021    0.0816   0.0003
           GAMMA     2    0.3797    0.0933   0.0754
    K INT CON ELECT       0.2830    0.0836   0.0504
    L INT CON ELECT       0.0379    0.0922   0.0074
    M INT CON ELECT       0.0126    0.0932   0.0025
           GAMMA     3    0.2388    0.1846   0.0939
    K INT CON ELECT       0.0026    0.1749   0.0009
    L INT CON ELECT       0.0004    0.1835   0.0001
           GAMMA     4    0.0247    0.2090   0.0110
           GAMMA     5    0.1613    0.3002   0.1031
    K INT CON ELECT       0.0005    0.2905   0.0003
           GAMMA     6    0.0429    0.3936   0.0359
           GAMMA     7    0.0009    0.4943   0.0010
           GAMMA     8    0.0001    0.7036   0.0002
           GAMMA     9    0.0006    0.7947   0.0010
           GAMMA    10    0.0015    0.8880   0.0029
    K ALPHA-1 X-RAY       0.3075    0.0086   0.0056
    K ALPHA-2 X-RAY       0.1534    0.0086   0.0028
     K BETA-1 X-RAY       0.0553    0.0095   0.0011
    KLL AUGER ELECT       0.5185    0.0075   0.0083
    KLX AUGER ELECT       0.1410    0.0085   0.0025
    KXY AUGER ELECT       0.0067    0.0094   0.0001
    LMM AUGER ELECT       1.7722    0.0008   0.0033
    MXY AUGER ELECT       3.7779    0.0000   0.0006
```

GALLIUM-68

ELECTRON CAPTURE AND
BETA-PLUS DECAY

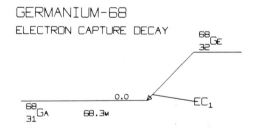

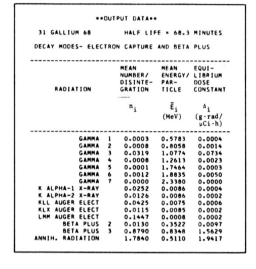

```
                        ••OUTPUT DATA••

        31 GALLIUM 68        HALF LIFE = 68.3 MINUTES

      DECAY MODES- ELECTRON CAPTURE AND BETA PLUS

      --------------------------------------------------
                          MEAN      MEAN     EQUI-
                          NUMBER/   ENERGY/  LIBRIUM
                          DISINTE-  PAR-     DOSE
             RADIATION    GRATION   TICLE    CONSTANT

                          n         Ē        Δ
                           i         i        i
                                    (MeV)    (g-rad/
                                             μCi-h)
      --------------------------------------------------
              GAMMA   1   0.0003    0.5783   0.0004
              GAMMA   2   0.0008    0.8058   0.0014
              GAMMA   3   0.0319    1.0774   0.0734
              GAMMA   4   0.0008    1.2613   0.0023
              GAMMA   5   0.0001    1.7464   0.0003
              GAMMA   6   0.0012    1.8835   0.0050
              GAMMA   7   0.0000    2.3380   0.0000
       K ALPHA-1 X-RAY    0.0252    0.0086   0.0004
       K ALPHA-2 X-RAY    0.0126    0.0086   0.0002
       KLL AUGER ELECT    0.0425    0.0075   0.0006
       KLX AUGER ELECT    0.0115    0.0085   0.0002
       LMM AUGER ELECT    0.1447    0.0008   0.0002
              BETA PLUS 2 0.0130    0.3522   0.0097
              BETA PLUS 3 0.8790    0.8348   1.5629
      ANNIH. RADIATION    1.7840    0.5110   1.9417
```

GERMANIUM-68

ELECTRON CAPTURE DECAY

```
                        ••OUTPUT DATA••

        32 GERMANIUM 68      HALF LIFE = 287. DAYS

      DECAY MODE- ELECTRON CAPTURE

      --------------------------------------------------
                          MEAN      MEAN     EQUI-
                          NUMBER/   ENERGY/  LIBRIUM
                          DISINTE-  PAR-     DOSE
             RADIATION    GRATION   TICLE    CONSTANT

                          n         Ē        Δ
                           i         i        i
                                    (MeV)    (g-rad/
                                             μCi-h)
      --------------------------------------------------
       K ALPHA-1 X-RAY    0.2491    0.0092   0.0049
       K ALPHA-2 X-RAY    0.1241    0.0092   0.0024
        K BETA-1 X-RAY    0.0463    0.0102   0.0010
       KLL AUGER ELECT    0.3646    0.0080   0.0062
       KLX AUGER ELECT    0.1020    0.0091   0.0019
       KXY AUGER ELECT    0.0059    0.0101   0.0001
       LMM AUGER ELECT    1.3000    0.0009   0.0026
       MXY AUGER ELECT    2.7714    0.0001   0.0006

      ------------
      DAUGHTER NUCLIDE, GALLIUM 68  IS RADIOACTIVE
      AND MAY CONTRIBUTE TO THE DOSE.
```

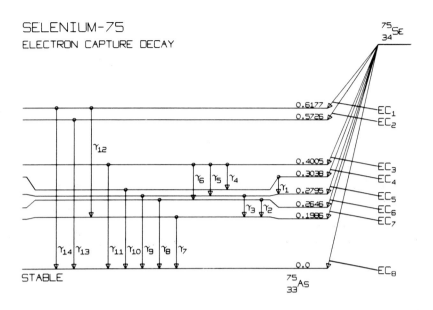

SELENIUM-75
ELECTRON CAPTURE DECAY

OUTPUT DATA

34 SELENIUM 75   HALF LIFE = 120. DAYS

DECAY MODE- ELECTRON CAPTURE

RADIATION		MEAN NUMBER/ DISINTE- GRATION n_i	MEAN ENERGY/ PAR- TICLE $\overline{E}_i$ (MeV)	EQUI- LIBRIUM DOSE CONSTANT Δ_i (g-rad/ μCi-h)
GAMMA	1	0.0002	0.0244	0.0000
K INT CON ELECT		0.0418	0.0125	0.0011
L INT CON ELECT		0.0094	0.0230	0.0004
M INT CON ELECT		0.0031	0.0242	0.0001
GAMMA	2	0.0100	0.0660	0.0014
K INT CON ELECT		0.0026	0.0541	0.0003
GAMMA	3	0.0000	0.0810	0.0000
GAMMA	4	0.0291	0.0848	0.0060
K INT CON ELECT		0.0256	0.0848	0.0046
L INT CON ELECT		0.0031	0.0953	0.0006
M INT CON ELECT		0.0010	0.0965	0.0002
GAMMA	5	0.1563	0.1211	0.0403
K INT CON ELECT		0.0063	0.1092	0.0014
L INT CON ELECT		0.0005	0.1197	0.0001
GAMMA	6	0.5393	0.1360	0.1562
K INT CON ELECT		0.0154	0.1241	0.0040
L INT CON ELECT		0.0014	0.1346	0.0004
M INT CON ELECT		0.0004	0.1358	0.0001
GAMMA	7	0.0135	0.1986	0.0057
K INT CON ELECT		0.0002	0.1867	0.0001
GAMMA	8	0.5710	0.2646	0.3218
K INT CON ELECT		0.0035	0.2527	0.0019
L INT CON ELECT		0.0002	0.2632	0.0001
GAMMA	9	0.2388	0.2795	0.1421
K INT CON ELECT		0.0018	0.2676	0.0010
L INT CON ELECT		0.0001	0.2781	0.0001
GAMMA	10	0.0123	0.3038	0.0080
K INT CON ELECT		0.0005	0.2919	0.0003
GAMMA	11	0.1164	0.4005	0.0993
K INT CON ELECT		0.0001	0.3886	0.0001
GAMMA	12	0.0001	0.4193	0.0001
GAMMA	13	0.0003	0.5726	0.0004
GAMMA	14	0.0000	0.6177	0.0000
K ALPHA-1 X-RAY		0.3175	0.0105	0.0071
K ALPHA-2 X-RAY		0.1581	0.0105	0.0035
K BETA-1 X-RAY		0.0625	0.0117	0.0015
KLL AUGER ELECT		0.3394	0.0091	0.0065
KLX AUGER ELECT		0.0994	0.0103	0.0021
KXY AUGER ELECT		0.0076	0.0115	0.0001
LMM AUGER ELECT		1.3522	0.0010	0.0031
MXY AUGER ELECT		2.9144	0.0001	0.0008

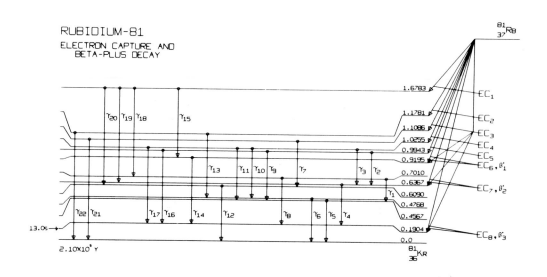

RUBIDIUM-81
ELECTRON CAPTURE AND
BETA-PLUS DECAY

```
**OUTPUT DATA**

37 RUBIDIUM 81        HALF LIFE = 4.58 HOURS

DECAY MODES- ELECTRON CAPTURE AND BETA PLUS
```

RADIATION		n_i	$\bar{E}_i$ (MeV)	Δ_i (g-rad/ μCi-h)
		MEAN NUMBER/ DISINTE- GRATION	MEAN ENERGY/ PAR- TICLE	EQUI- LIBRIUM DOSE CONSTANT
GAMMA	1	0.0026	0.2443	0.0013
GAMMA	2	0.0068	0.3576	0.0051
GAMMA	3	0.0049	0.3888	0.0040
GAMMA	4	0.2315	0.4463	0.2200
GAMMA	5	0.0315	0.4567	0.0306
GAMMA	6	0.0051	0.4768	0.0051
GAMMA	7	0.0024	0.4996	0.0025
GAMMA	8	0.0022	0.5106	0.0023
GAMMA	9	0.0233	0.5376	0.0266
GAMMA	10	0.0042	0.5487	0.0049
GAMMA	11	0.0055	0.5688	0.0066
GAMMA	12	0.0031	0.6090	0.0040
GAMMA	13	0.0009	0.7013	0.0013
GAMMA	14	0.0029	0.7291	0.0045
GAMMA	15	0.0005	0.7588	0.0008
GAMMA	16	0.0079	0.8039	0.0135
GAMMA	17	0.0078	0.8351	0.0138
GAMMA	18	0.0049	0.9773	0.0102
GAMMA	19	0.0050	1.0416	0.0110
GAMMA	20	0.0007	1.0693	0.0015
GAMMA	21	0.0006	1.1086	0.0014
GAMMA	22	0.0001	1.1783	0.0002
K ALPHA-1 X-RAY		0.2326	0.0126	0.0062
K ALPHA-2 X-RAY		0.1160	0.0125	0.0031
K BETA-1 X-RAY		0.0493	0.0141	0.0014
K BETA-2 X-RAY		0.0048	0.0143	0.0001
KLL AUGER ELECT		0.1575	0.0108	0.0036
KLX AUGER ELECT		0.0497	0.0123	0.0013
KXY AUGER ELECT		0.0048	0.0138	0.0001
LMM AUGER ELECT		0.7586	0.0013	0.0021
MXY AUGER ELECT		1.6583	0.0002	0.0007
BETA PLUS	2	0.0199	0.2635	0.0111
BETA PLUS	3	0.2877	0.4572	0.2801
ANNIH. RADIATION		0.6154	0.5110	0.6698

```
DAUGHTER NUCLIDE, KRYPTON 81M IS RADIOACTIVE
AND MAY CONTRIBUTE TO THE DOSE.
BRANCHING TO 0.1910 MEV, 13.0 SECOND HALF LIFE,
   ISOMERIC LEVEL IN KRYPTON-81 IS 0.960 PER
   DISINTEGRATION OF RUBIDIUM-81
```

KRYPTON-81M

ISOMERIC LEVEL DECAY

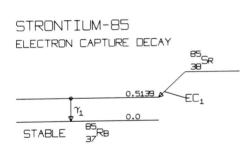

```
      81M
       36 KR                                   0.1900


                  γ₁

      81
       36 KR        2.10X10⁵ Y                 0.0
```

STRONTIUM-85

ELECTRON CAPTURE DECAY

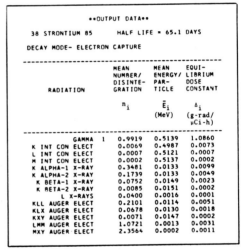

```
                                    85
                                     38 SR


                          0.5139 △    EC₁
                       γ₁        0.0

      STABLE     85
                  37 RB
```

STRONTIUM-87M

ELECTRON CAPTURE AND
ISOMERIC LEVEL DECAY

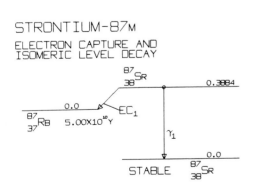

```
                          87
                           38 SR
                                                0.3884
           0.0
                    △   EC₁
      87
       37 RB   5.00X10¹⁰ Y
                                   γ₁

                                                0.0
               STABLE     87
                           38 SR
```

```
                    **OUTPUT DATA**

        36 KRYPTON 81M       HALF LIFE = 13.0 SECONDS

        DECAY MODE- ISOMERIC LEVEL

        ------------------------------------------------
                               MEAN      MEAN      EQUI-
                               NUMBER/   ENERGY/   LIBRIUM
                               DISINTE-  PAR-      DOSE
                 RADIATION     GRATION   TICLE     CONSTANT

                               n_i       Ē_i       Δ_i
                                         (MeV)     (g-rad/
                                                   μCi-h)
        ------------------------------------------------
                 GAMMA   1     0.6644    0.1910    0.2703
          K INT CON ELECT      0.2626    0.1766    0.0988
          L INT CON ELECT      0.0547    0.1892    0.0220
          M INT CON ELECT      0.0182    0.1907    0.0074
          K ALPHA-1 X-RAY      0.0993    0.0126    0.0026
          K ALPHA-2 X-RAY      0.0495    0.0125    0.0013
           K BETA-1 X-RAY      0.0210    0.0141    0.0006
          KLL AUGER ELECT      0.0672    0.0108    0.0015
          KLX AUGER ELECT      0.0212    0.0123    0.0005
          LMM AUGER ELECT      0.3489    0.0013    0.0009
          MXY AUGER ELECT      0.7730    0.0002    0.0003

        ------------
        DAUGHTER NUCLIDE, KRYPTON 81  IS RADIOACTIVE
        AND MAY CONTRIBUTE TO THE DOSE.
```

```
                    **OUTPUT DATA**

        38 STRONTIUM 85       HALF LIFE = 65.1 DAYS

        DECAY MODE- ELECTRON CAPTURE

        ------------------------------------------------
                               MEAN      MEAN      EQUI-
                               NUMBER/   ENERGY/   LIBRIUM
                               DISINTE-  PAR-      DOSE
                 RADIATION     GRATION   TICLE     CONSTANT

                               n_i       Ē_i       Δ_i
                                         (MeV)     (g-rad/
                                                   μCi-h)
        ------------------------------------------------
                 GAMMA   1     0.9919    0.5139    1.0860
          K INT CON ELECT      0.0069    0.4987    0.0073
          L INT CON ELECT      0.0007    0.5121    0.0007
          M INT CON ELECT      0.0002    0.5137    0.0002
          K ALPHA-1 X-RAY      0.3481    0.0133    0.0099
          K ALPHA-2 X-RAY      0.1739    0.0133    0.0049
           K BETA-1 X-RAY      0.0752    0.0149    0.0023
           K BETA-2 X-RAY      0.0085    0.0151    0.0002
             L X-RAYS          0.0400    0.0016    0.0001
          KLL AUGER ELECT      0.2101    0.0114    0.0051
          KLX AUGER ELECT      0.0678    0.0130    0.0018
          KXY AUGER ELECT      0.0071    0.0147    0.0002
          LMM AUGER ELECT      1.0721    0.0013    0.0031
          MXY AUGER ELECT      2.3564    0.0002    0.0011
```

```
                    **OUTPUT DATA**

        38 STRONTIUM 87M      HALF LIFE = 2.80 HOURS

        DECAY MODES- ELECTRON CAPTURE AND ISOMERIC LEVEL

        ------------------------------------------------
                               MEAN      MEAN      EQUI-
                               NUMBER/   ENERGY/   LIBRIUM
                               DISINTE-  PAR-      DOSE
                 RADIATION     GRATION   TICLE     CONSTANT

                               n_i       Ē_i       Δ_i
                                         (MeV)     (g-rad/
                                                   μCi-h)
        ------------------------------------------------
                 GAMMA   1     0.8319    0.3884    0.6882
          K INT CON ELECT      0.1380    0.3722    0.1095
          L INT CON ELECT      0.0202    0.3863    0.0166
          M INT CON ELECT      0.0067    0.3881    0.0055
          K ALPHA-1 X-RAY      0.0554    0.0141    0.0016
          K ALPHA-2 X-RAY      0.0277    0.0140    0.0008
           K BETA-1 X-RAY      0.0122    0.0158    0.0004
          KLL AUGER ELECT      0.0300    0.0120    0.0007
          KLX AUGER ELECT      0.0099    0.0138    0.0002
          LMM AUGER ELECT      0.1664    0.0014    0.0005
          MXY AUGER ELECT      0.3711    0.0002    0.0002
```

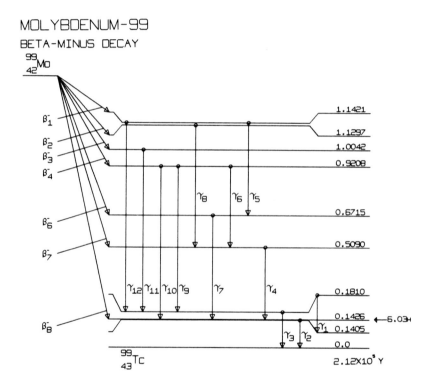

```
                        ••OUTPUT DATA••

        42 MOLYBDENUM 99      HALF LIFE = 66.7 HOURS

        DECAY MODE- BETA MINUS

   -------------------------------------------------------
                          MEAN        MEAN      EQUI-
                          NUMBER/     ENERGY/   LIBRIUM
                          DISINTE-    PAR-      DOSE
               RADIATION  GRATION     TICLE     CONSTANT

                          n_i         Ē_i       Δ_i
                                      (MeV)     (g-rad/
                                                μCi-h)
   -------------------------------------------------------
            BETA MINUS  1   0.0012    0.0658    0.0001
            BETA MINUS  3   0.0014    0.1112    0.0003
            BETA MINUS  4   0.1850    0.1401    0.0552
            BETA MINUS  6   0.0004    0.2541    0.0002
            BETA MINUS  7   0.0143    0.2981    0.0090
            BETA MINUS  8   0.7970    0.4519    0.7673
                GAMMA   1   0.0130    0.0405    0.0011
   K INT CON ELECT         0.0428    0.0195    0.0017
   L INT CON ELECT         0.0053    0.0377    0.0004
   M INT CON ELECT         0.0017    0.0401    0.0001
                GAMMA   2   0.0564    0.1405    0.0168
   K INT CON ELECT         0.0058    0.1194    0.0014
   L INT CON ELECT         0.0007    0.1377    0.0002
                GAMMA   3   0.0657    0.1810    0.0253
   K INT CON ELECT         0.0085    0.1600    0.0029
   L INT CON ELECT         0.0012    0.1782    0.0004
   M INT CON ELECT         0.0004    0.1806    0.0001
                GAMMA   4   0.0143    0.3664    0.0112
                GAMMA   5   0.0001    0.3807    0.0000
                GAMMA   6   0.0002    0.4115    0.0002
                GAMMA   7   0.0005    0.5289    0.0005
                GAMMA   8   0.0002    0.6207    0.0003
                GAMMA   9   0.1367    0.7397    0.2154
   K INT CON ELECT         0.0002    0.7186    0.0003
                GAMMA  10   0.0479    0.7782    0.0794
   K INT CON ELECT         0.0000    0.7571    0.0001
                GAMMA  11   0.0014    0.8231    0.0024
                GAMMA  12   0.0011    0.9610    0.0022
   K ALPHA-1 X-RAY         0.0253    0.0183    0.0009
   K ALPHA-2 X-RAY         0.0127    0.0182    0.0004
    K BETA-1 X-RAY         0.0060    0.0206    0.0002
   KLL AUGER ELECT         0.0087    0.0154    0.0002
   KLX AUGER ELECT         0.0032    0.0178    0.0001
   LMM AUGER ELECT         0.0615    0.0019    0.0002
   MXY AUGER ELECT         0.1403    0.0004    0.0001


   ------------
   DAUGHTER NUCLIDE, TECHNETIUM 99M IS
   RADIOACTIVE AND MAY CONTRIBUTE TO THE DOSE.
   BRANCHING TO 0.1426 MEV, 6.03 HOUR HALF LIFE,
       ISOMERIC LEVEL IN TECHNETIUM-99 IS 0.860 PER
       DISINTEGRATION OF MOLYBDENUM-99.
```

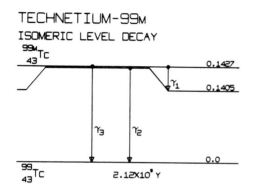

TECHNETIUM-99m
ISOMERIC LEVEL DECAY

```
**OUTPUT DATA**

43 TECHNETIUM 99M     HALF LIFE = 6.03 HOURS

DECAY MODE- ISOMERIC LEVEL
```

RADIATION	MEAN NUMBER/ DISINTE- GRATION n_i	MEAN ENERGY/ PAR- TICLE $\bar{E}_i$ (MeV)	EQUI- LIBRIUM DOSE CONSTANT Δ_i (g-rad/ μCi-h)
GAMMA 1	0.0000	0.0021	0.0000
M INT CON ELECT	0.9860	0.0016	0.0035
GAMMA 2	0.8787	0.1405	0.2630
K INT CON ELECT	0.0913	0.1194	0.0232
L INT CON ELECT	0.0118	0.1377	0.0034
M INT CON ELECT	0.0039	0.1400	0.0011
GAMMA 3	0.0003	0.1426	0.0001
K INT CON ELECT	0.0088	0.1215	0.0022
L INT CON ELECT	0.0035	0.1398	0.0010
M INT CON ELECT	0.0011	0.1422	0.0003
K ALPHA-1 X-RAY	0.0441	0.0183	0.0017
K ALPHA-2 X-RAY	0.0221	0.0182	0.0008
K BETA-1 X-RAY	0.0105	0.0206	0.0004
KLL AUGER ELECT	0.0152	0.0154	0.0005
KLX AUGER ELECT	0.0055	0.0178	0.0002
LMM AUGER ELECT	0.1093	0.0019	0.0004
MXY AUGER ELECT	1.2359	0.0004	0.0011

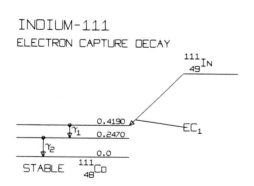

INDIUM-111
ELECTRON CAPTURE DECAY

```
**OUTPUT DATA**

49 INDIUM 111        HALF LIFE = 2.81 DAYS

DECAY MODE- ELECTRON CAPTURE
```

RADIATION	MEAN NUMBER/ DISINTE- GRATION n_i	MEAN ENERGY/ PAR- TICLE $\bar{E}_i$ (MeV)	EQUI- LIBRIUM DOSE CONSTANT Δ_i (g-rad/ μCi-h)
GAMMA 1	0.8959	0.1720	0.3282
K INT CON ELECT	0.0896	0.1452	0.0277
L INT CON ELECT	0.0108	0.1682	0.0038
M INT CON ELECT	0.0036	0.1713	0.0013
GAMMA 2	0.9395	0.2470	0.4942
K INT CON ELECT	0.0507	0.2202	0.0238
L INT CON ELECT	0.0073	0.2432	0.0037
M INT CON ELECT	0.0024	0.2463	0.0012
K ALPHA-1 X-RAY	0.4663	0.0231	0.0230
K ALPHA-2 X-RAY	0.2364	0.0229	0.0115
K BETA-1 X-RAY	0.1198	0.0260	0.0066
K BETA-2 X-RAY	0.0237	0.0267	0.0013
L X-RAYS	0.1108	0.0030	0.0007
KLL AUGER ELECT	0.1103	0.0192	0.0045
KLX AUGER ELECT	0.0441	0.0223	0.0021
KXY AUGER ELECT	0.0067	0.0254	0.0003
LMM AUGER ELECT	0.9867	0.0024	0.0052
MXY AUGER ELECT	2.2886	0.0006	0.0030

TIN-113
ELECTRON CAPTURE DECAY

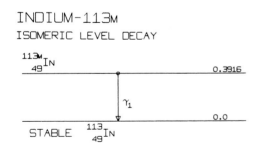

INDIUM-113M
ISOMERIC LEVEL DECAY

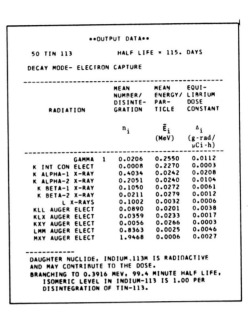

••OUTPUT DATA••

50 TIN 113   HALF LIFE = 115. DAYS

DECAY MODE- ELECTRON CAPTURE

RADIATION	MEAN NUMBER/ DISINTE- GRATION n_i	MEAN ENERGY/ PAR- TICLE $\bar{E}_i$ (MeV)	EQUI- LIBRIUM DOSE CONSTANT Δ_i (g-rad/ μCi-h)
GAMMA 1	0.0206	0.2550	0.0112
K INT CON ELECT	0.0008	0.2270	0.0003
K ALPHA-1 X-RAY	0.4034	0.0242	0.0208
K ALPHA-2 X-RAY	0.2051	0.0240	0.0104
K BETA-1 X-RAY	0.1050	0.0272	0.0061
K BETA-2 X-RAY	0.0211	0.0279	0.0012
L X-RAYS	0.1002	0.0032	0.0006
KLL AUGER ELECT	0.0890	0.0201	0.0038
KLX AUGER ELECT	0.0359	0.0233	0.0017
KXY AUGER ELECT	0.0056	0.0266	0.0003
LMM AUGER ELECT	0.8363	0.0025	0.0046
MXY AUGER ELECT	1.9468	0.0006	0.0027

DAUGHTER NUCLIDE, INDIUM-113M IS RADIOACTIVE
AND MAY CONTRIBUTE TO THE DOSE.
BRANCHING TO 0.3916 MEV, 99.4 MINUTE HALF LIFE,
    ISOMERIC LEVEL IN INDIUM-113 IS 1.00 PER
    DISINTEGRATION OF TIN-113.

••OUTPUT DATA••

49 INDIUM 113M   HALF LIFE = 99.4 MINUTES

DECAY MODE- ISOMERIC LEVEL

RADIATION	MEAN NUMBER/ DISINTE- GRATION n_i	MEAN ENERGY/ PAR- TICLE $\bar{E}_i$ (MeV)	EQUI- LIBRIUM DOSE CONSTANT Δ_i (g-rad/ μCi-h)
GAMMA 1	0.6206	0.3916	0.5178
K INT CON ELECT	0.2668	0.3637	0.2067
L INT CON ELECT	0.0503	0.3877	0.0415
M INT CON ELECT	0.0620	0.3910	0.0516
K ALPHA-1 X-RAY	0.1243	0.0242	0.0064
K ALPHA-2 X-RAY	0.0632	0.0240	0.0032
K BETA-1 X-RAY	0.0324	0.0272	0.0018
K BETA-2 X-RAY	0.0065	0.0279	0.0003
L X-RAYS	0.0325	0.0032	0.0002
KLL AUGER ELECT	0.0274	0.0201	0.0011
KLX AUGER ELECT	0.0110	0.0233	0.0005
LMM AUGER ELECT	0.2715	0.0025	0.0014
MXY AUGER ELECT	0.6846	0.0006	0.0009

IODINE-123
ELECTRON CAPTURE DECAY

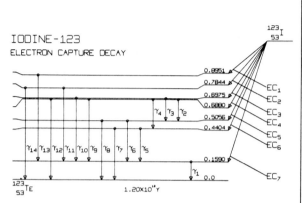

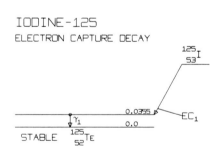

IODINE-125
ELECTRON CAPTURE DECAY

OUTPUT DATA

53 IODINE 123   HALF LIFE = 13.0 HOURS

DECAY MODE- ELECTRON CAPTURE

RADIATION		MEAN NUMBER/ DISINTE- GRATION n_i	MEAN ENERGY/ PAR- TICLE $\bar{E}_i$ (MeV)	EQUI- LIBRIUM DOSE CONSTANT Δ_i (g-rad/ μCi-h)
GAMMA	1	0.8356	0.1591	0.2831
K INT CON ELECT		0.1343	0.1272	0.0364
L INT CON ELECT		0.0174	0.1545	0.0057
M INT CON ELECT		0.0058	0.1582	0.0019
GAMMA	2	0.0002	0.1837	0.0000
GAMMA	3	0.0002	0.1927	0.0001
GAMMA	4	0.0006	0.2483	0.0003
GAMMA	5	0.0006	0.2810	0.0003
GAMMA	6	0.0010	0.3466	0.0007
GAMMA	7	0.0034	0.4404	0.0032
GAMMA	8	0.0026	0.5056	0.0028
GAMMA	9	0.0105	0.5290	0.0118
GAMMA	10	0.0026	0.5385	0.0030
GAMMA	11	0.0006	0.6249	0.0009
GAMMA	12	0.0002	0.6877	0.0003
GAMMA	13	0.0002	0.7361	0.0004
GAMMA	14	0.0004	0.7844	0.0007
K ALPHA-1 X-RAY		0.4715	0.0274	0.0275
K ALPHA-2 X-RAY		0.2419	0.0272	0.0140
K BETA-1 X-RAY		0.1273	0.0309	0.0084
K BETA-2 X-RAY		0.0264	0.0318	0.0017
L X-RAYS		0.1332	0.0037	0.0010
KLL AUGER ELECT		0.0877	0.0226	0.0042
KLX AUGER ELECT		0.0370	0.0264	0.0020
KXY AUGER ELECT		0.0059	0.0301	0.0003
LMM AUGER ELECT		0.9242	0.0029	0.0057
MXY AUGER ELECT		2.1864	0.0008	0.0038

OUTPUT DATA

53 IODINE 125   HALF LIFE = 60.2 DAYS

DECAY MODE- ELECTRON CAPTURE

RADIATION		MEAN NUMBER/ DISINTE- GRATION n_i	MEAN ENERGY/ PAR- TICLE $\bar{E}_i$ (MeV)	EQUI- LIBRIUM DOSE CONSTANT Δ_i (g-rad/ μCi-h)
GAMMA	1	0.0666	0.0354	0.0050
K INT CON ELECT		0.8000	0.0036	0.0062
L INT CON ELECT		0.1142	0.0309	0.0075
M INT CON ELECT		0.0190	0.0346	0.0014
K ALPHA-1 X-RAY		0.7615	0.0274	0.0445
K ALPHA-2 X-RAY		0.3906	0.0272	0.0226
K BETA-1 X-RAY		0.2056	0.0309	0.0135
K BETA-2 X-RAY		0.0426	0.0318	0.0028
L X-RAYS		0.2226	0.0037	0.0017
KLL AUGER ELECT		0.1416	0.0226	0.0068
KLX AUGER ELECT		0.0597	0.0264	0.0033
KXY AUGER ELECT		0.0096	0.0301	0.0006
LMM AUGER ELECT		1.5442	0.0029	0.0096
MXY AUGER ELECT		3.6461	0.0008	0.0063

IODINE-131
BETA-MINUS DECAY

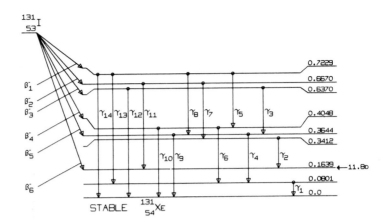

```
                    ••OUTPUT DATA••

        53  IODINE  131        HALF LIFE = 8.06 DAYS

     DECAY MODE- BETA MINUS
```

RADIATION		MEAN NUMBER/ DISINTE- GRATION n_i	MEAN ENERGY/ PAR- TICLE $\bar{E}_i$ (MeV)	EQUI- LIBRIUM DOSE CONSTANT Δ_i (g-rad/ uCi-h)
BETA MINUS	1	0.0200	0.0691	0.0029
BETA MINUS	2	0.0067	0.0867	0.0012
BETA MINUS	3	0.0664	0.0964	0.0136
BETA MINUS	5	0.8980	0.1916	0.3666
BETA MINUS	6	0.0080	0.2839	0.0048
GAMMA	1	0.0258	0.0801	0.0044
K INT CON ELECT		0.0343	0.0456	0.0033
L INT CON ELECT		0.0043	0.0751	0.0007
M INT CON ELECT		0.0014	0.0792	0.0002
GAMMA	2	0.0029	0.1772	0.0011
K INT CON ELECT		0.0004	0.1426	0.0001
GAMMA	3	0.0006	0.2723	0.0003
GAMMA	4	0.0578	0.2843	0.0350
K INT CON ELECT		0.0023	0.2497	0.0012
L INT CON ELECT		0.0004	0.2792	0.0002
GAMMA	5	0.0010	0.3180	0.0007
GAMMA	6	0.0003	0.3250	0.0002
GAMMA	7	0.0036	0.3257	0.0025
GAMMA	8	0.0001	0.3585	0.0001
GAMMA	9	0.8201	0.3644	0.6366
K INT CON ELECT		0.0147	0.3299	0.0103
L INT CON ELECT		0.0023	0.3594	0.0017
M INT CON ELECT		0.0007	0.3635	0.0006
GAMMA	10	0.0006	0.4048	0.0005
GAMMA	11	0.0029	0.5029	0.0031
GAMMA	12	0.0653	0.6367	0.0886
K INT CON ELECT		0.0002	0.6021	0.0003
GAMMA	13	0.0014	0.6430	0.0020
GAMMA	14	0.0173	0.7228	0.0267
K ALPHA-1 X-RAY		0.0249	0.0297	0.0015
K ALPHA-2 X-RAY		0.0128	0.0294	0.0008
K BETA-1 X-RAY		0.0068	0.0336	0.0004
K BETA-2 X-RAY		0.0014	0.0345	0.0001
KLL AUGER ELECT		0.0041	0.0244	0.0002
KLX AUGER ELECT		0.0018	0.0285	0.0001
LMM AUGER ELECT		0.0477	0.0031	0.0003
MXY AUGER ELECT		0.1147	0.0009	0.0002

```
     ------------
     DAUGHTER NUCLIDE, XENON 131M IS RADIOACTIVE
     AND MAY CONTRIBUTE TO THE DOSE.
     BRANCHING TO 0.1639 MEV, 11.8 DAY HALF LIFE,
        ISOMERIC LEVEL IN XENON-131 IS 0.0144 PER
        DISINTEGRATION OF IODINE-131.
```

XENON-133
BETA-MINUS DECAY

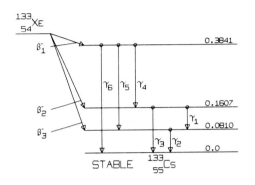

```
                    **OUTPUT DATA**

   54 XENON 133         HALF LIFE = 5.31 DAYS

 DECAY MODE- BETA MINUS
```

RADIATION		MEAN NUMBER/ DISINTE- GRATION n_i	MEAN ENERGY/ PAR- TICLE $\bar{E}_i$ (MeV)	EQUI- LIBRIUM DOSE CONSTANT Δ_i (g-rad/ µCi-h)
BETA MINUS	2	0.0163	0.0750	0.0026
BETA MINUS	3	0.9830	0.1006	0.2106
GAMMA	1	0.0061	0.0796	0.0010
K INT CON ELECT		0.0084	0.0436	0.0007
L INT CON ELECT		0.0012	0.0742	0.0001
GAMMA	2	0.3603	0.0809	0.0621
K INT CON ELECT		0.5261	0.0450	0.0504
L INT CON ELECT		0.0848	0.0756	0.0136
M INT CON ELECT		0.0282	0.0799	0.0048
GAMMA	3	0.0000	0.1606	0.0000
GAMMA	4	0.0000	0.2230	0.0000
GAMMA	5	0.0000	0.3028	0.0000
GAMMA	6	0.0002	0.3839	0.0001
K ALPHA-1 X-RAY		0.2552	0.0309	0.0168
K ALPHA-2 X-RAY		0.1321	0.0306	0.0086
K BETA-1 X-RAY		0.0712	0.0349	0.0053
K BETA-2 X-RAY		0.0150	0.0359	0.0011
L X-RAYS		0.0823	0.0043	0.0007
KLL AUGER ELECT		0.0402	0.0253	0.0021
KLX AUGER ELECT		0.0177	0.0296	0.0011
KXY AUGER ELECT		0.0029	0.0339	0.0002
LMM AUGER ELECT		0.4894	0.0033	0.0034
MXY AUGER ELECT		1.1847	0.0009	0.0025

CESIUM-137
BETA-MINUS DECAY

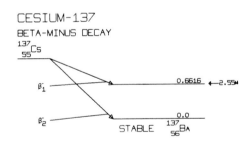

```
                    **OUTPUT DATA**

   55 CESIUM 137        HALF LIFE = 30.0 YEARS

 DECAY MODE- BETA MINUS
```

RADIATION		MEAN NUMBER/ DISINTE- GRATION n_i	MEAN ENERGY/ PAR- TICLE $\bar{E}_i$ (MeV)	EQUI- LIBRIUM DOSE CONSTANT Δ_i (g-rad/ µCi-h)
BETA MINUS	1	0.9460	0.1747	0.3520
BETA MINUS	2	0.0540	0.4269	0.0491

DAUGHTER NUCLIDE, BARIUM 137M IS RADIOACTIVE
AND MAY CONTRIBUTE TO THE DOSE.
BRANCHING TO 0.6616 MEV, 2.55 MINUTE HALF LIFE,
    ISOMERIC LEVEL IN BARIUM-137 IS 0.946 PER
    DISINTEGRATION OF CESIUM-137.

BARIUM-137M
ISOMERIC LEVEL DECAY

```
                    **OUTPUT DATA**

   56 BARIUM 137M       HALF LIFE = 2.55 MINUTES

 DECAY MODE- ISOMERIC LEVEL
```

RADIATION		MEAN NUMBER/ DISINTE- GRATION n_i	MEAN ENERGY/ PAR- TICLE $\bar{E}_i$ (MeV)	EQUI- LIBRIUM DOSE CONSTANT Δ_i (g-rad/ µCi-h)
GAMMA	1	0.8981	0.6616	1.2658
K INT CON ELECT		0.0820	0.6241	0.1091
L INT CON ELECT		0.0147	0.6560	0.0206
M INT CON ELECT		0.0049	0.6605	0.0069
K ALPHA-1 X-RAY		0.0392	0.0321	0.0026
K ALPHA-2 X-RAY		0.0203	0.0318	0.0013
K BETA-1 X-RAY		0.0110	0.0363	0.0008
K BETA-2 X-RAY		0.0023	0.0374	0.0001
L X-RAYS		0.0133	0.0044	0.0001
KLL AUGER ELECT		0.0059	0.0263	0.0003
KLX AUGER ELECT		0.0026	0.0308	0.0001
LMM AUGER ELECT		0.0756	0.0034	0.0005
MXY AUGER ELECT		0.1841	0.0010	0.0004

YTTERBIUM-169
ELECTRON CAPTURE DECAY

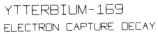

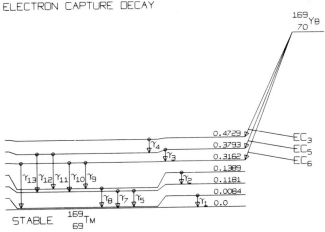

```
                    ••OUTPUT DATA••

        70 YTTERBIUM 169      HALF LIFE = 32.0 DAYS

        DECAY MODE- ELECTRON CAPTURE

    ------------------------------------------------
                          MEAN     MEAN     EQUI-
                          NUMBER/  ENERGY/  LIBRIUM
                          DISINTE- PAR-     DOSE
            RADIATION     GRATION  TICLE    CONSTANT

                            n        E        Δ
                             i        i        i
                                   (MeV)    (g-rad/
                                            μCi-h)
    ------------------------------------------------
                GAMMA  1   0.0000   0.0084   0.0000
    M INT CON ELECT        0.9540   0.0065   0.0132
                GAMMA  2   0.0021   0.0207   0.0000
    L INT CON ELECT        0.0921   0.0113   0.0022
    M INT CON ELECT        0.0307   0.0188   0.0012
                GAMMA  3   0.4516   0.0631   0.0607
    K INT CON ELECT        0.4080   0.0037   0.0032
    L INT CON ELECT        0.0722   0.0537   0.0082
    M INT CON ELECT        0.0240   0.0612   0.0031
                GAMMA  4   0.0078   0.0936   0.0015
    K INT CON ELECT        0.0240   0.0342   0.0017
    L INT CON ELECT        0.0038   0.0842   0.0006
    M INT CON ELECT        0.0953   0.0917   0.0186
                GAMMA  5   0.0382   0.1097   0.0089
    K INT CON ELECT        0.0788   0.0503   0.0084
    L INT CON ELECT        0.0117   0.1003   0.0025
    M INT CON ELECT        0.4711   0.1078   0.1082
                GAMMA  6   0.0004   0.1172   0.0001
                GAMMA  7   0.0190   0.1181   0.0048
    K INT CON ELECT        0.0132   0.0587   0.0016
    L INT CON ELECT        0.0140   0.1087   0.0032
    M INT CON ELECT        0.0046   0.1162   0.0011
                GAMMA  8   0.1142   0.1305   0.0317
    K INT CON ELECT        0.0628   0.0711   0.0095
    L INT CON ELECT        0.0539   0.1211   0.0139
    M INT CON ELECT        0.0179   0.1286   0.0049
                GAMMA  9   0.1731   0.1771   0.0653
    K INT CON ELECT        0.0831   0.1177   0.0208
    L INT CON ELECT        0.0136   0.1677   0.0048
    M INT CON ELECT        0.0801   0.1752   0.0299
                GAMMA 10   0.2616   0.1979   0.1103
    K INT CON ELECT        0.0915   0.1385   0.0270
    L INT CON ELECT        0.0150   0.1885   0.0060
    M INT CON ELECT        0.1506   0.1960   0.0629
                GAMMA 11   0.0012   0.2404   0.0006
                GAMMA 12   0.0174   0.2610   0.0097
    K INT CON ELECT        0.0004   0.2016   0.0002
                GAMMA 13   0.1104   0.3076   0.0724
    K INT CON ELECT        0.0054   0.2482   0.0028
    L INT CON ELECT        0.0015   0.2982   0.0010
    M INT CON ELECT        0.0005   0.3057   0.0003
    K ALPHA-1 X-RAY        0.7750   0.0507   0.0837
    K ALPHA-2 X-RAY        0.4154   0.0497   0.0440
     K BETA-1 X-RAY        0.2472   0.0575   0.0302
     K BETA-2 X-RAY        0.0569   0.0593   0.0072
            L X-RAYS       0.4027   0.0075   0.0064
    KLL AUGER ELECT        0.0626   0.0405   0.0054
    KLX AUGER ELECT        0.0322   0.0481   0.0033
    KXY AUGER ELECT        0.0055   0.0556   0.0006
    LMM AUGER ELECT        1.3635   0.0056   0.0163
    MXY AUGER FLECT        5.2840   0.0018   0.0212
```

MERCURY-197
ELECTRON CAPTURE DECAY

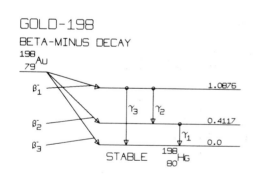

STABLE $^{197}_{79}Au$

```
                    **OUTPUT DATA**

      80 MERCURY 197        HALF LIFE = 65.0 HOURS

      DECAY MODE- ELECTRON CAPTURE
```

RADIATION		MEAN NUMBER/ DISINTE- GRATION n_i	MEAN ENERGY/ PAR- TICLE $\bar{E}_i$ (MeV)	EQUI- LIBRIUM DOSE CONSTANT Δ_i (g-rad/ µCi-h)
GAMMA	1	0.2535	0.0773	0.0417
L INT CON ELECT		0.5583	0.0639	0.0760
M INT CON ELECT		0.1861	0.0745	0.0295
GAMMA	2	0.0029	0.1915	0.0011
K INT CON ELECT		0.0023	0.1107	0.0005
L INT CON ELECT		0.0095	0.1781	0.0036
M INT CON ELECT		0.0031	0.1887	0.0012
GAMMA	3	0.0009	0.2680	0.0005
K INT CON ELECT		0.0003	0.1872	0.0001
K ALPHA-1 X-RAY		0.3609	0.0688	0.0529
K ALPHA-2 X-RAY		0.1980	0.0669	0.0282
K BETA-1 X-RAY		0.1250	0.0779	0.0207
K BETA-2 X-RAY		0.0335	0.0807	0.0057
L ALPHA X-RAYS		0.2434	0.0097	0.0050
L BETA X-RAYS		0.2280	0.0114	0.0055
L GAMMA X-RAYS		0.0307	0.0133	0.0008
KLL AUGER ELECT		0.0189	0.0540	0.0021
KLX AUGER ELECT		0.0107	0.0646	0.0014
KXY AUGER ELECT		0.0017	0.0752	0.0002
LMM AUGER ELECT		0.8736	0.0078	0.0146
MXY AUGER ELECT		2.6315	0.0027	0.0153

GOLD-198
BETA-MINUS DECAY

$^{198}_{79}Au$

β_1^-

β_2^-

β_3^-

γ_3 γ_2

1.0876

0.4117

γ_1 0.0

STABLE $^{198}_{80}Hg$

```
                    **OUTPUT DATA**

      79 GOLD 198          HALF LIFE = 2.69 DAYS

      DECAY MODE- BETA MINUS
```

RADIATION		MEAN NUMBER/ DISINTE- GRATION n_i	MEAN ENERGY/ PAR- TICLE $\bar{E}_i$ (MeV)	EQUI- LIBRIUM DOSE CONSTANT Δ_i (g-rad/ µCi-h)
BETA MINUS	1	0.0130	0.0811	0.0022
BETA MINUS	2	0.9860	0.3163	0.6643
BETA MINUS	3	0.0002	0.4648	0.0002
GAMMA	1	0.9555	0.4117	0.8380
K INT CON ELECT		0.0287	0.3286	0.0201
L INT CON ELECT		0.0095	0.3979	0.0081
M INT CON ELECT		0.0031	0.4089	0.0027
GAMMA	2	0.0107	0.6758	0.0154
K INT CON ELECT		0.0002	0.5927	0.0003
GAMMA	3	0.0022	1.0876	0.0053
K ALPHA-1 X-RAY		0.0139	0.0708	0.0021
K ALPHA-2 X-RAY		0.0076	0.0688	0.0011
K BETA-1 X-RAY		0.0048	0.0802	0.0008
K BETA-2 X-RAY		0.0013	0.0831	0.0002
L ALPHA X-RAYS		0.0060	0.0099	0.0001
L BETA X-RAYS		0.0056	0.0118	0.0001
LMM AUGER ELECT		0.0206	0.0081	0.0003
MXY AUGER ELECT		0.0622	0.0028	0.0003

MERCURY-203
BETA-MINUS DECAY

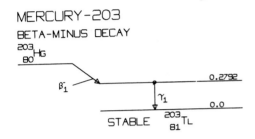

$^{203}_{80}\text{Hg}$

β_1^-

0.2792

γ_1

0.0

STABLE $^{203}_{81}\text{TL}$

```
                        ••OUTPUT DATA••

     80 MERCURY 203         HALF LIFE = 46.5 DAYS

     DECAY MODE- BETA MINUS
```

	MEAN NUMBER/ DISINTE- GRATION	MEAN ENERGY/ PAR- TICLE	EQUI- LIBRIUM DOSE CONSTANT
RADIATION	n_i	$\bar{E}_i$ (MeV)	Δ_i (g-rad/ µCi-h)
BETA MINUS 1	1.0000	0.0577	0.1229
GAMMA 1	0.8173	0.2792	0.4860
K INT CON ELECT	0.1332	0.1936	0.0549
L INT CON ELECT	0.0396	0.2649	0.0223
M INT CON ELECT	0.0097	0.2762	0.0057
K ALPHA-1 X-RAY	0.0638	0.0728	0.0099
K ALPHA-2 X-RAY	0.0352	0.0708	0.0053
K BETA-1 X-RAY	0.0224	0.0825	0.0039
K BETA-2 X-RAY	0.0063	0.0855	0.0011
L ALPHA X-RAYS	0.0275	0.0102	0.0006
L BETA X-RAYS	0.0258	0.0122	0.0006
L GAMMA X-RAYS	0.0034	0.0142	0.0001
KLL AUGER ELECT	0.0031	0.0569	0.0003
KLX AUGER ELECT	0.0018	0.0683	0.0002
LMM AUGER ELECT	0.0900	0.0083	0.0016
MXY AUGER ELECT	0.2717	0.0029	0.0017

RADIUM-224
ALPHA DECAY

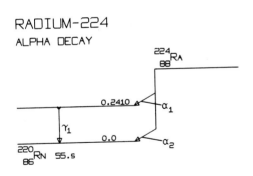

$^{224}_{88}\text{RA}$

0.2410 α_1

γ_1

0.0 α_2

$^{220}_{86}\text{RN}$ 55.s

```
                        ••OUTPUT DATA••

     88 RADIUM 224         HALF LIFE = 3.64 DAYS

     DECAY MODE- ALPHA
```

	MEAN NUMBER/ DISINTE- GRATION	MEAN ENERGY/ PAR- TICLE	EQUI- LIBRIUM DOSE CONSTANT
RADIATION	n_i	$\bar{E}_i$ (MeV)	Δ_i (g-rad/ µCi-h)
ALPHA 1	0.0520	5.4472	0.6033
RECOIL ATOM	0.0520	0.0990	0.0109
ALPHA 2	0.9480	5.6840	11.4773
RECOIL ATOM	0.9480	0.1033	0.2086
GAMMA 1	0.0400	0.2410	0.0205
K INT CON ELECT	0.0044	0.1425	0.0013
L INT CON ELECT	0.0056	0.2242	0.0026
M INT CON ELECT	0.0018	0.2374	0.0009
K ALPHA-1 X-RAY	0.0020	0.0837	0.0003
K ALPHA-2 X-RAY	0.0011	0.0810	0.0002
K BETA-1 X-RAY	0.0007	0.0948	0.0001
LMM AUGER ELECT	0.0052	0.0097	0.0001
MXY AUGER ELECT	0.0170	0.0035	0.0001

```
     ------------
     DAUGHTER NUCLIDE, RADON 220  IS RADIOACTIVE
     AND MAY CONTRIBUTE TO THE DOSE.
```

APPENDIX C

Properties of the Elements

Name	Symbol	At. No.	At. Wt.* (^{12}C scale)	Density* (g/cm^3)	K_B† (keV)
Actinium	Ac	89	~227	—	106.759
Aluminum	Al	13	26.982	2.702	1.559
Americium	Am	95	~243	—	125.030
Antimony	Sb	51	121.75	6.684	30.491
Argon	Ar	18	39.948	1.784‡	3.206
Arsenic	As	33	74.922	5.727	11.867
Astatine	At	85	~210	—	95.730
Barium	Ba	56	137.33	3.51	37.441
Berkelium	Bk	97	~247	—	131.590
Beryllium	Be	4	9.012	1.85	0.1117
Bismuth	Bi	83	208.981	9.80	90.526
Boron	B	5	10.81	(2.34—2.37)	0.192
Bromine	Br	35	79.904	3.119	13.475
Cadmium	Cd	48	112.41	8.642	26.712
Calcium	Ca	20	40.08	1.54	4.038
Californium	Cf	98	~251	—	135.960
Carbon	C	6	12.011	(1.8—3.5)	0.2847
Cerium	Ce	58	140.12	(6.657–6.757)	40.444
Cesium	Cs	55	132.905	1.879	35.985
Chlorine	Cl	17	35.453	3.214‡	2.823
Chromium	Cr	24	51.996	7.20	5.9908
Cobalt	Co	27	58.933	8.9	7.7114
Copper	Cu	29	63.546	8.92	8.980
Curium	Cm	96	~247	—	128.220
Dysprosium	Dy	66	162.50	8.550	53.789
Einsteinium	Es	99	~254	—	139.490
Erbium	Er	68	167.26	9.006	57.486
Europium	Eu	63	151.96	5.243	48.519
Fermium	Fm	100	~257	—	143.090
Fluorine	F	9	18.998	1.69‡	.6967
Francium	Fr	87	~223	—	101.140

Name	Symbol	At. No.	At. Wt.* (^{12}C scale)	Density* (g/cm^3)	K_B† (keV)
Gadolinium	Gd	64	157.25	7.900	50.239
Gallium	Ga	31	69.72	(5.9–6.1)	10.368
Germanium	Ge	32	72.59	5.35	11.103
Gold	Au	79	196.967	19.3	80.722
Hafnium	Hf	72	178.49	13.31	65.351
Helium	He	2	4.003	0.179‡	0.0246
Holmium	Ho	67	164.930	8.795	55.618
Hydrogen	H	1	1.008	0.090‡	0.0136
Indium	In	49	114.82	7.30	27.940
Iodine	I	53	126.905	4.93	33.120
Iridium	Ir	77	192.20	22.421	76.111
Iron	Fe	26	55.847	7.86	7.111
Krypton	Kr	36	83.80	3.736‡	14.326
Lanthanum	La	57	138.905	(6.145–6.17)	38.925
Lawrencium	Lr	103	~257	—	154.380
Lead	Pb	82	207.2	11.344	88.005
Lithium	Li	3	6.939	0.534	0.055
Lutetium	Lu	71	174.97	9.840	63.314
Magnesium	Mg	12	24.312	1.74	1.303
Manganese	Mn	25	54.938	7.20	6.5382
Mendelevium	Md	101	~256	—	146.780
Mercury	Hg	80	200.59	13.594	83.103
Molybdenum	Mo	42	95.94	10.2	20.002
Neodymium	Nd	60	144.24	(6.80–7.004)	43.569
Neon	Ne	10	20.179	0.900‡	0.8704
Neptunium	Np	93	237.00	(18.0–20.5)	118.680
Nickel	Ni	28	58.71	8.90	8.3324
Niobium	Nb	41	92.906	8.57	18.983
Nitrogen	N	7	14.007	1.251	0.4099
Nobelium	No	102	~259	—	150.540
Osmium	Os	76	190.2	22.48	73.871
Oxygen	O	8	15.999	1.429‡	0.5431
Palladium	Pd	46	106.4	(11.4–12.0)	24.350
Phosphorus	P	15	30.974	(2.34–2.70)	2.149
Platinum	Pt	78	195.09	21.45	78.395
Plutonium	Pu	94	239.05	(15.9–19.8)	121.820
Polonium	Po	84	210.05	9.4	93.105
Potassium	K	19	39.098	0.86	3.6084
Praseodymium	Pr	59	140.908	6.773	41.991
Promethium	Pm	61	~145	7.22	45.185
Protactinium	Pa	91	231.10	15.37	112.600
Radium	Ra	88	226.025	5	103.920
Radon	Rn	86	~222	9.73‡	98.400
Rhenium	Re	75	186.2	20.53	71.675
Rhodium	Rh	45	102.906	12.4	23.220
Rubidium	Rb	37	85.468	1.532	15.201
Ruthenium	Ru	44	101.07	12.30	22.118
Samarium	Sm	62	150.35	7.520	46.846
Scandium	Sc	21	44.956	2.989	4.496
Selenium	Se	34	78.96	4.81	12.658
Silicon	Si	14	28.086	(2.32–2.34)	1.838
Silver	Ag	47	107.868	10.5	25.514
Sodium	Na	11	22.990	0.97	1.0717
Strontium	Sr	38	87.62	2.6	16.106

Properties of the Elements (continued)

Name	Symbol	At. No.	At. Wt.* (^{12}C scale)	Density* (g/cm³)	K_B† (keV)
Sulfur	S	16	32.06	2.07	2.472
Tantalum	Ta	73	180.948	(14.4–16.6)	67.413
Technetium	Tc	43	98.906	—	21.044
Tellurium	Te	52	127.60	6.25	31.814
Terbium	Tb	65	158.925	8.229	51.996
Thallium	Tl	81	204.37	11.85	85.529
Thorium	Th	90	232.038	11.7	109.650
Thulium	Tm	69	168.934	9.321	59.390
Tin	Sn	50	118.69	(5.75–7.28)	29.200
Titanium	Ti	22	47.90	4.5	4.9658
Tungsten	W	74	183.85	19.35	69.523
Uranium	U	92	238.029	19.05	115.610
Vanadium	V	23	50.941	5.96	5.4657
Xenon	Xe	54	131.30	5.887‡	34.566
Ytterbium	Yb	70	173.04	6.965	61.332
Yttrium	Y	39	88.906	4.469	17.039
Zinc	Zn	30	65.38	7.14	9.660
Zirconium	Zr	40	91.22	6.49	18.000

*Reprinted with permission from The Handbook of Chemistry and Physics (ed. 60). Copyright CRC Press, Inc., Boca Raton, FL, 1979–1980. Density values in parentheses are given for elements that may exist in different crystalline forms.

†From Lederer, C.M., and Shirley, V.S.: Table of Isotopes. 7th ed. New York, Wiley-Interscience, 1978.

‡Densities for gases in g/l.

APPENDIX D

THE GREEK ALPHABET

Alpha	A	α
Beta	B	β
Gamma	Γ	γ
Delta	Δ	δ
Epsilon	E	ε
Zeta	Z	ζ
Eta	H	η
Theta	Θ	θ
Iota	I	ι
Kappa	K	κ
Lambda	Λ	λ
Mu	M	μ
Nu	N	ν
Xi	Ξ	ξ
Omicron	O	o
Pi	Π	π
Rho	P	ρ
Sigma	Σ	σ
Tau	T	τ
Upsilon	Υ	υ
Phi	Φ	φ
Chi	X	χ
Psi	Ψ	ψ
Omega	Ω	ω

APPENDIX E

UNIVERSAL DECAY TABLE

The following table can be used to determine the fraction of activity remaining of any radionuclide, from 0.001 half-life to 1.00 half-life. To use the table:

1. Divide elapsed time by the known physical half-life of the radionuclide under consideration $(t/T_{1/2})$. Note that the same time unit must be used in each instance.
2. Use this answer (to three significant figures) to locate the fraction of the original activity remaining. The first two significant figures are listed in the vertical column at the left of the table; the third significant figure is listed horizontally, across the top of the table.
3. Multiply original activity by this decimal fraction to obtain the activity remaining.

Example: What amount of activity remains of 20 mCi of Tc-99m after 5 hr?

1. $t/T_{1/2} = 5/6 = 0.833$
2. Fraction remaining from decay table $= 0.56136$
3. 20 mCi × 0.56136 = 11.23 mCi

Activity Remaining for $t/T_{1/2}$

	.000	.001	.002	.003	.004	.005	.006	.007	.008	.009
	1.00000	.99931	.99861	.99792	.99723	.99654	.99585	.99516	.99447	.99378
.01	.99309	.99240	.99172	.99103	.99034	.98966	.98897	.98829	.98760	.98692
.02	.98623	.98555	.98487	.98418	.98350	.98282	.98214	.98146	.98078	.98010
.03	.97942	.97874	.97806	.97739	.97671	.97603	.97536	.97468	.97400	.97333
.04	.97265	.97198	.97131	.97063	.96996	.96929	.96862	.96795	.96728	.96661
.05	.96594	.96527	.96460	.96393	.96326	.96259	.96193	.96126	.96059	.95993
.06	.95926	.95860	.95794	.95727	.95661	.95595	.95528	.95462	.95396	.95330
.07	.95264	.95198	.95132	.95066	.95000	.94934	.94868	.94803	.94737	.94671
.08	.94606	.94540	.94475	.94409	.94344	.94278	.94213	.94148	.94083	.94017
.09	.93952	.93887	.93822	.93757	.93692	.93627	.93562	.93498	.93433	.93368
.10	.93303	.93239	.93174	.93109	.93045	.92980	.92916	.92852	.92787	.92723
.11	.92659	.92595	.92530	.92466	.92402	.92338	.92274	.92210	.92146	.92083
.12	.92019	.91955	.91891	.91828	.91764	.91700	.91637	.91573	.91510	.91447
.13	.91383	.91320	.91257	.91193	.91130	.91067	.91004	.90941	.90878	.90815
.14	.90752	.90689	.90626	.90563	.90501	.90438	.90375	.90313	.90250	.90188
.15	.90125	.90063	.90000	.89938	.89876	.89813	.89751	.89689	.89627	.89565
.16	.89503	.89440	.89379	.89317	.89255	.89193	.89131	.89069	.89008	.88946
.17	.88884	.88823	.88761	.88700	.88638	.88577	.88515	.88454	.88393	.88332
.18	.88270	.88209	.88148	.88087	.88026	.87965	.87904	.87843	.87782	.87721
.19	.87661	.87600	.87539	.87478	.87418	.87357	.87297	.87236	.87176	.87115
.20	.87055	.86995	.86934	.86874	.86814	.86754	.86694	.86634	.86574	.86514
.21	.86454	.86394	.86334	.86274	.86214	.86155	.86095	.86035	.85976	.85916
.22	.85857	.85797	.85738	.85678	.85619	.85559	.85500	.85441	.85382	.85323
.23	.85263	.85204	.85145	.85086	.85027	.84968	.84910	.84851	.84792	.84733
.24	.84675	.84616	.84557	.84499	.84440	.84382	.84323	.84265	.84206	.84148
.25	.84090	.84031	.83973	.83915	.83857	.83799	.83741	.83683	.83625	.83567
.26	.83509	.83451	.83393	.83335	.83278	.83220	.83162	.83105	.83047	.82989
.27	.82932	.82874	.82817	.82760	.82702	.82645	.82588	.82531	.82473	.82416
.28	.82359	.82302	.82245	.82188	.82131	.82074	.82017	.81960	.81904	.81847
.29	.81790	.81734	.81677	.81620	.81564	.81507	.81451	.81394	.81338	.81282

Activity Remaining for t/T½ (continued)

	.000	.001	.002	.003	.004	.005	.006	.007	.008	.009
.30	.81225	.81169	.81113	.81057	.81000	.80944	.80888	.80832	.80776	.80720
.31	.80664	.80608	.80552	.80497	.80441	.80385	.80329	.80274	.80218	.80163
.32	.80107	.80051	.79996	.79941	.79885	.79830	.79775	.79719	.79664	.79609
.33	.79554	.79499	.79443	.79388	.79333	.79278	.79223	.79169	.79114	.79059
.34	.79004	.78949	.78895	.78840	.78785	.78731	.78676	.78622	.78567	.78513
.35	.78458	.78404	.78350	.78295	.78241	.78187	.78133	.78079	.78025	.77970
.36	.77916	.77862	.77809	.77755	.77701	.77647	.77593	.77539	.77486	.77432
.37	.77378	.77325	.77271	.77218	.77164	.77111	.77057	.77004	.76950	.76897
.38	.76844	.76791	.76737	.76684	.76631	.76578	.76525	.76472	.76419	.76366
.39	.76313	.76260	.76207	.76154	.76102	.76049	.75996	.75944	.75891	.75838
.40	.75786	.75733	.75681	.75628	.75576	.75524	.75471	.75419	.75367	.75315
.41	.75262	.75210	.75158	.75106	.75054	.75002	.74950	.74898	.74846	.74794
.42	.74742	.74691	.74639	.74587	.74536	.74484	.74432	.74381	.74329	.74278
.43	.74226	.74175	.74123	.74072	.74021	.73969	.73918	.73867	.73816	.73765
.44	.73713	.73662	.73611	.73560	.73509	.73458	.73408	.73357	.73306	.73255
.45	.73204	.73154	.73103	.73052	.73002	.72951	.72900	.72850	.72799	.72749
.46	.72699	.72648	.72598	.72548	.72497	.72447	.72397	.72347	.72297	.72247
.47	.72196	.72146	.72096	.72047	.71997	.71947	.71897	.71847	.71797	.71747
.48	.71698	.71648	.71598	.71549	.71499	.71450	.71400	.71351	.71301	.71252
.49	.71203	.71153	.71104	.71055	.71005	.70956	.70907	.70858	.70809	.70760
.50	.70711	.70662	.70613	.70564	.70515	.70466	.70417	.70368	.70320	.70271
.51	.70222	.70174	.70125	.70076	.70028	.69979	.69931	.69882	.69834	.69786
.52	.69737	.69689	.69641	.69592	.69544	.69496	.69448	.69400	.69352	.69304
.53	.69255	.69208	.69160	.69112	.69064	.69016	.68968	.68920	.68873	.68825
.54	.68777	.68729	.68682	.68634	.68587	.68539	.68492	.68444	.68397	.68349
.55	.68302	.68255	.68207	.68160	.68113	.68066	.68019	.67971	.67924	.67877
.56	.67830	.67783	.67736	.67689	.67642	.67596	.67549	.67502	.67455	.67408
.57	.67362	.67315	.67268	.67222	.67175	.67129	.67082	.67036	.66989	.66943
.58	.66896	.66850	.66804	.66757	.66711	.66665	.66619	.66573	.66526	.66480
.59	.66434	.66388	.66342	.66296	.66250	.66204	.66159	.66113	.66067	.66021
.60	.65975	.65930	.65884	.65838	.65793	.65747	.65702	.65656	.65611	.65565
.61	.65520	.65474	.65429	.65384	.65338	.65293	.65248	.65203	.65157	.65112
.62	.65067	.65022	.64977	.64932	.64887	.64842	.64797	.64752	.64707	.64662
.63	.64618	.64573	.64528	.64483	.64439	.64394	.64349	.64305	.64260	.64216
.64	.64171	.64127	.64082	.64038	.63994	.63949	.63905	.63861	.63816	.63772
.65	.63728	.63684	.63640	.63596	.63552	.63508	.63464	.63420	.63376	.63332
.66	.63288	.63244	.63200	.63156	.63113	.63069	.63025	.62982	.62938	.62894

.67	.62460	.62503	.62546	.62590	.62633	.62677	.62720	.62764	.62807	.62851
.68	.62028	.62071	.62114	.62157	.62201	.62244	.62287	.62330	.62373	.62417
.69	.61600	.61643	.61685	.61728	.61771	.61814	.61857	.61900	.61942	.61985
.70	.61174	.61217	.61259	.61302	.61344	.61387	.61429	.61472	.61515	.61557
.71	.60752	.60794	.60836	.60878	.60921	.60963	.61005	.61047	.61090	.61132
.72	.60332	.60374	.60416	.60458	.60500	.60542	.60584	.60626	.60668	.60710
.73	.59915	.59957	.59999	.60040	.60082	.60123	.60165	.60207	.60249	.60290
.74	.59502	.59543	.59584	.59625	.59667	.59708	.59750	.59791	.59832	.59874
.75	.59091	.59132	.59173	.59214	.59255	.59296	.59337	.59378	.59419	.59460
.76	.58682	.58723	.58764	.58805	.58845	.58886	.58927	.58968	.59009	.59050
.77	.58277	.58317	.58358	.58398	.58439	.58479	.58520	.58561	.58601	.58642
.78	.57875	.57915	.57955	.57995	.58035	.58075	.58116	.58156	.58196	.58237
.79	.57475	.57515	.57554	.57594	.57634	.57674	.57714	.57754	.57794	.57834
.80	.57078	.57117	.57157	.57197	.57236	.57276	.57316	.57355	.57395	.57435
.81	.56683	.56723	.56762	.56801	.56841	.56880	.56920	.56959	.56999	.57038
.82	.56292	.56331	.56370	.56409	.56448	.56487	.56527	.56566	.56605	.56644
.83	.55903	.55942	.55981	.56019	.56058	.56097	.56136	.56175	.56214	.56253
.84	.55517	.55555	.55594	.55632	.55671	.55710	.55748	.55787	.55826	.55864
.85	.55133	.55172	.55210	.55248	.55287	.55325	.55363	.55402	.55440	.55478
.86	.54753	.54791	.54829	.54867	.54905	.54943	.54981	.55019	.55057	.55095
.87	.54374	.54412	.54450	.54488	.54525	.54563	.54601	.54639	.54677	.54715
.88	.53999	.54036	.54074	.54111	.54149	.54186	.54224	.54261	.54299	.54337
.89	.53626	.53663	.53700	.53737	.53775	.53812	.53849	.53887	.53924	.53961
.90	.53255	.53292	.53329	.53366	.53403	.53440	.53477	.53514	.53552	.53589
.91	.52888	.52924	.52961	.52998	.53034	.53071	.53108	.53145	.53182	.53218
.92	.52522	.52559	.52595	.52632	.52668	.52705	.52741	.52778	.52814	.52851
.93	.52159	.52196	.52232	.52268	.52304	.52340	.52377	.52413	.52449	.52486
.94	.51799	.51835	.51871	.51907	.51943	.51979	.52015	.52051	.52087	.52123
.95	.51441	.51477	.51513	.51548	.51584	.51620	.51656	.51692	.51727	.51763
.96	.51086	.51121	.51157	.51192	.51228	.51263	.51299	.51334	.51370	.51406
.97	.50733	.50768	.50803	.50839	.50874	.50909	.50945	.50980	.51015	.51051
.98	.50383	.50418	.50453	.50488	.50523	.50558	.50593	.50628	.50663	.50698
.99	.50035	.50069	.50104	.50139	.50174	.50208	.50243	.50278	.50313	.50348
100										.50000

APPENDIX F

COMMON ABBREVIATIONS

Ab—Antibody

ACPC—Aminocyclopentane carboxylic acid

ACTH—Adrenocorticotropic hormone

ADC—Analog to digital converter

Ag—Antigen

ALARA—As low as reasonably achievable

ART—Algebraic reconstruction technique

ATP—Adenosine triphosphate

BCD—Binary coded decimal

BDDTC—Bis-diethyldithiocarbamate

BEI—Butanol-extractable iodine

BLEDTA—1-(p-bromoacetamidophenyl) ethylenedinitrilotetracetic acid

BLIP—Brookhaven Linac Isotope Producer

BMR—Basal metabolic rate

cAMP—Cyclic adenosine monophosphate

CAT—Computerized axial tomography

CEA—Carcinoembryonic antigen

CFR—Code of Federal Regulations

CPB—Competitive protein binding

CPK—Creatine phosphokinase

CPU—Central processing unit

CRT—Cathode-ray tube

CSF—Cerebrospinal fluid

CT—Computed tomography

CTT—Computerized transaxial tomography

DAC—Digital to analog converter

DADS—N,N'bis(mercaptoacetamido)-ethylenediamine

DDTC—Diethyldithiocarbamate

DFP—Diisopropylfluorophosphate

DHTA—Dihydrothioctic acid

DIDA—Diethyliminodiacetic acid

DISIDA—Diisopropyliminodiacetic acid

DIT—Diiodotryosine

DMA—Direct memory access

DMSA—Dimercaptosuccinic acid

DNA—Deoxyribonucleic acid

DOS—Disk operating system

DSA—Digital subtraction angiography

DTA—Diethylenetriamine

DTPA—Diethylenetriaminepentaacetic acid

EDTA—Ethylenediaminetetraacetic acid

EHDP—Ethane-1-hydroxy-1,1-diphosphonate

EIDA—Diethyliminodiacetic acid

FDA—Food and Drug Administration

FDG—2-fluoro-2-deoxy-D-glucose

FSH—Follicle stimulating hormone

FTI—Free thyroxine index

FWHM—Full width at half maximum
Ge(Li)—Germanium-lithium (drifted
    detector)
GFR—Glomerular filtration rate
GHA—Glucoheptonate
GM—Geiger-Müller
GSD—Genetically significant dose
HAA—Human Australian Antigen
HAM—Human albumin microspheres
HCAT—Homotaurocholate
HCG—Human chorionic gonadotropin
HEDP—Hydroxyethylidene
    diphosphonate
HEDSPA—1-hydroxy-ethylidene-1,1-
    disodium phosphonate
HEDTA—N-
    hydroxyethylethylenediamine-
    tetraacetic acid
HGH—Human growth hormone
HIDA—Dimethyliminodiacetic acid
HIPDM—2-hydroxyl-3-methyl-5-
    iodobenzyl-1,3-propanediamine
HMDP—Hydroxymethylene
    diphosphonate
HPLC—High pressure liquid
    chromatography
HSA—Human serum albumin
HVL—Half-value layer
IgG—Gamma G immunoglobulin
I/O—Input/Output
IAEA—International Atomic Energy
    Agency
IC—Integrated circuit
IDA—Iminodiacetic acid
IND—Investigational new drug
    (application)
IRMA—Immunoradiometric analysis
ITLC—Instant thin-layer chromatography
KTS—Kethoxal-bis(thiosemicarbazone)
LAMPH—Los Alamos Meson Physics
    Facility
LATS—Long-acting thyroid stimulator
LDH—Lactic dehydrogenase
LED—Light-emitting diode
LET—Linear energy transfer
LFOV—Large field of view
LSB—Least significant bit
LSF—Line spread function
MAA—Macroaggregated albumin

MCA—Multichannel analyzer
MDP—Methylenediphosphonate
MEK—Methylethyl ketone
MIRD—Medical Internal Radiation Dose
    (committee)
MIT—Monoiodotyrosine
MNG—Multinodular goiter
MPBB—Maximum permissible body
    burden
MPC—Maximum permissible
    concentration
MR—Magnetic resonance
MSB—Most significant bit
MTF—Modulation transfer function
MWPC—Multiwire proportional counter
NCRP—National Council on Radiation
    Protection
NDA—New drug application
NEMA—National Electrical
    Manufacturers Association
NF—National Formulary
NMR—Nucler magnetic resonance
NRC—Nuclear Regulatory Commission
NTA—Nitrilotriacetic acid
PAC—Penicillamine-acetazolamide
    complex
PBI—Protein-bound iodine
PBNAA—Partial body neutron activation
    analysis
PETT—Positron-emission transaxial
    tomography
PG—Pyridoxylidene glutamate
PGNAA—Prompt gamma neutron
    activation analysis
PHA—Pulse height analyzer
PIPIDA—N-(para-isopropyl)
    iminodiacetic acid
PLES—Parallel line equal space
    (phantom)
PM—Photomultiplier (tube)
Poly—Polyphosphate
POP—2,5-Diphenyloxazole
POPOP—1,4-Bis-(5-phenoxazole)benzene
PPi—(Tc)pyrophosphate
PPx—(Tc)polyphosphate
PSF—Point spread function
PTH—Parathyroid hormone
PTU—Propylthiouracil
PVP—Polyvinyl pyrrolidone

PYP—Pyrophosphate
RAI—Radioactive iodine (uptake)
RAM—Random access memory
RBE—Relative biologic effectiveness
RDP—Radiopharmaceutical drug product
RF—Radiofrequency
RIA—Radioimmunoassay
RNA—Ribonucleic acid
ROC—Receiver operating curve
ROI—Region of interest
ROM—Read-only memory
SC—Sulfur colloid
SGOT—Serum glutamic oxaloacetic
    transaminase
SGPT—Serum glutamic pyruvic
    transaminase
SNR—Signal-to-noise ratio
SSKI—Saturated solution of potassium
    iodide
T3—Triiodothyronine
T4—Thyroxine, levothyroxine
TAC—Time-activity curve
TBG—Thyroxine-binding globulin
TBNAA—Total body neutron activation
    analysis
TBPA—Thyroxine binding prealbumin

TcPen—Tc-99m penicillamine
TLC—Thin-layer chromatography
TLD—Thermoluminescent detector
TRH—Thyrotropin-releasing hormone
TSH—Thyroid-stimulating hormone
USP—United States Pharmacopoeia

The appendices in *Textbook of Nuclear Medicine, Volume II: Clinical Applications* contain many useful tables, which are listed here for reference:

A. Radiation Absorbed Dose Estimates
B. Common Abbreviations
C. Reference Man
   1. Masses of organ and tissues for reference adult and other anatomic values
   2. Total body content for some elements
   3. Organ weights in children
   4. Nomogram for determining surface area
   5. Predicted "normal" blood volumes
D. Selected Units and Conversion Factors

INDEX

Page numbers in *italics* indicate figures; page numbers followed by "t" indicate tables.